TREATMENT
of
HEART DISEASES

TREATMENT
of
HEART DISEASES

EDITOR

James T. Willerson, MD

Professor of Medicine
Chairman, Department of Internal Medicine
University of Texas Medical School at Houston
Director, Cardiology Research
Texas Heart Institute
Houston, Texas

ASSOCIATE EDITORS

Donald S. Baim, MD

Denton A. Cooley, MD

O. Howard Frazier, MD

Scott M. Grundy, MD, PhD

Norman M. Kaplan, MD

Milton Packer, MD

Michael S. Sweeney, MD

Douglas P. Zipes, MD

New York • **Gower Medical Publishing** • London

Library of Congress Cataloging-in-Publication Data
Treatment of heart diseases / editor, James T. Willerson; associate
    editors, Donald Baim...[et al.]; with illustrations by Laura
    Pardi Duprey.
            p. cm.
        Includes bibliographic references and index.
        ISBN 0-397-44695-0
        1. Heart--Disease--Treatment.   I. Willerson, James T., 1939-
    II. Baim, Donald S.
        [DNLM: 1. Heart Diseases--therapy. 2. Hyperlipidemia--etiology.
    3. Hyperlipidemia--therapy.   4. Hypertension--etiology.
    5. Hypertension--therapy.   WG 200 T784]
    RC683.8.T74 1992
    DNLM/DLC
    for Library of Congress   92-1450
                                                                          CIP

British Library Cataloguing-in-Publication Data
A catalogue record for this book is available from the British Library.

10 9 8 7 6 5 4 3 2 1

Distributed in the USA and Canada by: Distributed in the rest of the world by:
Raven Press   *Gower Medical Publishing*
1185 Avenue of the Americas   Middlesex House
New York, NY 10036   34-42 Cleveland Street
USA   London W1P 5FB
                                            United Kingdom

Distributed in Japan by:
Nankodo Company Ltd.
42-6 Hongo 3-Chome
Bunkyo-Ku
Tokyo 113
Japan

                        editorial director: Leah Kennedy
                       cover illustration: Laura Pardi Duprey
                             illustrators: Laura Pardi Duprey
                                               Bill Andrews (chapter 6)
                                               Precision Graphics (charts)
              cover and interior design: Kathryn Greenslade
                       design assistants: Jennifer Bergamini
                                               Talar Agasyan
                                printed in: Hong Kong by Imago

Contributors

Donald S. Baim, MD
Associate Professor of Medicine
Harvard Medical School
Director, Invasive Cardiology
Beth Israel Hospital
Boston, Massachusetts

Denton A. Cooley, MD
Clinical Professor of Surgery
University of Texas Medical School
in Houston
Surgeon-in-Chief
Texas Heart Institute
Houston, Texas

O. Howard Frazier, MD
Professor of Surgery
Chief, Division of Cardiovascular
and Thoracic Surgery
University of Texas Medical School
in Houston
Chief, Transplant Service
Co-Director, Cullen Cardiovascular
Research Laboratories
Texas Heart Institute
Houston, Texas

Scott M. Grundy, MD, PhD
Professor of Medicine
Director, Center for Human Nutrition
Chairman, Department of Clinical
Nutrition
University of Texas Southwestern
Medical Center at Dallas
Dallas, Texas

Norman M. Kaplan, MD
Professor of Internal Medicine
Chief, Hypertension Division
University of Texas Southwestern
Medical Center at Dallas
Dallas, Texas

Milton Packer, MD
Chief, Division of Circulatory
Physiology
Head, Center for Heart Failure
Research
Columbia Presbyterian Medical Center
New York, New York

Branislav Radovancevic, MD
Director, Transplant Research
Texas Heart Institute
Houston, Texas

Michael S. Sweeney, MD
Associate Professor of Surgery
University of Texas Medical School
at Houston
Director, Cardiovascular
and Thoracic Surgery
Hermann Hospital
Houston, Texas

James T. Willerson, MD
Professor of Medicine
Chairman,
Department of Internal Medicine
University of Texas Medical School
at Houston
Director, Cardiology Research
Texas Heart Institute
Houston, Texas

Douglas P. Zipes, MD
Professor of Medicine
Indiana University School of Medicine
Senior Research Associate
Krannert Institute of Cardiology
Indianapolis, Indiana

Acknowledgments

- The authors wish to acknowledge Gower Medical Publishing, especially Laura Pardi Duprey for her outstanding artwork that is included in the book, and our secretaries, Susan Beaubien, Marianne Mallia, Shirley Myers, Myrtle M. Skinner, Vanessa Smith, Sharon Washington, for their outstanding and dedicated secretarial assistance in the preparation of this book.

Preface

● Treatment of heart diseases is an art and one that the physician acquires during a lifetime of experience. However, the most effective treatment comes from an understanding of basic mechanisms responsible for heart disease and an appreciation of the relative benefits of various interventions and patient prognosis with and without specific treatment. In this book, we have addressed the major cardiac problems that patients experience and have provided comprehensive discussions of mechanisms of disease, options for and types of specific therapy, and a discussion of results that may be expected. Each chapter contains a summary of the authors' preferences for specific therapies, with an emphasis on therapy based on insight into specific mechanisms responsible for heart disease.

● We believe that this book will be useful to all who help to care for patients with cardiac disease. It is our intention to update this book at regular intervals to introduce new advances in insight and specific therapies with the expectation that this book might provide a useful reference for years to come.

Contents

3

Treatment of Arrhythmias and Abnormalities in Conduction

Douglas P. Zipes, MD

Antiarrhythmic Options in the Future   *3.71*

Etiologies and Treatment of Hyperlipidemia

Scott M. Grundy, MD, PhD

Percutaneous Transluminal Coronary Angioplasty and Newer Treatments for Coronary Heart Disease

Donald S. Baim, MD

Surgical Treatment of Heart Diseases

O. Howard Frazier, MD • Michael S. Sweeney, MD
Branislav Radovancevic, MD
Denton A. Cooley, MD

7
Etiologies and Treatment of Systemic Arterial Hypertension

Norman M. Kaplan, MD

1

MEDICAL TREATMENT OF CORONARY HEART DISEASE

JAMES T. WILLERSON, MD

Synopsis of Chapter One

CORONARY ARTERY DISEASE SYNDROMES

STABLE ANGINA

Angina pectoris is the clinical term for chest pain resulting from a relative oxygen deficiency in heart muscle (Table 1.1). Heberden assigned the name, based on the "strangling and anxiety" associated with the condition, which he described as a "disorder of the breast marked with strong and peculiar symptoms and considerable for the kind of danger belonging to it."[1] This description was enlarged upon by Herrick in 1912.[2]

Angina is usually described by the patient as a left precordial tightness or ache provoked by exercise or emotion and relieved by rest. Angina occurs when the oxygen demand of the myocardium exceeds the oxygen supply.[3-7] Most individuals with angina have underlying atherosclerotic coronary artery disease. However, angina may also develop in some patients with ventricular hypertrophy, left ventricular outflow obstruction, severe aortic valvular regurgitation and/or stenosis, cardiomyopathy, or dilated ventricles in whom coronary artery stenoses are not present. The explanation for angina occurring under circumstances when coronary heart disease is not present is that even normal coronary arteries may not adequately supply oxygen to hypertrophied, dilated, or failing heart muscle. A limited coronary vasodilator reserve may also explain angina, especially in some patients with left ventricular outflow obstruction, including valvular aortic stenosis, idiopathic hypertrophic subaortic stenosis, and/or marked ventricular hypertrophy.[8,9] Coronary artery vasoconstriction occurring with exercise or stress may also be a contributing factor.[10,11] The reason normal individuals without coronary heart disease do not develop angina is probably because other factors that limit physical activity, such as dyspnea and fatigue, protect the heart from a marked imbalance between oxygen delivery and demand.

The pathologic alteration in coronary arteries that predisposes to angina is atherosclerosis and/or neointimal fibrotic proliferation (Figure 1.1). Severe narrowing of the coronary artery lumen restricts oxygen delivery, especially when oxygen demand in the heart is increased, such as during increases in heart rate, during marked increases in myocardial contractility, and/or with increases in myocardial wall tension.[3-7] Therefore, angina may develop during exercise, cold exposure, emotional stress, or after eating a large meal. It may also occur because of extracardiac influences. In particular, severe anemia or carbon monoxide exposure limits the capacity of blood to carry or release oxygen, and may cause angina under conditions that the subject would otherwise tolerate well. Increases in systemic arterial pressure and consequent dilatation of the heart may result in angina. Increases in heart rate or contractile state, such those associated with hyperthyroidism, pheochromocytoma, and exogenous administration or endogenous release of catecholamines, may also result in angina.

UNSTABLE ANGINA

Angina at rest and/or with limited physical activity, that occurs in a crescendo pattern, is known as unstable angina. Generally, unstable angina results from primary decreases in coronary blood flow and myocardial oxygen delivery (Figure 1.2). Examples of this decrease include:
- Progressive coronary artery atherosclerosis.
- Transient platelet aggregation and coronary artery thrombosis.
- Coronary artery spasm.
- Coronary vasoconstriction upon adrenergic stimulation.
- Probably at sites of endothelial injury upon the accumulation of potent vasoconstrictors, including thromboxane A_2, serotonin (5HT), selected leukotrienes, prostaglandin D_2, thrombin, platelet activating factor (PAF), and possibly endothelin (Figure 1.3).[12-20]

TABLE 1.1 • CORONARY HEART DISEASE SYNDROMES

Stable angina pectoris

Unstable angina pectoris

Variant angina (Prinzmetal's angina)

Acute myocardial infarction
- Non-Q-wave (usually nontransmural infarcts)
- Q-wave (usually transmural myocardial infarcts)

Coronary artery spasm leads to abrupt and dynamic decreases in myocardial oxygen delivery[21–22] (Figures 1.4, 1.5). With a primary decrease in coronary blood flow, there is no association between symptoms and exertion. The majority of anginal episodes occur during limited activity and at rest. These patients usually have little change in heart rate or blood pressure prior to the onset of pain. The pain occurs first, and may be followed later by increased blood pressure and/or heart rate. Continuous electrocardiographic monitoring may document transient ST-segment changes with the onset of pain. There may be either ST-segment elevation indicating transmural ischemia and involvement of a major epicardial coronary artery or, more commonly, ST-segment depression when subendocardial ischemia develops and smaller caliber coronary arteries are involved (refer to Figure 1.5). ST-segment alterations may also occur in the absence of chest pain, suggesting the presence of "silent ischemia."[23–25]

VARIANT ANGINA OR PRINZMETAL'S ANGINA

Patients with variant angina pectoris—Prinzmetal's angina—have angina at rest, often in the early morning hours, associated with ST-segment elevation on the electrocardiogram and the presence of coronary artery spasm, which is a focal obliteration of a coronary artery lumen[21–22] (refer to Figures 1.4, 1.5).

Early descriptions of typical angina by Latham[26] and Osler[27] suggested that this entity was due to periodic spasm of a large coronary artery. Subsequently, clinical studies with anatomic correlations suggested that fixed atherosclerotic coronary artery disease was responsible for typical angina and myocardial infarction. In 1959, Prinzmetal et al[28] revived interest in coronary arterial spasm when they described a group of individuals with "variant angina."

The clinical features of this syndrome are distinctly different from those of typical angina:[21,28–37]

• The patients described by Prinzmetal et al usually had chest pain at rest rather than with physical exertion or emotional stimulation.
• The episodes of pain tended to recur at roughly the same time every day—often during the early morning hours—awakening the patient from sleep.
• Patients usually had ST-segment elevations on electrocardiograms recorded during chest pain (refer to Figures 1.4, 1.5).
• The episodes of chest pain were sometimes accompanied by atrioventricular block and/or ventricular ectopic activity, and occasionally the patients had transient ventricular tachycardia.
• Chest discomfort was relieved quickly by nitroglycerin, after which the ST-segment elevation resolved.

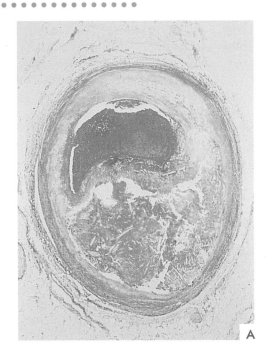
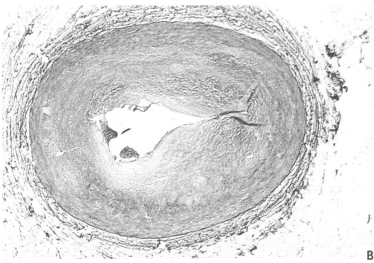

FIGURE 1.1 • Histologic section of coronary artery showing occlusive thrombus adherent to intact fibrous cap covering classic atheroma (A). Neointimal proliferation occurs with restenosis after coronary artery angioplasty, leading to coronary artery luminal diameter narrowing and the need for some additional revascularization procedure (B). Patients who develop coronary heart disease following cardiac transplantation also demonstrate this same alteration in their coronary arteries—a neointimal proliferation. Recently, it has become apparent that even native atheromata have substantial fibroproliferative alterations. (Reproduced with permission. **1A** Becker AE, Anderson RH: *Cardiac Pathology* London, England: Gower Medical Publishing; 1988:3.7. **1B** Hurst JW, Anderson RH, Becker AE, et al: *Atlas of the Heart* New York, NY: Gower Medical Publishing; 1988:6.3.)

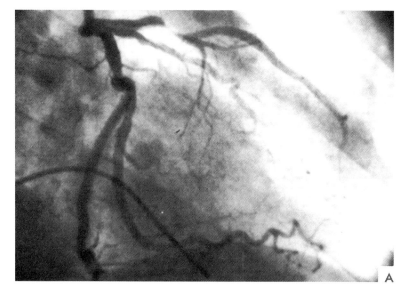

FIGURE 1.2 • Right anterior oblique projections of the left coronary artery in a 61-year old patient with unstable angina shows an severe concentric stenosis of the left anterior descending artery (A). The guidewire is in the distal artery and the inflated balloon is positioned across the stenosis (B). Immediate postangioplasty angiogram shows successful dilation (C). (Reproduced with permission. Hall DP, Gruentzig AR: Technique of percutaneous transluminal angioplasty of the coronary, renal, mesenteric, and peripheral arteries. In: Hurst JW, ed. *The Heart* 6th ed. New York, NY: McGraw-Hill; 1986:1902 and Hurst JW, Anderson RH, Becker AE, et al: *Atlas of the Heart* New York, NY: Gower Medical Publishing; 1988:6.29.)

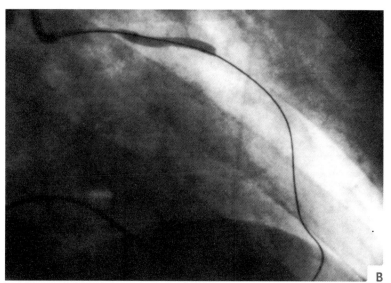

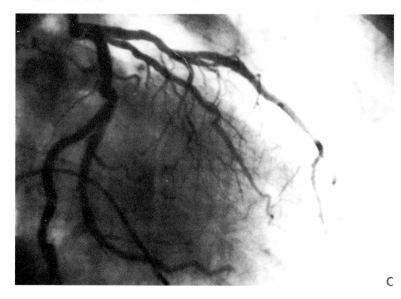

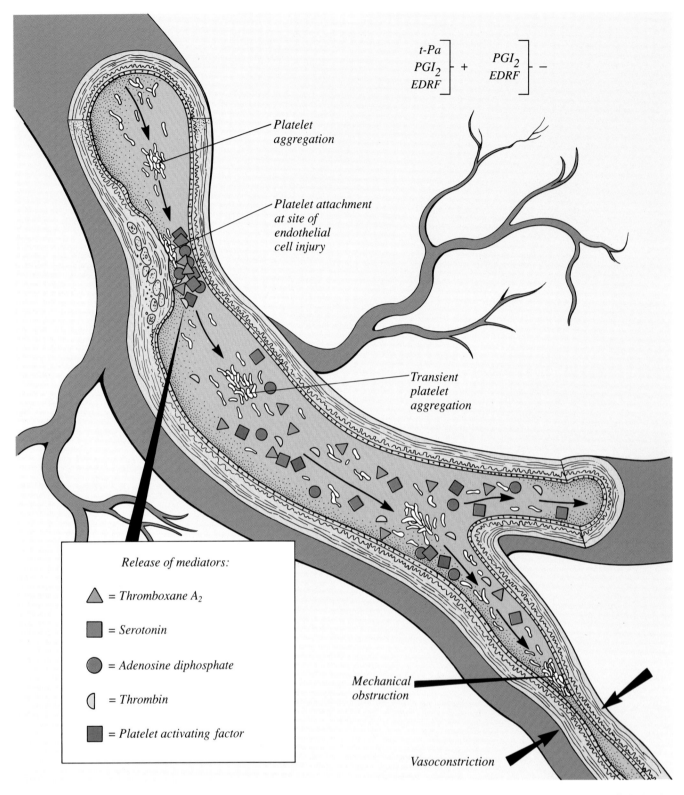

$$\begin{matrix} t\text{-}Pa \\ PGI_2 \\ EDRF \end{matrix} \Bigg] + \begin{matrix} PGI_2 \\ EDRF \end{matrix} \Bigg] -$$

Platelet aggregation

Platelet attachment at site of endothelial cell injury

Transient platelet aggregation

Release of mediators:

△ = *Thromboxane A$_2$*

▢ = *Serotonin*

● = *Adenosine diphosphate*

◖ = *Thrombin*

▢ = *Platelet activating factor*

Mechanical obstruction

Vasoconstriction

FIGURE 1.3 • Possible mechanism responsible for the conversion from chronic coronary heart disease to acute coronary artery disease syndromes is shown. Endothelial injury, usually at sites of atherosclerotic plaques, is associated with platelet attachment and aggregation, as well as the release of selected mediators—including thromboxane A$_2$, serotonin and adenosine diphosphate (ADP). Endothelial injury may occur as a consequence of atherosclerotic plaque fissuring or ulceration leading to this sequence of events—the local accumulation of thromboxane A$_2$, serotonin, and/or ADP promotes platelet aggregation. Thromboxane A$_2$ and serotonin are vasoconstrictors at sites of endothelial injury. Thus, the conversion from chronic stable to acute unstable coronary heart disease syndromes may be the result of en-

dothelial injury, platelet aggregation, platelet and other cell-derived mediator accumulation, further platelet aggregation and vasoconstriction with a consequent dynamic narrowing in coronary artery lumen. Additional potential causes of endothelial injury may be:

- Flow shear stress
- Hypertension
- Immune complex deposition and complement activation
- Mechanical and/or immunologic injury to the endothelium as it occurs with coronary artery angioplasty and following heart transplantation. (Adapted with permission. Willerson JT, Golino P, Eidt J, et al: *Circulation* 1989;80:198.)

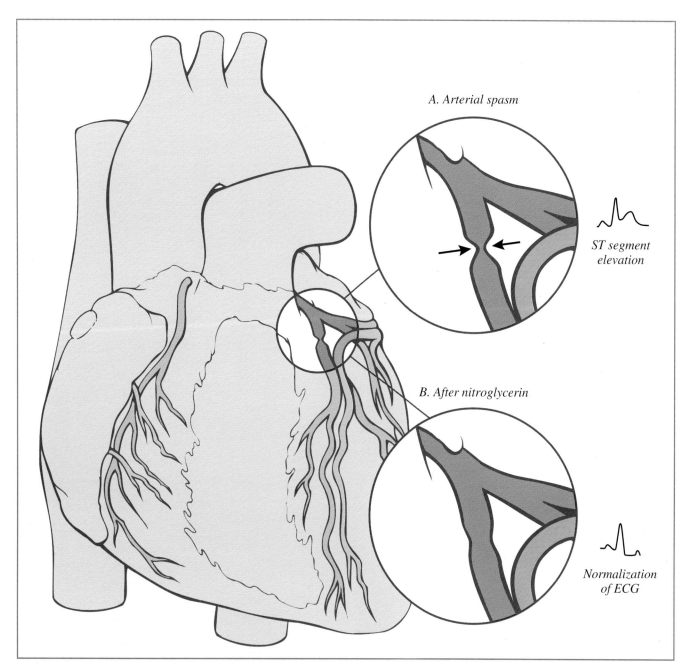

FIGURE 1.4 • Scattered atherosclerotic plaques with focal obliteration of the coronary artery lumen caused by coronary artery spasm at a spot (arrows) (A). The associated ST-segment elevation that occurs with coronary artery spasm is demonstrated in the upper inset. The resolution of the coronary artery spasm following administration of nitroglycerin (B). The normalization of the ECG is shown.

Patients with Prinzmetal's angina did not undergo selective coronary arteriography, but Prinzmetal and his colleagues hypothesized that patients with variant angina had severe proximal stenoses of one or more large coronary arteries that developed spasm periodically.

Since the original description of variant angina by Prinzmetal's group, many observers have confirmed the existence of this syndrome and have shown the presence of coronary artery spasm at sites of fixed coronary artery stenosis and in regions of the coronary vasculature where no obvious stenosis ex-

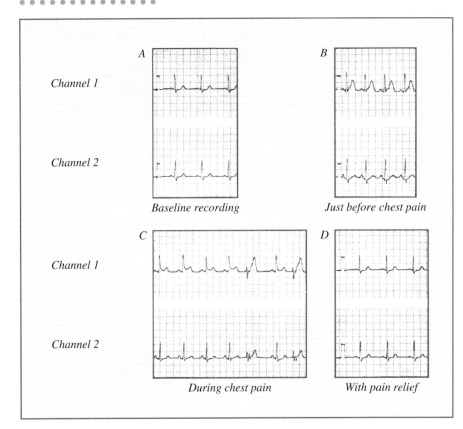

FIGURE 1.5 • A continuous 24-hr Holter recording in a patient with coronary artery spasm was performed prior to chest pain (A), as chest pain began (B), during chest pain (C), and with pain relief (D). Note the T-wave prominence and ST-segment elevation that occur with coronary artery spasm.

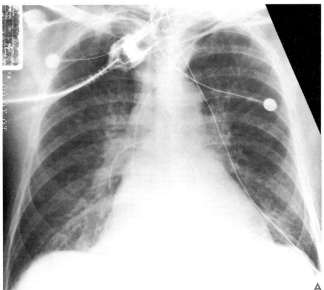
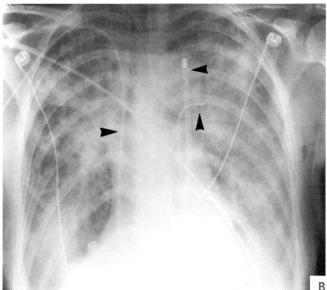

FIGURE 1.6 • Acute myocardial infarction. Supine portable chest film demonstrates mild left ventricular enlargement and moderate pulmonary edema—note the perihilar haze (A). A Swan-Ganz catheter was inserted. its tip is in the right lower lobe artery. The supine portable chest film (B) of this patient with extensive myocardial damage with papillary muscle dysfunction shows bilateral alveolar pulmonary edema. The heart is not significantly enlarged and there is no left atrial enlargement. A Swan-Ganz catheter (arrow 1) was placed with its tip in a branch of the left pulmonary artery. An intra-aortic counterpulsion balloon catheter (arrow 2) is alo present with its tip at the level of the aortic arch. This patient had an acute myocardial infarction with left ventricular failure and mitral insufficiency. (Reproduced with permission. Soto B, Kassner EG, Baxley WA: *Imaging of cardiovascular Disorders* New York, NY: Gower Medical Publishing; 1992:132.)

ists.[28–39] In patients with coronary artery spasm, Prinzmetal's angina may sometimes be induced by ergonovine maleate.[40–50] Maneuvers that have produced coronary artery spasm in susceptible patients include hyperventilation with the administration of an alkaline buffer, cold-pressor testing, and the administration of methacholine, a parasympathomimetic agent.[45,48,50–55] We have speculated that endothelial and/or adventitial injury, often in association with coronary artery stenosis, leads to the accumulation of platelets and white blood cells, mononuclear cells, and T cells, and to the release of humoral mediators, including serotonin, thromboxane A_2, prostaglandin D_2, thrombin, platelet activating function, leukotrienes, and/or histamine, which either singly or in combination may cause coronary artery spasm.[15–17] This is especially likely to be true when endothelial injury decreases vascular concentrations of endothelially derived relaxing factors, tissue plasminogen activator, and/or prostacyclin[17] (refer to Figure 1.3). It is also possible that the endothelially derived vasoconstrictor—endothelin—may be primarily responsible for coronary artery spasm in some patients.[15–17]

ACUTE MYOCARDIAL INFARCTION

Acute myocardial infarction may occur when regional myocardial oxygen delivery is inadequate for a period of more than 20 minutes (Figures 1.6, 1.7). Herrick in 1912 described acute myocardial infarction caused by coronary artery thrombosis.[2] Subsequently, the role of coronary artery thrombosis in causing myocardial infarction was debated,[56] until studies by DeWood and colleagues demonstrated, by coronary arteriography, that coronary artery thrombosis is virtually always the cause of acute Q-wave myocardial infarcts.[57] Others have confirmed the association between thrombosis of the infarct-related coronary artery and the development of acute Q-wave (transmural) myocardial infarction by using detailed clinicopathologic correlates.[58] Thus, acute Q-wave myocardial infarction is usually caused by a reduction in coronary blood flow and, consequently, reduced myocardial oxygen delivery[56–58] (Figure 1.8). Occasionally, myocardial oxygen demand exceeds the ability of stenotic coronary arteries to deliver oxygen, leading to acute myocardial infarction.

After 20 min to 2 hrs of inadequate myocardial oxygen delivery, acute myocardial infarction is usually confined to the in-

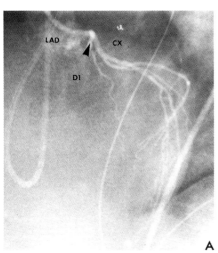
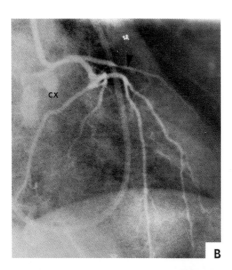

FIGURE 1.7 • The left coronary arteriogram in the left anterior oblique (LAO) (A) and right anterior oblique (RAO) (B) projection of this patient with an acute myocardial infarction demonstrate occlusion (arrow) of the proximal segment of the left anterior descending artery (LAD) just beyond the origin of the first diagonal branch (D1). The proximal margin of the occlusion has a smooth, triangular configuration. The distal segment of the left anterior descending artery is not opacified—the absence of collaterals suggests the occlusion is acute. The circumflex artery (CX) is patent. (Reproduced with permission. Soto B, Kassner EG, Baxley WA: *Imaging of Cardiovascular Disorders* New York, NY: Gower Medical Publishing; 1992:166.)

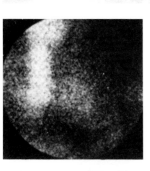
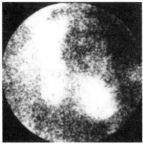
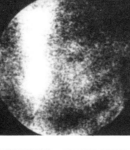
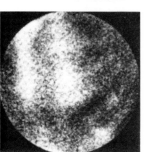
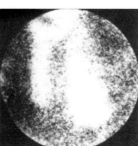
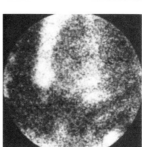

FIGURE 1.8 • The increased intensity of a technetium-99m pyrophosphate (Tc-99m-PPi) myocardial scintigram occurs with time in patients with acute transmural myocardial infarction. The left panels demonstrate the faintly positive radioisotope uptake approximately 10 hrs after myocardial infarction. The center panels show increased uptake 3 days after infarction. The right panels reveal marked resolution in Tc-99m-PPi uptake approximately 7 days after infarction. (Reproduced with permission. Buja LM, Willerson JT: Measurement of myocardial infarction size. In: Chatterjee K, Cheitlin MD, Karliner J, et al. eds. *Cardiology. An Illustrated Text* New York, NY: Gower Medical Publishing; 1992:7.135.)

ner one third of the myocardial wall, resulting in a subendo-cardial or "non-Q-wave" infarct (Figures 1.9, 1.10 and refer to Figure 1.3). Approximately 30% of patients with non-Q-wave infarcts have occlusive thrombus in the infarct-related artery.[58] Most non-Q-wave myocardial infarcts are due to transient coronary artery occlusion, perhaps linked to platelet aggrega-tion and vasoconstriction.[59]

When critical reductions in myocardial blood flow persist for more than 2 hrs, the resultant infarct is usually a transmural or Q-wave infarct (Figures 1.11, 1.12). Factors that may lead to coronary artery thrombosis include endothelial injury associated with the fissuring or ulceration of atherosclerotic plaque, and the release from the aggregating platelets of selective mediators, including thromboxane A_2, adenosine diphosphate (ADP), and serotonin (refer to Figure 1.3).[15–17] Thrombin activation at sites of endothelial injury contributes to dynamic vasoconstriction and platelet aggregation.[19] Increases in systemic and local cat-echolamine concentrations associated with the development of unstable angina and myocardial infarction may increase platelet aggregation and contribute to coronary vasoconstriction. Re-ductions in fibrinolytic capability at sites of endothelial injury associated with a decrease in prostacyclin, tissue plasmino-gen activating factor, and/or endothelial relaxing factors, may also contribute to coronary artery thrombosis and vasocon-striction (refer to Figure 1.3).[15–17]

We have suggested that unstable angina, non-Q-wave my-ocardial infarction, and Q-wave myocardial infarction represent a continuum. The process begins with endothelial injury to a

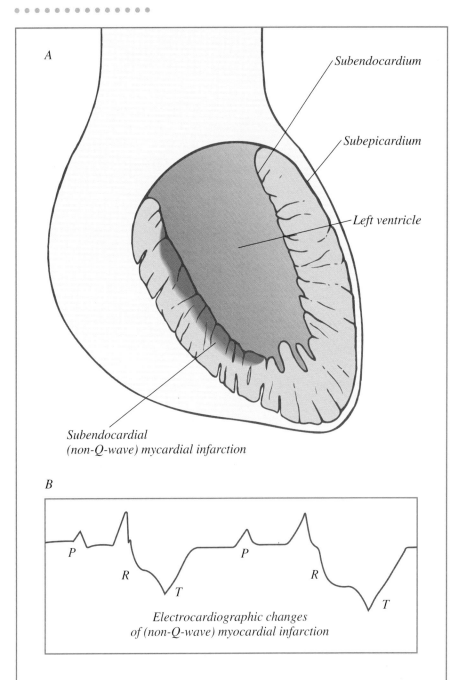

A

Subendocardium

Subepicardium

Left ventricle

Subendocardial
(non-Q-wave) mycardial infarction

B

P

R

T

P

R

T

Electrocardiographic changes
of (non-Q-wave) myocardial infarction

FIGURE 1.9 • The location of myocardial necrosis with subendocardial or non-Q-wave myocardial infarcts (A). The shaded area represents the region of subendocardial (non-Q-wave) myocardial infarction. Note the electrocardiographic changes associated with this type of myocardial infarction (B).

coronary artery, usually at sites of coronary artery stenosis, and leads to:
- Platelet aggregation.
- Mediator release from the aggregating platelets.
- Incorporation of white and red blood cells.
- Formation of a platelet–white cell–red cell thrombus.[15–17]

I believe that when the platelet–fibrin thrombus persists for periods of less than 20 minutes, the syndrome of unstable angina develops.[15–17] However, as stated above, when reduction in coronary blood flow and oxygen delivery to the heart is more prolonged—lasting 20 minutes to 2 hrs—a non-Q-wave or subendocardial myocardial infarction occurs.[15–17] When the period of inadequate myocardial oxygen delivery persists for more than 2 hours, a Q-wave infarct results.[15–17] Approximately 90% of patients with acute Q-wave myocardial infarcts have occlusive coronary thrombi at sites of coronary artery stenosis, as well as atherosclerotic plaque fissuring and/or ulceration (refer to Figure 1.1).[57,58,60,61] It seems likely that this same sequence of events can be induced by causes of endothelial injury other than atherosclerotic plaque fissuring and/or ulceration. Additional possibilities include endothelial injury associated with systemic arterial hypertension, flow shear stress, smoking, diabetes, infection, aging, immune-complex deposition, substance abuse (for example, cocaine), and the placement of a catheter into a coronary artery, especially during the process of percutaneous transluminal coronary artery angioplasty (PTCA).[15–17]

TREATING THE PATIENT WITH STABLE ANGINA

Patients with stable angina usually have angina during effort, exercise, or other circumstances that raise myocardial oxygen demand by increasing the heart rate, contractile state, and/or ventricular wall tension. Therapy for stable angina is directed at reducing the heart rate, blood pressure, and contractile responses to exercise, thus reducing myocardial oxygen demand. Increasing coronary blood flow and oxygen delivery may also be useful.

In individual patients, stable angina often develops in a predictable manner and at a level of activity or stress associated with a particular systolic blood pressure and heart rate. Indeed, the product of heart rate multiplied by systolic blood pressure provides an estimate of myocardial oxygen demand. The following are the recommended pharmacologic therapies for patients with stable angina.

NITRATES
Angina may be relieved within 3 to 7 minutes by rest or nitroglycerin.[62–65] The beneficial effects of nitroglycerin and other nitrates are the result of:
- A dilation of the systemic veins and a decrease in venous return to the right heart, that reduces myocardial wall tension and oxygen demand.

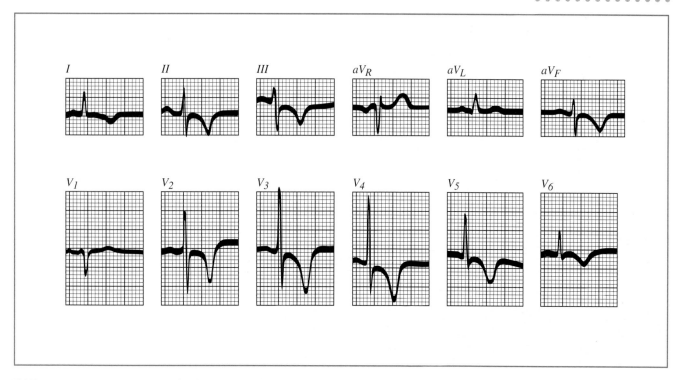

FIGURE 1.10 • A typical ECG found in the patient with an acute non-Q-wave myocardial infarct (top row). With these infarcts, the ECG is unable to provide specific evidence of the presence of the infarct, but ST-segment depression of varying magnitude and T-wave abnormalities, usually T-wave flattening or inversion, often develop (bottom row). The only evolution of the electrocardiographic abnormalities is a return to the normal pattern.

• Vasodilation of large and medium-sized coronary arteries, with a concomitant increase in coronary blood flow to the subendocardial region, where the imbalance between oxygen supply and demand exists[62–65] (Figure 1.13).

Nitrates increase oxygen delivery to the subendocardial region supplied by a severely narrowed coronary artery. Most other coronary vasodilators increase coronary blood flow and oxygen delivery to the epicardium and/or midmyocardium

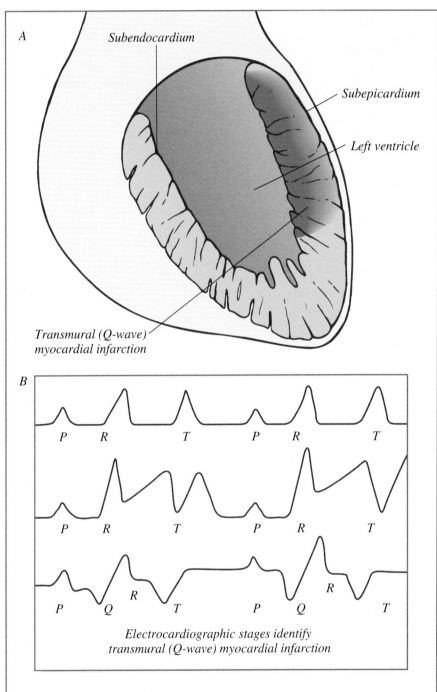

A

Subendocardium

Subepicardium

Left ventricle

Transmural (Q-wave) myocardial infarction

B

P R T P R T

P R T P R T

P Q R T P Q R T

Electrocardiographic stages identify transmural (Q-wave) myocardial infarction

FIGURE 1.11 • The topographic location of myocardial necrosis with transmural Q-wave myocardial infarction (A). The shaded area represents the region of transmural Q-wave myocardial infarction. The ECG stages identify this type of myocardial infarction (B).

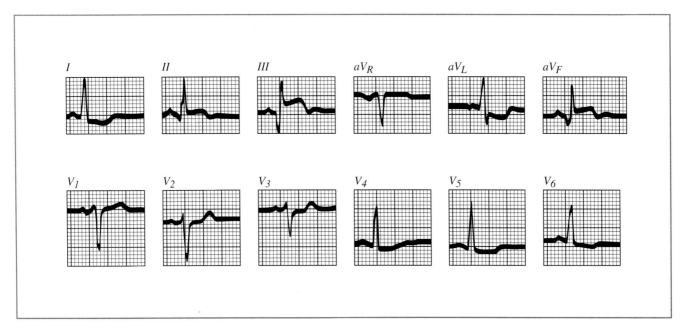

FIGURE 1.12 • These sequential ECG alterations document the development of a new inferior Q-wave infarct beginning with T-wave prominence followed by hyperacute ST-segment elevation, T-wave inversion and the development of a significant Q-wave—0.04 seconds in duration.

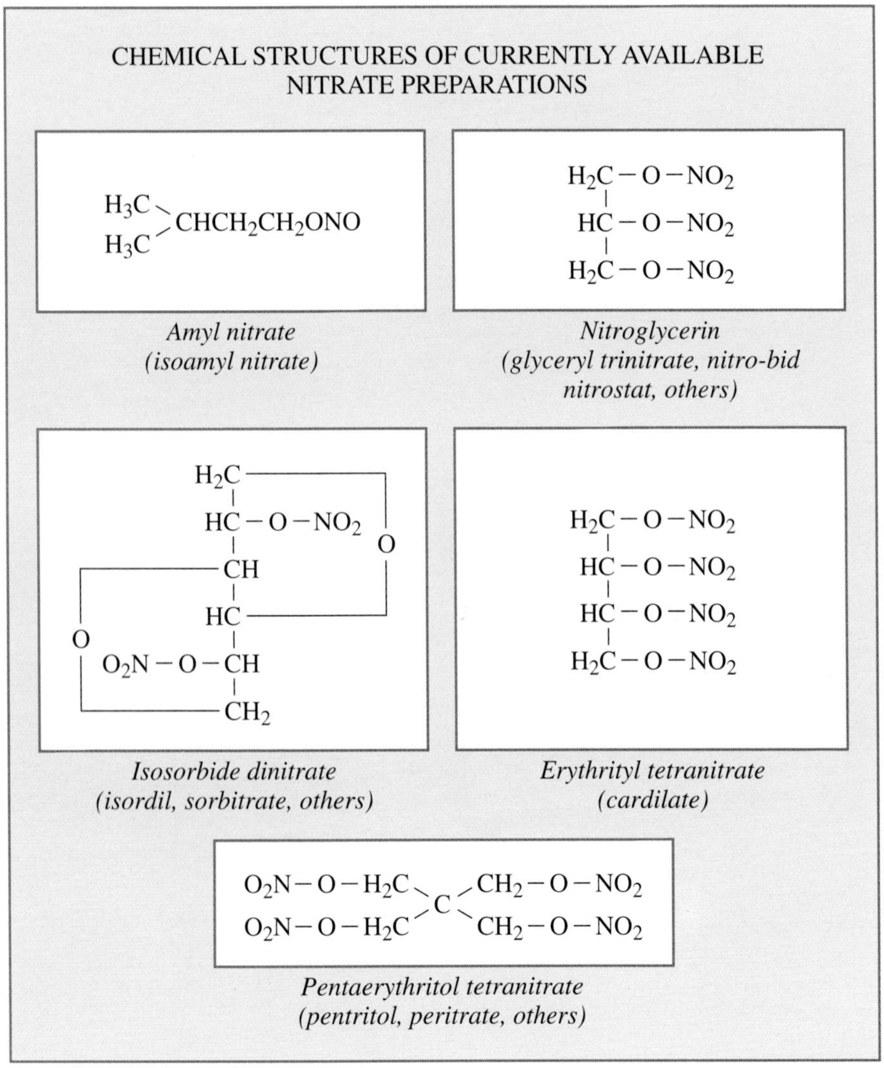

FIGURE 1.13 • The chemical structures for the various nitrate preparations.

CHEMICAL STRUCTURES OF CURRENTLY AVAILABLE NITRATE PREPARATIONS

$$H_3C$$
$$>CHCH_2CH_2ONO$$
$$H_3C$$

Amyl nitrate
(isoamyl nitrate)

$$H_2C-O-NO_2$$
$$HC-O-NO_2$$
$$H_2C-O-NO_2$$

Nitroglycerin
(glyceryl trinitrate, nitro-bid nitrostat, others)

$$H_2C-$$
$$HC-O-NO_2$$
$$-CH \quad\quad O$$
$$HC-$$
$$O_2N-O-CH$$
$$-CH_2$$

Isosorbide dinitrate
(isordil, sorbitrate, others)

$$H_2C-O-NO_2$$
$$HC-O-NO_2$$
$$HC-O-NO_2$$
$$H_2C-O-NO_2$$

Erythrityl tetranitrate
(cardilate)

$$O_2N-O-H_2C \quad\quad CH_2-O-NO_2$$
$$>C<$$
$$O_2N-O-H_2C \quad\quad CH_2-O-NO_2$$

Pentaerythritol tetranitrate
(pentritol, peritrate, others)

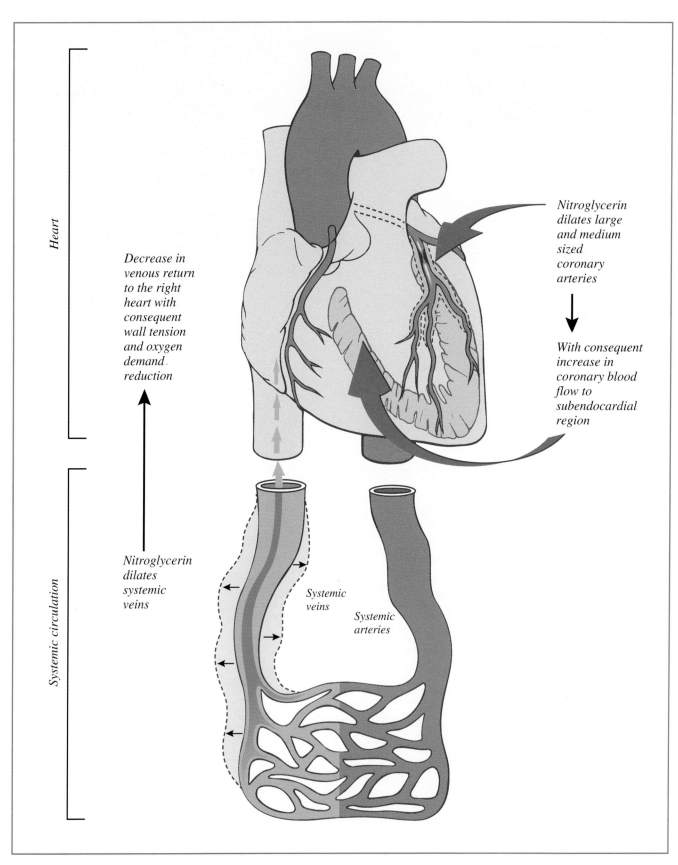

Heart

Systemic circulation

Decrease in venous return to the right heart with consequent wall tension and oxygen demand reduction

Nitroglycerin dilates systemic veins

Nitroglycerin dilates large and medium sized coronary arteries

With consequent increase in coronary blood flow to subendocardial region

Systemic veins

Systemic arteries

FIGURE 1.14 • Nitroglycerin's physiologic effects in the heart and in the peripheral venous system. Nitroglycerin dilates large and medium-sized coronary arteries and improves myocardial blood flow to the subendocardial region. In the systemic circulation, nitro- glycerin is a venodilator. Thus, it decreases venous return to the right heart and diminishes preload and wall tension thereby decreasing myocardial oxygen demand.

without directly changing oxygen availability within the subendocardial region itself (Figure 1.14). The coronary-vasodilator effect of nitroglycerin is associated with an increase in endothelial guanylate cyclase activity and consequent increase in cyclic guanosine monophosphate (GMP), and is independent of the endothelium[66,67] (Figure 1.15). An increase in myocardial oxygen availability and decrease in oxygen demand usually relieve angina promptly.

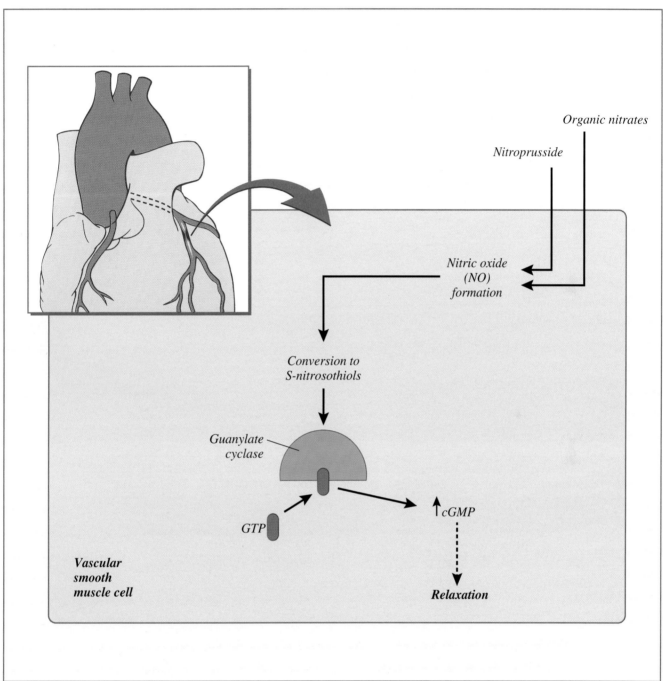

FIGURE 1.15 • The cellular biochemical effects of nitrates that correlate with its properties as a coronary artery vasodilator. The nitrates increase guanylate cyclase activity resulting in an increase in cyclic GMP which is associated with vasodilation. It is believed that nitroglycerin exerts its endothelium-independent vasodilating effect through the activation of guanylate cyclase and the cellular increases in cyclic GMP.

The most commonly used oral nitrate preparations are listed in Table 1.2. Typically, relatively long-acting and orally administered nitrates, such as isosorbide dinitrate, are given at 6- to 8-hour intervals during the day and a nitroglycerin patch or paste is applied during the night, which is then removed the following morning after the patient arises.[68–70] This approach currently provides the best opportunity for using the "nitrate effect" to its maximal potential and for avoiding the tolerance and loss of nitrate effect associated with continuous administration of the same preparation.[71,72]

TABLE 1.2 • NITRATE PREPARATIONS USED IN THE TREATMENT OF ANGINA PECTORIS

Preparation	Dosage	Duration of effect	Frequency of administration
Sublingual nitroglycerin	0.3–0.5 mg	15–30 min	For individual episodes
Sublingual or chewable isosorbide dinitrate	2.5–10 mg	30 min to 1 hr	May be used instead of nitroglycerin
Oral isosorbide dinitrate (Isordil)	5–30 mg	2 hr	Every 2–3 hr while patient is awake
Oral isosorbide dinitrate (Tembid) longer-acting preparation	40 mg	6–8 hr	Every 6–8 hr
Pentaerythritol tetranitrate (Peritrate)			
Oral	10–40 mg	3–4 hr	Every 3–4 hr
Sustained	80 mg	8–10 hr	Every 8–10 hr
Sustained release oral nitroglycerin (Nitro-Bid)	2.5–6.5 mg	6 hr	Every 6 hr
Nitroglycerin ointment	Thin film over 1–2-inch area of anterior chest	4–6 hr	Every 4–6 hr
Nitroglycerin patches (sustained release)	5–20 mg	6 hr	Every 12–24 hr

(Modified from Willerson JT, Hillis LD, Buja LM: In: *Ischemic Heart Disease: Clinical and Pathophysiological Aspects*. New York, NY: Raven Press;1982:189.)

TABLE 1.3 • β-ADRENERGIC ANTAGONISTS

Name	ß-blockade potency ratio (propranolol=1.0)	Cardio-selective[1]	Usual therapeutic dose range (mg/d)	Elimination half-life	Route of excretion
Propranolol (nonspecific)	1.0	0	80–480	2.5–6.0 hr	Urine
Timolol	6.0	0	5–40	4–5 hr	Urine
Oxprenelol	0.5–1.0	0	40–360	2 hr	Urine
Sotalol	0.3	0	80–480	5–13 hr	Urine
Metoprolol (ß$_1$)	1.0	+	100–800	3–4 hr	Urine
Pindolol	6.0	0	2.5–30.0	3–4 hr	Urine
Atenolol (ß$_1$)	1.0	+	100–400	6–9 hr	Approximately 40% of unchanged drug in urine
Alprenolol (ß$_1$)	0.3	0	200–800	2–3 hr	Urine
Acebutolol	0.3	+	400–800	8 hr	Uncertain

[1]Seen only at low dosage. (Reproduced with permission. Hillis LD, Firth BG, Willerson JT: *Manual of Clinical Problems in Cardiology 2nd Edition* Boston, MA: Little, Brown and Company; 1984:285.)

ADRENERGIC ANTAGONISTS

Beta-adrenergic antagonists attenuate heart rate, systolic blood pressure, and contractile responses at rest and with exercise.[73-80] Reductions in the heart rate–systolic blood pressure may reduce myocardial oxygen demand enough to allow a patient to engage in a particular activity without angina, whereas previously that was not possible.

The ß-blockers used in the treatment of stable angina are listed in Table 1.3. Beta-blockers are classified as ß₁- or "selective" ß-blockers, ß₂-blockers, and nonspecific ß-blockers (Figures 1.16–1.18) (Table 1.3). Beta₁ blockers, such as metoprolol, alter heart rate and myocardial contractile responses, but at low doses may not interfere with bronchial smooth-muscle dilation. At higher doses, the selective ß-blockers have physiologic ef-

CHEMICAL STRUCTURES OF SOME OF THE CURRENTLY USED β-ADRENERGIC ANTAGONISTS

Acebutolol

Alprenolol (β₁)

Atenolol (β₁)

Metoprolol (β₁)

Oxprenolol

Pindolol

Propranolol (nonspecific)

Sotalol

Timolol

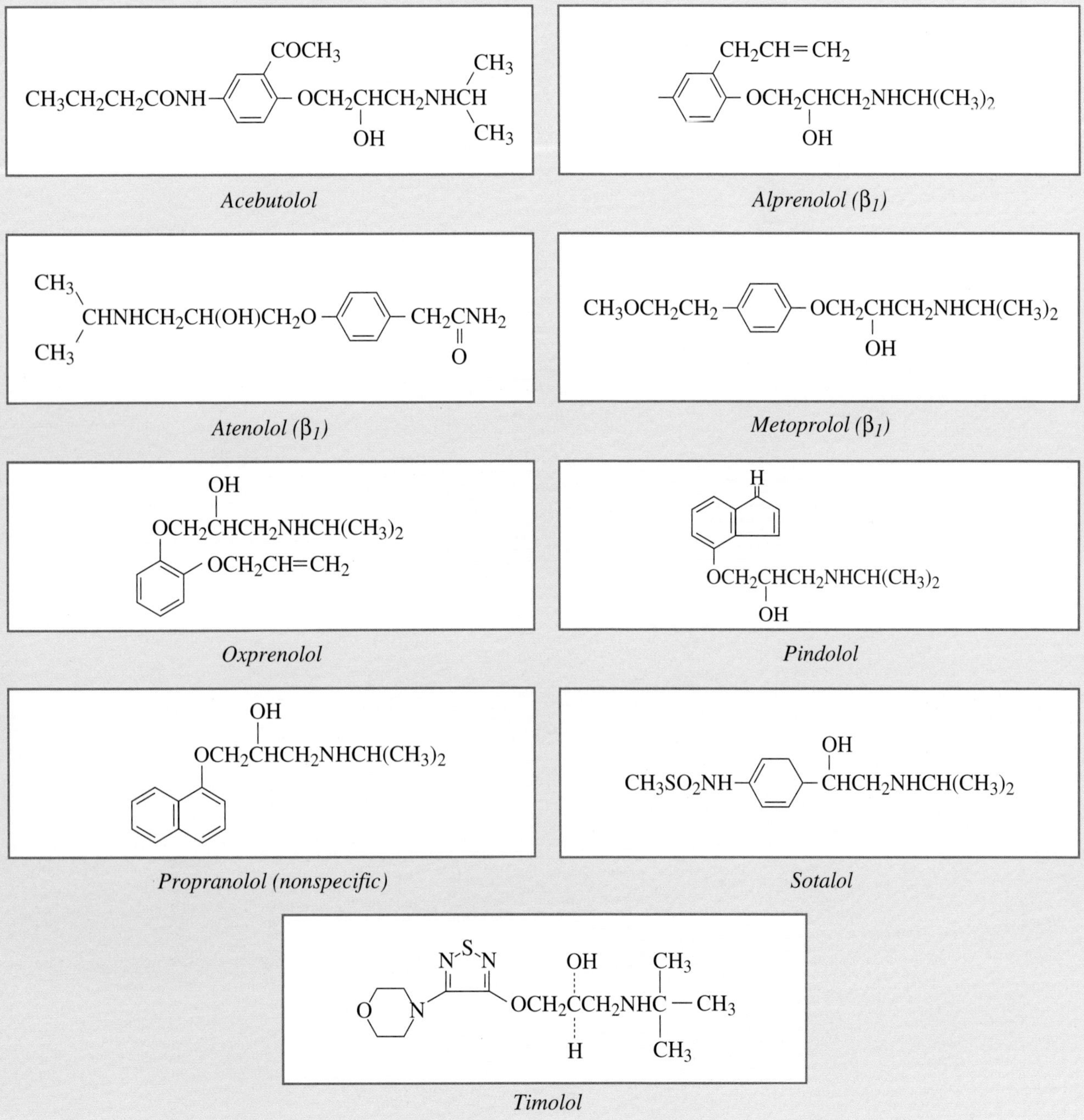

FIGURE 1.16 • The chemical structures for the ß-blockers currently in use.

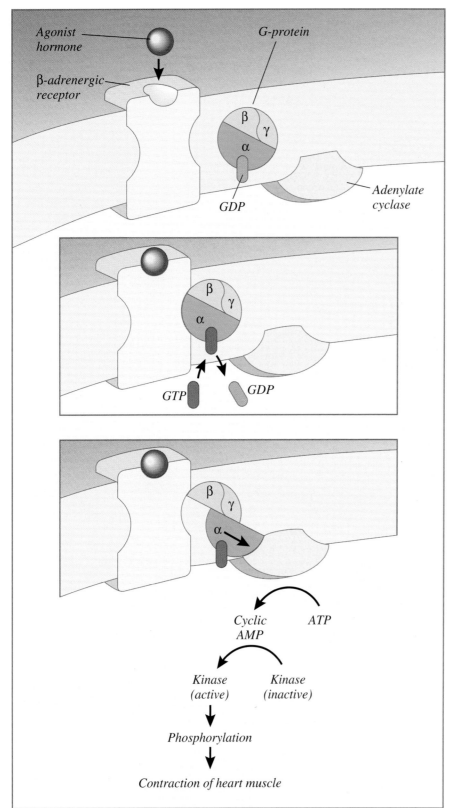

FIGURE 1.17 • The cellular basis for the ability of ß-adrenergic antagonists to interfere with agonist stimulation of ß-adrenergic receptors. Released form synaptic terminals, catacholamines enhance cardiac output and maintain arterial diffusion pressure. Beta-adrenergic receptor binds the catacholamines. The following is how catacholamines are released at the synapse leading to enhanced heart rate and contractile force:

• Sympathetic nerve terminals release norepinephrine, which binds to the ß-adrenergic receptor, activating adenylate cyclase.
• The increase in intracellular cyclic AMP leads to activation of protein kinase A.
• Protein kinase A phosphorylates a variety of proteins that enhance their catalytic activity, promoting a calcium-dependent increase in cardiac contractility.

fects more like those of the nonspecific ß-blockers, and may attenuate bronchial and smooth-muscle dilation and exacerbate bronchospasm. Nonspecific ß-blockers, such as propranolol, reduce heart rate and myocardial contractile state, and interfere with bronchial and vascular smooth-muscle dilation. Thus, reducing the dosage of β_1-blockers may be preferable in patients with chronic obstructive pulmonary diseases. Selective ß-blockers may also reduce insulin release less than nonspecific ß-blockers, and may therefore provide an advantage in the treatment of selected patients with insulin-dependent diabetes.

Side effects of the ß-blockers are listed in Table 1.4. Additionally, ß-blockers cause bradycardia, hypotension, and atrioventricular (AV) block, and may depress myocardial contractility. They may also exacerbate coronary artery spasm and make it more severe and frequent. Therefore, they should not be used in patients with bradycardia, hypotension, AV block, severe bronchopulmonary lung disease, coronary artery spasm, and/or clinically important heart failure. They should be used cautiously in patients with important peripheral vascular disease and insulin-dependent diabetes mellitus, particularly

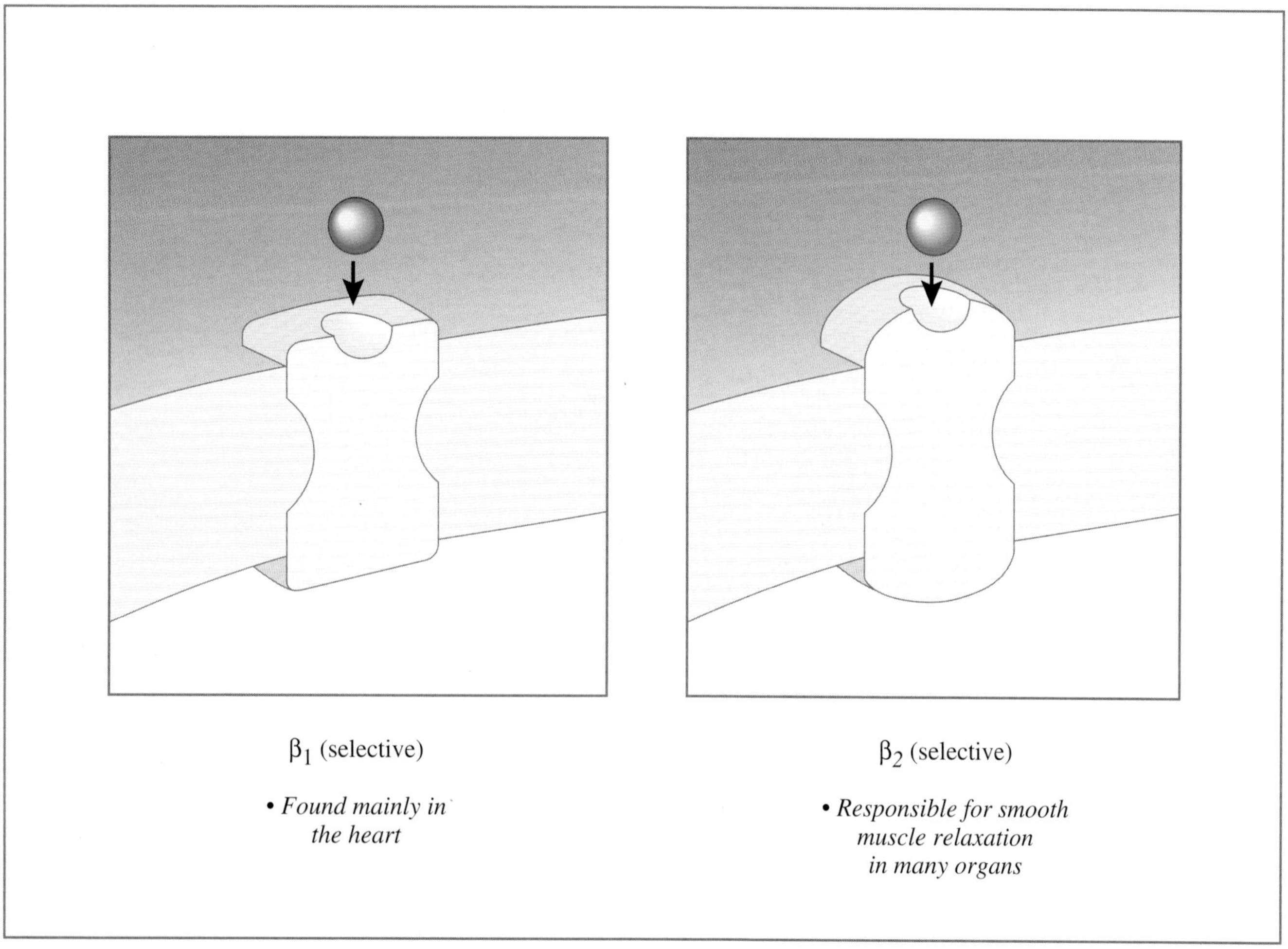

β_1 (selective)

• *Found mainly in the heart*

β_2 (selective)

• *Responsible for smooth muscle relaxation in many organs*

FIGURE 1.18 • The specific site of action for the β_1- and nonspecific ß-blockers.

TABLE 1.4 • SIDE EFFECTS OF ß-ADRENERGIC ANTAGONISTS		
Easy fatigability	Dyspnea with effort	Bradycardia
Insomnia	Sexual impotence	Heart block
Dizziness or syncope	Bronchospasm	Hypotension

when the blood sugar concentration has been labile and difficult to control.

Indications for ß-blocker administration are shown in Table 1.5. Contraindications to the administration of ß-blockers are listed in Table 1.6. Increasing in popularity are ß-blockers that may be administered once a day and have a sustained release into the systemic circulation, resulting in attenuation of ß-adrenergic responses throughout the day (Table 1.3). A ß-blocker should be considered for the patient who experiences angina at a relatively low level of physical activity or stress. Beta blockers are often used in conjunction with nitrates to treat exercise or stress-related angina.

CALCIUM ANTAGONISTS

Slow-channel calcium antagonists alter slow-channel calcium transport into the cell (Figures 1.19–1.23) (Table 1.7).[81–104] As a result, these agents cause vasodilation of vascular smooth muscle and increase coronary blood flow. Two of the slow-channel calcium antagonists, verapamil and diltiazem, slow the heart rate by decreasing sinus node impulse formation and atrioventricular (AV) conduction. Thus, verapamil and diltiazem have some of the same hemodynamic effects as ß-blockers in that they reduce myocardial oxygen demand at both rest and during exercise by attenuating the heart rate and contractile responses. However, they also increase coronary blood flow, primarily to epicardial regions supplied by severely narrowed coronary arteries.

Nifedepine, a dihydropyridine-derived slow-channel calcium antagonist, does not decrease impulse formation in the sinus node or delay AV conduction. Therefore, it does not decrease heart rate, but may actually increase it by producing systemic arterial vasodilation. Nifedepine dilates vascular smooth muscle, including coronary arteries, leading to increased coronary blood flow to the epicardial regions supplied by significantly narrowed coronary arteries (refer to Figures 1.19–1.23). Nitrendipine has physiologic actions similar to those of nifedepine.

TABLE 1.5 • INDICATIONS FOR ß-ADRENERGIC ANTAGONISTS IN PATIENTS WITH STABLE ANGINA
Prevent angina developing at relatively low-heart-rate–systolic blood pressure products
Treat exercise—induced ventricular arrhythmias
Treat systemic arterial hypertension

TABLE 1.6 • CONTRAINDICATIONS TO THE ADMINISTRATION OF ß-ADRENERGIC ANTAGONISTS
Severe congestive heart failure[1]
Marked bradycardia—heart rates < 55 beats/min
Advanced atrioventricular block— second or third degree
Systemic arterial hypotension— systolic blood pressure < 90 mm Hg
Severe peripheral vascular disease
Insulin-dependent diabetes mellitus that is poorly controlled and labile
Sexual impotence

[1]Selected patients with severe heart failure treated chronically with low doses of B-blockers are symptomatic during the course of months to years.

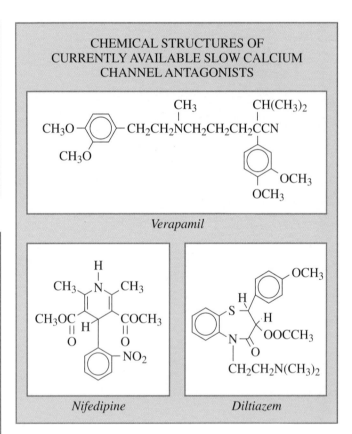

CHEMICAL STRUCTURES OF CURRENTLY AVAILABLE SLOW CALCIUM CHANNEL ANTAGONISTS

Verapamil

Nifedipine   *Diltiazem*

FIGURE 1.19 • The chemical structures for the slow-channel calcium antagonists that are currently available.

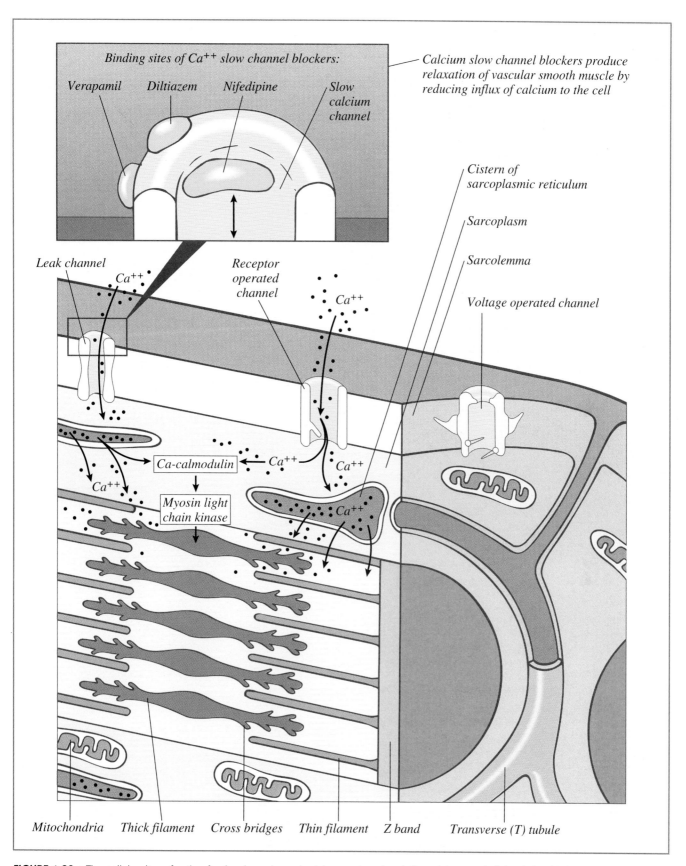

FIGURE 1.20 • The cellular sites of action for the slow-channel calcium antagonists. When the concentration of free intracellular calcium increases, a complex is formed between calcium and a specific calcium-binding protein, calmodulin. The calcium/calmodulin complex activates an enzyme—myosin light chain kinase—which promotes phosphorylation of the myosin light chain. This brings about the formation of cross bridges between actin and myosin. The inset shows the binding sites for the slow calcium-channel blockers. These slow calcium-channel blockers cause a relaxation of the vascular smooth muscle by reducing the influx of calcium to the cell.

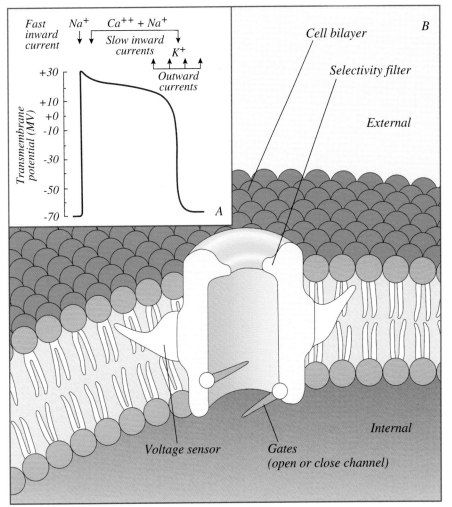

FIGURE 1.21 • The ionic movements associated with this ventricular action potential demonstrates the first current is carried by Na^+ and Ca^{++} is the second (A). Ca^{++}, which is a relatively slowly activated current, traverses the membrane through voltage-sensitive, gated, and ionic-sensitive channels. There seems to be a selectivity filter at the orifice of the channel because certain divalent cations cannot pentrate through it (B). The channel contains voltage sensors with gates opening to allow for the influx of Ca^{++}.

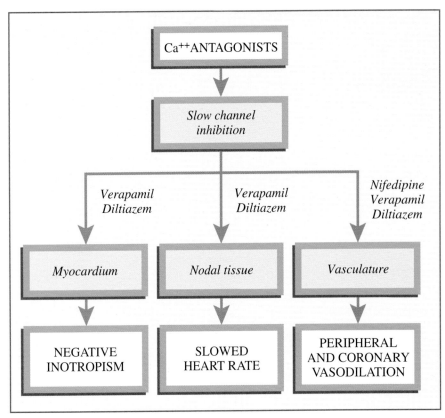

FIGURE 1.22 • The location and type of effect produced by each of the slow-channel calcium antagonists.

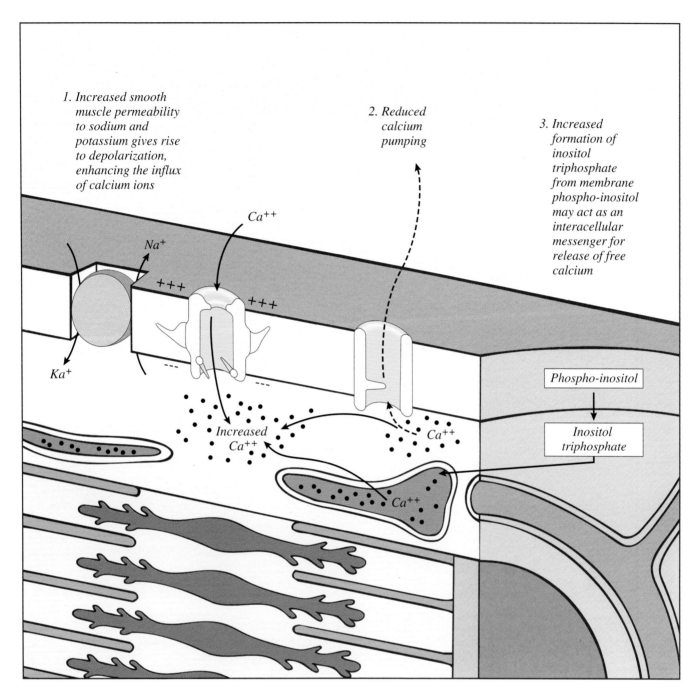

1. Increased smooth muscle permeability to sodium and potassium gives rise to depolarization, enhancing the influx of calcium ions

2. Reduced calcium pumping

3. Increased formation of inositol triphosphate from membrane phospho-inositol may act as an interacellular messenger for release of free calcium

Ca^{++}

Na^+

$+++$

$+++$

Ka^+

$- - -$

$- - -$

Increased Ca^{++}

Ca^{++}

Ca^{++}

Phospho-inositol

Inositol triphosphate

FIGURE 1.23 • Mechanisms by which membrane alterations may modify vascular smooth-muscle contraction.

Table 1.8 lists clinical indications for the administration of slow-channel calcium antagonists. Verapamil has a marked negative inotropic effect on the heart, and should not be given to patients with clinically important heart failure. Diltiazem has a smaller negative inotropic effect, but should neither be given to patients with severe heart failure nor be combined with another negative inotropic agent, such as a ß-blocker, in the patient with clinically important heart failure. Nifedepine may be given relatively safely to patients with important heart failure. Its negative inotropic effect is masked by its ability to reduce systemic vascular resistance, which allows the heart to contract against a reduced afterload.

Each of the slow-channel calcium antagonists has important side effects (Table 1.9). Nifedepine is probably the least well-tolerated of the calcium antagonists. Many patients describe a flushing sensation, dizziness, and palpitations that are consequences of its systemic vasodilating effect. Peripheral edema occurs in many who receive nifedepine, and is probably the result of venodilation.

Constipation is the major side effect noted by patients taking verapamil, although symptoms related to congestive heart failure, bradycardia, and/or advanced AV block may also occur. The combination of verapamil with a ß-blocker is particularly potent in reducing heart rate, systemic blood pressure, and

TABLE 1.7 • CALCIUM CHANNEL BLOCKERS

	Dosage		Onset of action		Therapeutic plasma concentration	Metabolism	Excretion
	Oral	IV	Oral	IV			
Diltiazem	30–90 mg q 6–8 hr	75–150 µg/kg ``(10–20 mg)	>30 min	<10 min	50-200 ng/mL	Deacetylation N-demethylation O-demethylation	60% fecal
Nifedipine	10–40 mg q 6–8 hr	5–15 µg/kg	>20 min	>5 min (3 min sublingual)	25-100 ng/mL	A hydroxycarboxylic acid and a lactone with no known activity	20–40% fecal 50–80% renal
Verapamil	80–120 mg q 6–12 hr	150 µg/kg ``(10–20 mg)	>30 min	>5 min	<100 ng/mL	N-dealkylation N-demethylation Major hepatic first pass effect	15% fecal 70% renal

(Reproduced with permission. Packer M, Firshman WH: *Calcium Channel Antagonists in Cardiovascular Disease* East Norwalk, CT: Appleton-Century-Crofts; 1984:8.)

TABLE 1.8 • CLINICAL INDICATIONS FOR THE ADMINISTRATION OF SLOW-CHANNEL CALCIUM ANTAGONISTS TO PATIENTS WITH STABLE ANGINA

Treat the patient with chest pain at a relatively low level of exercise or stress. A calcium antagonist may be used alone or in combination with nitrates and/or a ß- blocker.[1]

Treat the patient with systemic arterial hypertension.

Treat the patient with atrial arrhythmias.[2]

Treat the patient with exercise-induced ventricular tachycardia.[3]

[1]The safest calcium antagonist to combine with a ß-blocker is nifedipine, Verapamil and a ß-blocker given together may lead to marked bradycardia, hypotension, congestive heart failure, or atrioventricular block. Diltiazem and a ß-blocker may lead to similar clinical problems. Therefore, verapamil and diltiazem should be used with caution when either is combined with a ß-blocker.

[2]Verapamil may convert paroxysmal atrial tachycardia to sinus rhythm when given intravenously, and verapamil or diltiazem may prevent its recurrence and/or control the ventricular rate in patient in whom the arrhythmia recurs. Verapamil and diltiazem help control the ventricular rate in the patient with an atrial arrhythmia, such as atrial fibrillation or atrial flutter. Nifedipine has no protective effect against the atrial arrhythmias.

[3]The slow-channel calcium antagonists often prevent exercise-induced ventricular tachycardia.

contractile state. It should be used very carefully and not given to patients with heart failure, AV block, hypotension, or bradycardia.

Diltiazem is the best tolerated of the slow-channel calcium antagonists. When side effects occur, they are usually related to bradycardia or increasing heart failure. A suitable calcium antagonist may be used as an alternative to a ß-blocker in the treatment of patients with stable angina.

COMBINED THERAPY WITH A CALCIUM ANTAGONIST, NITRATE, AND ß-BLOCKER

A calcium antagonist may be combined with a nitrate and a ß-blocker in the treatment of patients with angina at low levels of effort. This combination of pharmacologic agents may be useful in allowing individual patients to be more active without inducing angina.

Clinically, nifedipine is safest to combine with a ß-blocker as a calcium antagonist. The next safest clinical combination is a ß-blocker with diltiazem. Combined therapy with a ß-blocker and diltiazem or verapamil should be initiated using relatively small doses of the calcium antagonist and gradually increasing them as the patient demonstrates hemodynamic responses consistent with the safety of the combined regimen.

PLATELET ANTAGONISTS

When endothelial injury occurs, platelets aggregate after attaching to the subendothelial collagen exposed by the injury. Platelet aggregation may mechanically obstruct severely narrowed coronary arteries, and is associated with the release of mediators that promote further platelet aggregation and dynamic vasoconstriction (refer to Figure 1.3).

Patients at increased risk for myocardial infarction with known or suspected coronary heart disease may have their risk of future myocardial infarction reduced by the administration of aspirin.[105,106] Aspirin is an inhibitor of platelet and endothelial cyclooxygenase, and thus reduces platelet thromboxane and endothelial-cell prostacyclin formation (Figure 1.24). Its effect on platelet cyclooxygenase is irreversible and persists for the lifetime of exposed platelets—approximately 11

days. With initial therapy, higher doses of aspirin are required to decrease endothelial cell cyclooxygenase activity. Therefore, aspirin in low doses tends to reduce thromboxane more than prostacyclin concentrations. However, chronic administration of aspirin even in low doses may reduce prostacyclin concentrations as well. Inhibiting the release of thromboxane attenuates platelet aggregation *in vivo*.

The amount of aspirin required to protect patients is not well established. The Harvard Physicians Study suggested that one aspirin every other day reduces the risk for myocardial infarction in male physicians believed to be at increased risk,[106] but a British study, in which one aspirin per day was administered, failed to show protection against myocardial infarction.[107]

The administration of aspirin to patients following myocardial infarction reduces the risk of recurrent infarction and death, especially in patients with non-Q-wave infarcts.[108] While the most protective dose of aspirin in patients with coronary disease is not known, many physicians recommend a dosage that ranges from the administration of one aspirin—325 mg—every other day to one aspirin daily in persons believed to be at risk for future coronary events. Ten large trials using platelet-inhibitor drugs in postmyocardial infarction patients have been reported.[105–108] In eight of these trials, aspirin at a dose of 300 to 1500 mg daily was used alone or in combination with dipyridamole. Pooled analyses suggest a significant reduction in mortality and reinfarction rates, of 15% and 31% respectively, in the aspirin-treatment groups.[105,108]

The chronic administration of aspirin, even in a low dose, may decrease vascular prostacyclin concentrations. This may be disadvantageous over time because prostacyclin is an endogenous endothelial vasodilator and inhibitor of platelet aggregation (refer to Figure 1.3).[15–17] We recommend a dosage of from one aspirin every other day to one aspirin per day in patients believed to be at increased risk for future coronary events and in whom there is no contraindication to such therapy. However, a dose as small as 80 mg of aspirin per day has been shown to reduce the frequency of vascular events and a sustained release form of aspirin also appears to be effective.[108a,108b]

· · · · · · · · · · · · · · · ·

TABLE 1.9 • SIDE EFFECTS OF SLOW CHANNEL CALCIUM ANTAGONISTS

Verapamil or Diltiazem	Nifedipine
• Marked bradycardia	• Flushing sensation
• Hypotension	• Dizziness
• Constipation	• Hypotension
• Congestive heart failure	• Peripheral edema
• Skin rash	• Tachycardia
• Heart block	• Skin rash

The side effects of aspirin therapy are listed in Table 1.10. Administration of aspirin with consequent cyclooxygenase inhibition and reduction in prostacyclin concentration may be associated with a reduction in renal blood flow and an increase in the serum blood urea nitrogen (BUN) and creatinine concentrations. Nonsteroidal anti-inflammatory agents that are cyclooxygenase inhibitors may also result in a reduction of renal blood flow and declining renal function. Periodic measurements of the BUN and creatinine concentrations are advised once aspirin therapy is begun. There is a risk of gastritis and gastrointestinal ulceration and bleeding when aspirin is administered. Some patients develop asthma. Thus, one needs to select patients carefully for the administration of aspirin, with the realization that more specific and potent antagonists of platelets and platelet-derived mediators should be available in the future.

Figure 1.25 demonstrates selected options for the treatment of patients with stable angina. It must be emphasized that when angina occurs at relatively low levels of effort or stress, or limits the lifestyle a patient wishes to lead while receiving appropriate medical intervention, the patient should be referred for coronary arteriography and subsequently for coronary artery revascularization, if the patient's coronary anatomy is suitable. The same is true for the patient with objective evidence of myocardial ischemia who is receiving appropriate medical intervention—classic ST-segment alteration and/or reversible alterations in myocardial perfusion or function—at low or moderate levels of stress. This can be seen on myocardial scintigraphy during exercise or with dipyridamole.[109-113] The life of a patient with a significant left main coronary artery stenosis—≥50% luminal-diameter narrowing—and of one with significant three-vessel coronary heart disease and depressed left ventricular function may be prolonged by coronary artery revascularization.[114-117]

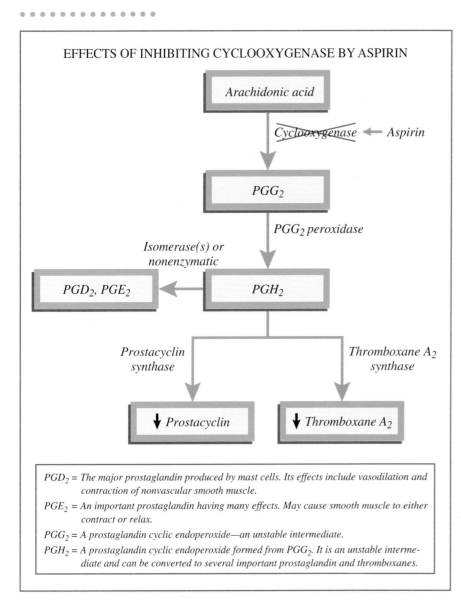

EFFECTS OF INHIBITING CYCLOOXYGENASE BY ASPIRIN

Arachidonic acid

Cyclooxygenase ← Aspirin

PGG_2

PGG_2 peroxidase

Isomerase(s) or nonenzymatic

PGD_2, PGE_2 ← PGH_2

Prostacyclin synthase

Thromboxane A_2 synthase

↓ Prostacyclin

↓ Thromboxane A_2

PGD_2 = The major prostaglandin produced by mast cells. Its effects include vasodilation and contraction of nonvascular smooth muscle.
PGE_2 = An important prostaglandin having many effects. May cause smooth muscle to either contract or relax.
PGG_2 = A prostaglandin cyclic endoperoxide—an unstable intermediate.
PGH_2 = A prostaglandin cyclic endoperoxide formed from PGG_2. It is an unstable intermediate and can be converted to several important prostaglandin and thromboxanes.

FIGURE 1.24 • The synthesis of thromboxane A_2 (TXA_2) and prostacyclin (PGI_2) from arachidonic acid in platelets and endothelial cells. Aspirin's inhibitory effect is at the cyclooxygenase step where it inhibits this enzyme and thereby diminishes the synthesis of both thromboxane A_2 and prostacyclin. Thromboxane TXA_2 synthesis inhibitors interfere with the conversion of PGH_2 to TXA_2 through thromboxane A_2 synthase. TXA_2 receptor antagonists antagonize the effects of TXA_2 on platelets and vascular tissue.

TABLE 1.10 • SIDE EFFECTS OF ASPIRIN		
Gastritis	Gastrointestinal bleeding	Asthma
Stomach or gastrointestinal ulceration	Easy bruising and bleeding with minor trauma	Decline in renal function Thrombocytopenia

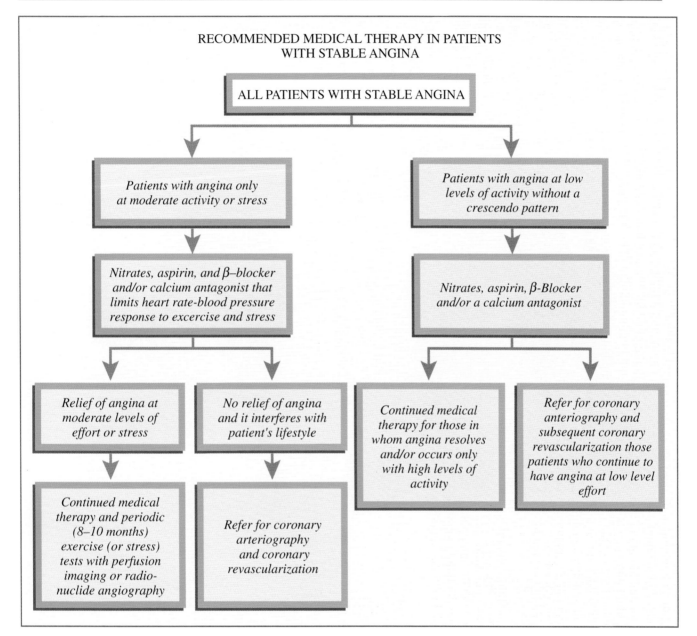

RECOMMENDED MEDICAL THERAPY IN PATIENTS
WITH STABLE ANGINA

ALL PATIENTS WITH STABLE ANGINA

Patients with angina only
at moderate activity or stress

Patients with angina at low
levels of activity without a
crescendo pattern

Nitrates, aspirin, and β–blocker
and/or calcium antagonist that
limits heart rate-blood pressure
response to excercise and stress

Nitrates, aspirin, β-Blocker
and/or a calcium antagonist

Relief of angina at
moderate levels of
effort or stress

No relief of angina
and it interferes with
patient's lifestyle

Continued medical
therapy for those in
whom angina resolves
and/or occurs only
with high levels of
activity

Refer for coronary
anteriography and
subsequent coronary
revascularization those
patients who continue to
have angina at low level
effort

Continued medical
therapy and periodic
(8–10 months)
exercise (or stress)
tests with perfusion
imaging or radio-
nuclide angiography

Refer for coronary
arteriography
and coronary
revascularization

FIGURE 1.25 • Therapeutic options for the treatment of the patient with stable angina.

TREATING THE PATIENT WITH UNSTABLE ANGINA

The development of unstable angina should be considered a relative medical emergency that warrants hospitalization to rule out recent myocardial infarction and to initiate therapy that might prevent infarction.

NITRATES

Pain relief for patients with unstable angina often occurs with complete bed rest and the institution of oral or transdermal nitrate therapy (refer to Table 1.2). Patients who continue to have unstable angina are given IV nitrates. Intravenous nitroglycerin is given beginning at a dose of 5 μg/min and increased in 5 μg/min doses until the patient's systolic blood pressure decreases by at least 10 mm Hg and the heart rate increases by 7 to 10 beats/min. The object of therapy is to relieve resting angina without causing tachycardia or hypotension. Irrespective of the route of their administration, tolerance to nitrates—lack of a hemodynamic response—may develop within 24 to 36 hrs unless there is a nitrate-free interval.[70,72]

We recommend the administration of isosorbide dinitrate (Isordil) every 8 hrs while the patient is awake, and the use of nitroglycerin transdermally only during the night and early morning hours—from bedtime to 9 am. This approach helps to reduce the development of tolerance to nitrates. Experimentally, the administration of N-acetylcysteine has been shown to promote and sustain the nitrate effect.[66,118]

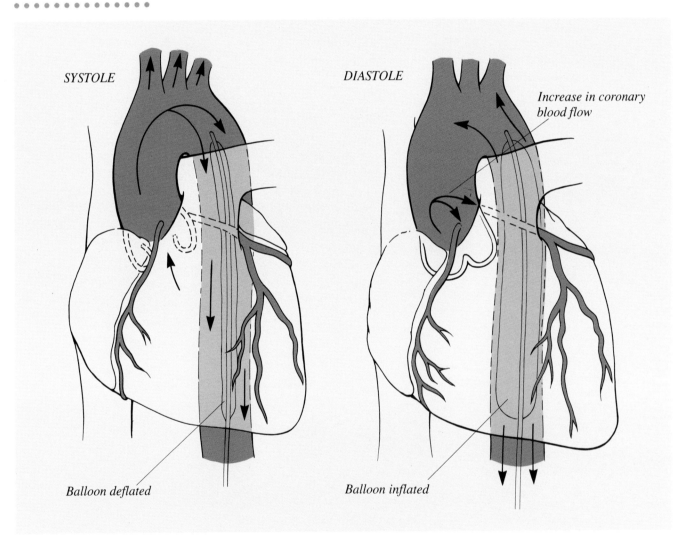

SYSTOLE

DIASTOLE

Increase in coronary blood flow

Balloon deflated

Balloon inflated

FIGURE 1.26 • The position in which the intraaortic balloon pump is placed in the aorta. The balloon deflates during cardiac systole and inflates during cardiac diastole. The net results of this filling and collapsing action are to increase the diastolic blood pressure in the proximal aorta and consequently increase coronary blood flow. The systolic collapse of the balloon reduces the work of the heart.

CALCIUM ANTAGONIST OR ß-BLOCKER

If unstable angina persists, a slow-channel calcium antagonist may be administered [81–96,119–121] (refer to Table 1.7). In the patient with a well-maintained blood pressure and heart rate in whom coronary artery spasm (Prinzmetal's angina) is not considered to be the pathophysiologic mechanism of unstable angina, a ß-blocker may be administered [75–77,79,80,122] (refer to Table 1.3). In the patient believed to have coronary artery spasm—the patient with angina at rest and ST-segment elevation during the pain without a preceding increase in heart rate or blood pressure—a calcium antagonist rather than a ß-blocker should be used [82–92] (refer to Table 1.7).

THE POSSIBILITY OF CARDIAC CATHETERIZATION OR CORONARY ARTERY REVASCULARIZATION

In the patient with persistent resting angina, cardiac catheterization and coronary artery revascularization become neces-sary. Intra-aortic balloon counterpulsation may be necessary to stabilize the patient prior to coronary arteriography and revascularization [123–125] (Figures 1.26, 1.27).

PLATELET ANTAGONISTS

A dose of one to four (325 mg) aspirin tablets/d reduces the risk of death and myocardial infarction in the patient with unstable angina [126–128] (Figure 1.28). Aspirin interferes with platelet aggregation and thromboxane A_2 release, thereby improving myocardial perfusion. If pain relief does not occur with bed rest and the use of appropriate medication, the risk of subsequent myocardial infarction, sudden death, and ventricular arrhythmias is increased. In the patient requiring urgent coronary artery revascularization, it is advisable to begin aspirin therapy immediately within 1 to 3 hrs after coronary artery bypass surgery to reduce the risk of prolonged bleeding while attenuating platelet aggregation on the newly established coronary artery grafts.

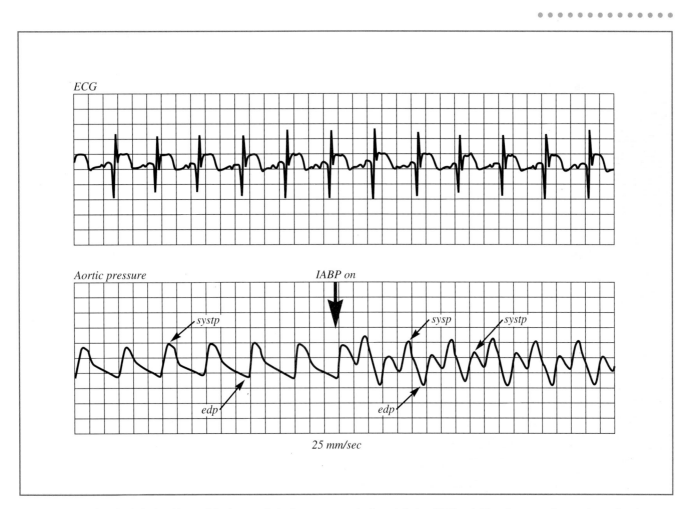

FIGURE 1.27 • The physiologic effects of the intraaortic balloon. Note the increase in aortic diastolic blood pressure associated with balloon inflation (IABP on). The electrocardiogram is used to time cardiac systole and diastole.

HEPARIN AND/OR OTHER THROMBIN ANTAGONISTS

Heparin and/or other thrombin antagonists should be given intravenously to the patient with persistent resting angina despite bed rest, nitrates, a calcium antagonist, and/or a ß-blocker.[128] Theroux et al.[128] have shown that the administration of heparin to these patients often relieves angina and reduces the risk of subsequent myocardial infarction and death (refer to Figure 1.28). The combination of aspirin and heparin in Theroux's study was no more effective than aspirin or heparin alone, and increased the risk of bleeding. We recommend the addition of IV bolus or continuous infusion heparin, in amounts sufficient to maintain serum partial thromboplastin time (PTT) values in the 48 to 60-sec range, for the patient with persistent resting angina despite appropriate medical intervention as described above.

CORONARY ARTERIOGRAPHY AND OTHER RECOMMENDED PROCEDURES

Coronary arteriography is often recommended for the patient with unstable angina without other severe and life-threatening medical disease or very advanced age, once the angina is controlled medically and a myocardial infarction is excluded (Figure 1.29). However, medical therapy with subsequent referral for coronary arteriography and coronary

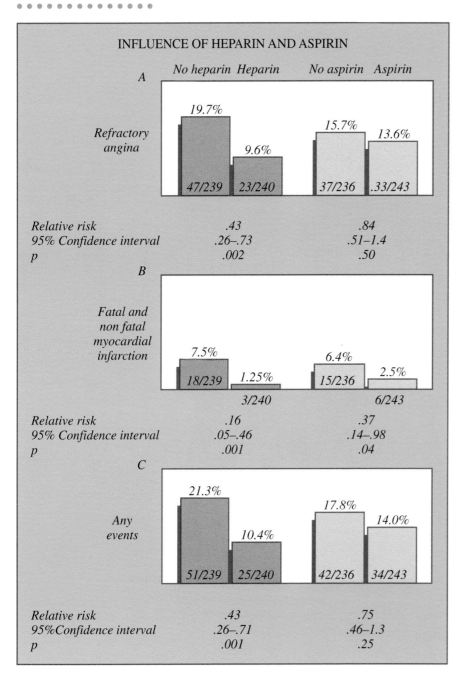

FIGURE 1.28 • Both aspirin and heparin reduce the risk of fatal and nonfatal myocardial infarction (B). Heparin also reduces the frequency of important coronary events, including death, fatal and nonfatal myocardial infarction and continuing angina (A–C). The combination of heparin and aspirin was no more successful than heparin alone in this study. (Reproduced with permission. Theroux P, Ouimet H, McCann J, et al: *N Engl J Med* 1988, 319:1105.)

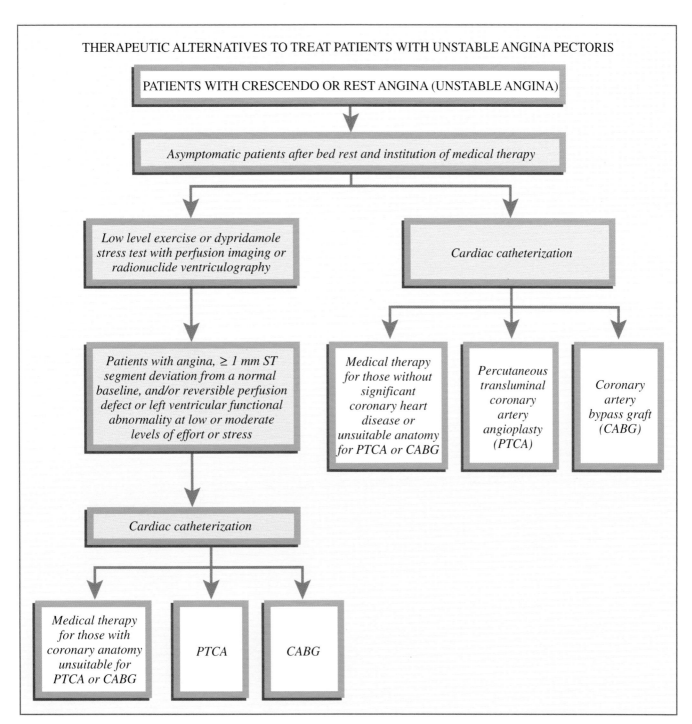

FIGURE 1.29 • Therapeutic alternatives for the treatment of patients with unstable angina pectoris.

revascularization is a reasonable alternative for patients who experience myocardial ischemia at low levels of effort (Figures 1.30, 1.31).

In the patient with recurrent resting angina despite an appropriate medical regimen, coronary arteriography becomes mandatory. Ten to fifteen percent of patients with unstable angina have significant stenoses—$\geq$ 50% luminal diameter narrowing—of the main left coronary artery.[129] Coronary artery bypass surgery prolongs the lives of these patients.[114–117] Furthermore, approximately 10% of patients with unstable angina

have no angiographic evidence of significant coronary disease,[129] and in 25% of these patients, the angiographic findings help in selecting an appropriate therapeutic approach. In the remaining patients, identifying the location and extent of coronary artery disease is useful prognostically. In the patient with continuing angina at rest, the arteriographic findings allow the physician to consider coronary artery bypass surgery or percutaneous transluminal coronary artery angioplasty (PTCA).

For the patient whose angina is controlled medically and a conservative regimen is chosen, and for the patient

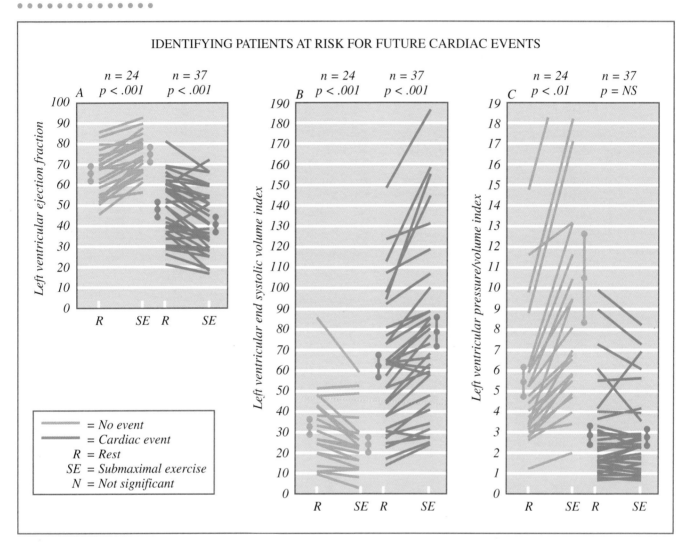

FIGURE 1.30 • Radionuclide ventriculography may be used at rest (R) and with low-level exercise (SE) at the time of hospital discharge after myocardial infarction to identify patients at risk for future cardiac events. Note the alterations in left ventricular ejection fraction (LVEF) (A), left ventricular end systolic volume indexed for body surface area (LVESVI) (B), and the left ventricular pressure volume index (LVPV index—the systolic blood pressure divided by the left ventric-

ular end systolic volume) (C). Patients who had future cardiac events, including death, recurrent myocardial infarction, unstable angina, and new congestive heart failure generally had abnormal submaximal exercise responses in their LVEFs, LVESVIs, and LVPV index and could be identified prospectively. (Reproduced with permission. Corbett J, Dehmer GJ, Lewis SE, et al: *Circulation* 1981;64:535.)

whose coronary angiographic findings do not suggest a need for immediate coronary artery revascularization, exercise or some form of stress testing should be done. Submaximal exercise tests may be done several days after the relief of chest pain, followed after several weeks by maximal exercise tests. The addition of some form of nuclear cardiology testing to the exercise test improves its sensitivity and specificity in the identification of patients with physiologically important coronary heart disease [109-113] (refer to Figures 1.30, 1.31).

Patients with continuing angina and/or objective evidence of myocardial ischemia at rest or with low levels of activity despite a good medical regimen, and those with significant three-vessel coronary stenoses and depressed left ventricular function—left ventricular ejection fraction greater than 25% and less than 50%—should undergo coronary artery revascularization.[114-117,129] Coronary artery revascularization relieves or markedly reduces the frequency of angina in the first group of patients, and prolongs the lives of patients in the second group (Figure 1.32).[114-117,129]

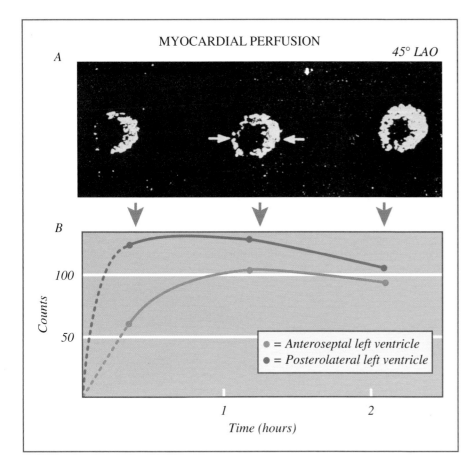

MYOCARDIAL PERFUSION

45° LAO

A

B

Counts

100

50

● = *Anteroseptal left ventricle*
● = *Posterolateral left ventricle*

1

2

Time (hours)

FIGURE 1.31 • Myocardial perfusion as evaluated by thallium-201 myocardial scintigraphy (A). Thallium-201 exercise scintigraphic studies are from a patient with an exercise-induced anteroseptal perfusion defect that reperfuses 1–2 hrs later (middle and far right). The images left-to-right, anterior, modified slight left anterior oblique and a 45° left anterior oblique image. Data from thallium-201 counts from the anteroseptal, and the posterolateral portions of the heart confirm the visual impression by demonstrating reduced thallium-201 uptake in the anteroseptal region and a delayed wash-out of thallium-201 from that same region in comparison to the posterolateral area (B).

In the patient with unstable angina, coronary artery bypass surgery or PTCA usually relieves angina. Coronary artery bypass surgery is associated with a reduced future risk of recurrent unstable angina as compared with continuing medical therapy.[129] However, coronary artery revascularization does not appear to reduce the risk of myocardial infarction or prolong the lives of patients with unstable angina who do not have a significant left main coronary artery stenosis and/or three-vessel coronary heart disease and reduced left ventricular function.

TREATING PATIENTS WITH CORONARY ARTERIAL SPASM (VARIANT ANGINA OR PRINZMETAL'S ANGINA)

Coronary artery spasm should be treated initially with nitrates and/or a selected calcium antagonist.[63–65,82–96] Beta-blockers are to be avoided in patients with suspected or documented coronary artery spasm since they may increase the frequency and severity of the spasm. Patients with variant angina generally respond well to medical therapy with nitrates and/or one of the selected calcium antagonists (Figure 1.33).

Episodes of coronary artery spasm tend to be intermittent, disappearing after a few days or weeks and sometimes recur-

ring months or years later. In general, coronary artery revascularization and percutaneous transluminal coronary angioplasty (PTCA) are not as useful in these patients as in those with other coronary heart disease syndromes. PTCA may cause immediate and recurrent spasms in individuals with coronary artery spasm. The exceptions are patients with extensive coronary stenoses and superimposed coronary artery spasm—it may be necessary to treat both of these pathophysiologic mechanisms of coronary heart disease. Coronary artery revascularization may be necessary in the patient with angina associated with low-level exercise or stress, an increased myocardial oxygen demand, and relative inability of the stenotic artery to deliver oxygen.[130] A calcium antagonist and/or nitrates are used to treat primary coronary blood flow decreases caused by coronary artery spasm, even if they are exercise-provoked.

TREATING PATIENTS WITH ACUTE Q-WAVE MYOCARDIAL INFARCTS

THROMBOLYTIC THERAPY

The patient with proven or suspected myocardial infarction should be admitted to a coronary care unit (CCU) where the heart rate and rhythm are monitored continuously. Unless there is some important contraindication (Table 1.11),

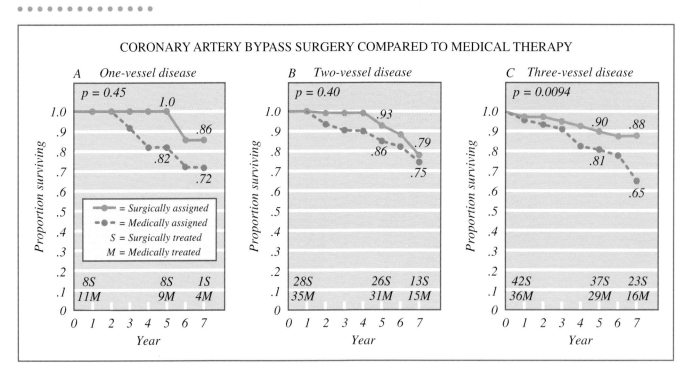

FIGURE 1.32 • The influence of coronary artery bypass surgery as compared to medical therapy in patients with significant single-vessel disease (A), two-vessel disease (B), and three-vessel disease (C). Survival is better in patients with three-vessel coronary disease who have coronary artery surgery. (Reproduced with permission. Passamani E, Davis KB, Gillespie MJ, et al: *N Engl J Med* 1985;312:1665.)

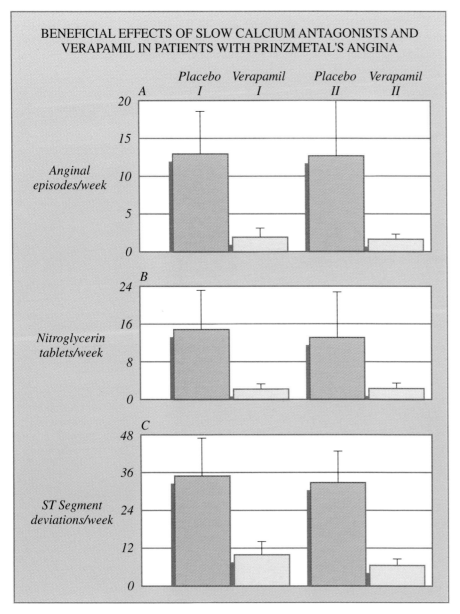

BENEFICIAL EFFECTS OF SLOW CALCIUM ANTAGONISTS AND
VERAPAMIL IN PATIENTS WITH PRINZMETAL'S ANGINA

FIGURE 1.33 • The beneficial effect of the slow-channel calcium antagonist—verapamil—in patients with Prinzmetal's angina. Verapamil reduced the:
• Number of anginal episodes per week (A).
• Number of nitroglycerin tablets consumed/week (B).
• Electrocardiographic alterations detected by continuous 24-hr Holter monitoring (C). (Reproduced with permission. Johnson SM, Mauritson DR, Willerson JT et al: *N Engl J Med* 1981;304:862.)

TABLE 1.11 • CONTRAINDICATIONS TO THROMBOLYTIC THERAPY

Active bleeding

Prolonged or traumatic cardiopulmonary resuscitation

Recent head trauma or known intracranial neoplasm

Intracerebral hemorrhage in the past

Pregnancy

Systemic arterial hypertension

Diabetic hemorrhagic retinopathy

Recent surgery within the previous 4 weeks

Active peptic ulcer

Known bleeding diathesis

Previous allergic reaction to streptokinase, is the only thrombolytic intervention available

Severe liver dysfunction

patients with anterior Q-wave infarcts evaluated within 6 hrs of symptom onset should receive thrombolytic therapy as soon as possible [131-189] (Tables 1.12, 1.13 and Figures 1.34–1.36). Patients with continuing or recurrent chest pain believed to represent angina and Q-wave infarction should probably receive thrombolytic therapy—even 6 to 24 hrs af-

TABLE 1.12 • CURRENTLY AVAILABLE THROMBOLYTIC INTERVENTIONS

Streptokinase

Acylated streptokinase (APSAC)

Urokinase

Zymogen precursor of urokinase (prourokinase; SCUPA)

Tissue plasminogen activator (t-PA)

New Fibrinolytic Agents Under Development

Mutant tissue plasminogen activators that have prolonged clearance, do not bind to their endogenous inhibitor, etc.

Monoclonal antibody to fibrin, coupled to plasminogen activators

Hybrid thrombolytic interventions combining the active regions of urokinase and rt-PA in one molecule.

TABLE 1.13 • CONTROLLED TRIALS USING THROMBOLYTIC THERAPY

Trial	Patients (n)	Mortality treatment	Control	Follow-up interval	Percent reduction	Percent reduction in mortality in subgroups by time to treatment
Gruppo Italiano perlo Studio della Streptochinasi nell'Infarto Miocardio (GISSI-1)—streptokinase	11,712	10.7%	13.0%	21 days	18%	6–12 hr (-3%) 3–6 hr (17%) 0–3 hr (23%) <1 hr (47%)
International Study of Infarct Survival-2 (ISIS-2)—streptokinase with/without aspirin	17,187	9.1%	11.8%	35 days	23%	12–24 hr (19%) 4–12 hr (13%) <4 hr (32%) <1 hr (42
Anglo-Scandinavian Study of Early Thrombolysis (ASSET)—recombinant tissue-plasminogen activator	5,011	7.2%	9.8%	30 days	26%	3–5 hr (24%) <3 hr (26%)
Eur Coll—recombinant tissue-/plasminogen activator and aspirin	721	2.8%	5.7%	14 days	51%	3–5 hr (8%) <3 hr (82%)
APSAC Interventional Mortality Study (AIMS)—Acylated streptokinase (APSAC)	1,258	6.0%	12.0%	30 days	47%	4–6 hr (52%) <4 hr (41%)
Gruppo Italiano perlo Studio della Streptochinasi nell'Infarto Mio-cardio (GISSI-2)—Streptokinase and tissue plasminogen activator	20,749	SK:8.5% t-PA:8.9%		13 days		All patients treated ≤ 6 hrs
International Study of Infarct Survival (ISIS-3)	46,092	SK:10.5% t-PA:10.3% APSAC:10.6%		35 days		All patients treated ≤ 24 hrs

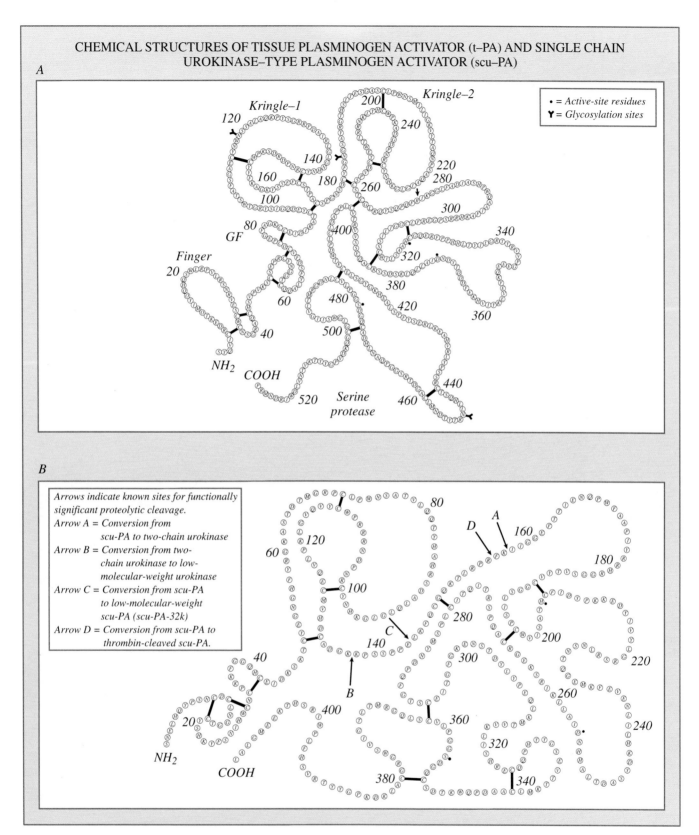

CHEMICAL STRUCTURES OF TISSUE PLASMINOGEN ACTIVATOR (t–PA) AND SINGLE CHAIN UROKINASE–TYPE PLASMINOGEN ACTIVATOR (scu–PA)

FIGURE 1.34 • Primary and secondary structure of tissue plaminogen activator (t-PA) (A), as well as the single chain urokinase-type plasminogen activator (scu-PA) (B). The scu-PA molecule is a single chain polypeptide of 411 amino acids. (Adapted with permission. Holmes WE, et al: *Biotechnology* 1985;3:923.)

ter myocardial infarction[160] (Figures 1.37, 1.38). Thrombolytic therapy should be given in association with a thrombin antagonist, IV heparin, presently, and aspirin during the first 24 hrs [160,184,185] (Figures 1.39, 1.40). Aspirin should be continued, one tablet every day or every other day for at least the next 6 months. Patients with inferior Q-wave infarcts should also receive thrombolytic therapy when they seek medical attention within the first 4 hrs after a myocardial infarction, especially if the infarct includes multiple surfaces of the heart—the right ventricle and/or lateral or true posterior wall of the left ventricle[134] (refer to Figures 1.36–1.38).

THROMBOLYTIC AGENTS

Thrombolytic agents currently available for the treatment of acute myocardial infarction are shown in Table 1.12 and Figures 1.34–1.36. Streptokinase is antigenic and was isolated originally from streptococci. This agent activates plasminogen to plasmin in the systemic circulation, as well as activating plasminogen bound to fibrin in the interstices of the thrombus. Plasmin is a serine protease that degrades fibrin, thrombin, and clotting factors V, VIII, IX, and XII.

• • • • • • • • • • • • • •

MOLECULAR STRUCTURE OF ANISTREPLASE

Streptokinase

Lys-plasminogen

Lys 78

p-Anisoyl group

O
CO

OCH₃

Catalytic center

Fibrin binding site (kringles)

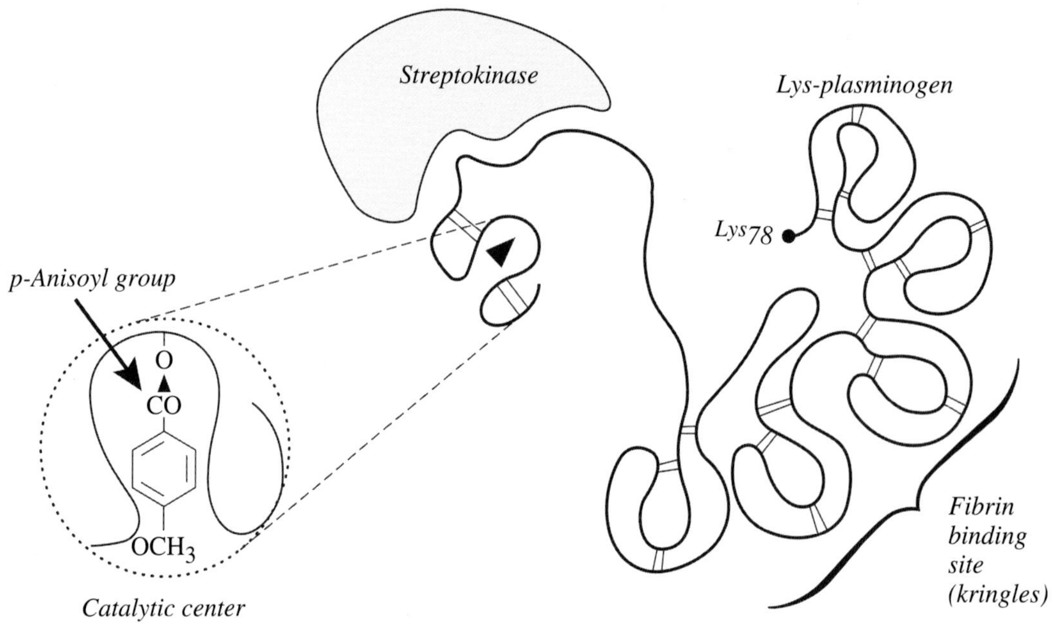

FIGURE 1.35 • Molecular structure of anistreplase. (Modified with permission. Haber E, Braunwald E, eds. *Thrombolysis. Basic Contributions and Clinical Progress* St. Louis, Mo: Mosby Year Book; 1991:266.)

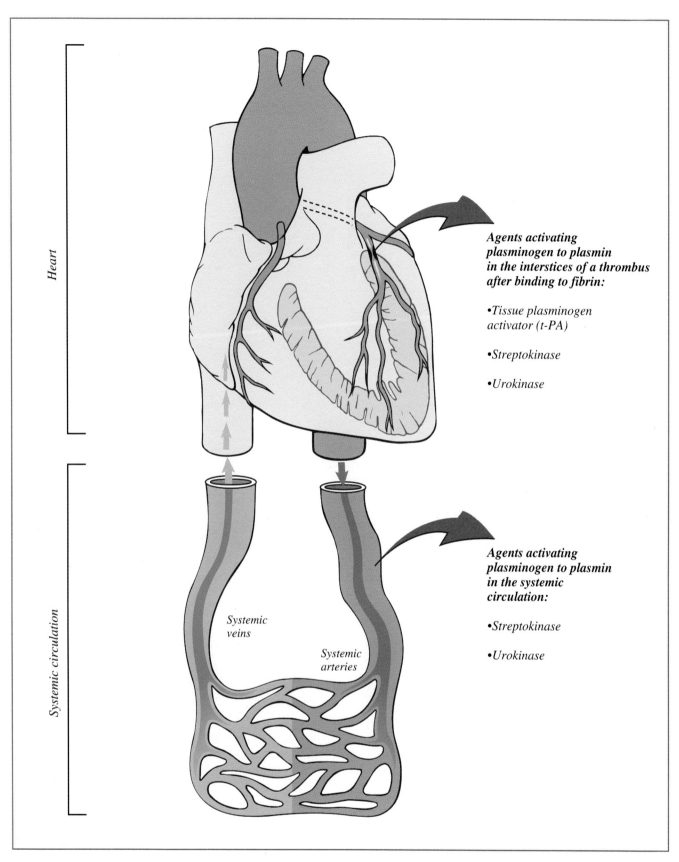

*Agents activating
plasminogen to plasmin
in the interstices of a thrombus
after binding to fibrin:*

*•Tissue plasminogen
activator (t-PA)*

•Streptokinase

•Urokinase

*Agents activating
plasminogen to plasmin
in the systemic
circulation:*

•Streptokinase

•Urokinase

Heart

Systemic circulation

*Systemic
veins*

*Systemic
arteries*

FIGURE 1.36 • The sites of action of currently available thrombolytic interventions. Tissue plasminogen activator (t-PA) activates plasminogen to plasmin in the interstices of a thrombus after binding to fibrin. Streptokinase and urokinase activate plasminogen to plasmin in the systemic circulation and in the interstices of a thrombus. t-PA is a more slective activator of plasminogen to plasmin compared to streptokinase and urokinase.

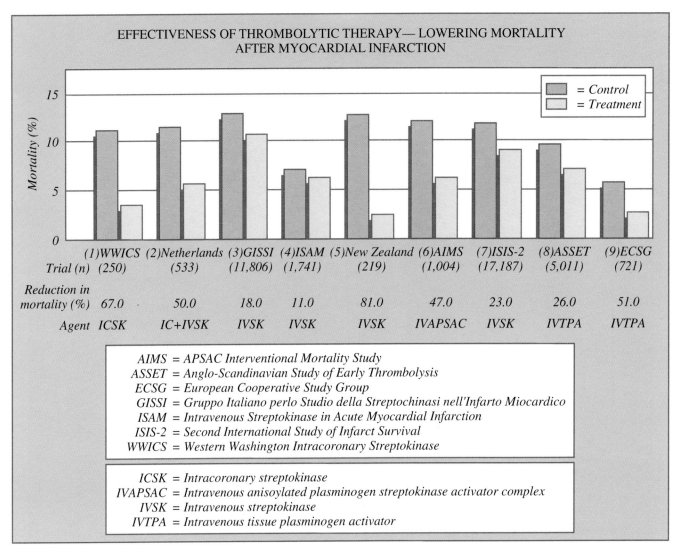

FIGURE 1.37 • Reductions in mortality associated with the administration of thrombolytic therapy in several different studies. (Modified with permission. Agress C: *Primary Cardiology* 1989;15:44 and Rich MW, ed. *Coronary Care for the House Officer* Baltimore, Md: Williams and Wilkins Co; 1989:79.)

References (1) Kennedy JW, Ritchie JL, Davis KB, et al: The Western Washington randomized trial of intracoronary streptokinase in acute myocardial infarction. *N Engl J Med* 1985;312:1073. (2) Netherlands trial. (3) Gruppo Italiano perlo Studio della Streptochinasi nell'Infarto Miocardico (GISSI): Effectiveness of intravenous thrombolytic treatment in acute myocardial infarction. *Lancet* 1986;1:397. (4) The ISAM Study Group: Intravenous streptokinase in acute myocardial infarction: Preliminary results of a prospective controlled trial (ISAM). *Circulation* 1985;72(Suppl 3):III-223 and ISAM Study Group: A prospective trial of intravenous streptokinase in acute myocardial infarction (ISAM): Mortality, morbidity, and infarct size at 21 days. *N Engl J Med* 1986;314:1465. (5) New Zealand trial. (6) AIMS Trial Study Group: Effect of intravenous APSAC on mortality after acute myocardial infarction: Preliminary report of a placebo-controlled trial. *Lancet* 1988;1:545. (7) ISIS-2 (Second International Study of Infarct Survival) Collaborative Group: Randomised trial of intravenous streptokinase, oral aspirin, both, or neither among 17,187 cases of suspected acute myocardial infarction. *Lancet* 1988;2:349. (8) Wilcox RG, von der Lippe G, Olsson CG, et al: Trial of tissue plasminogen activator for mortality reduction in acute myocardial infarction: Anglo-Scandinavian Study of Early Thrombolysis (ASSET). *Lancet* 1988;2:525. (9) de Bono DP: The European Cooperative Study Group trial of intravenous recombinant tissue-type activator (rt-PA) and conservative therapy versus rt-PA and immediate coronary angioplasty. *J Am Coll Cardiol* 1988;12(Suppl 6A):20A.

Urokinase is nonantigenic and was isolated originally from fetal kidney tissue. It also activates plasminogen to plasmin in the circulation and plasminogen bound to fibrin within a thrombus. Thus, both streptokinase and urokinase may reduce the systemic fibrinogen concentration as a result of their nonselective thrombolytic effects.

The decrease in systemic fibrinogen concentration persists for approximately 24 hrs. Streptokinase should not be

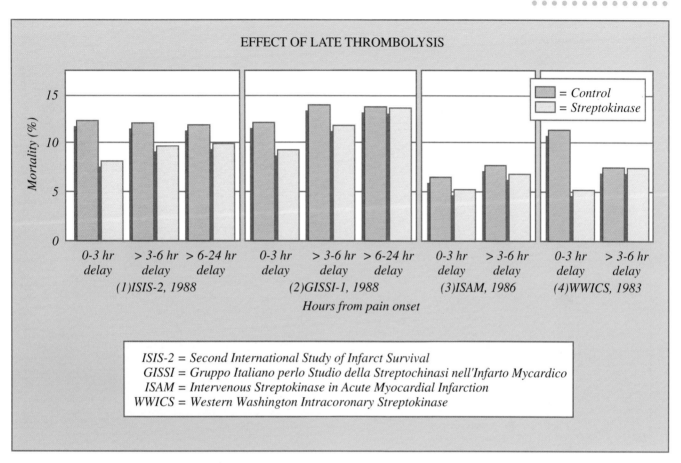

FIGURE 1.38 • The influence of the various forms of thrombolytic therapy on mortality reduction in patients with acute myocardial infarcts when streptokinase is used as a thrombolytic agent. The greatest reduction in mortality is associated with the earliest administration of streptokinase. (Modified with permission. Agress C: *Primary Cardiology* 1989;15:44 and ISIS-2 (Second International Study of Infarct Survival) Collaborative: *Lancet* 1988;2:349.)

References (1) ISIS-2 (Second International Study of Infarct Survival) Collaborative Group: Randomised trial of intravenous streptokinase, oral aspirin, both, or neither among 17,187 cases of suspected acute myocardial infarction. *Lancet* 1988;2:349. (2) Gruppo Italiano perlo Studio della Streptochinasi nell'Infarto Miocardico (GISSI): Effectiveness of intravenous thrombolytic treatment in acute myocardial infarction. *Lancet* 1986;1:397. (3) The ISAM Study Group: Intravenous streptokinase in acute myocardial infarction: Preliminary results of a prospective controlled trial (ISAM). *Circulation* 1985;72(Suppl 3):III-223 and ISAM Study Group: A prospective trial of intravenous streptokinase in acute myocardial infarction (ISAM): Mortality, morbidity, and infarct size at 21 days. *N Engl J Med* 1986;314:1465. (4) Kennedy JW, Ritchie JL, Davis KB, et al: The Western Washington randomized trial of intracoronary streptokinase in acute myocardial infarction. *N Engl J Med* 1985;312:1073.

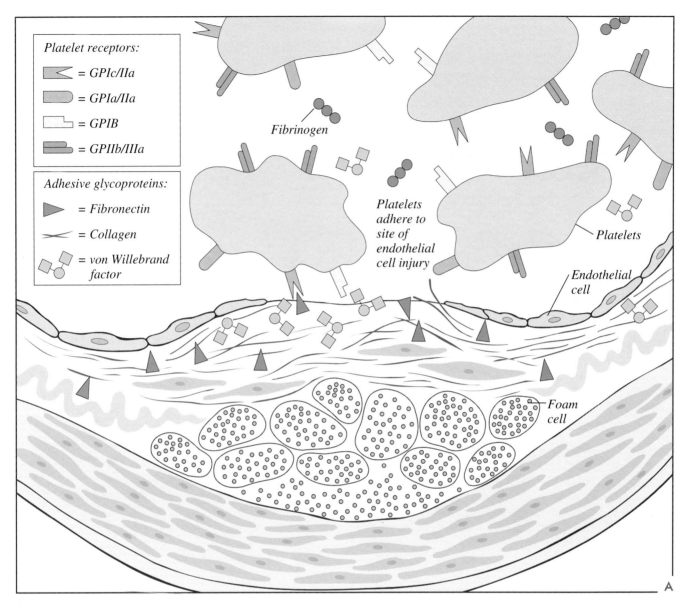

Platelet receptors:

= GPIc/IIa

= GPIa/IIa

= GPIB

= GPIIb/IIIa

Adhesive glycoproteins:

= Fibronectin

= Collagen

= von Willebrand factor

Fibrinogen

Platelets adhere to site of endothelial cell injury

Platelets

Endothelial cell

Foam cell

A

FIGURE 1.39 • Platelet adhesion and aggregation (A). The major physiologic role of platelets is to prevent damage from damaged cells. Complex adaptations have enabled them to adhere to sites of vascular damage followed by the formation of a hemostatic plug. Finally, the acceleration of the deposition of insoluble fibrin strands stabilizes the repair.

The endothelium is a nonthrombogenic surface, but when it is damaged, adhesive glycoproteins, such as collagen, von Willebrand factor, and fibronectin are exposed to flowing blood. Platelets contain a number of different receptors on their surface that have a high affinity for the adhesive glycoproteins in the subendothelium—GPIb, GPIa/IIa, and GPIc/IIa. After platelets adhere to the surface, their GPIb/IIIa receptors undergo a transition that increases their affinity for several adhesive glycoproteins. Most evidence points to important roles for fibrinogen and von Willebrand factor—depending on shear forces. At present, it appears that all platelet aggregation is mediated by the GPIIb/IIIa receptor.

Formation of platelet-fibrin thrombi (B). Von Willebrand factor serves as an anchor to mediate adhesion of platelets to the zone of vascular injury. Fibrinogen plays a dual role, it is:

• An adhesive molecule bridging the GPIIb/IIIa receptor on activated platelets.

• A substrate for thrombin.

The resulting fibrin meshwork constitutes an integral structure of the platelet-fibrin thrombus.

Disintegration of a platelet-fibrin thrombus and of hemostatic plug during lysis mediated by plasmin (C). Plasminogen activators—tissue plasminogen activator (t-PA), steptokinase, and urokinase—induce activation of plasminogen to plasmin. Plasmin breaks down the fibrin scaffolding of pathologic thrombi or of a hemostatic plug. Reopening of the occluded blood vessels in one location may be accompanied by disruption of recently formed hemostatic plugs sealing off breaks elsewhere in the vasculature. (Modified and reproduced with permission. Haber E, Braunwald E, eds. *Thrombolysis. Basic Contributions and Clinical Progress* St. Louis, Mo: Mosby Year Book; 1991:157,134,135.)

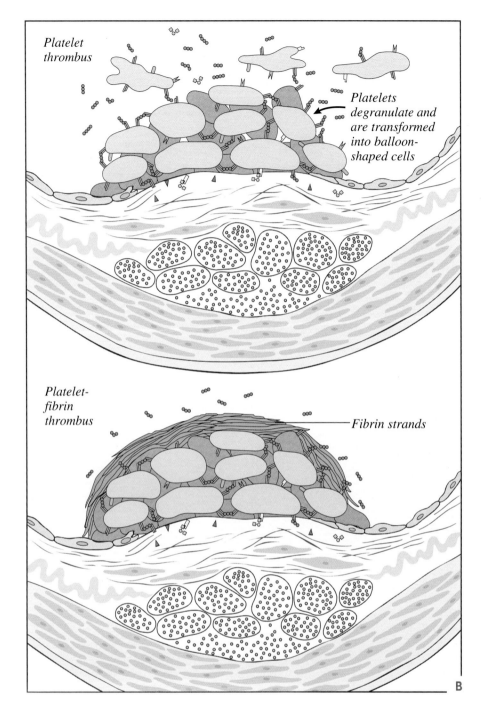

Platelet thrombus

Platelets degranulate and are transformed into balloon-shaped cells

Platelet-fibrin thrombus

Fibrin strands

B

FIGURE 1.39 CONT'D • Formation of platelet-fibrin thrombi (B). Von Willebrand factor serves as an anchor to mediate adhesion of platelets to the zone of vascular injury. Fibrinogen plays a dual role, it is:
• An adhesive molecule bridging the GPIIb/IIIa receptor on activated platelets.
• A substrate for thrombin.
The resulting fibrin meshwork constitutes an integral structure of the platelet-fibrin thrombus.

given again within 1 year after its initial administration, since it may cause an allergic response and be less effective the second time because of the development of systemic antibodies to it. Acylated streptokinase, also known as anisoylated plasminogen streptokinase activator complex (APSAC), may be more thrombus-selective than streptokinase in its plasminogen activation. Tissue plasminogen ac- tivating factor (t-PA) exerts an even more selective thrombolytic effect than APSAC, converting plasminogen to plasmin primarily within the t-PA/fibrin complex of a thrombus. In the doses usually administered—80 to 100 mg—t-PA does not significantly activate plasminogen to plasmin in the systemic circulation. When given intravenously 5 hrs after the onset of myocardial infarction symptoms, t-PA is supe-

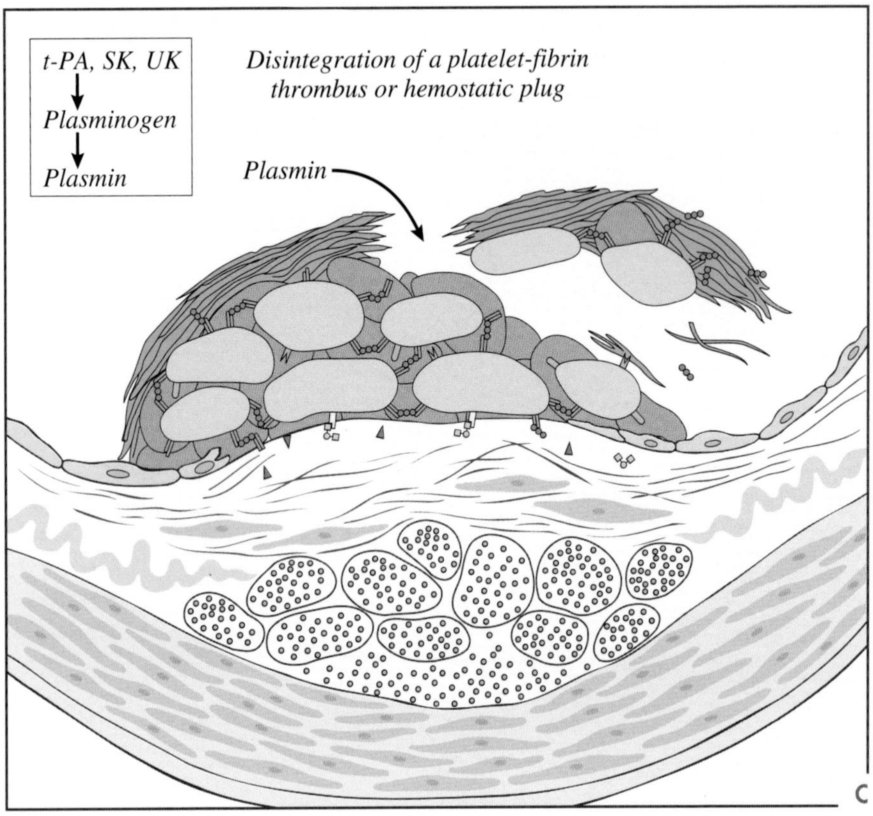

t-PA, SK, UK
↓
Plasminogen
↓
Plasmin

Disintegration of a platelet-fibrin thrombus or hemostatic plug

Plasmin

C

FIGURE 1.39 CONT'D • Disintegration of a platelet-fibrin thrombus and of hemostatic plug during lysis mediated by plasmin (C). Plasminogen activators—tissue plasminogen activator (t-PA), steptokinase, and urokinase—induce activation of plasminogen to plasmin. Plasmin breaks down the fibrin scaffolding of pathologic thrombi or of a hemostatic plug. Reopening of the occluded blood vessels in one location may be accompanied by disruption of recently formed hemostatic plugs sealing off breaks elsewhere in the vasculature. (Modified and reproduced with permission. Haber E, Braunwald E, eds. *Thrombolysis. Basic Contributions and Clinical Progress* St. Louis, Mo: Mosby Year Book; 1991:157,134,135.)

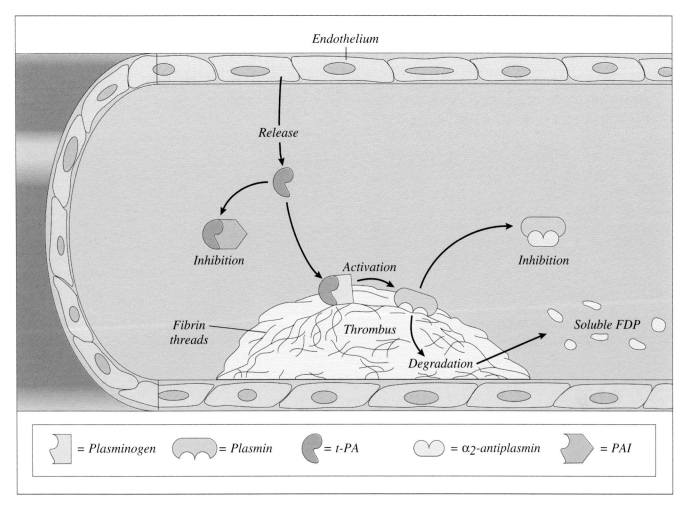

Endothelium

Release

Inhibition

Activation

Inhibition

Fibrin threads

Thrombus

Soluble FDP

Degradation

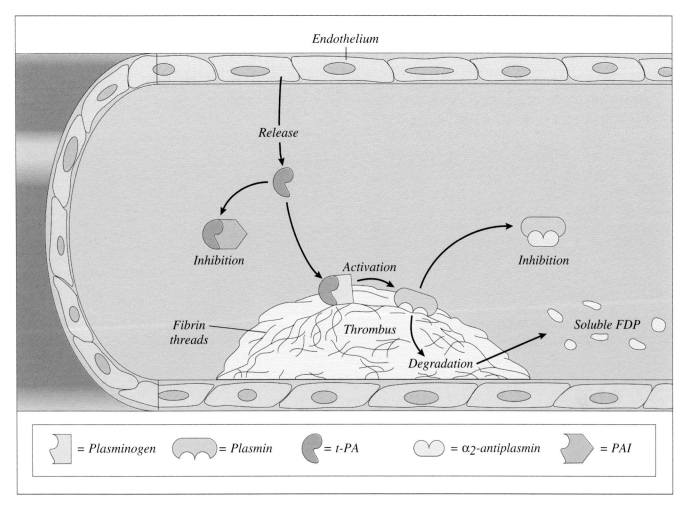 = *Plasminogen*   = *Plasmin*   = *t-PA*   = *α₂-antiplasmin*   = *PAI*

FIGURE 1.40 • Some of the important interactions for regulation of the fibrinolytic enzyme system. Crucial in the regulation of fibrinolytic activity in the circulation is the vessel wall. Tissue plasminogen activator (t-PA) is secreted when stimulated from the vascular endothelium. Also, PAI-1 inactivates some of the t-PA. Protolytic enzyme, plasmin, is the central component of the fibrinolyic system. Activation of plasminogen occurs at the fibrin site due to the affinity for fibrin of t-PA and plasminogen. Plasmin attached to fibrin is protected against inactivation by A₂-antiplasmin assuring a localized action of the fibrinolytic enzyme system. (Modified with permission: Haber E, Braunwald E, eds. *Thrombolysis. Basic Contributions and Clinical Progress* St. Louis, Mo: Mosby Year Book; 1991:124.)

rior to streptokinase in achieving relatively rapid thrombolysis[152] (Figures 1.41, 1.42), but by 24 to 48 hrs later, essentially the same number of coronary arteries are patent in patients treated with streptokinase or t-PA (Figure 1.43).

THROMBOLYTIC THERAPY—EFFECTS ON VENTRICULAR FUNCTION AND MORTALITY

Successful thrombolytic therapy within the first 1 to 2 hrs after infarction may reduce infarct size and preserve segmen-

tal and global left ventricular function (Figures 1.44–1.46 and Table 1.14). Successful thrombolytic therapy within the initial 6 hours reduces mortality in patients with anterior Q-wave infarcts[133,134,160] (refer to Figures 1.37, 1.38).

The second International Study of Infarct Survival (ISIS-2) provided evidence that aspirin alone at a dose of 160 mg, streptokinase alone and, even more potently, combined aspirin and streptokinase, reduce mortality in patients with suspected myocardial infarction treated within 24 hrs

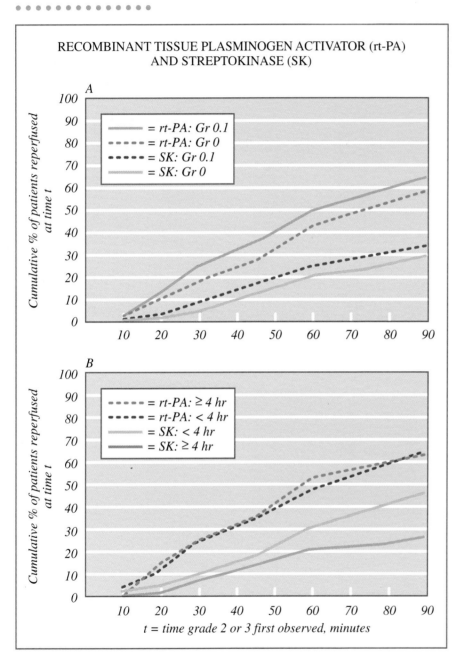

FIGURE 1.41 • Recombinant tissue plasminogen activator (rt-PA) is superior to streptokinase (SK) in opening the infarct-related artery when both are given intravenously approximately 5 hrs after symptom onset suggestive of myocardial infarction (A,B). (Reproduced with permission. Chesebro JH, Knatterud G, Roberts R: *J Am Coll Cardiol* 1985;6:518)

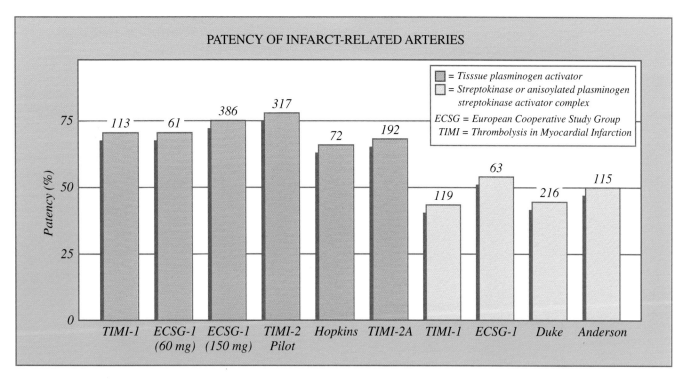

FIGURE 1.42 • Patency of infarct-related areteries in patients treated with streptokinase, tissue plasminogen activator (t-PA), or anisoylated plasminogen streptokinase activator complex (APSAC) in trials in which angiographic endpoints were employed. Patency rates were substantially higher for patients treated with t-PA compared to those treated with other agents. (Reproduced with permission. Sobel BE: *J Am Coll Cardiol* 1989:14:850.)

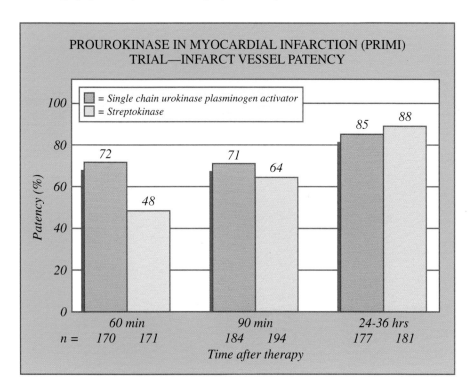

FIGURE 1.43 • Data from the Prourokinase in Myocardial Infarction (PRIMI) trial—angiographic infarct vessel patency. Early patency was superior for prourokinase compared to streptokinase, but at 24 hrs, both were equal. (Reproduced with permission. PRIMI Trial Study Group: *Lancet* 1989;2:863.)

REPERFUSION TO IMPROVE SEGMENTAL
LEFT VENTRICULAR FUNCTION

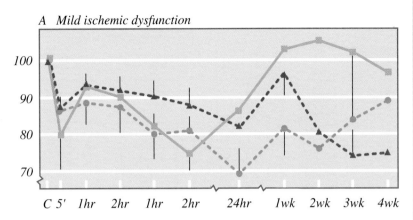

A *Mild ischemic dysfunction*

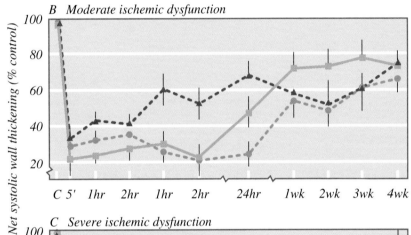

B *Moderate ischemic dysfunction*

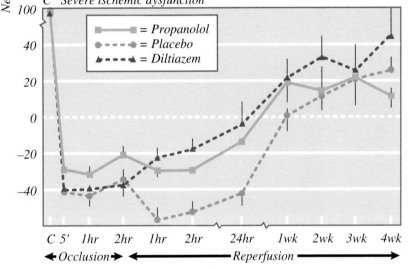

C *Severe ischemic dysfunction*

FIGURE 1.44 • The influence of reperfusion to improve segmental left ventricular function at sites of:
• Mild dysfunction (class I segments) (A).
• Moderate ischemic dysfunction (class II segments) (B).
• Severe ischemic dysfunction (class III segments) (C). Net systolic wall thickening as monitored by ultrasonic crystals placed across the left ventricular wall at sites of mild, moderate, and severe ischemia. Reperfusion occurred as a result of releasing a ligature around a canine left anterior descending coronary artery at 2 hrs after coronary artery occlusion and the animals were followed for a subsequent 4 weeks. Reperfusion with an infarct duration of 2 hrs was associated with important segmental functional recovery at sites of moderate and severe left ventricular dysfunction. (Reproduced with permission. *Circ Res* 1983;53:248.)

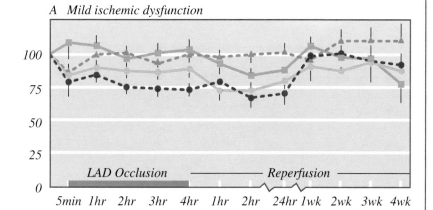

REPERFUSION TO IMPROVE SEGMENTAL LEFT VENTRICULAR FUNCTION

A Mild ischemic dysfunction

LAD Occlusion — Reperfusion

5min 1hr 2hr 3hr 4hr 1hr 2hr 24hr 1wk 2wk 3wk 4wk

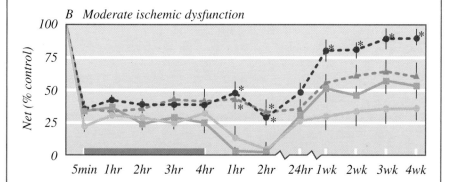

B Moderate ischemic dysfunction

Net (% control)

5min 1hr 2hr 3hr 4hr 1hr 2hr 24hr 1wk 2wk 3wk 4wk

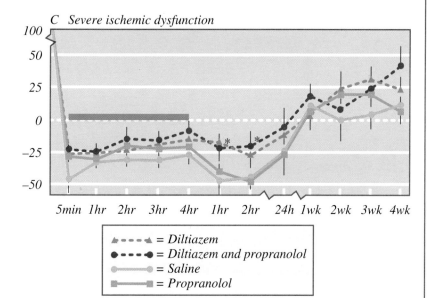

C Severe ischemic dysfunction

5min 1hr 2hr 3hr 4hr 1hr 2hr 24h 1wk 2wk 3wk 4wk

▲----▲ = *Diltiazem*
●----● = *Diltiazem and propranolol*
○——○ = *Saline*
■——■ = *Propranolol*

FIGURE 1.45 • This study is similar to the one in Figure 1.44, but the coronary occlusion lasted 4 hrs prior to reperfusion. In animals that did not receive any pharmacologic therapy— saline-treated animals—there was no important recovery of segmental function at sites of mild (A), moderate (B), and severe (C) ischemic dysfunction during the coronary artery occlusion. However, in animals that received a ß-blocker (propranolol), a calcium antagonist (diltiazem), or the combination of propranolol and diltiazem, there was improvement in segmental ventricular function associated with the reperfusion at left ventricular sites of moderate (B) and severe left ventricular dysfunction. (Reproduced with permission. *Circulation* 1985;72:413–430.)

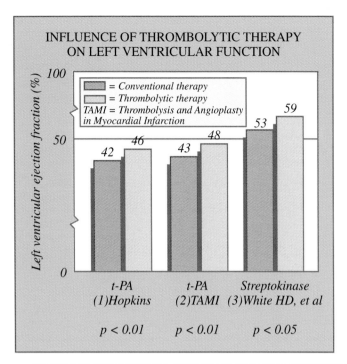

INFLUENCE OF THROMBOLYTIC THERAPY
ON LEFT VENTRICULAR FUNCTION

FIGURE 1.46 • The influence of various forms of thrombolytic thera-py on left ventricular function evaluated as left ventricular ejection fraction (LVEF). When thrombolytic therapy is given within 3 hrs of symptom onset, there is usually an improvement in global and seg-mental ventricular function. When thrombolytic therapy is delayed for more than 4 hrs, its impact to improve global ventricular function is much reduced.

References (1) Guerci AD, Gerstenblith G, Brinker JA, et al: A randomized trial of intravenous tissue plasminogen activator for acute myocardial infarction with subse-quent randomization to elective coronary angioplasty. *N Engl J Med* 1987; 317:1613. (2) Topol EJ: Selective thrombolytic agents for clinical use. In: Haber E, Braunwald E, eds. *Thrombolysis: Basic Contibutions and Clinical Progress* St. Louis, Mo: Mosby Year Book; 1991:301. (3) White HD, Norris RM, Brown MA, et al: Effect of intravenous streptokinase on left ventricular function and early survival after acute myocardial infarction. *N Engl J Med* 1987;317:850.

TABLE 1.14 • GLOBAL VENTRICULAR FUNCTION AND EARLY MORTALITY IN CONTROLLED STUDIES WITH STREPTOKINASE AND RECOMBINANT TISSUE PLASMINOGEN ACTIVATOR (RT-PA)

Study	Patients (n)	Percent global ejection fraction			
		Placebo	Strepto-kinase	rt-PA	p
Streptokinase compared with placebo					
Intravenous Streptokinase in Acute Myocardial Infarction (ISAM), 1986[1]	1741	53.9 ± 0.7	56.8 ± 0.7		<0.005
White HD, et al, 1987[2]	219	50.7	54.0		0.09
	172*	53.0 ± 13.5	59 ± 10.5		<0.005
Western Washington Trial, 1988[3]	368	50.7 ± 12.6	54.3 ± 12.2		0.056
rt-PA compared with placebo					
Guerci AD, et al, 1987[4]	138	46.4 ± 15.3		53.2 ± 15.5	<0.02
O'Rourke M, et al, 1988[5]	145	54.0 ± 14		61.0 ± 13	0.0006
National Heart Foundation of Australia (NHFA), 1988 [6]	144	51.7 ± 15.1		57.7 ± 15.7	0.04
European Cooperative Study Group-5 (ECSG-5), 1988[7]	721	48.5 ± 11.3		50.7 ± 10.9	<0.04
>3 hr	386	49.8		50.8	NS
<3 hr	335	46.8		50.7	<0.01
Streptokinase compared with rt-PA					
White HJ, et al, 1989[8]	270		58 ± 12	58.0 ± 12	NS
Plasminogen Activator Italian Multicenter Study (PAIMS)[9]	171		56 ± 10	56.0 ± 10	NS

Medical Treatment of Coronary Heart Disease

Study	Patients (n)	Percent early mortality			
		Placebo	Strepto-kinase	rt-PA	p
Streptokinase compared with placebo					
Intravenous Streptokinase in Acute Myocardial Infarction (ISAM), 1986[1]	1741	7.1	6.3		NS
White HD, et al, 1987[2]	219	12.5	3.7		<0.05
	172*	12.9	2.5		0.012
Western Washington Trial, 1988[3]	368	9.6	6.3		0.23
rt-PA compared with placebo					
Guerci AD, et al, 1987[4]	138	7.6		5.6	NS
O'Rourke M, et al, 1988[5]	145	5.5		5.4	NS
National Heart Foundation of Australia (NHFA), 1988 [6]	144	4 7		9.6	0.22
European Cooperative Study Group-5 (ECSG-5), 1988[7]	721			2.8	0.053
<3 hr	386			1.1	0.009
>3 hr	335			4.5	NS
Streptokinase compared with rt-PA					
White HJ, et al, 1989[8]	270		7.4	3.7	NS
Plasminogen Activator Italian Multicenter Study (PAIMS)[9]	171		8.2	4.6	NS

p = Level of significance of the difference between groups

NS = Not significant

* = Patients with first infarction only

(Reproduced with permission. In:Haber E, Braunwald E, ed. *Thrombolysis. Basic Contributions and Clinical Progress* St. Louis, Mo: Mosby Year Book;1991:324.)

[1]ISAM Group: A prospective trial of intravenous streptokinase in acute myocardial infarction (ISAM): Mortality, morbidity and infarct size at 21 days. *N Engl J Med* 1986;314:1465.

[2]White HD, Norris RM, Brown MA, et al: Effect of intravenous streptokinase on left ventricular function and early survival after acute myocardial infarction. *N Engl J Med* 1987;317:850.

[3]Kennedy JW, Martin GV, Davis KB, et al: The Western Washington intravenous streptokinase in acute myocardial infarction randomized trial. *Circulation* 1988;77:345.

[4]Guerci AD, Gerstenblith G, Brinker JA, et al: A randomized trial of intravenous tissue plasminogen activator for acute myocardial infarction with subsequent randomization to elective coronary angioplasty. *N Engl J Med* 1987;317:1613.

[5]O'Rourke M, Baron D, Keogh A, et al: Limitation of myocardial infarction by early infusion of recombinant tissue-type plasminogen activator. *Circulation* 1988; 77:1311.

[6]National Heart Foundation of Australia Coronary Thrombolysis Group: Coronary Thrombolysis and myocardial salvage by tissue plasminogen activator given up to 4 hours after onset of myocardial infarction. *Lancet* 1988;1:203.

[7]Van de Werf F, Arnold AER, for the European Cooperative Study Group for Recombinant Tissue Type Plasminogen Activator. Intravenous tissue plasminogen activator and size of infarct, left ventricular function, and survival in acute myocardial infarction. *Br Med J* 1988;287:1374.

[8]White HJ, Rivers JT, Maslowski AH, et al: Effect of intravenous streptokinase as compared with that of tissue plasminogen activator on left ventricular function after first myocardial infarction. *N Engl J Med* 1989;320:817.

[9]Magnani B, for the PAIMS Investigators: Plasminogen Activator Italian Multicenter Study (PAIMS): Comparison of intravenous recombinant single-chain human tissue-type plasminogen activator (rt-PA) with intravenous streptokinase in acute myocardial infarction. *J Am Coll Cardiol* 1989;13:19.

of symptom onset—independent of infarct location[160] (Figure 1.47).

The APSAC Interventional Mortality Study (AIMS) has shown in 1,258 patients that anisoylated plasminogen streptokinase activator complex (APSAC) reduced mortality in patients with suspected myocardial infarction treated within 6 hrs of symptom onset and this survival benefit was still evident at 12 months[190] (Figure 1.48 and refer to Table 1.13).

The Second Gruppo Italiano perlo Studio della Streptochinasi nel Infarto Miocardico (GISSI-2) study demonstrated that recombinant tissue plasminogen activator (rt-PA) and

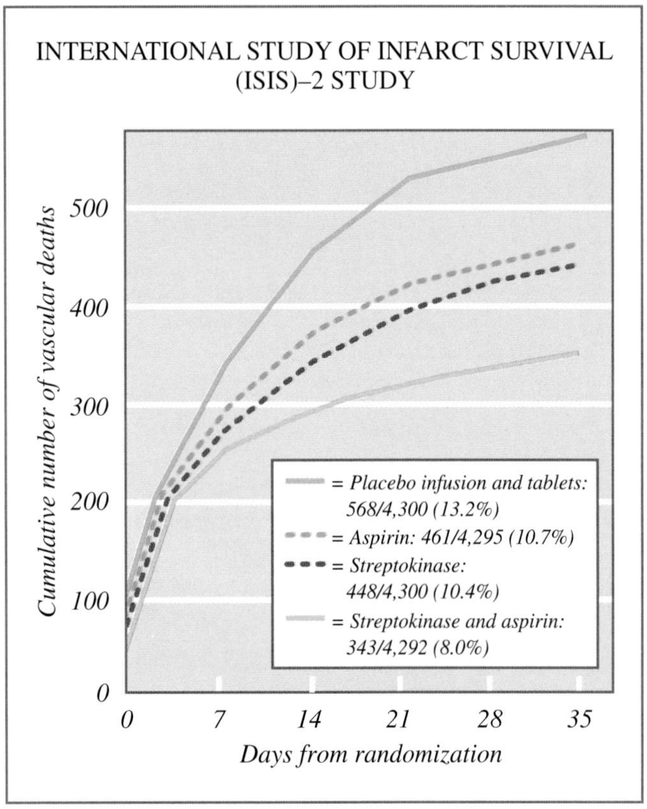

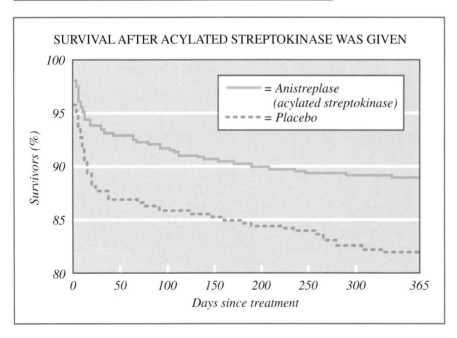

INTERNATIONAL STUDY OF INFARCT SURVIVAL (ISIS)–2 STUDY

Cumulative number of vascular deaths

= Placebo infusion and tablets: 568/4,300 (13.2%)
= Aspirin: 461/4,295 (10.7%)
= Streptokinase: 448/4,300 (10.4%)
= Streptokinase and aspirin: 343/4,292 (8.0%)

Days from randomization

FIGURE 1.47 • Data from the ISIS-2 Trial demonstrates that the combination of aspirin and streptokinase was superior to streptokinase alone, aspirin alone, and placebo in reducing mortality in patients with acute myocardial infarcts. (Reproduced with permission. ISIS-2 (Second International Study of Infarct Survival) Collaborative Group: *Lancet* 1988;1:349.)

SURVIVAL AFTER ACYLATED STREPTOKINASE WAS GIVEN

Survivors (%)

= Anistreplase (acylated streptokinase)
= Placebo

Days since treatment

FIGURE 1.48 • Life–table survival curves up to 1 year after APSAC (acylated streptokinase or antistreplase) or placebo were given in the APSAC Interventional Mortality Study (AIMS) trial. (Reproduced with permission. AIMS Trial Study Group: *Lancet* 1990;335:427.)

streptokinase have similar efficacies in reducing mortality in patients with acute Q-wave myocardial infarcts treated within 4 hours of symptom onset[184] (Figures 1.49, 1.50 and refer to Table 1.13). However, these patients also received a ß-blocker and aspirin, and heparin was given subcutaneously and delayed for at least 12 hrs after symptom onset.[184] Failure to give heparin with the thrombolytic intervention may have limited the efficacy of the latter, since thrombin exerts an important effect in:

• Promoting platelet aggregation.
• Producing vasoconstriction in the early hours of thrombus development.

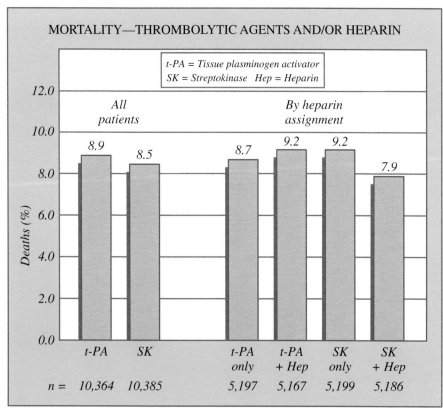

FIGURE 1.49 • Mortality data from the Second Gruppo Italiano perlo Studio della Streptochinasi nell'Infarto Miocardico (GISSI-2) and the International t-PA/SK Thrombolysis trials—assigned by either thrombolytic agent or by heparin. (Reproduced with permission. The International t-PA/SK Mortality Trial Study Group: *Lancet* 1990;2:336.)

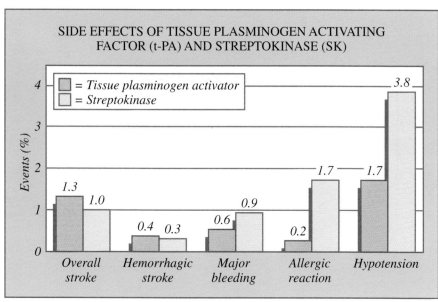

FIGURE 1.50 • Side effects of tissue plasminogen activator (t-PA) and streptokinase taken from the Second Gruppo Italiano perlo Studio della Streptochinasi nell'Infarto Miocardico (GISSI-2) and the International t-PA/SK Thrombolysis trials. (Reproduced with permission. The International t-PA/SK Mortality Trial Study Group: *Lancet* 1990;2:336.)

Heparin, as well as other more specific thrombin antagonists currently under development, should antagonize these effects (Table 1.15).

The Heparin-Aspirin Rethrombosis Trial (HART), conducted by Ross et al., established that heparin potentiates the thrombolytic efficacy of rt-PA in patients with infarcts.[185] We have demonstrated that thrombin antagonists shorten the time to thrombolysis with t-PA and delay reocclusion following thrombolytic therapy in experimental animal models.[187]

Finally, a critical review of eight randomized, controlled trials of rt-PA and 10 such trials of APSAC have shown that the likelihood of early death is reduced by either agent (Figure 1.43).[189]

RETHROMBOSIS AFTER THROMBOLYTIC THERAPY

Between 10% and 20% of patients develop rethrombosis of an infarct-related artery after successful thrombolytic therapy, despite the administration of heparin during the initial 3 to 4

TABLE 1.15 • PERCENTAGE OF EARLY MORTALITY IN PATIENTS WITH THROMBOLYTIC DRUGS WITH OR WITHOUT INTRAVENOUS HEPARIN

Study	Percent
Without intravenous heparin	
Gruppo Italiano perlo Studio della Streptochinasi nell'Infarto Miocardio-1 (GISSI-1)	10.2
Gruppo Italiano perlo Studio della Streptochinasi nell'Infarto Miocardio (GISSI-2)—International trial[1]	8.7
International Study of Infarct Survival-2 (ISIS-2)— all streptokinase-treated patients[1]	9.2
With intravenous heparin	
European Cooperative Study Group-4 (ECSG-4)— (tissue plasminogen activator and placebo	1.8
European Cooperative Study Group (ECSG)—tissue plasminogen activator and streptokinase	4.7
Thrombolysis in Myocardial Infarction-2 (TIMI-2)[2]	5.0
International Study of Infarct Survival-2 (ISIS-2) — streptokinase plus planned heparin	6.4
Heparin-Aspirin Rethrombosis Trial (HART)	3.0
Anglo-Scandinavian Study of Early Thrombolysis (ASSET)	7.2
Australian National Heart Foundation Trial	3.5

[1]t-PA as the active thrombolytic drug.
[2]With streptokinase as the active thrombolytic drug.

days after such therapy and coumadin or platelet-active agents thereafter. Rethrombosis appears to occur in patients with the most severe persistent residual coronary artery stenoses of their infarct-related arteries, especially those with residual coronary luminal diameters of less than 0.4 mm.[188]

Rethrombosis may occur slightly less frequently when either streptokinase, anisoylated plasminogen streptokinase activator complex (APSAC), urokinase, or combinations of thrombolytic interventions—such as rt-PA and urokinase—is given (Table 1.16). This may indicate that a decrease in the fibrinogen concentration may be useful in decreasing the risk of rethrombosis. A combination of nonfibrin-specific (urokinase) and a fibrin-specific thrombolytic intervention (t-PA) may reduce rethrombosis after thrombolytic therapy more than t-PA, streptokinase, or urokinase alone. The relative efficacies of streptokinase and t-PA in achieving thrombolysis are shown in Tables 1.13, 1.17–1.19. The major risk of thrombolytic therapy is hemorrhage (Table 1.20).

TABLE 1.16 • COMBINATION THROMBOLYTIC THERAPY

Combined therapy	n	Dose	Urokinase or streptokinase	Patency (90 min)	Reoc-clusion
Tissue plasminogen activator and urokinase (t-PA and UK)					
TAMI-2, 1988[1]	112	1 mg/kg over 60 min	0.5-2.0 million U/60 min	76%	9%
TAMI-5, 1990[2]	191	1 mg/kg over 60 min	1.5 million U/60 min	78%	2%
TAMI-7, 1990[3]	40	1 mg/kg over 30 min	1.5 million U/60 min	85%	3%
URALMI, 1990[4]	129	20mg-1g/kg over 60 min	1.0-2.0 million U/60 min	81%	9%
Tissue plasminogen activator and streptokinase (t-PA and SK)					
KAMIT, 1990[5]	109	50 mg/60 min	1.5 million U/60 min	78%	3%
KAMIT Pilot, 1989[6]	40	50 mg/60 min	1.5 million U/60 min	75%	8%

TAMI = Thrombolysis and Angioplasty in Myocardial Infarction

URALMI= Urokinase and Alteplase in the Treatment of Myocardial Infarction

[1]Topol EJ, Califf RM, George BS, et al, and the TAMI Study Group: Coronary arterial thrombolysis with combined infusion of recombinant tissue-type plasminogen activator and urokinase in patients with acute myocardial infarction. *Circulation* 1988;77:1100.

[2]Califf RM, Topol EJ, Harrelson L, et al, and the TAMI Study Group: In-hospital clinical outcomes in the TAMI 5 study. *J Am Coll Cardiol* 1990;15:76A. Abstract.

[3]Wall TC, Topol EJ, George BS, et al: The TAMI-7 trial of accelerated plasminogen activator dose regimens for coronary thrombolysis: Preliminary data. *Circulation* 1990. In press. Abstract

KAMIT = Kentucky Acute Myocardiol Infarction Trial

[4]URALMI Collaborative Group: Combination of urokinase and alteplase in the treatment of myocardial infarction. *J Am Coll Cardiol* 1990. In press. Abstract.

[5]Grines CL, Nissen SE, Booth DC, et al, and the KAMIT Study Group. A prospective, randomized trial comparing combination half dose t-PA with streptokinase to full dose t-PA in acute myocardial infarction: Preliminary report. *J Am Coll Cardiol* 1990;15:4A. Abstract.

[6]Grines CL, Nissen SE, Booth DC, et al, and the KAMIT Study Group: A new thrombolytic regimen for acute myocardial infarction using combination half dose tissue-type plasminogen activator with full dose streptokinase: A pilot study. *J Am Coll Cardiol* 1989;14:573.

TABLE 1.17 • INTRAVENOUS STREPTOKINASE: ANGIOGRAPHICALLY DOCUMENTED REPERFUSION RATES IN PATIENTS WITH TOTAL CORONARY OCCLUSIONS

Study	Recanalization rate		Streptokinase dose X 10³	Time from onset of pain to streptokinase (hr)	Reperfusion (min)
Rogers WJ, et al, 1983[1]	8/26	31%	500–1,000	6.8	38
TIMI, 1985[2]	40/115	35%	1,500	4.8	
TIMI, 1985[3]	11/34	32%	1,500	4.5	
Blunda M, et al, 1984[4]	6/12	50%	478	4.0	54
Schroder R, et al, 1983[5]	11/21	52%	500	3.8	
Spann JF, et al, 1984[6]	21/43	49%	850–1,500	3.5	
Neuhaus KL et al, 1983[7]	24/40	60%	1,700	3.4	48
Alderman EL et al, 1984[8]	8/13	62%	725	3.4	39
Overall	129/304	42%			Avg = 45 min

Time to streptokinase:

> 4 hr	59/175	34%
< 4 hr	70/129	54%

TIMI = Multicenter evaluation of Thrombolysis in Myocardial Infarction

(Reproduced with permission. Willerson JT, Winniford M, Buja LM: *Am J Med Sci* 1987;293:187.)

[1]Rogers WJ, Mantle JA, Hood WP, et al: Prospective randomized trial of intravenous and intracoronary streptokinase in acute myocardial infarction. *Circulation* 1983;68:1051.

[2,3]TIMI Study Group: The thrombolysis in myocardial infarction (TIMI) trial: Phase 1 findings. *N Engl J Med* 1985;312:932.

[4]Blunda M, Meiser SG, Schechter JA, et al: Intravenous versus intracoronary streptokinase for acute transmural myocardial infarction. *Cathet Cardiovasc Diagn* 1984;10:319.

[5]Schroder R, Biamino G, v Leitner ER, et al: Intravenous short-term infusion of streptokinase in acute myocardial infarction. *Circulation* 1983;67:536.

[6]Spann JF, Sherry S, Carabello BA, et al: Coronary thrombolysis by intravenous streptokinase in acute myocardial infarction: Acute and follow-up studies. *Am J Cardiol* 1984;5/3:655.

[7]Neuhaus KL, Tebbe U, Sauer G, et al: High dose intravenous streptokinase in acute myocardial infarction. *Clin Cardiol* 1983;6:426.

[8]Alderman EL, Jutzy KR, Berte LE, et al: Randomized comparison of intravenous versus intracoronary streptokinase for myocardial infarction. *Am J Cardiol* 1984;6:426.

TABLE 1.18 • EFFICACY OF TISSUE PLASMINOGEN ACTIVATING FACTOR IN ACHIEVING CORONARY THROMBOLYSIS

Author	Recanalization rate	Time from onset of pain to tissue-plasminogen activator (t-PA)	Mean time to reperfusion (Minutes)
Collen D, et al, 1985[1]	25/33 (75%)	< 6 hr	90 min
Thrombolysis in Myocardial Infaction (TIMI) trial: Phase I[2]	78/118 (66%)	5 hr	60 min

(Reproduced with permission. Willerson JT, Winniford M, Buja LM: *Am J Med Sci* 1987;293:187.)

[1]Collen D, Stump D, Van de Werf F, et al: Coronary thrombolysis in dogs with intravenously administered human pro-urokinase. *Circulation* 1985;72:384.

[2]TIMI Study Group: The thrombolysis in myocardial infarction (TIMI) trial: Phase 1 findings. *N Engl J Med* 1985;312:932.

TABLE 1.19 • INTRACORONARY STREPTOKINASE: REPERFUSION RATES IN PATIENTS WITH TOTAL CORONARY OCCLUSIONS

Study	Recanalization rate		Time from onset of pain to streptokinase (hr)	Time to reperfusion (min)
Rogers WJ, et al, 1983[1]	19/25	76%	6.5	31
Rentrop P, et al, 1981[2]	32/43	74%	5.9	
Tennant SN, et al, 1984[3]	20/35	57%	5.7	45
Raizner AE, et al, 1985[4]	8/16	50%	5.6	
Khaja F, et al, 1983[5]	12/20	60%	5.4	
Kennedy JW, et al, 1985[6]	73/108	68%	4.6	
Blunda M, et al, 1984[7]	8/13	62%	4.4	
Anderson JL, et al, 1984[8]	18/21	86%	4.3	23
DeCoster PM, et al, 1985[9]	18/21	86%	4.1	
Anderson JL, et al, 1984[10]	15/20	75%	4.0	30
Leiboff RH, et al, 1984[11]	15/22	68%	4.0	44
Valentine RP, et al, 1985[12]	50/85	59%	4.0	
Taylor GJ, et al, 1984[13]	44/63	70%	3.6	20
Cribier A, et al, 1983[14]	39/61	64%	3.6	
Ganz W, et al, 1983[15]	64/74	86%	3.4	25
Alderman EL, et al, 1984[16]	11/15	73%	3.3	28
Cowley M, et al, 1983[17]	16/18	89%		
Rentrop P, et al, 1984[18]	17/20	85%		
Smalling RW, et al, 1983[19]	73/100	73%		
Overall	522/780	71%		Avg = 30 min

Time to streptokinase:

4.5 hr	282/395	71%
≤ 4 hr	164/247	66%

(Reproduced with permission. Willerson JT, Winniford M, Buja LM: *Am J Med Sci* 1987;293:187.)

[1]Rogers WJ, Mantle JA, Hood WP, et al: Prospective randomized trial of intravenous and intracoronary streptokinase in acute myocardial infarction. *Circulation* 1983;68:1051.

[2]Rentrop P, Blanke H, Karsch KR, et al: Selective intracoronary thrombolysis in acute myocardial infarction and unstable angina pectoris. *Circulation* 1981;63:307.

[3]Tennant SN, Dixon J, Venable TC, et al: Intracoronary thrombolysis in patients with acute myocardial infarction: Comparison of the efficacy of urokinase with streptokinase. *Circulation* 1984;69:756.

[4]Raizner AE, Tortoledo FA, Verni MS, et al: Intracoronary thrombolytic therapy in acute myocardial infarction: a prospective, randomized, controlled trial. *Am J Cardiol* 1985;55:301.

[5]Khaja F, Walton JA, Brymer JF, et al: Intracoronary fibrinolytic therapy in acute myocardial infarction. *N Engl J Med* 1983;308:1305.

[6]Alderman EL, Jutzy KR, Berte LE, et al: Randomized comparison of intravenous versus intracoronary streptokinase for myocardial infarction. *Am J Cardiol* 1984;54:14.

[7]Blunda M, Meiser SG, Schechter JA, et al: Intravenous versus intracoronary streptokinase for acute transmural myocardial infarction. *Cathet Cardiovasc Diagn* 1984;10:319.

[8]Kennedy JW,, Gensini GG, Timmis GC, et al: Acute myocardial infarction treated with intracoronary streptokinase: A report for the Society for Cardiac Angiography. *Am J Cardiol* 1985;55:871.

[9]De Coster PM, Melin JA, Detry JMR, et al: Coronary artery reperfusion in acute myocardial infarction: Assessment by pre- and postintervention thallium-201 myocardial perfusion imaging. *Am J Cardiol* 1985;55:889.

[10]Anderson JL, Marshall HW, Askins JC, et al: A randomized trial of intravenous and intracoronary streptokinase in patients with acute myocardial infarction. *Circulation* 1984;70:606.

[11]Leiboff RH, Katz RJ, Wasserman AG, et al: A randomized, angiographically controlled trial of intracoronary streptokinase in acute myocardial infarction. *Am J Cardiol* 1984;53:404.

[12]Valentine RP, Pitts DE, Brooks-Brunn JA, et al: Intravenous versus intracoronary streptokinase in acute myocardial infarction. *Ann J Cardiol* 1985;55:309.

[13]Taylor GJ, Mikell FL, Moses HW, et al: Intravenous versus intracoronary streptokinase therapy for acute myocardial infarction. *Cathet Cardiovasc Diagn* 1984;10:319.

[14]Criber A, Berland J, Champoud O, et al: Intracoronary thrombolysis in evolving myocardial infarction. *Br Heart J* 1983;50:401.

[15]Ganz W, Geft I, Maddahi J, Berman D, et al: Nonsurgical reperfusion in evolving myocardial infarction. *J Am Coll Cardiol* 1983;1247.

[17]Cowley M, Hastillo A, Vetrovec GW, et al: Fibrinolytic effects of intracoronary streptokinase administration in patients with acute myocardial infarction and coronary insufficiency. *Circulation* 1983;67:1031.

[18]Rentrop KP, Feit F, Blanke H, et al: Effects of intracoronary streptokinase and intracoronary nitroglycerin infusion on coronary angiographic patterns and mortality in patients with acute myocardial infarction. *N Engl J Med* 1984;311:1457.

[19]Smalling RW, Fuentes F, Matthews MW, et al: Sustained improvement in left ventricular function and mortality by intracoronary streptokinase administration during evolving myocardial infarction. *Circulation* 1983;68:131.

TABLE 1.20 • HEMORRHAGE AFTER THROMBOLYTIC THERAPY

	Study	Total Patients	Number of bleeds
Intracoronary	Merx W, et al, 1981[1]	204	12 (7%)
	Rentrop KP, et al, 1984[2]	29	2 (7%)
	Schwarz F, et al, 1984[3]	101	6 (6%) (1 fatal)
	Rogers WJ, et al, 1983[4]	25	1 (4%)
	Smalling RW, et al, 1983[5]	136	5 (4%)
	Mathey DG, et al, 1981[6]	41	0
	Anderson JL, et al, 1983[7]	24	0
	Khaja F, et al, 1983[8]	20	0
	Kennedy JW, et al, 1985[9]	134	7 (5%)
Intravenous	Rogers WJ, et al, 1983[4]		
	Neuhaus KL, et al, 1983[11]	26	1 (4%)
	Schroder R, et al, 1983[12]	40	0
	Spann SF, et al, 1984[13]	93	0
	Anderson JL, et al, 1984[14]	43	0
	Taylor GJ, et al, 1984[15]	27	4 (15%)
		121	6 (5%)

(Reproduced with permission. Willerson JT, Winniford M, Buja LM: *Am J Med Sci* 1987;293:187.)

[1] Merx W, Dorr R, Rentrop P, et al. Evaluation of the effectiveness of intracoronary streptokinase infusion in an acute myocardial infarction: Post-procedure management and hospital course in 204 patients. *Am Heart J* 1981;102:1181.

[2] Rentrop KP, Feit F, Blanke H, Stecy P, et al. Effects of intracoronary streptokinase and intracoronary nitroglycerin infusion on coronary angiographic patterns and mortality in patients with acute myocardial infarction. *N Engl J Med* 1984;311:1457.

[3] Schwarz F, Hofmann M, Schuler G, et al: Thrombolysis in acute myocardial infarction: Effect of intravenous followed by intracoronary streptokinase application on estimates of infarct size. *Am J Cardiol* 1984;53:1505.

[4] Rogers WJ, Mantle JA, Hood WP, et al: Prospective randomized trial of intravenous and intracoronary streptokinase in acute myocardial infarction. *Circulation* 1983;68:1051.

[5] Smalling RW, Fuentes F, Matthews MW, et al. Sustained improvement in left ventricular function and mortality by intracoronary streptokinase administration during evolving myocardial infarction. *Circulation* 1983;68:131.

[6] Mathey DG, Kuck K-H, Tilsner V, et al. Nonsurgical coronary artery recanalization in acute transmural myocardial infarction. *Circulation* 1983;68:131.

[7] Anderson JL, Marshall HW, Bray BE, et al: A randomized trial of intracoronary streptokinase in the treatment of acute myocardial infarction. *New Engl J Med* 1983;308:1312.

[8] Khaja F, Walton JA, Brymer JF, et al. Intracoronary fibrinolytic therapy in acute myocardial infarction. *N Engl J Med* 1983;308:1305.

[9] Kennedy JW, Gensini GG, Timmis GC, et al: Acute myocardial infarction treated with intracoronary streptokinase: A report for the Society of Cardia Angiography. *Am J Cardiol* 1985;55:871.

[11] Nehaus KL, Tebbe U, Sauer G, et al: High dose intravenous streptokinase in acute myocardial infarction. *Clin Cardiol* 1983;6:426.

[12] Schroder R, Biamino G, v Leitner ER, et al. Intravenous short-term infusion of streptokinase in acute myocardial infarction. *Circulation* 1983;67:536.

[13] Spann JF, Sherry S, Carabello BA, et al: Coronary thrombolysis by intravenous streptokinase in acute myocardial infarction: Acute and follow-up studies. *Am J Cardiol* 1984;53:655.

[14] Anderson JL, Marshall HW, Askins JC, et al: A randomized trial of intravenous and intracoronary streptokinase therapy for acute myocardial infarction in community hospitals. *Am J Cardiol* 1984;54:256.

[15] Taylor GJ, Mikell FL, Moses HW, et al: Intravenous versus intracoronary streptokinase therapy for acute myocardial infarction in community hospitals. *Am J Cardiol* 1984;54:256.hj

Recommended Dosages and Methods of Administration

We recommend that t-PA be given in total intravenous doses of 80 to 100 mg. At present, optimal thrombolytic efficacy appears to be obtained with a "front-loading" dose of 10 to 15 mg, followed by the remainder of the dose as a sustained infusion, with an additional 60 mg given during the initial hour and the remainder over a total of 3 hrs. A t-PA dose of 150 mg is associated with increased risk of intracranial hemorrhage.[171] Recommendations for other dosages and methods of administration for available thrombolytic interventions are shown in Table 1.21.

COMPARISONS OF THROMBOLYTIC INTERVENTIONS IN THEIR INFLUENCE TO REDUCE MORTALITY

Two large, randomized, prospective trials have compared the ability of streptokinase and tissue plasminogen activator to reduce mortality in patients with acute myocardial infarction (refer to Figures 1.49, 1.50). The Second Gruppo Italiano per lo Studio della Streptochinasi nell' Infarto Miocardico (GISSI-2) trial[134] compared these thrombolytic interventions directly in approximately 21,000 patients. The International Study of Infarct-3 (ISIS-3) trial[191] compared streptokinase, acylated streptokinase (APSAC) and tissue plasminogen activator with and

TABLE 1.21 • RECOMMENDED DOSAGES AND METHODS FOR ADMINISTRATION OF AVAILABLE THROMBOLYTIC INTERVENTIONS

Streptokinase

Give 1.5 million U intravenously during the first 30 minutes for a total dosage of 1.5 million U.

APSAC

Give 30 U IV during 5 min.

Urokinase

Give 2 million U IV during 30 min.

Tissue Plasminogen Activator

Give 10 mg as initial loading dose IV, followed by 50 mg in the first hr— total of 60 mg—and 20 mg during each of the subsequent 2 hrs— total of 100 mg.

Current Adjunctive Therapy

These agents are to be given simultaneously with or immediately prior to the thrombolytic therapy.

Aspirin

160–325 mg—chewed or taken orally initially—and continued daily for 6–12 months.

Heparin

Give as 1,000 U hr IV and adjust to maintain PTT at 1.5–2 times the upper limit of normal. Continue heparin for 48–72 hrs.

without heparin given subcutaneously 4 hrs after symptom onset, in approximately 46,000 patients with suspected myocardial infacrtion. No differences in mortality rates were found among the different thrombolytic interventions, although neither trial optimized the administration of heparin to maximally potentiate the individual thrombolytic agents' effects. Currently underway is another very large, multicenter trial—Global Utilization of Streptokinase and Tissue Plasminogen Activator for Occluded Coronaries (GUSTO)—that will compare streptokinase and tissue plasminogen activator with heparin. It is hoped that this trial will determine whether there is any reduction in mortality when more fibrin-specific thrombolytic agents are given to patients with evolving Q-wave infarcts. Other comparisons between nonfibrin-specific and fibrin specific thrombolytic interventions are shown in Figures 1.51 and 1.52.

PERCUTANEOUS TRANSLUMINAL CORONARY ARTERY ANGIOPLASTY

Percutaneous transluminal coronary artery angioplasty (PTCA) represents an alternative to thrombolytic therapy for restoring blood flow through an infarct-related artery. Alternatively, it may be used either immediately or several days after thrombolytic therapy.[139,153,154,158,159,168–171] Recent data suggest there is no advantage to combining PTCA and thrombolytic therapy in the first 1 to 3 days after thrombolytic therapy for patients with acute Q-wave myocardial infarct [139,159,171,186] (refer to Figure 1.53).

Percutaneous transluminal coronary angioplasty may be used to dilate the infarct-related artery as an alternative to or following thrombolytic therapy in patients at increased risk of reocclusion of the infarct-related artery, but emergency PTCA is not usually necessary following thrombolytic therapy[159,172,186] (Figure 1.53). PTCA with or without thrombolytic therapy should be strongly considered in the patient seen within 2 hrs of an acute anterior Q-wave infarct who presents with cardiogenic shock, severe left ventricular failure, the acute development of bilateral bundle-branch block, and/or refractory ventricular arrhythmias. In some patients, rapid and early—less than 2 hrs from symptom onset—opening of the infarct-related artery with PTCA or thrombolytic therapy may reverse cardiogenic shock and/or severe left heart failure.

TREATING PATIENTS WITH NON-Q-WAVE INFARCTS

Since the pathophysiology of non-Q-wave infarcts is one of transient coronary artery occlusion followed by reperfusion, it seems logical to employ interventions that hinder platelet aggregation and improve coronary blood flow. Thus, a combination of nitrates, selected calcium antagonists, and aspirin are often administered. There are almost certainly subsets of patients with non-Q-wave infarcts who will benefit from thrombolytic therapy, specifically the patient with a persistent oc-

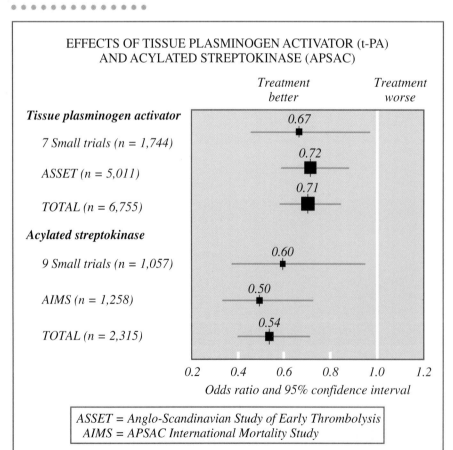

EFFECTS OF TISSUE PLASMINOGEN ACTIVATOR (t-PA) AND ACYLATED STREPTOKINASE (APSAC)

Treatment better   *Treatment worse*

Tissue plasminogen activator

7 Small trials (n = 1,744)   0.67

ASSET (n = 5,011)   0.72

TOTAL (n = 6,755)   0.71

Acylated streptokinase

9 Small trials (n = 1,057)   0.60

AIMS (n = 1,258)   0.50

TOTAL (n = 2,315)   0.54

0.2   0.4   0.6   0.8   1.0   1.2

Odds ratio and 95% confidence interval

ASSET = Anglo-Scandinavian Study of Early Thrombolysis
AIMS = APSAC International Mortality Study

FIGURE 1.51 • The effects of recombinant tissue plasminogen activator (rt-PA) and APSAC (acylated streptokinase or antistreplase) on mortality in 8 different randomized controlled trials with r-tPA and 10 different trials with APSAC. (Reproduced with permission. Held PH, Teo K, Yusuf S: *Circulation* 1990;82:1668.)

clusion of the infarct-related artery. When it is possible to identify this subset of patients prospectively, it should be possible to treat them more effectively.

GENERAL THERAPY OF ACUTE MYOCARDIAL INFARCTS

Since many of the complications of acute myocardial infarction occur within the first 96 hrs, the patient should remain in a coronary care unit for some part of this time. Complete bed rest is recommended initially, followed by gradual mobilization of patients who are clinically stable so that they are beginning to walk and sit in chairs within 2 to 3 days after the infarct. Emotional stimulation and strenuous physical effort should be avoided. Chest pain during the initial 24 hrs is treated with opiates, usually IV morphine or meperidine. Thereafter, recurrent chest pain believed to represent angina is treated with nitrates, a calcium antagonist, aspirin, and/or ß-blockers, whichever is most appropriate for the individual patient.

Recent data suggest that in-hospital infarct extension may be reduced in selected patients with non-Q-wave infarction by treatment with the calcium antagonist, diltiazem.[192] The patient who experiences angina while at rest or during low-level effort despite nitrates, calcium antagonists, and/or ß-blockers, should be referred for coronary arteriography (Figure 1.54) and, subsequently, coronary artery revascularization. Intravenous nitroglycerin may be used to relieve the chest pain and stabilize the patient prior to angiography.[193–200]

During the initial hours after myocardial infarction, oxygen is administered by mask or nasal cannula and the patient's vital signs are checked frequently. Reassurance that the chest pain will be relieved and that survival is insured is important. Some physicians use low-dose heparin to prevent complications related to prolonged bed rest and relative inactivity following a

ADVANTAGES/DISADVANTAGES OF THE CURRENTLY AVAILABLE THROMBOLYTIC AGENTS

Agent	Price	Saves lives	Bleeding	Patency	Advantages	Disadvantages
Streptokinase	$76	◉	⊖	⊖	• Low reocclusion	• Allergy, Abs • Hypotension
Tissue plasminogen activator	$2,200	◉	⊖	◉	• No allergy • No hypotension	• ↑Reocclusion, need heparin
Anisoylated plasminogen streptokinase activator complex	$1,700	◉	⊖	⊖	• Low reocclusion • Bolus	• Allergy, Abs • Hypotension

◉ Good   ⊖ Fair

FIGURE 1.52 • Advantages and disadvantages among the various thrombolytic agents. (Adapted with permission. Haber E, Braunwald E, eds. *Thrombolysis. Basic Contributions and Clinical Progress* St. Louis, Mo: Mosby Year Book; 1991:311.)

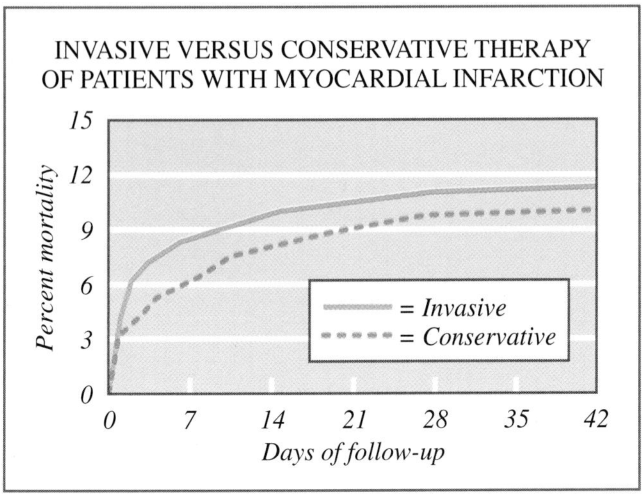

INVASIVE VERSUS CONSERVATIVE THERAPY OF PATIENTS WITH MYOCARDIAL INFARCTION

= Invasive
= Conservative

FIGURE 1.53 • Conservative strategy of thrombolytic therapy is found to be just as effective as an invasive strategy that consists of thrombolytic therapy and mandatory coronary arteriography and coronary artery revascularization if the coronary anatomy is appropriate 24 to 48 hrs following thrombolytic therapy. (Reproduced with permission. The TIMI Study Group: *N Engl J Med* 1989;320:618.)

myocardial infarction. Full anticoagulation with intravenously administered heparin for 7 to 10 days, followed by coumadin for 3 to 6 months, is given to patients with an acute left ventricular thrombus complicating myocardial infarction. In patients with anterior Q-wave infarcts, development of left ventricular thrombi is a 10% to 40% risk.[201–203] Recently developed left ventricular thrombi are more likely to embolize when they protrude into the left ventricular cavity and/or appear mobile upon echocardiographic evaluation.

ß-BLOCKERS

Several studies have shown that ß-blockers without an intrinsic sympathomimetic effect reduce the risk of future myocardial infarction and death in patients who are older, or have:
• Anterior Q-wave infarcts.
• Reversible left ventricular failure.
• Moderately depressed left ventricular ejection fractions.
• Continuing myocardial ischemia at low levels of effort [204–208] (Figures 1.55–1.57).

• • • • • • • • • • • • • •

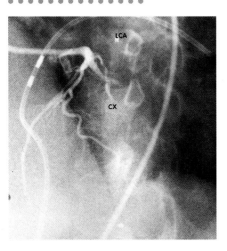 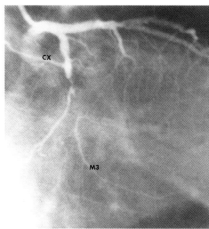

FIGURE 1.54 • Occlusion of the circumflex artery just beyond the origin of the small second marginal artery is seen in this patient with an acute myocardial infarction. Note the irregular outline of the circumflex artery—proximal to the occlusion. This suggests the presence of thrombus. (CX = circumflex artery; LCA = left main artery; M3 = distal portion.) Reproduced with permission. Soto B, Kassner EG, Baxley WA: *Imaging of Cardiac Disorders* New York, NY: Gower Medical Publishing; 1992:A-2.)

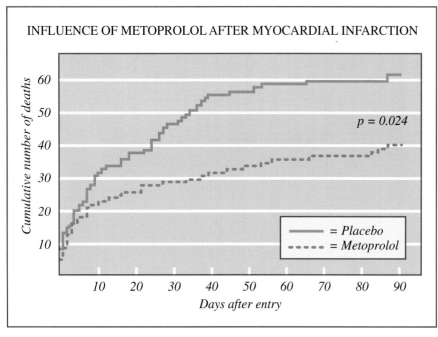

INFLUENCE OF METOPROLOL AFTER MYOCARDIAL INFARCTION

$p = 0.024$

Cumulative number of deaths

= Placebo
= Metoprolol

Days after entry

FIGURE 1.55 • The influence of metoprolol administration on the cumulative number of deaths in patients after myocardial infarction. Metoprolol reduced mortality in patients after myocardial infarction. (Reproduced with permission. Hjalmarson A, Herlitz J, Malek I, et al: *Lancet* 1981;2:825.)

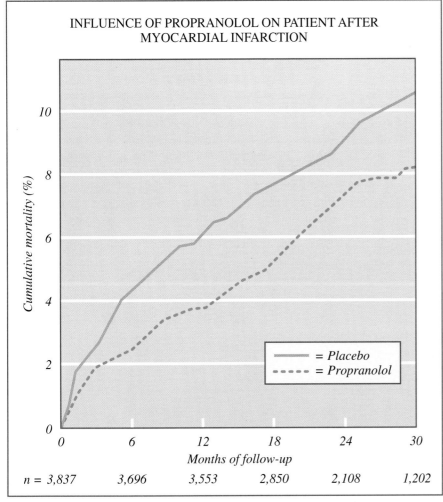

INFLUENCE OF PROPRANOLOL ON PATIENT AFTER MYOCARDIAL INFARCTION

FIGURE 1.56 • The influence of propanolol in reducing mortality in patients after myocardial infarction is shown in this figure. (Reproduced with permission. ß-Blocker Heart Attack Study Group: *JAMA* 1981;246:2073.)

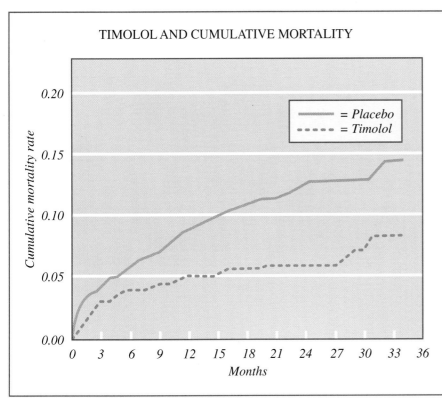

TIMOLOL AND CUMULATIVE MORTALITY

FIGURE 1.57 • The influence of the nonspecific ß-blocker, timolol, on cumulative mortality in patients after myocardial infarction is shown. The administration of timolol significantly reduced mortality among the patients for more than 30 months after myocardial infarction. (Reproduced with permission. The Norwegian Multicenter Study Group: *N Engl J Med* 1981;304:806.)

Specifically, timolol, metoprolol, and propranolol reduce the risk of recurrent myocardial infarction and death in patients at risk during follow-up periods of up to 6 years (refer to Figures 1.55–1.57). Beta-blockers with intrinsic sympathomimetic activity do not appear to reduce mortality and the risk of reinfarction. Acute administration of a relatively selective ß-blocker—metoprolol—reduces the frequency of recurrent myocardial ischemia and reinfarction during the first 6 days after Q-wave infarction in patients who receive t-PA and heparin as a thrombolytic intervention[171] (Table 1.22). Beta-blockers should not be given to patients with acute myocardial infarction accompanied by marked bradycardia, atrioventricular (AV) block, clinically important congestive heart failure, bronchospasm, and/or systemic arterial hypotension. They should be used very carefully in the patient with insulin-dependent diabetes mellitus. The recommended management of patients with acute myocardial infarction is shown in Figure 1.58.

THERAPY OF SPECIFIC COMPLICATIONS RELATED TO MYOCARDIAL INFARCTION

CARDIOGENIC SHOCK

Cardiogenic shock is defined as systemic arterial hypotension caused by extensive infarction of the left ventricle with the amount of irreversible myocardial damage usually equaling or exceeding 40% of the muscle mass[209] (Figures 1.59, 1.60). Prompt opening of the infarct-related artery may be accomplished with percutaneous transluminal coronary angioplasty (PTCA) and/or thrombolytic therapy. Thrombolytic therapy or PTCA within 2 hrs of symptom onset may reverse cardiogenic shock, if the infarct-related artery opens as a result[210](Figures 1.61, 1.62). If the infarct-related artery is not

● ● ● ● ● ● ● ● ● ● ● ● ● ● ● ●

TABLE 1.22 • CLINICAL EVENTS IN PATIENTS RECEIVING IMMEDIATE AND DEFERRED ß-BLOCKER THERAPY

Event	ß-blockade Group				p Value
	Immediate (n = 696)		Deferred (n = 694)		
Within the first 6 days					
Death	17	2.4	17	2.4	0.99
Fatal or nonfatal reinfarction	18	2.6	31	4.5	0.06
Nonfatal reinfarction	16	2.3	31	4.5	0.02
Death or reinfarction	33	4.7	48	6.9	0.08
Recurrent ischemia	107	15.4	147	21.2	0.005
Within the first 42 days					
Death	26	3.7	25	3.6	0.90
Fatal or nonfatal reinfarction	30	4.3	44	6.3	0.09
Nonfatal reinfarction	27	3.9	42	6.1	0.06
Death or reinfarction	51	7.3	66	9.5	0.14
Recurrent ischemia	217	31.2	235	33.9	0.29

(Reproduced with permission. *N Engl J Med* 1989;320:618.)

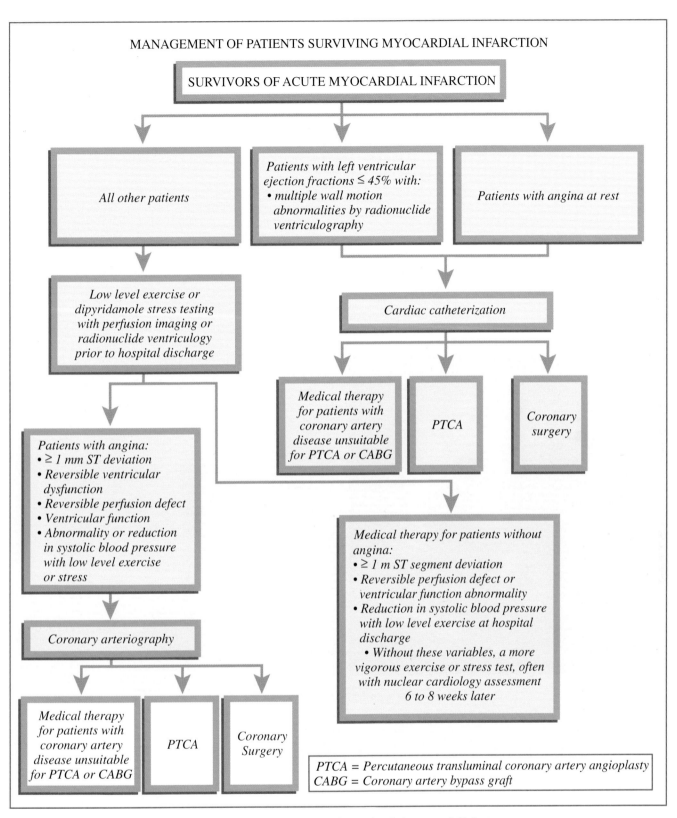

MANAGEMENT OF PATIENTS SURVIVING MYOCARDIAL INFARCTION

SURVIVORS OF ACUTE MYOCARDIAL INFARCTION

All other patients

Patients with left ventricular ejection fractions ≤ 45% with:
• *multiple wall motion abnormalities by radionuclide ventriculography*

Patients with angina at rest

Low level exercise or dipyridamole stress testing with perfusion imaging or radionuclide ventriculogy prior to hospital discharge

Cardiac catheterization

Medical therapy for patients with coronary artery disease unsuitable for PTCA or CABG

PTCA

Coronary surgery

Patients with angina:
• *≥ 1 mm ST deviation*
• *Reversible ventricular dysfunction*
• *Reversible perfusion defect*
• *Ventricular function*
• *Abnormality or reduction in systolic blood pressure with low level exercise or stress*

Medical therapy for patients without angina:
• *≥ 1 m ST segment deviation*
• *Reversible perfusion defect or ventricular function abnormality*
• *Reduction in systolic blood pressure with low level exercise at hospital discharge*
  • *Without these variables, a more vigorous exercise or stress test, often with nuclear cardiology assessment 6 to 8 weeks later*

Coronary arteriography

Medical therapy for patients with coronary artery disease unsuitable for PTCA or CABG

PTCA

Coronary Surgery

PTCA = Percutaneous transluminal coronary artery angioplasty
CABG = Coronary artery bypass graft

FIGURE 1.58 • A suggested scheme for the management of patients who survive their myocardial infarcts.

opened promptly, the risk of death is substantial. Some patients may be saved by an aggressive regimen that includes inotropic agents, such as dobutamine, dopamine, or norepinephrine; diuresis; and/or mechanical circulatory assistance.[124,211–216] However, most patients die as a result of extensive heart muscle damage in the absence of an intervention that restores coronary blood flow acutely or the gift of a new heart—either an artificial heart device or a successful heart transplant.

The development of artificial heart devices that may be used indefinitely, and/or the ability to utilize cardiac transplantation rapidly or following a longer period of cardiac assistance with an artificial heart device, should enhance the survival of patients with extensive myocardial infarcts. Most patients with cardiogenic shock resulting from left ventricular infarction have either anterior Q-wave infarcts or have had several previous infarcts, making the location of the most recent infarcts relatively less important.

RIGHT VENTRICULAR INFARCTS

Cardiogenic shock may occur in patients with extensive right ventricular infarction.[217–226] In most instances, these patients have:

- Inferior Q-wave infarcts.
- Elevated right ventricular end-diastolic and right atrial pressures.
- Low or normal mean pulmonary capillary wedge pressures.
- Preserved left ventricular function.

Clinically, these patients present with systemic arterial hypotension, tachycardia, elevated venous pressure, clinical evidence of right ventricular dysfunction, clear lungs, and mean pulmonary capillary wedge pressures within normal limits. These patients may be stabilized by prompt intravascular volume expansion with saline, and by raising their mean pulmonary capillary wedge pressures to values of 16 to 20 mm Hg, if necessary, to restore adequate systemic arterial blood pres-

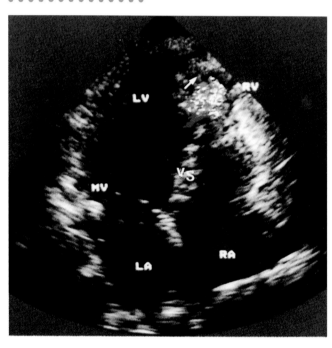

FIGURE 1.59 • The portable chest film from a patient with extensive myocardial infarction shows a normal-sized heart and bilateral pulmonary alveolar edema. The diagnosis: acute myocardial infarction with cardiogenic shock. Note the Swan-Ganz catheter and the intraaortic balloon catheter (Reproduced with permission. Kassner EG: *Atlas of Radiologic Imaging* New York, NY: Gower Medical Publishing; 1989:4.7.)

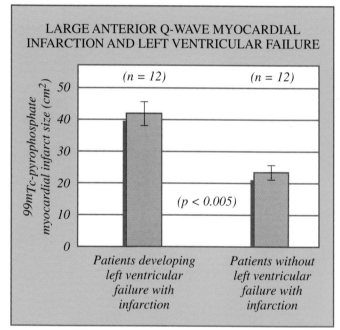

FIGURE 1.60 • The consequences of a large anterior Q-wave myocardial infarct in leading to left ventricular failure. Patients with the largest anterior infarcts, as identified by pyrophosphate scintigraphy, have the highest incidence of left ventricular failure. (Reproduced with permission. Buja LM, Willerson JT: *Prog Cardiovasc Dis* 1987;4:272).

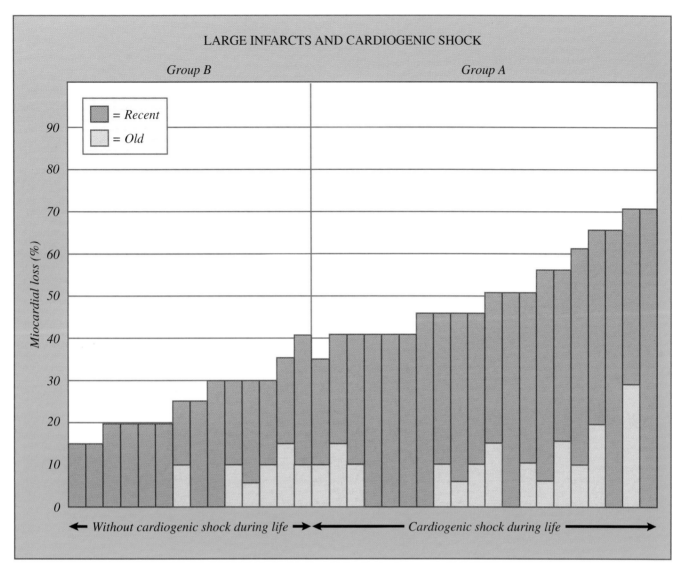

LARGE INFARCTS AND CARDIOGENIC SHOCK

Group B   Group A

= Recent
= Old

Miocardial loss (%)

◄— *Without cardiogenic shock during life* —►◄— *Cardiogenic shock during life* —►

FIGURE 1.61 • Patients with the largest infarcts will most likely develop cardiogenic shock following infarction. Patients generally had 40% or more of their left ventricular muscle mass irreversibly damaged (A) and the other patients generally had less than 40% of their left ventricular muscle mass irreversibly damaged (B). The contributions of recent and old infarcts are shown. (Reproduced with permission. Hjalmarson A, Herlitz J, Malek I, et al: *Lancet* 1981;2:825.)

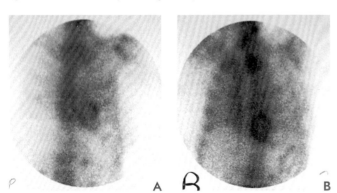

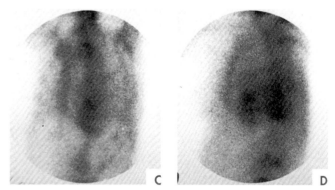

FIGURE 1.62 • Acute myocardial infarction demonstrated by pyrophosphate scintigraphy. This 36-year old woman presented with acute cardiogenic shock. The ECG showed evidence of extensive anterior wall infarction—consistent with occlusion of the left anterior descending artery. Pyrophosphate scan obtained 24 hrs after the onset of symptoms in anterior (A); 30° left anterior oblique (LAO) (B); 60° LAO (C); and left lateral projections (D) shows 4+ uptake—significantly greater than bone uptake in the ribs and sternum—in a large "doughnut"-shaped lesion. The lesion migrates with the sternum, indicating its anterior location. The doughnut configuration indicates absence of flow in the center of the infarcted region with abnormal uptake by the compromised myocardium at the periphery of the lesion. This scintigraphic pattern connotes a poor prognosis. (Reproduced with permission. Soto B, Kassner EG, Baxley WA: *Imaging of Cardiovascular Disorders* New York, NY: Gower Medical Publishing; 1992:133.)

sure. If hypotension is corrected rapidly, most of these patients survive.

An alternative or adjunctive therapy includes the administration of a thrombolytic agent or the use of percutaneous transluminal coronary angioplasty (PTCA) to open the infarct-related artery promptly. Right ventricular infarction may be identified in patients with inferior Q-wave infarcts by obtaining right precordial leads that show ST-segment elevation in leads V_4R or V_4R to V_6R[224] (Figure 1.63). Right ventricular infarction may be suggested by a two-dimensional echocardiogram or radionuclide ventriculogram that shows relatively selective right ventricular dysfunction in the patient with an inferior infarct.

ACUTE VENTRICULAR SEPTAL DEFECTS

Acute ventricular septal defects (VSDs) usually occur in patients with Q-wave infarcts that are often anterior Q-wave infarcts.[227–233] A new systolic murmur located at the lower left sternal border suggests the development of a VSD or acute mitral insufficiency, which may occur within hours to 12 days after myocardial infarction. If the VSD is large enough to allow a left-to-right shunt of 1.5:1 or greater, pressure and volume loads are imposed on the heart and ventricular failure often ensues. Acute VSDs are usually associated with a palpable systolic thrill and a holosystolic murmur located at the left sternal border. A flow-directed catheter demonstrates an oxygen step-up in the right heart and, with pulmonary-to-systemic flow ratios of approximately 2:1 or greater, there is a future risk of pulmonary hypertension. Defects of this size must be surgically closed.[227–233] Subacute bacterial endocarditis is an additional risk in the patient with a VSD. With the development of a murmur consistent with possible VSD, a flow-directed catheter should be inserted so that an oxygen step-up in the right heart may be identified if it is present. Alternatively, a two-dimensional echocardiogram with Doppler ultrasonography may be used to identify the location and presence of a VSD (Figure 1.64).

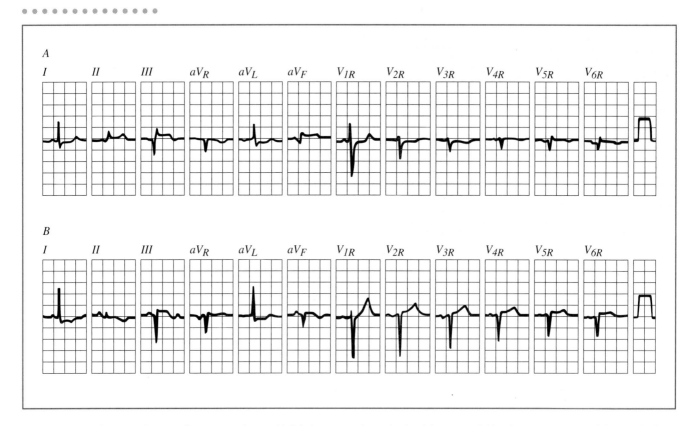

FIGURE 1.63 • Electrocardiograms from two patients with inferior myocardial infarcts are shown. The right precordial leads (V_1R-V_6R) do not show important ST elevation (A). ST-segment elevation is shown in the right precordial leads (V_3R-V_6R) (B). A right ventricular infarction was evident from the patient's ECG (B).

Patients with a VSD are placed on a diuretic and an unloading agent, such as IV nitroprusside and/or an angiotensin converting enzyme (ACE) inhibitor if their blood pressures allow. However, with the development of heart failure, the VSD should be closed surgically following left ventricular angiography and coronary arteriography. Coronary artery bypass grafting of the infarct-related artery and other importantly narrowed coronary arteries is usually accomplished at the same time (refer to Chapter 6). The operative risk for correcting a VSD immediately after myocardial infarction is substantial, but failing to correct the defect and allowing congestive heart failure to progress is often fatal.[227–232]

ACUTE MITRAL INSUFFICIENCY

Acute mitral insufficiency may occur as a consequence of papillary muscle rupture or dysfunction.[234–241] With papillary muscle rupture, severe mitral insufficiency develops. Papillary muscle dysfunction usually leads to mild or moderate mitral insufficiency. In both circumstances, severe congestive heart failure may ensue. With mitral papillary muscle rupture, prompt surgical correction of the mitral insufficiency, by either primary repair or replacement with a new valve, is mandatory if the patient is to survive.[234–241]

Papillary muscle rupture may produce a soft systolic murmur or no audible murmur. With papillary muscle dysfunction, there is typically a late-peaking systolic murmur heard at the cardiac apex. Third heart sounds are usually heard with moderate or severe mitral insufficiency, and the patient ordinarily develops heart failure. Two-dimensional echocardiography with Doppler imaging allows one to detect and estimate the severity of mitral insufficiency (Figures 1.65, 1.66). A flow-directed catheter should demonstrate prominent V waves in the pulmonary capillary wedge tracing in the patient with acute mitral insufficiency (refer to Figure 1.66). Medical therapy, including diuretics and/or systemic unloading interventions (for example, IV nitroprusside), may resolve the congestive heart failure in patients with papillary muscle dysfunction.

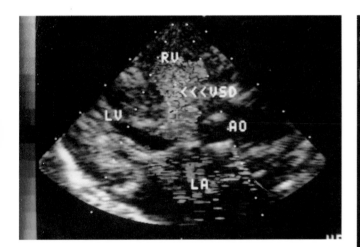

FIGURE 1.64 • A two-dimensional electrocardiogram (a color Doppler image) shows a ventricular septal defect. (Reproduced with permission. Soto B, Kassner EG, Baxley WA: *Imaging of Cardiac Disorders* New York, NY: Gower Medical Publishing; 1992:A-2.)

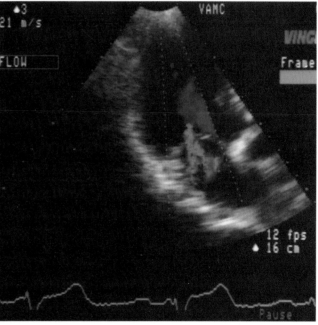

FIGURE 1.65 • Two-dimensional echocardiogram with Doppler flow pattern demonstrating mitral insufficiency.

VENTRICULAR ANEURYSMS

A ventricular aneurysm is identified by the presence of systolic thinning of the infarcted segment during systole (Figures 1.67, 1.68).[242-247] With large ventricular aneurysms, congestive heart failure may develop. Sustained ventricular tachycardia or embolic events may also result from left ventricular mural thrombi within the aneurysm.[248-252] Congestive heart failure is treated in a standard manner, including diuretics, digoxin, and unloading therapy.

Sustained ventricular tachycardia is treated by invasive electrophysiologic evaluation and the selection of an antiarrhythmic agent that is protective, or by ECG-guided sur-

gical endocardial resection and revascularization.[251,252] Implantable automatic defibrillators are inserted in patients with recurrent ventricular tachycardia for whom no effective pharmacologic therapy has been identified and no completely successful surgical procedure can be employed.[253] Systemic embolic events in patients with recently developed ventricular aneurysms are treated with heparin and later coumadin. Several months after left ventricular thrombi form in ventricular aneurysms, they firmly adhere to the left ventricular endocardium and the risk of systemic embolization is small. At this point, anticoagulation is usually no longer necessary.

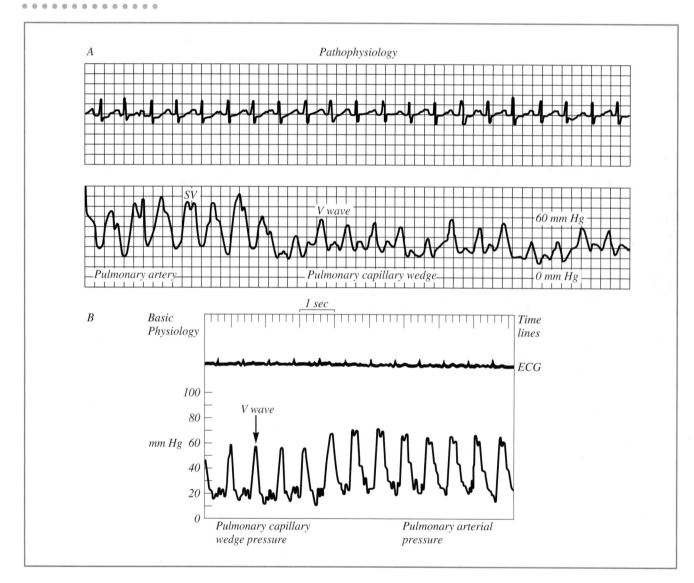

FIGURE 1.66 • The prominent V-waves developing in the pulmonary capillary wedge tracing in a patient with acute mitral insufficiency (A,B).

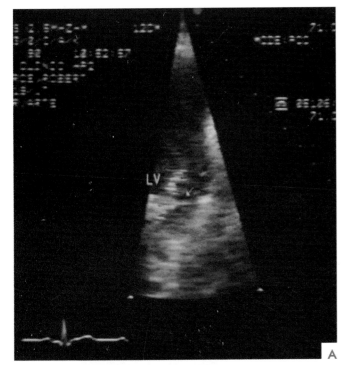

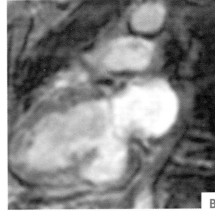

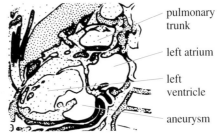

pulmonary trunk

left atrium

left ventricle

aneurysm

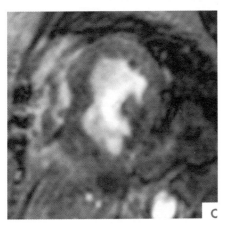

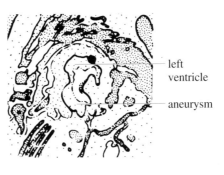

left ventricle

aneurysm

FIGURE 1.67 • A two-dimensional echocardiogram demonstrates a left ventricular aneurysm (A). Long axial view via apical window shows deformity of the inferolateral segment of the left ventricle (LV). Flowing blood can be seen entering the mouth of the aneurysm (arrow) during systole.

The long (B) and short axis (C) sections through the left ventricle of this patient's gradient-echo study (cine MRI) revealed an aneurysm of the posterolateral segment. The aneurysm communicates widely with the left ventricular cavity, which is only minimally enlarged. (Reproduced with permission. Soto B, Kassner EG, Baxley WA: *Imaging of Cardiovascular Disorders* New York, NY: Gower Medical Publishing; 1992:A.11 and 136.)

FIGURE 1.68 • Left ventricular aneurysm with mural thrombus. This right anterior oblique (RAO) projection of the left ventriculogram in systole (A) and diastole (B) demonstrates an area of dyskinesis (brace) in the anterolateral aspect of the left ventricle. The large filling defect (arrows) at the apex represents a mural thrombus. The patient had recently sustained an acute anterolateral myocardial infarction secondary to occlusion of the left anterior descending artery. (Reproduced with permission. Soto B, Kassner EG, Baxley WA: *Imaging of Cardiovascular Disorders* New York, NY: Gower Medical Publishing; 1992:168.)

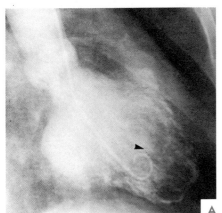

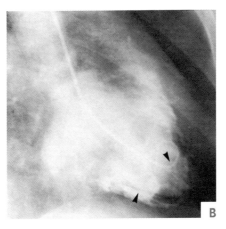

False ventricular aneurysms represent a partial rupture of the heart[242–247,254–256] (Figures 1.69, 1.70). The outer border of the aneurysm is the partial rupture and pericardium. There is a serious risk of rupturing the false ventricular aneurysm, and it must be corrected surgically as soon as possible. Partial rupture of the heart is recognized by identifying the development of an enlarging pericardial effusion or pericardial tamponade in the patient after infarction. A two-dimensional echocardiogram with Doppler imaging, a radionuclide ventriculogram, or a left ventricular angiogram often identifies a false ventricular aneurysm, which typically communicates with the left ventricular cavity through a narrow neck.[242,243]

PERICARDITIS

Acute pericarditis occurs commonly in patients with acute Q-wave myocardial infarcts[257,258] (Figure 1.71). Histologic evidence of pericarditis is found in most patients who succumb after Q-wave myocardial infarction. Chest pain that occurs with pericarditis may be mistaken for angina and/or a continuing myocardial infarction. However, if the patient is ques-

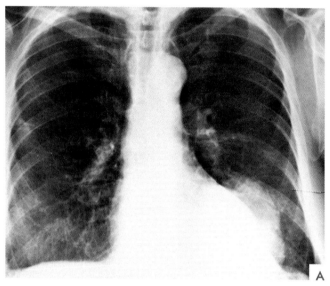
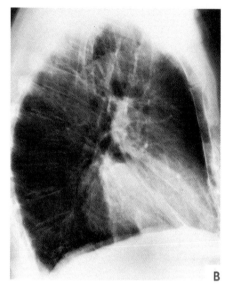
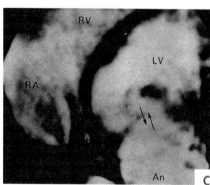

FIGURE 1.69 • A patient with a history of previous myocardial infarction presented with symptoms of congestive heart failure. This patient was found to have a pseudoaneurysm of the left ventricle. Posteroanterior chest film shows a mass adjacent to the left heart border. The left ventricle is only minimally enlarged (A). The large pseudoaneurysm projects posteriorly on the lateral view (B). In another patient, the axial section through the left ventricle shows a large pseudoaneurysm (an) arising from the upper posterior aspect of the left ventricle (LV). Note the narrow neck (arrows) at the site of ventricular rupture. The filling defects within the pseudoaneurysm and along its margin represent thrombus. (C). (Figure 1.69 A,B reproduced with permission from Soto B, Kassner EG, Baxley WA: Imaging of Cardiac Disorders. Volume 2 New York, NY: Gower Medical Publishing; 1992:138. Figure 1.69 C reproduced with permission from Lackner K, Thurn P: Radiology 1981;140:413.)

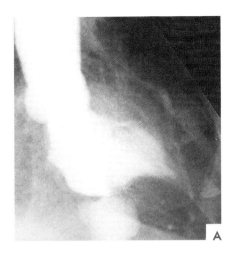
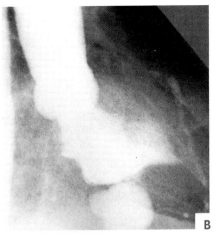

FIGURE 1.70 • Early (A) and late phases (B) of a left ventriculogram (right anterior oblique (RAO) projection) in a patient with a recent myocardial infarction involving the inferior wall revealed a psuedoaneurysm of the left ventricle. The pseudoaneurysm appears as a sac connected to the ventricular cavity by a narrow tract. The coronary arteries are related to the neck of the aneurysm and do not course over the surface. The filling defects within the pseudoaneurysm represent thrombus. DA = descending artery. (Reproduced with permission. Soto B, Kassner EG, Baxley WA: *Imaging of Cardiovascular Disorders* New York, NY: Gower Medical Publishing; 1992:168.)

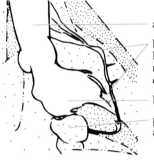

aorta

left anterior DA reaching neck of pseudoaneurysm

left ventricle

pseudoaneurysm

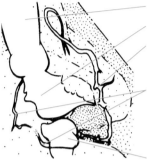

aorta

left ventricle

left anterior DA reaching neck of pseudoaneurysm

branches of posterior DA reaching neck of pseudoaneurysm thrombus

pseudoaneurysm

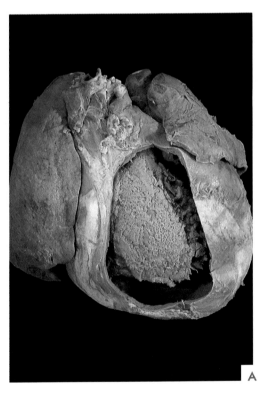

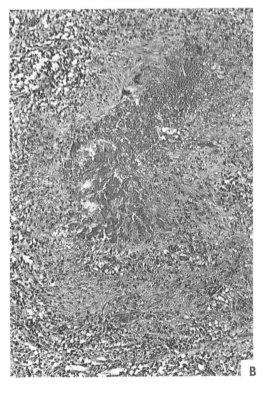

FIGURE 1.71 • The gross (A) and histologic (B) patterns found in patients with pericarditis. (Reproduced with permission. Hurst JW, Anderson RH, Becker AE, et al: *Atlas of the Heart* New York, NY: Gower Medical Publishing; 1988:7.4.)

tioned thoroughly, it is generally learned that the quality of the pain has changed to a pleuritic quality. It is made worse by assuming the supine position and is partially relieved by sitting up. On occasion, a pericardial friction rub, consisting of a two- or three-component, leathery, harsh sound, is audible over the left precordium and persists when the patient holds his/her breath. It is important not to mistake the pain of pericarditis for continuing angina after myocardial infarction. In general, the chest pain associated with pericarditis responds well to small doses of indomethacin or, on occasion, to moderate or large doses of aspirin.[257,259] Steroid therapy is sometimes necessary. It is desirable to avoid multidose and large-dose steroid therapy in patients soon after myocardial infarction, since it interferes with infarct healing, leading to a thinner scar and an increased risk of heart rupture.[260] There is evidence in experimental animal models that selected nonsteroidal anti-inflammatory agents—including indomethacin—interfere with wound healing and adversely alter infarct size.[259]

The patient with active pericarditis should not receive anticoagulant therapy unless it is required for a life-threatening condition. There is a substantial risk of hemopericardium in the patient who receives anticoagulant therapy during active pericarditis. The pericardial effusion may be large and cardiac tamponade may develop (Figures 1.72, 1.73). The development of pericardial tamponade requires pericardiocentesis, and usually an indwelling pericardial catheter, for at least several days so that reaccumulation of the pericardial effusion with pericardial tamponade does not occur. In some patients, pericarditis recurs after myocardial infarction, requiring the use of steroid therapy and/or a pericardial resection.[258]

INFARCT EXTENSION

Infarct extension results when there is reinfarction after the acute event.[261–264] Patients with systemic arterial hypertension, tachycardia, hypotension, and metabolic abnormalities, including hypoglycemia, are at risk for infarct extension (Figure 1.74). In addition, patients who receive pharmacologic agents

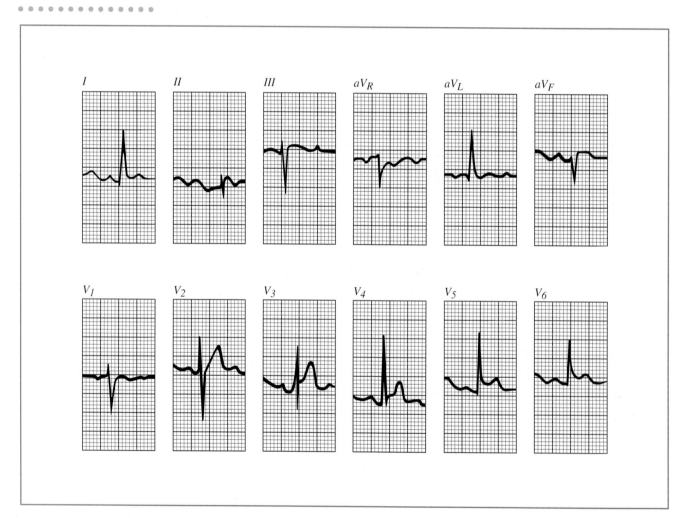

FIGURE 1.72 • PR segment depression and ST segmental elevation on the ECG are commonly found in patients with pericarditis. (Re-drawn from Hurst JW, Anderson RH, Becker AE, et al: *Atlas of the Heart* New York, NY: Gower Medical Publishing; 1988:7.4.)

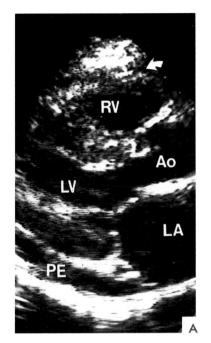 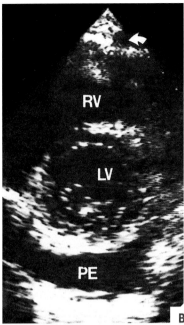 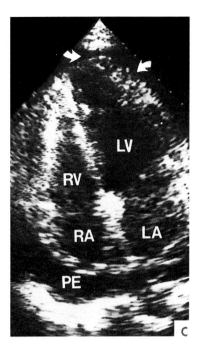

FIGURE 1.73 • Parasternal long axis (A) and short axis (B) cross-sectional echocardiograms demonstrate a moderate-sized posterior (PE) and small anterior pericardial effusions. The apical four chamber view (C) shows fluid completely surrounding the heart. (Reproduced with permission. Hurst JW, Anderson RH, Becker AE, et al: *Atlas of the Heart* New York, NY: Gower Medical Publishing; 1988:7.7.)

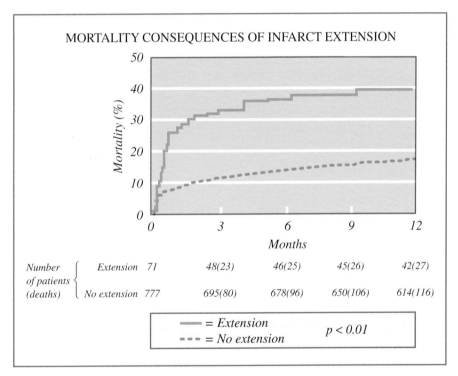

MORTALITY CONSEQUENCES OF INFARCT EXTENSION

Number of patients (deaths)						
	Extension	71	48(23)	46(25)	45(26)	42(27)
	No extension	777	695(80)	678(96)	650(106)	614(116)

―――― = Extension
‐ ‐ ‐ = No extension   p < 0.01

FIGURE 1.74 • The mortality consequences of infarct extension in patients with new my-ocardial infarcts are shown and those individuals most at risk for infarct extension are identified. (Reproduced with permission. Hutchins GM, Bulkley BH: *Am J Cadiol* 1978;41:227.)

that increase myocardial oxygen demand without increasing oxygen delivery are at risk for infarct extension. Thus, one attempts to avoid the use of powerful inotropic interventions that substantially increase the heart rate and/or contractile state of the nonfailing heart. Table 1.23 summarizes some of the clinical factors associated with infarct extension.

INFARCT EXPANSION

Infarct expansion is caused by stress and strain relationships within the infarct area.[265–268] The result is a topographic enlargement of the infarct area without any change in the extent of infarction. This is most likely to occur in the patient with systemic arterial hypertension, and is associated with progressive cardiac enlargement and deterioration of ventricular function, with increased morbidity and mortality.[262,265–268]

In experimental animal models, angiotensin converting enzyme (ACE)inhibitors attenuate or prevent infarct expansion.[267,268] Limited clinical studies have suggested the same potential utility for ACE inhibitors in patients with anterior Q-wave infarcts[267] (Figure 1.75).

Control of systemic arterial hypertension is important in the patient with myocardial infarction for reducing the risk of infarct expansion or extension and rupture of the heart.[268] Rupture of the heart occurs most commonly in women with their first infarcts and in patients who have systemic arterial hypertension during and following infarction.[269] Blood pressure control is also important in these patients to prevent the worsening of heart failure as a result of the increased afterload that exists in hypertension.

Agents chosen to treat systemic arterial hypertension during and after infarction should be those that do not importantly depress ventricular function or increase heart rate. Angiotensin converting enzyme inhibitors, selected calcium antagonists, nitrates—including IV nitroglycerin and nitroprusside and, on occasion, ß-blockers—may be used in selected patients to control blood pressure and prevent the complications mentioned above.

HEART BLOCK

Heart block occurs as a consequence of chronic coronary heart disease and with myocardial infarction. Chapter 3 provides a detailed discussion of the mechanisms, recognition, and treatment of heart block. First-degree heart block alone requires no therapy, although one should avoid the administration of an agent that might further delay atrioventricular conduction. Second-degree heart block of the Mobitz I ("Wenckebach") type occurs primarily in patients with an acute inferior myocardial infarction or chronic inferior ischemia associated with a sig-

TABLE 1.23 • UNIVARIATE ANALYSIS OF POSSIBLE RISK FACTORS FOR INFARCT EXTENSION

Risk Factor	Extension		P Value
	Yes	No	
Angina on the second hospital day	27/71(38%)	177/777(23%)	< 0.01
ST-segment depression on initial electrocardiogram	16/67(24%)	97/755(13%)	< 0.02
Previous myocardial infarction	24/71(34%)	175/776(23%)	< 0.04
Early peaking of MB creatine kinase (≤ 15 hr)	25/70(36%)	193/775(25%)	< 0.05
History of diabetes mellitus	19/71(27%)	138/770(18%)	< 0.07
Obesity—body mass index (> upper 25th percentile)	14/71(20%)	197/773(26%)	NS
Inferior ST-segment elevation or infarction on initial electrocardiogram	28/67(42%)	388/755(51%)	NS
Pretreatment left ventricular ejection fraction < 40%	28/62(45%)	238/652(37%)	NS
Angina < 3 weeks before this episode	36/71(51%)	344/777(44%)	NS
Systolic pressure ≥ 150 mm Hg in first 48 hrs	51/71(72%)	508/766(66%)	NS
Anterior ST-segment elevation or infarction on initial electrocardiogram	27/67(40%)	337/755(45%)	NS
Diastolic pressure ≥ 90mm Hg in first 48 hrs	59/70(84%)	664/769(86%)	NS
Heart rate > 100 in first 48 hrs	31/71(44%)	325/769(42%)	NS
Male sex	52/71(73%)	564/777(73%)	NS
Age, *years*	58.5 ± 1.1	56.7 ± 0.4	NS

NS = not significant

(Reproduced with permission. Muller JE, Rude RE, Braunwald E, et al: *Ann Intern Med* 1988;108:1.)

Medical Treatment of Coronary Heart Disease

nificant right or circumflex coronary artery stenosis: It also develops in patients who have degenerative conduction-system disease and those given excessive amounts of a cardiac glycoside. It is usually an infrajunctional (atrioventricular (AV) nodal) form of heart block.

Mobitz I heart block requires pacing only if the ventricular rate is slow enough to cause hemodynamic or electrical problems, including dizziness or syncope, progressive angina or congestive heart failure, or if it predisposes to enhanced reentry mechanisms and frequent or complex ventricular premature beats.

Mobitz II heart block is an intraventricular block that is unstable and usually associated with an acute anterior myocardial infarction or degenerative conduction-system disease. A temporary pacemaker should be inserted when this form of heart block develops, usually followed at a later date by the implantation of a permanent pacemaker.

Complete heart block may develop for many reasons, including:

• Acute myocardial infarction.
• Cardiac glycoside excess.
• Degenerative conduction-system disease.

When heart block complicates acute myocardial infarction, a temporary pacemaker should be inserted, followed at a later date by a permanent pacemaker if the heart block fails to resolve. In the patient with an acute inferior infarct, complete heart block almost always resolves within 2 weeks. With anterior infarcts, complete heart block may not resolve.

BUNDLE-BRANCH BLOCK

Acute left bundle-branch block occurs in patients who experience large myocardial infarcts and often in cases of infarction complicated by heart failure and/or shock. The risk of developing complete heart block is from 20% to 40%, and insertion of a temporary pacemaker prophylactically is recommended. If atrioventricular (AV) block does not develop within a week, the pacemaker may be removed. The development of acute right bundle-branch block should be monitored carefully, but the risk of developing complete heart block is only approximately 10%.

The acute development of bilateral bundle-branch block—left axis deviation and right bundle-branch block, right axis deviation and right bundle-branch block, first-degree atrioventricular block and left-bundle branch block, or alternating left and right bundle-branch block on the ECG—is associated with a large infarct. These infarcts are often complicated by heart failure, complete heart block, shock, and/or death. Complete heart block develops in 40% to 60% of patients not receiving thrombolytic therapy, and requires the prophylactic insertion of a temporary pacemaker. Early thrombolytic therapy or percutaneous transluminal coronary angioplasty (PTCA) in these patients sometimes reverses the bilateral bundle-branch block and reduces the ultimate infarct size, thus altering the otherwise expected adverse outcome. A permanent pacemaker should be inserted in patients who develop atrioventricular block with bilateral bundle-branch block.

When left, right, or bilateral bundle-branch block precedes an infarct, prophylactic pacemaker insertion is not recom-

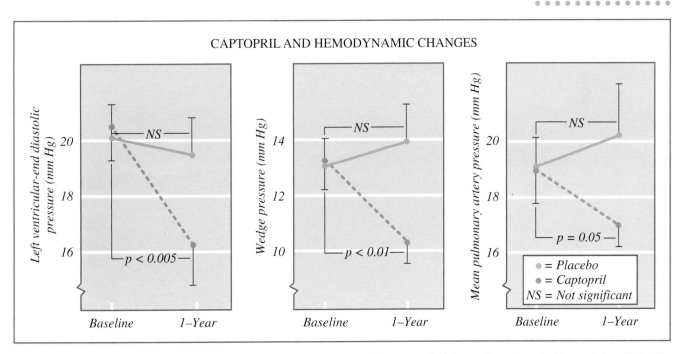

FIGURE 1.75 • An angiotensin-converting enzyme inhibitor—captopril—may attenuate infarct expansion in selected patients with acute anterior myocardial infarcts. (Reproduced with permission. Pfeffer M, Corbett J, Leachman R: *N Engl J Med* 1988;319:83.)

mended unless other clinical indications suggest the need for this form of therapy.

RECURRENT MYOCARDIAL ISCHEMIA

Patients who have had a myocardial infarction and experience recurrent myocardial ischemia at rest or during low levels of activity while on an appropriate medical regimen should be referred for coronary arteriography and revascularization if their coronary artery anatomy is suitable (refer to Chapter 6).[110,112,270–279] Submaximal exercise tests should be obtained from 5 to 10 days after infarction in patients who can exercise, so as to identify individuals with angina, ST-segment deviation, and/or life-threatening ventricular arrhythmias at low-level effort.[110,112,277–280]

Low-level exercise-induced arrhythmias are treated with appropriate antiarrhythmic agents, possibly including a ß-blocker. Patients with left ventricular ejection fractions of 40% or less, and more than 8 to 10 ventricular premature beats/hr, ventricular premature beat couplets, or runs of ventricular tachycardia, have an increased risk of sudden death in the 6 months after myocardial infarction.[280] A reduction in systemic arterial blood pressure developing with low-level exercise in the patient who has had an infarction, and/or a 3 mm or greater ST-segment depression from a relatively normal ECG baseline, suggest significant left main and/or important three-vessel coronary heart disease.[110,112,277–279] These findings should prompt an evaluation of the patient by coronary arteriography, since patients with significant left main and/or three-vessel coronary heart disease have their lives prolonged by coronary artery revascularization. The additional use of nuclear cardiology procedures, including perfusion scintigraphy with thallium-201 or technetium-labeled isonitriles (RP30), or the assessment of ventricular function by radionuclide ventriculography with low-level exercise testing after infarction, allows one to identify most patients at risk for future important coronary events (refer to Figures 1.30, 1.31).[110,112,277–280]

CONCLUSIONS

It is very important to treat coronary artery disease syndromes using mechanistic pathophysiologic insight that allows one to focus medical therapy on specific vascular and myocardial alterations that are responsible for stable angina, unstable angina, coronary artery spasm (Prinzmetal's angina), and acute myocardial infarction. The therapy of myocardial infarction depends on the type of myocardial infarction—non-Q wave or Q wave myocardial infarction—and recognizing the importance of the restoring blood flow at a very early stage in myocardial infarction development with acute Q-wave myocardial infarcts. It is anticipated that development of thrombolytic interventions that have a more rapid thrombolytic effect and a delayed continuing action will enhance the protective effect and reduce the risk of reocclusion of the infarct-related artery. Specifically, I believe that a combination of platelet active agents and selected thrombin antagonist with effective thrombolytic agents will decrease the time to thrombolysis and delay or prevent coronary artery reocclusion following thrombolytic therapy in many patients that are treated in the future.

Specific complications of myocardial infarction can be reduced in frequency and severity by more effective treatment for myocardial infarcts. Correction of secondary risk factors, including reductions in serum cholesterol, low-density lipoprotein (LDL), avoidance of smoking, control of blood pressure, and appropriate medication, including platelet active agents, should minimize the progression of future coronary artery disease, decreasing the frequency of clinical appearance of unstable angina and myocardial infarction. These advances in clinical care will come from constantly improving mechanistic insight into the most critical pathophysiologic alterations that cause the conversion from chronic to acute coronary artery disease syndromes.

REFERENCES

1. Heberden W: Some account of a disorder of the breast. *Med Trans. R. Coll. Physicians* II. London: 1786:59.

2. Herrick, JB: Clinical features of sudden obstruction of the coronary ateries. *JAMA* 1912;59:2015.

3. Sarnoff SJ, Braunwald E, Welch GH Jr, et al: Hemodynamic determinants of oxygen consumption of the heart, with special reference to the tension-time index. *Am J Physiol* 1958;192:148.

4. Rude RE, Izquierdo C, Buja LM, Willerson JT: Effects of inotropic and chronotropic stimuli on acute myocardial ischemic injury. I. Studies with dobutamine in the barbiturate-anesthetized dog. *Circulation* 1982;65:1321.

5. Rude RE, Izquierdo C, Bush LR, et al: Effects of inotropic and chronotropic stimuli on acute myocardial ischemic injury. II. Studies with dopamine and ouabain in the barbiturate-anesthetized dog. *J Cardiovasc Pharmacol* 1983;5:717.

6. Rude RE, Bush LR, Izquierdo C, et al: Effects of inotropic and chronotropic stimuli on acute myocardial ischemic injury. III. Influences of basal heart rate. *Am J Cardiol* 1984;53:1688.

7. Sonnenblick EH, Ross J Jr, Braunwald E: Oxygen consumption of the heart: Newer concepts of its multifactoral determination. *Am J Cardiol* 1969;22:328.

8. Marcus ML, Doty DB, Hiratzka LF, et al: Decreased coronary reserve—A mechanism for angina pectoris in patients with aortic stenosis and normal coronary arteries. *N Engl J Med* 1982;307:1362.

9. Marcus ML, Mueller TM, Eastham CL: Effects of short- and long-term left ventricular hypertrophy on coronary circulation. *Am J Physiol* 1981;24:H358.

10. Berkenboom GM, Abramowicz M, Vandermoten P, Degre SG: Role of alpha-adrenergic coronary tone in exercise-induced angina pectoris. *Am J Cardiol* 1986;57:195.

11. Gage JE, Hess OM, Murakami T, et al: Vasoconstriction of stenotic coronary arteries during dynamic exercise in patients with classic angina pectoris: reversibility by nitroglycerin. *Circulation* 1986;73:865.

12. Ashton JH, Ogletree ML, Michel IM, et al: Serotonin and thromboxane A_2/prostaglandin H_2 receptor activation cooperatively mediate cyclic flow variations in dogs with severe coronary artery stenoses. *Circulation* 1987;76:952.

13. Golino P, Ashton JH, Buja LM, et al: Local platelet activation causes vasoconstriction of large epicardial canine coronary arteries *in vivo*: Thromboxane A_2 and serotonin are possible mediators. *Circulation* 1989;79:154.

14. Bush LR, Campbell WB, Kern K: The effects of alpha$_2$ adrenergic and serotonergic receptor blockade on platelet aggregation in stenosed canine coronary arteries. *Circ Res* 1984;55:642.

15. Willerson JT, Hillis LD, Winniford M, Buja LM: Speculation regarding mechanisms responsible for acute ischemic heart disease syndromes. *J Am Coll Cardiol* 1986;8:245.

16. Willerson JT, Campbell WB, Winniford MD, et al: Conversion from chronic to acute ischemic heart disease: Speculation regarding mechanisms (editorial). *Am J Cardiol* 1984;54:1349.

17. Willerson JT, Golino P, Eidt J, et al: Specific platelet mediators and unstable coronary artery lesions. Experimental evidence and potential clinical implications. *Circulation* 1989;80:198.

18. Hirsh PD, Hillis LD, Campbell WB, et al: Release of prostaglandins and thromboxane into the coronary circulation in patients with ischemic heart disease. *N Engl J Med* 1981;304:685.

19. Eidt JF, Allison P, Noble S, et al: Thrombin is an important mediator of platelet aggregation in stenosed and endothelially-injured canine coronary arteries. *J Clin Invest* 1989;84:18.

20. van den Berg EK, Schmitz JM, Benedict CR, Malloy CR, Willerson JT, Dehmer GJ: Transcardiac serotonin concentration is increased in selected patients with limiting angina and complex coronary lesion morphology. *Circulation* 1989;49:116.

21. Maseri A, Severi S, De Nes M, et al: "Variant" angina: one aspect of a continuous spectrum of vasospastic myocardial ischemia; pathogenic mechanisms, estimated incidence and clinical and coronary arteriographic findings in 138 patients. *Am J Cardiol* 1978;42:1019.

22. Dalen JE, Ockene IS, Alpert JS: Coronary spasm, coronary thrombosis and myocardial infarction. *Am Heart J* 1982;104:1119.

23. Gottlieb SO, Weisfeldt ML, Ouyang P, et al: Silent ischemia as a marker for early unfavorable outcomes in patients with unstable angina. *N Engl J Med* 1986;314:1214.

24. Fleg JL, Gerstenblith G, Zonderman AB, et al: Prevalence and prognostic significance of exercise-induced silent myocardial ischemia detected by thallium scintigraphy and electrocardiography in asymptomatic volunteers. *Circulation* 1990;81:428.

25. Weiner DA, Ryan TJ, McCabe CH, et al: Significance of silent myocardial ischemia during exercise testing in patients with coronary artery disease. *Am J Cardiol* 1987;59:725.

26. Latham P: *Collected Works, Vol 1. New Sydenham Society*, London, 1876.

27. Osler W: The Lumleian lectures on angina pectoris. *Lancet* 1910;1:697.

28. Prinzmetal M, Kennamer R, Merliss R, et al: Angina pectoris. I. a variant form of angina pectoris. *Am J Med* 1959;27:375.

29. Hillis LD, Braunwald E: Coronary artery spasm. *N Engl J Med* 1978;299:695.

30. Silverman ME, Flamm MD Jr: Variant angina pectoris: Anatomic findings and prognostic implications. *Ann Intern Med* 1971;75:339.

31. Cheng TO, Bashour R, Kelser GA, et al: Variant angina of Prinzmetal with normal coronary arteriograms. A variant of the variant. *Circulation* 1973;47:476.

32. Wiener L, Kasparian H, Duca PR, et al: Spectrum of coronary arterial spasm: Clinical, angiographic, and myocardial metabolic experience in 29 cases. *Am J Cardiol* 1976;38:945.

33. Dhurandhar RW, Watt DL, Silver MD, et al: Prinzmetal's variant form of angina with arteriographic evidence of coronary arterial spasm. *Am J Cardiol* 1972;30:902.

34. Oliva PB, Potts DE, Pluss RG: Coronary arterial spasm in Prinzmetal angina: Documentation by coronary arteriography. *N Engl J Med* 1973;288:745.

35. Maseri A, Mimmo R, Chierchia S: Coronary artery spasm as a cause of acute myocardial ischemia in man. *Chest* 1975;68:625.

36. Higgins CB, Wexler L, Silverman JF, et al: Clinical and arteriographic features of Prinzmetal's variant angina: Documentation of etiologic factors. *Am J Cardiol* 1976;37:831.

37. Maseri A, Parodi O, Severi S, et al: Transient transmural reduction of myocardial blood flow, demonstrated by thallium-201 scintigraphy, as a cause of variant angina. *Circulation* 1976;54:280.

38. McLaughlin PR, Doherty PW, Martin RP, et al: Myocardial imaging in a patient with reproducible variant angina. *Am J Cardiol* 1977;39:126.

39. Berman ND, McLaughlin PR, Huckell VF, et al: Prinzmetal's angina with coronary artery spasm: Angiographic, pharmacologic, metabolic, and radionuclide perfusion studies. *Am J Med* 1976;60:727.

40. Ricci DR, Orlick AE, Doherty PW, et al: Reduction of coronary blood flow during coronary artery spasm occurring spontaneously and after provocation by ergonovine maleate. *Circulation* 1978;57:392.

41. Nelson C, Nowak B, Childs H, et al: Provocative testing for coronary arterial spasm: Rationale, risk, and clinical illustrations. *Am J Cardiol* 1977;40:624.

42. Schroeder JS, Bolen JL, Quint RA, et al: Provocation of coronary spasm with ergonovine maleate: New test with result in 57 patients undergoing coronary arteriography. *Am J Cardiol* 1977;40:487.

43. Curry RC Jr, Pepine CJ, Sabom MB, et al: Effects of ergonovine in patients with and without coronary artery disease. *Circulation* 1977;56:803.

44. Heupler FA, Proudfit WL, Razavi M, et al: Ergonovine maleate provocative test for coronary arterial spasm. *Am J Cardiol* 1978;41:631.

45. Helfant R: Coronary arterial spasm and provocative testing in ischemic heart disease. *Am J Cardiol* 1978;41:787.

46. Buxton A, Goldberg S, Hirshfeld JW, et al: Refractory ergonovine-induced coronary vasospasm: Importance of intracoronary nitroglycerin. *Am J Cardiol* 1980;46:329.

47. Scherf D, Perlman A, Schlachman M: Effect of dihydroergonovine on the heart. *Proc Soc Exp Biol Med* 1949;71:420.

48. Heupler FA Jr: Provocative testing for coronary arterial spasm: Risk, method, and rationale. *Am J Cardiol* 1980;46:335.

49. Fester A: Provocative testing for coronary arterial spasm with ergonovine maleate. *Am J Cardiol* 1980;46:338.

50. Cipriano PR, Guthaner DF, Orlick AE, et al: The effects of ergonovine maleate on coronary arterial size. *Circulation* 1979;59:82.

51. Endo M, Hirosawa K, Kaneko N, et al: Prinzmetal's variant angina: Coronary arteriogram and left ventriculogram during angina attack induced by methacholine. *N Engl J Med* 1976;294:252.

52. Yasue H, Horio Y, Imoto N, et al: Induction of coronary artery spasm by acetylcholine in patients with variant angina: Possible role of the parasympathetic nervous system in the pathogenesis of coronary artery spasm. *Circulation* 1986;74:955.

53. Raizner AE, Chahine RA, Ishimori T, et al: Provocation of coronary artery spasm by the cold pressor test: Hemodynamic, arteriographic, and quantitative angiographic observations. *Circulation* 1980;62:925.

54. Mudge GH Jr, Grossman W, Mills RM Jr, et al: Reflex increase in coronary vascular resistance in patients with ischemic heart disease. *N Engl J Med* 1976;295:1333.

55. Hasue H, Nagao M, Omote S, et al: Coronary arterial spasm and Prinzmetal's variant form of angina induced by hyperventilation and tris-buffer infusion. *Circulation* 1978;58:56.

56. Chandler AB, Chapman I, Erhardt LR, et al: Coronary thrombosis in myocardial infarction. Report of a workshop on the role of coronary thrombosis in the pathogenesis of acute myocardial infarction. *Am J Cardiol* 1974;34:823.

57. DeWood MA, Spores J, Notske R: Prevalence of total coronary occlusion during the early hours of transmural myocardial infarction. *N Engl J Med* 1980;303:897.

58. Buja LM, Willerson JT: Clinicopathologic findings in 100 episodes of acute ischemic heart disease (acute myocardial infarction or coronary insufficiency) in 83 patients. *Am J Cardiol* 1981;47:343.

59. Gibson RS, Beller GA, Gheorghiade M, et al: The prevalence and clinical significance of residual myocardial ischemia 2 weeks after uncomplicated non-Q wave infarction: A prospective natural history study. *Circulation* 1986;73:1186.

60. Falk E: Plaque rupture with severe preexisting stenosis precipitating coronary thrombosis: Characteristics of coronary atherosclerotic plaques. *Br Heart J* 1983;50:127.

61. Davies MJ, Thomas AC. Plaque fissuring—the cause of acute myocardial infarction, sudden ischemic death, and crescendo angina. *Br Heart J* 1985;53:363.

62. Mason DT, Braunwald E: The effects of nitroglycerin and amyl nitrate on arteriolar and venous tone in the human forearm. *Circulation* 1965;32:755.

63. Reichek N, Priest C, Zimrin D, et al: Antianginal effects of nitroglycerin patches. *Am J Cardiol* 1984;54:1.

64. Parker JO, VanKoughnett KA, Fung HL: Transdermal isosorbide dinitrate in angina pectoris: Effect of acute and sustained therapy. *Am J Cardiol* 1984;54:8.

65. Glancy DL, Richter MA, Ellis EV, et al: Effect of swallowed isosorbide dinitrate on blood pressure, heart rate, and exercise capacity in patients with coronary artery disease. *Am J Med* 1977;62:39.

66. Horowitz JD, Antman EM, Lorell BH, et al: Potentiation of the cardiovascular effects of nitroglycerin by N-acetylcysteine. *Circulation* 1983;68:1247.

67. Murad F, Arnold WP, Mittal CK, Braughler JM: Properties and regulation of guanylate cyclase and some proposed functions of cyclic GMP. *Cyclic Nucleotide Res* 1979;11:175.

68. Markis JE, Gorlin R, Mills RM, et al: Sustained effect of orally administered isosorbide dinitrate on exercise performance of patients with angina pectoris. *Am J Cardiol* 1979;43:265.

69. Danahy DT, Aronow WS: Hemodynamics and antianginal effects of high dose oral isosorbide dinitrate after chronic use. *Circulation* 1977;56:205.

70. Thadani U, Fung H-L, Darke AC, et al: Oral isosorbide dinitrate in angina pectoris: Comparison of duration of action and dose-response relation during acute and sustained therapy. *Am J Cardiol* 1982;49:411.

71. Needleman P, Johnson EM, Jr: Mechanism of tolerance development to organic nitrates. *J Pharmacol Exp Ther* 1973;184:709.

72. Abrams J: Nitrate tolerance and dependence. *Am Heart J* 1980;99:113.

73. Frishman W: Clinical pharmacology of the new beta-adrenergic blocking drugs. IX. Nadolol: A new long-acting beta-adrenoceptor blocking drug. *Am Heart J* 1980;99:124.

74. Moses JW, Borer JS: Beta-adrenergic antagonists in the treatment of patients with heart disease. *DM* 1981;27:1.

75. Koch-Weser J: Metoprolol. *N Engl J Med* 1979;301:698.

76. Frishman WH: ß-adrenoceptor antagonists: New drugs and new indications. *N Engl J Med* 1981;305:500.

77. Opie LH: Drugs and the heart. I. Beta-blocking agents. *Lancet* 1980;1:693.

78. Dreyfuss J, Brannick LJ, Vukovich RA, et al: Metabolic studies in patients with nadolol: Oral and intravenous administration. *J Clin Pharmacol* 1977;17:300.

79. Frishman W: Clinical pharmacology of the new beta-adrenergic blocking drugs. I. Pharmacodynamic and pharmacokinetic properties. *Am Heart J* 1979;97:663.

80. Conolly ME, Kersting F, Dollery CT: The clinical pharmacology of beta-adrenoceptor-blocking drugs. *Prog Cardiovasc Dis* 1976;19:203.

81. Forman R, Eng C, Kirk ES: Comparative effect of verapamil and nitroglycerin on collateral blood flow. *Circulation* 1983;67:1200.

82. Muller JE, Gunther SJ: Nifedipine therapy for Prinzmetal's angina. *Circulation* 1978;57:137.

83. Hugenholtz PG, Michels HR, Serruys PW, et al: Nifedipine in the treatment of unstable angina, coronary spasm and myocardial ischemia. *Am J Cardiol* 1981;47:163.

84. Gunther S, Green L, Muller JE, et al: Prevention by nifedipine of abnormal coronary vasoconstriction in patients with coronary artery disease. *Circulation* 1981;63:849.

85. Solberg LE, Nissen RG, Vlietstra RE, et al: Prinzmetal's variant angina—response to verapamil. *Mayo Clin Proc* 1978;53:256.

86. Johnson SM, Mauritson DR, Willerson JT, Hillis LD: A controlled trial of verapamil for Prinzmetal's variant angina. *N Engl J Med* 1981;304:862.

87. Freedman B, Dunn RF, Richmond DR, et al: Coronary artery spasm during exercise: Treatment with verapamil. *Circulation* 1981;64:68.

88. Hansen JF, Sando E: Treatment of Prinzmetal's angina due to coronary artery spasm using verapamil: A report of three cases. *Eur J Cardiol* 1978;7:327.

89. Schroeder JS, Lamb IH, Ginsburg R, et al: Diltiazem for long-term therapy of coronary arterial spasm. *Am J Cardiol* 1982;49:533.

90. Johnson SM, Mauritson DR, Willerson JT, et al: A comparison of verapamil and nifedipine in the treatment of variant angina pectoris. *Am J Cardiol* 1981;47(6):1295.

91. Winniford MD, Johnson SM, Mauritson DR, et al: Verapamil therapy for Prinzmetal's variant angina: Comparison with placebo and nifedipine. *Am J Cardiol* 1982;50:913.

92. Hillis LD: The new coronary vasodilators: Calcium blockers. *J Cardiovasc Med* 1980;5:583.

93. Theroux P, Waters DD, Affaki GS, et al: Provocative testing with ergonovine to evaluate the efficacy of treatment with calcium antagonists in variant angina. *Circulation* 1979;60:504.

94. Nagao T, Ikeo T, Sato M: Influence of calcium ions on responses to diltiazem in coronary arteries. *Jpn J Pharmacol* 1977;27:330.

95. Weishaar R, Ashikawa K, Bing RJ: Effect of diltiazem, a calcium antagonist, on myocardial ischemia. *Am J Cardiol* 1979;43:1137.

96. Previtali M, Salerno JA, Tavazzi L, et al: Treatment of angina at rest with nifedipine: A short-term controlled study. *Am J Cardiol* 1980;45:825.

97. Heng MK, Singh BN, Roche AHG, et al: Effects of intravenous verapamil on cardiac arrhythmias and on the electrocardiogram. *Am Heart J* 1975;90:487.

98. Schamroth L, Krinkler DM, Garreet C: Immediate effects of intravenous verapamil in cardiac arrhythmias. *Cardiovasc Res* 1971;5:419.

99. Andreasen F, Boye E, Christoffersen E, et al: Assessment of verapamil in the treatment of angina pectoris. *Eur J Cardiol* 1975;2:443.

100. Neumann M, Luisada AA: Double blind evaluation of orally administered iproveratril in patients with angina pectoris. *Am J Med Sci* 1966;251:552.

101. Sandler G, Clayton GA, Thronicroft S: Clinical evaluation of verapamil in angina pectoris. *Br Med J* 1968;3:224.

102. Livesley B, Catley PF, Campbell RC, et al: Double-blind evaluation of verapamil, propranolol, and disosorbide dinitrate against a placebo in the treatment of angina pectoris. *Br Med J* 1973;1:375.

103. Balasubramian V, Khanna PK, Naryanan GR, et al: Verapamil in ischemic heart disease—quantitative assessment by serial multistage treadmill exercise. *Postgrad Med J* 1976;52:143.

104. Johnson SM, Mauritson DR, Corbett JR, et al: Double-blind, randomized, placebo-controlled comparison of propranolol and verapamil in the treatment of patients with stable angina pectoris. *Am J Med* 1981;71:443.

105. Klimt CR, Knatterud GL, Stamler J, Meier P: Persantine-aspirin reinfarction study. II. Secondary coronary prevention with persantine and aspirin. *J Am Coll Cardiol* 1986;7:251.

106. Steering Committee of the Physicians' Health Study Research Group: Final report on the aspirin component of the ongoing physicians' health study. *N Engl J Med* 1989;321:129.

107. Peto R, Gray R, Collins R, et al: Randomised trial of prophylactic daily aspirin in British male doctors. *Br Med J* 1988;296:13.

108. Secondary prevention of vascular disease by prolonged antiplatelet treatment: Antiplatelet trialists' collaboration. *Br Med J* 1988;296:320.

108ª. Clarke RJ, Mayo G, Price P, et al: Suppression of thromboxane A_2 but not of systemic prostacyclin by controlled release aspirin. *N Engl J Med* 1991;325:1137.

108ᵇ. Reilly IAG, Fitzgerald GA: Aspirin in cardiovascular disease. *Drugs* 1988;35:154.

109. Borer J, Bacharach SL, Green MV, et al: Real time radionuclide cineangiography in the noninvasive evaluation of global and regional left ventricular function at rest and during exercise in patients with coronary artery disease. *N Engl J Med* 1977;296:839.

110. Gibson RS, Watson DD, Craddock GB, et al: Prediction of cardiac events after uncomplicated myocardial infarction. Prospective study comparing predischarge exercise thallium-201 scintigraphy and coronary angiography. *Circulation* 1983;68:321.

111. Ritchie JL, Trobaugh GB, Hamilton GW, et al: Myocardial imaging with thallium-201 at rest and during exercise: comparison with coronary arteriography and resting and stress electrocardiography. *Circulation* 1977;56:66.

112. Corbett J, Dehmer GJ, Lewis SE, et al: The prognostic value of submaximal exercise testing with radionuclide ventriculography prior to hospital discharge in patients with recent myocardial infarction. *Circulation* 1981;64(3):535-544.

113. Dehmer GJ, Lewis SE, Hillis LD, et al: Exercise induced alterations in left ventricular volumes in man: usefulness in predicting the relative extent of coronary artery disease. *Circulation* 1981;63:1008.

114. Veterans Administration Coronary Artery Bypass Surgery Cooperative Study Group: Eleven-year survival in the Veterans Administration randomized trial of coronary bypass surgery for stable angina. *N Engl J Med* 1984;311:1333.

115. Passamani E, Davis KB, Gillespie MJ, Killip T, and the CASS principal investigators and their associates: A randomized trial of coronary artery bypass surgery. Survival of patients with a low ejection fraction. *N Engl J Med* 1985;312:1665.

116. CASS principal investigators and their associates: Coronary artery surgery study (CASS): A randomized trial of coronary artery bypass surgery; survival data. *Circulation* 1983;68:939.

117. European Coronary Surgery Study Group: Coronary-artery bypass surgery in stable angina pectoris: Survival at two years. *Lancet* 1979;1:889.

118. Winniford MD, Kennedy P, Wells P, Hillis LD: Potentiation of nitroglycerin induced coronary dilatation by N-acetylcysteine. *Circulation* 1986;73:138.

119. Parodi O, Maseri A, Simonetti I: Management of unstable angina at rest by verapamil: A double-blind crossover study in coronary care unit. *Br Med J* 1979;41:167.

120. Mauritson DR, Johnson SM, Winniford MD, et al: Verapamil for unstable angina pectoris: A short-term randomized, double-blind study. *Am Heart J* 1983;106:652.

121. Moses JW, Wertheimer JH, Bodenheimer MM, et al: Efficacy of nifedepine in rest angina refractory to propranolol and nitrates in patients with obstructive coronary artery disease. *Ann Intern Med* 1981;94:425.

122. Moses JW, Borer JS: Beta-adrenergic antagonists in the treatment of patients with heart disease. *DM* 1981;27:1.

123. Gold HK, Leinbach RC, Buckley MJ, et al: Refractory angina pectoris: follow-up after intraaortic balloon pumping and surgery. *Circulation* 1976;54 (Suppl 3):41.

124. McEnany MT, Kay HR, Buckley MJ, et al: Clinical experience with intraaortic balloon pump support in 723 patients. *Circulation* 1978;58 (Suppl 1):124.

125. Gold HK, Leinbach RC, Mundth ED, et al: Reversal of myocardial ischemia complicating acute infarction by intraaortic balloon pumping (IABP). *Circulation* 1972;45–46 (Suppl II):22.

126. Lewis HD Jr, Davis JW, Archibald DG, et al: Protective effects of aspirin against acute myocardial infarction and death in men with unstable angina. *N Engl J Med* 1983;309:396.

127. Cairns JA, Gent M, Singer J, et al: Aspirin, sulfinpyrazone, or both in unstable angina. *N Engl J Med* 1985;313:1369.

128. Theroux P, Ouimet H, McCann J, et al: Aspirin, heparin, or both to treat acute unstable angina. *N Engl J Med* 1988;319:1105.

129. Pugh B, Platt MR, Mills LJ, et al: Unstable angina pectoris: A randomized study of patients treated medically and surgically. *Am J Cardiol* 1978;41:1291.

130. DiPaolo C, Kerin NZ, Rubenfire M, Levine F: Surgical treatment of medically refractory variant angina pectoris: Segmental coronary resection with aortocoronary bypass and plexectomy. *Am J Cardiol* 1985;56:792.

131. Maroko PR, Kjekshus JK, Sobel BE, et al: Factors influencing infarct size following experimental coronary artery occlusion. *Circulation* 1971;43:67.

132. Chazov EL, Mateera LS, Masaev AV, et al: Intracoronary administration of fibrinolysis in acute myocardial infarction. *Ter Arkh* 1976;48:8.

133. Kennedy JW, Ritchie JL, Davis FB, et al: Western Washington randomized trial of intracoronary streptokinase in acute myocardial infarction. *N Engl J Med* 1983;309:1477.

134. Gruppo Italiano per lo Studio della Streptochinasi nel-infarto miocardico (GISSI): effectiveness of intravenous thrombolytic treatment in acute myocardial infarction. *Lancet* 1986;1:397.

135. Stack RS, Phillips HR, Grierson DS, et al: Functional improvement of jeopardized myocardium following intracoronary streptokinase infusion in acute myocardial infarction. *J Clin Invest* 1983;72:84.

136. Sheehan RH, Braunwald E, Canner P, et al: The effect of intravenous thrombolytic therapy on left ventricular function: A report on tissue-type plasminogen activator and streptokinase from the Thrombolysis in Myocardial Infarction (TIMI Phase I) Trial. *Circulation* 1987;75:817.

137. Serruys PW, Simoons ML, Suryapranata H, et al: Preservation of global and regional left ventricular function after early thrombolysis in acute myocardial infarction. *J Am Coll Cardiol* 1986;7:729.

138. Simoons ML, Serruys PW, van den Brand M, et al: Early thrombolysis in acute myocardial infarction: Reduction of infarct size, preservation of left ventricular function and improved survival. *J Am Coll Cardiol* 1986;7:718.

139. O'Neill W, Timmis GC, Bourillon P, et al: A prospective randomized clinical trial of intracoronary streptokinase versus coronary angioplasty for acute myocardial infarction. *N Engl J Med* 1986;314:812.

140. Hillis LD, Borer J, Braunwald E, et al: High-dose intravenous streptokinase for acute myocardial infarction: Preliminary results of a multicenter trial. *J Am Coll Cardiol* 1985;6:957.

141. Anderson JL, Marshall HW, Bray BE, et al: A randomized trial of intracoronary streptokinase in the treatment of acute myocardial infarction. *N Engl J Med* 1983;308:1312.

142. Rentrop P, Blanke H, Karsch KR, et al: Changes in left ventricular function after intracoronary streptokinase infusion in clinically evolving myocardial infarction. *Am Heart J* 1981;102:1188.

143. Sherman CT, Litvak F, Grundfest W, et al: Coronary angioscopy in patients with unstable angina pectoris. *N Engl J Med* 1986;315:913.

144. Rentrop KP: Thrombolytic therapy in patients with acute myocardial infarction. *Circulation* 1985;71:627.

145. The Multicenter Postinfarction Research Group. Risk stratification and survival after myocardial infarction. *N Engl J Med* 1983;309:331.

146. Mathey DG, Kuck K-H, Tilsner V, et al: Nonsurgical coronary artery recanalization in acute transmural myocardial infarction. *Circulation* 1981;63:489.

147. Ganz W, Buchbinder M, Marcus H, et al: Intracoronary thrombolysis in evolving myocardial infarction. *Am Heart J* 1981;101:4.

148. Markis JE, Malagold M, Parker JA, et al: Myocardial salvage after intracoronary thrombolysis with streptokinase in acute myocardial infarction: Assessment by intracoronary thallium-201. *N Engl J Med* 1981;305:777.

149. Simoons ML, Serruys PW, v/d Brand M, et al: Improved survival after early thrombolysis in acute myocardial infarction: A randomized trial by the Interuniversity Cardiology Institute in The Netherlands. *Lancet* 1985;2:578.

150. The ISAM-Study Group: Intravenous streptokinase in acute myocardial infarction: Preliminary results of a prospective controlled trial (ISAM). *Circulation* 1985;72 (Suppl 3):III-223.

151. Bergman SR, Fox KAA, Ter-Pogossian MM, et al: Clot selective coronary thrombolysis with tissue-type plasminogen activator. *Science* 1983;220:1181.

152. The TIMI Study Group: Thrombolysis in myocardial infarction (TIMI trial). Phase I findings. *N Engl J Med* 1985;312:932.

153. Meyer J, Merx W, Schmitz H, et al: Percutaneous transluminal coronary angioplasty immediately after intracoronary streptolysis of transmural myocardial infarction. *Circulation* 1982;66:905.

154. Lee G, Amsterdam EA, Low R, et al: Efficacy of percutaneous transluminal coronary recanalization utilizing streptokinase thrombolysis in patients with acute myocardial infarction. *Am Heart J* 1981;102:1159.

155. Rutsch W, Schartl M, Mathey D, et al: Percutaneous transluminal coronary recanalization: procedures, results, and acute complications. In *Transluminal Coronary Angioplasty and Intracoronary Thrombolysis: Coronary Heart Disease IV*. Edited by M Kaltenbach, A Gruntzig, K Rentrop, et al (eds): Berlin: Springer-Verlag, 1982, p. 233.

156. Schroder R, Vohringer H, Linderer T, et al: Follow-up after coronary arterial reperfusion with intravenous streptokinase in relation to residual myocardial infarct artery narrowings. *Am J Cardiol* 1985;55:313.

157. Harrison DG, Ferguson DW, Collins SM, et al: Rethrombosis after reperfusion with streptokinase: Importance of geometry of residual lesions. *Circulation* 1984;69:991.

158. Pitt B, Topol EJ, O'Neill WW: Role of percutaneous transluminal coronary angioplasty in acute myocardial infarction. *Am J Cardiol* 1987;60:155.

159. Topol EJ, Califf RM, George BS, et al: A randomized trial of immediate versus delayed elective angioplasty after intravenous tissue plasminogen activator in acute myocardial infarction. *N Engl J Med* 1987;317:581.

160. ISIS-2 (Second International Study of Infarct Survival) Collaborative Group. Randomized trial of intravenous streptokinase, oral aspirin, both, or neither among 17,187 cases of suspected acute myocardial infarction: ISIS-2. *Lancet* 1988;1:349.

161. Yusef S, Collins R, Peto R, et al: Intravenous and intracoronary fibrinolytic therapy in acute myocardial infarction: Overview of results on mortality, reinfarction and side-effects from 33 randomized controlled trials. *Eur Heart J* 1985;6:556.

162. Laffel GL, Braunwald E: Thrombolytic therapy: A new strategy for the treatment of acute myocardial infarction. *N Engl J Med* 1984;311:710.

163. ISAM Study Group: A prospective trial of intravenous streptokinase in acute myocardial infarction (ISAM): Mortality, morbidity and infarct size at 21 days. *N Engl J Med* 1986;314:1465.

164. Verstraete M, Bernard R, Bory M, et al: Randomized trial of intravenous recombinant tissue-type plasminogen activator versus intravenous streptokinase in acute myocardial infarction. Report from the European Cooperative Study Group for Recombinant Tissue-Type Plasminogen Activator. *Lancet* 1985;1:842.

165. Mathey DG, Sheehan FH, Schofer J, Dodge HT: Time from onset of symptoms to thrombolytic therapy: A major determinant of myocardial salvage in patients with acute transmural infarction. *J Am Coll Cardiol* 1985;6:518.

166. Schwarz F, Schuler G, Katus H, et al: Intracoronary thrombolysis in acute myocardial infarction: duration of ischemia as a major determinant of late results after recanalization. *Am J Cardiol* 1982;50:933.

167. Vermeer F, Simoons ML, Bar FW, et al: Which patients benefit most from early thrombolytic therapy with intracoronary streptokinase? *Circulation* 1986;74:1379.

168. O'Neill W, Timmis GC, Bourdillon PD, et al: A prospective randomized clinical trial of intracoronary streptokinase versus coronary angioplasty for acute myocardial infarction. *N Engl J Med* 1986;314:812.

169. Fung AY, Lai P, Topol EJ, et al: Value of percutaneous transluminal coronary angioplasty after unsuccessful intravenous streptokinase therapy in acute myocardial infarction. *Am J Cardiol* 1986;58:868.

170. Kereiakes DJ, Selmon MR, McAuley BJ, et al: Angioplasty in total coronary artery occlusion: Experience in 76 consecutive patients. *J Am Coll Cardiol* 1985;6:526.

171. The TIMI Study Group: Comparison of invasive and conservative strategies after treatment with intravenous tissue plasminogen activator in acute myocardial infarction: Results of the thrombolysis in myocardial infarction—(TIMI) phase II trial. *N Engl J Med* 1989;320:618.

172. ISIS Pilot Study Investigators: Randomized factorial trial of high-dose intravenous streptokinase, of oral aspirin and of intravenous heparin in acute myocardial infarction. *Eur Heart J* 1987;8:634.

173. Passamani E, Hodges M, Herman M, et al: The thrombolysis in myocardial infarction (TIMI) phase II pilot study: Tissue plasminogen activator followed by percutaneous transluminal coronary angioplasty. *J Am Coll Cardiol* 1987;10:51B.

174. European Cooperative Study Group for Recombinant Tissue-type Plasminogen Activator: Randomized trial of intravenous recombinant tissue-type plasminogen activator versus intravenous streptokinase in acute myocardial infarction. *Lancet* 1985;1:842.

175. Chesebro JH, Knatterud G, Roberts R: Thrombolysis in myocardial infarction (TIMI) trial, phase I: A comparison between intravenous tissue plasminogen activator and intravenous streptokinase. *Circulation* 1987;76:142.

176. Mueller HS, Rao AK, Forman SA, and the TIMI investigators: Thrombolysis in myocardial infarction (TIMI): Comparative studies of coronary reperfusion and systemic fibrinogenolysis with two forms of recombinant tissue-type plasminogen activator. *J Am Coll Cardiol* 1987;10:479.

177. Van de Werf F, Arnold AER. Intravenous tissue plasminogen activator and size of infarct, left ventricular function and survival in acute myocardial infarction. *Br Med J* 1988;297:1374.

178. White HD, Rivers JT, Maslowski AH, et al: Effect of intravenous streptokinase as compared with that of tissue plasminogen activator on left ventricular function after first myocardial infarction. *N Engl J Med* 1989;320:817.

179. Hogg KJ, Gemmill JD, Lifson K, et al: Comparative effects of anistreplase and streptokinase on coronary artery patency in acute myocardial infarction (abstr). *Circulation* 1989;80 (Suppl II):II-419.

180. Pacouret G, Charbonnier B, Trousseau CHU: Multicenter European randomized trial of anistreplase versus streptokinase in acute myocardial infarction (abstr). *Circulation* 1989;80 (Suppl II):II-420.

181. Anderson JL, Hackworthy RA, Sorensen SG, et al: Comparison of intravenous antistreplase (APSAC) and streptokinase in acute myocardial infarction: Interim report of a randomized, double-blind patency study (abstr). *Circulation* 1989;80 (Suppl II):II-420.

182. AIMS Trial Study Group: Effect of intravenous APSAC on mortality after acute myocardial infarction: Preliminary report of a placebo-controlled clinical trial. *Lancet* 1988;1:545.

183. White HD, Norris RM, Brown MA, et al: Effect of intravenous streptokinase on left ventricular function and early survival after acute myocardial infarction. *N Engl J Med* 1987;317:850.

184. The International Study Group. In-hospital mortality and clinical course of 20,891 patients with suspected myocardial infarction randomized between alteplase and streptokinase with and without heparin. *Lancet* 1990;336:71.

185. Hsia J, Hamilton WP, Kleiman N, Roberts R, Chaitman BC, Ross AM: A comparison between heparin and low dose aspirin as adjunctive therapy with tissue plasminogen activator for acute myocardial infarction. *N Engl J Med* 1990;323:1433.

186. Guerci AD, Gerstenblith G, Brinker JA, et al: A randomized trial of intravenous tissue plasminogen activator for acute myocardial infarction with subsequent randomization to elective angiography. *N Engl J Med* 1987;317:1613.

187. Yao S, McNatt J, Anderson HV, Eidt J, Cui K, Maraganore JM, Buja LM, Willerson JT: Thrombin inhibitors enhance recombinant tissue-type plasminogen activator-induced thrombolysis and delay reocclusion. *Am J Phys*, in press, 1992.

188. Harrison DG, Ferguson DW, Collins SM, Skorton DJ, Ericksen EE, Kioschos JM, Marcus ML, White CW: Rethrombosis after reperfusion with streptokinase: importance of geometry of residual lesions. *Circulation* 1984;69:991.

189. Held PH, Teo K, Yusuf S: Effects of tissue-type plasminogen activator and anisoylated plasminogen streptokinase complex on mortality in acute myocardial infarction. *Circulation* 1990;82:1668.

190. AIMS Trial Study Group: Long-term effects of intravenous antistreplase in acute myocardial infarction; Final Report of the AIMS Study. *Lancet* 1990;335:427.

191. *International Study of Infarct Survival, Phase 3 (ISIS-3)* Presented at the American College of Cardiology. Atlanta, GA, March 5, 1991.

192. Gibson RS, Boden WE, Theroux P, et al, and the diltiazem reinfarction study group: Diltiazem and reinfarction in patients with non-Q-wave myocardial infarction. Results of a double-blind, randomized, multicenter trial. *N Engl J Med* 1986;315:423.

193. Gunnar RM, Lambrew CT, Abrams W, et al: Task Force IV: Pharmacologic interventions. *Am J Cardiol* 1982;50:393.

194. Bussmann WD, Passek D, Seidel W, Kaltenbach M: Reduction of CK and CK-MB indexes of infarct size by intravenous nitroglycerin. *Circulation* 1981;63:615.

195. Jugdutt BI, Warnica JW: Intravenous nitroglycerin therapy to limit myocardial infarct size, expansion and complications. Effect of timing, dosage and infarct location. *Circulation* 1988;78:906.

196. Stockman MB, Verrier RL, Lown B: Effect of nitroglycerin on vulnerability to ventricular fibrillation during myocardial ischemia and reperfusion. *Am J Cardiol* 1979;43:233.

197. Flaherty JT, Reid PR, Kelly DT, et al: Intravenous nitroglycerin in acute myocardial infarction. *Circulation* 1975;51:132.

198. Borer JS, Redwood DR, Levit B, et al: Reduction in myocardial ischemia with nitroglycerin or nitroglycerin plus phenylephrine administered during acute myocardial infarction. *N Engl J Med* 1975;293:1008.

199. Cottrell JE, Turndorf H: Intravenous nitroglycerin. *Am Heart J* 1978;96:550.

200. Flaherty JT: Intravenous nitroglycerin. *Johns Hopkins Med J* 1982;151:36.

201. Visser CA, Kan G, Lie KI, Durrer D: Incidence and one-year follow-up of left ventricular thrombus following acute myocardial infarction. An echocardiographic study. *J Am Coll Cardiol* 1983;1:648.

202. Asinger RW, Mikell FE, Elspeyer J, Hodges M: Incidence of left ventricular thrombosis after acute tramsmural myocardial infarction. Serial evaluation of two-dimensional echocardiography. *N Engl J Med* 1981;305:297.

203. Meltzor RS, Visser CA, Fuster V: Intracardiac thrombi and systemic embolization. *Ann Intern Med* 1986;104:689.

204. The Norwegian multicenter study group: Timolol-induced reduction in mortality and reinfarction in patients surviving acute myocardial infarction. *N Engl J Med* 1981;304:801.

205. Frishman WH, Furberg CD, Friedewald WT: ß-adrenergic blockade for survivors of acute myocardial infarction. *N Engl J Med* 1984;310:830.

206. Pederson TR for the Norwegian multicenter study group: Six-year follow-up of the Norwegian multicenter study on timolol after acute myocardial infarction. *N Engl J Med* 1985;313:1055.

207. Hjalmarson A, Herlitz J, Malek I, et al: Effect on mortality of metoprolol in acute myocardial infarction. *Lancet* 1981;2:823.

208. Beta-Blocker Heart Attack Study Group: The beta-blocker heart attack trial. *JAMA* 1981;246:2073.

209. Page DL, Caulfield JB, Kastor JA, et al: Myocardial changes associated with cardiogenic shock. *N Engl J Med* 1971;285:133.

210. Lee L, Bates ER, Pitt B, et al: Percutaneous transluminal coronary angioplasty improves survival in acute myocardial infarction complicated by cardiogenic shock. *Circulation* 1988;78:1345.

211. Willerson JT, Curry GC, Watson JT, et al: Intraaortic balloon counterpulsation in patients in cardiogenic shock, medically refractory left ventricular failure, and/or recurrent ventricular tachycardia. *Am J Med* 1975;58:183.

212. Gutovitz AL, Sobel BE, Roberts R: Progressive nature of myocardial injury in selected patients with cardiogenic shock. *Am J Cardiol* 1978;41:469.

213. Resnekov L: Cardiogenic shock. *Chest* 1983;83:893.

214. Gunnar RM, Cruz A, Boswell J, et al: Tobin JR: Myocardial infarction in shock: Hemodynamic studies and results of therapy. *Circulation* 1966;33:753.

215. Johnson SA, Scanlon PJ, Loeb HS, et al: Treatment of cardiogenic shock in myocardial infarction by intraaortic balloon counterpulsation and surgery. *Am J Med* 1977;62:687.

216. Alonso DR, Scheidt S, Post M, Killip T: Pathophysiology of cardiogenic shock; quantification of myocardial necrosis, clinical, pathologic, and electrocardiographic correlation. *Circulation* 1973;48:588.

217. Gewirtz H, Gold HK, Fallon JT, et al: Role of right ventricular infarction in cardiogenic shock associated with inferior myocardial infarction. *Br Heart J* 1979;42Z:719.

218. Sharpe DN, Botvinick EH, Shames DM, et al: The noninvasive diagnosis of right ventricular infarction. *Circulation* 1978;57:483.

219. Dell'Italia LD, Starling MR, Crawford MH, et al: Right ventricular infarction: Identification by hemodynamic measurements before and after volume loading and correlation with noninvasive techniques. *J Am Coll Cardiol* 1984;4:931.

220. Isner JM, Roberts WC: Right ventricular infarction complicating left ventricular infarction secondary to coronary heart disease: Frequency, location, associated findings, and significance from analysis of 236 necropsy patients with acute or healed myocardial infarction. *Am J Cardiol* 1978;42:885.

221. Cohn JN, Guiha NH, Broder MI, et al: Right ventricular infarction. Clinical and hymodynamic features. *Am J Cardiol* 1974;33:209.

222. Lorell B, Leinbach RC, Pohost GM, et al: Right ventricular infarction: clinical diagnosis and differentiation from cardiac tamponade and pericardial constriction. *Am J Cardiol* 1979;43:465.

223. Coma-Canella L, Lopez-Sendon J, Gamallo C: Low output syndrome in right ventricular infarction. *Am Heart J* 1979;98:613.

224. Croft CH, Nicod P, Corbett JR, et al: Detection of acute right ventricular infarction by right precordial electrocardiography. *Am J Cardiol* 1982;50:421.

225. Lorell B, Leinbach RC, Pohost GM, et al: Right ventricular infarction: Clinical diagnosis and differentiation from cardiac tamponade and pericardial constriction. *Am J Cardiol* 1979;43:465.

226. Roberts N, Harrison DG, Reimer KA, et al: Right ventricular infarction with shock but without significant left ventricular infarction: A new clinical syndrome. *Am Heart J* 1985;110:1047.

227. Radford MJ, Johnson RA, Daggett WM, et al: Ventricular septal rupture: A review of clinical and physiologic features and an analysis of survival. *Circulation* 1981;64:454.

228. Matsui K, Kay JH, Mendez M, et al: Ventricular septal rupture secondary to myocardial infarction. Clinical approach and surgical results. *JAMA* 1981;245:1537.

229. Edwards BS, Edwards WD, Edwards JE: Ventricular septal rupture complicating acute myocardial infarction: Identification of simple and complex types in 53 autopsied hearts. *Am J Cardiol* 1984;54:1201.

230. Moore CA, Nygaard TW, Kaiser DL, et al: Post infarction ventricular septal rupture: The importance of location of infarction and right ventricular function in determining survival. *Circulation* 1986;74:45.

231. Nishimura RA, Schaft HV, Gersh BJ, et al: Early repair of mechanical complications after acute myocardial infarction. *JAMA* 1986;356:47.

232. Montoya A, McKeever L, Scanlon P, Sullivan HJ, Gunnar RM, Pifarre R: Early repair of ventricular septal rupture after infarction. *Am J Cardiol* 1980;45:345.

233. Vlodaver Z, Edwards JE: Rupture of ventricular septum or papillary muscle complicating myocardial infarction. *Circulation* 1977;55:815.

234. Roberts WC, Cohen LD: Left ventricular papillary muscles. Description of the normal and a survey of conditions causing them to be abnormal. *Circulation* 1972;46:138.

235. Wei JY, Hutchins GM, Bulkley BH: Papillary muscle rupture in fatal acute myocardial infarction. *Ann Intern Med* 1979;90:149.

236. Sanders CA, Armstrong PW, Willerson JT, et al: Etiology and differential diagnosis of acute mitral regurgitation. *Prog Cardiovasc Dis* 1971;14:129.

237. Nichimura RA, Schaft HV, Shub C, et al: Papillary muscle rupture complicating acute myocardial infarction: Analysis of 17 patients. *Am J Cardiol* 1983;51:373.

238. Barbour DJ, Roberts WC: Rupture of a left ventricular papillary muscle during acute myocardial infarction: Analysis of 22 necropsy patients. *J Am Coll Cardiol* 1986;8:558.

239. Cheng TO: Some new observations on the syndrome of papillary muscle dysfunction. *Am J Med* 1969;47:924.

240. Tepe NA, Edmunds LH: Operation for acute postinfarction mitral insufficiency and cardiogenic shock. *J Thorac Cardiovasc Surg* 1985;89:525.

241. Connolly MW, Gelbfish JS, Jacobowitz IJ, et al: Surgical results for mitral regurgitation from coronary artery disease. *J Thorac Cardiovasc Surg* 1986;91:379.

242. Vlodaver Z, Coe JJ, Edwards JE: True and false aneurysms: Propensity for the latter to rupture. *Circulation* 1975;51:567.

243. Martin RH, Almond CH, Saab S, Watson LE: True and false aneurysms of the left ventricle following myocardial infarction. *Am J Med* 1977;62:418.

244. Catherwood E, Mintz GS, Kotler MN, et al: Two-dimensional echocardiographic recognition of left ventricular pseudoaneurysm. *Circulation* 1980;62:294.

245. Roelandt J, vandenBrand M, Vletter WB, Nauta J, Hugenholtz PG: Echocardiographic diagnosis of pseudoaneurysm of the left ventricle. *Circulation* 1975;52:466.

246. Gueron M, Wanderman KL, Hirsch M, Borman J: Pseudoaneurysm of the left ventricle after myocardial infarction: A curable form of myocardial rupture. *J Thorac Caradiovasc Surg* 1975;69:736.

247. Roberts WC, Morrow AG: Pseudoaneurysm of the left ventricle: An unusual sequel of myocardial infarction and rupture of the heart. *Am J Med* 1967;43:639.

248. Stratton JR, Resnick AD: Increased embolic risk in patients with left ventricular thrombi. *Circulation* 1987;75:1004.

249. Weinrich DJ, Burke JF, Pauletto FJ: Left ventricular mural thrombi complicating acute myocardial infarction: long-term follow-up with serial echocardiography. *Ann Intern Med* 1984;100:789.

250. Asinger RW, Mikell FL, Elsperger J, et al: Incidence of left ventricular thrombosis after acute transmural myocardial infarction: Serial evaluation by two-dimensional echocardiography. *N Engl J Med* 1981;305:297.

251. Josephson ME, Harken AH, Horowitz LN: Endocardial excision: A new surgical technique for the treatment of recurrent ventricular tachycardia. *Circulation* 1979;60:1430.

252. Miller JM, Marchlinski FE, Harken AH, et al: Subendocardial resection for sustained ventricular tachycardia in the early period after acute myocardial infarction. *Am J Cardiol* 1985;55:980.

253. Mirowski M, Reid PR, Winkle RA, et al: Mortality in patients with implanted automatic defibrillators. *Ann Intern Med* 1983;98:585.

254. Van Tassel RA, Edwards JE: Rupture of the heart complicating myocardial infarction; analysis of 40 cases including nine examples of left ventricular false aneurysms. *Chest* 1972;61:104.

255. Lewis AJ, Burchell HB, Titus JL: Clinical and pathologic features of postinfarction cardiac rupture. *Am J Cardiol* 1969;23:43.

256. Feneley MP, Chang VP, O'Rourke MF: Myocardial rupture after acute myocardial infarction. Ten year review. *Br Heart J* 1983;49:550.

257. Berman J, Haffajee CL, Alpert JS: Therapy of symptomatic pericarditis after myocardial infarction. Retrospective and prospective studies of aspirin, indomethacin, prednisone, and spontaneous resolution. *Am Heart J* 1981;101:750.

258. Fowler NO, Harbin AD III: Recurrent acute pericarditis: Follow-up study of 31 patients. *J Am Coll Cardiol* 1986;7:300.

259. Hannerman H, Kloner RA, Schoen FJ, et al: Indomethacin-induced scar thinning following experimental myocardial infarction. *Circulation* 1983;67:1290.

260. Roberts R, deMello V, Sobel BE: Deleterious effects of methylprednisolone in patients with myocardial infarction. *Circulation* 1976;53 (Suppl I):204.

261. Rothkopf M, Boerner J, Stone MJ, et al: Detection of myocardial infarct extension by CK-B radioimmunoassay. *Circulation* 1979;59:268.

262. Hutchins GM, Bulkley BH: Infarct expansion versus extension: Two different complications of acute myocardial infarction. *Am J Cardiol* 1978;41:227.

263. Muller JE, Rude RE, Braunwald E, et al: Myocardial infarct extension: incidence, outcome, and risk factors in the MILIS study. *Ann Intern Med* 1988;108:1.

264. Marmor A, Sobel BE, Roberts R: Factors presaging early recurrent myocardial infarction ("extension"). *Am J Cardiol* 1981;48:603.

265. Hammerman H, Schoen FJ, Braunwald E, et al: Drug-induced expansion of infarct: Morphologic and functional correlations. *Circulation* 1984;69:611.

266. Eaton LW, Weiss JL, Bulkley BH, et al: Regional cardiac dilatation after acute myocardial infarction. Recognition by two-dimensional echocardiography. *N Engl J Med* 1979;300:57.

267. McKay RG, Pfeffer MA, Pasternak RC, et al: Left ventricular remodeling after myocardial infarction. A corollary to infarct expansion. *Circulation* 1986;74:693.

268. Pfeffer M, Lamas GA, Vaughan DE, et al: Effect of captoporil on progressive ventricular dilatation. *N Engl J Med* 1988;319:80.

269. Nicod P, Corbett J, Leachman R, et al: Myocardial rupture after myocardial infarction: Detection by multigated image acquisition scintigraphy. *Am J Med* 1982;73:765.

270. DeBusk RF, Blomqvist CG, Kouchoukos NT, et al: Identification and treatment of low-risk patients after acute myocardial infarction and coronary artery bypass graft surgery. *N Engl J Med* 1986;314:161.

271. Rapaport E, Remedios P: The high-risk patient after recovery from myocardial infarction: Recognition and management. *J Am Coll Cardiol* 1983;1:391.

272. Norris RM, Brandt PWT, Caughey DE, et al: A new coronary prognostic index. *Lancet* 1969;1:274.

273. Tofler GH, Stone PH, Muller JE, et al: Effects of gender and race on prognosis after acute myocardial infarction: Adverse prognosis for women, particularly black women. *J Am Coll Cardiol* 1987;9:473.

274. Moss AJ, Bigger JT, Odoroff CL: Postinfarction risk stratification. *Prog Cardiovasc Dis* 1987;29:389.

275. Norris RM, Barnaby PF, Brandt PWT, et al: Prognosis after recovery from first acute myocardial infarction: Determinants of reinfarction and sudden death. *Am J Cardiol* 1984;53:408.

276. Smith J, Marcus FI, Serkoman R, with the Multicenter Postinfarction Research Group: Prognosis of patients with diabetes mellitus after acute myocardial infarction. *Am J Cardiol* 1984;54:718.

277. Weiner DA, McCabe CH, Ryan TJ: Identification of patients with left main and three vessel coronary disease with clinical and exercise test variables. *Am J Cardiol* 1980;46:21.

278. Hung J, Goris M, Nash E, et al: Comparative value of maximal treadmill testing, exercise thallium myocardial perfusion scintigraphy and exercise radionuclide ventriculography for distinguishing high- and low-risk patients soon after acute myocardial infarction. *Am J Cardiol* 1984;53:1221.

279. Corbett JR, Nicod P, Lewis SE, Rude RE, Willerson JT: Prognostic value of submaximal exercise radionuclide ventriculography following acute transmural and nontransmural myocardial infarction. *Am J Cardiol* 1983;52:82A.

280. Mukharji J, Rude RE, Poole WK, et al. (Milis Study Group): Risk factors for sudden death after acute myocardial infarction: Two-year follow-up. *Am J Cardiol* 1984;54:31.

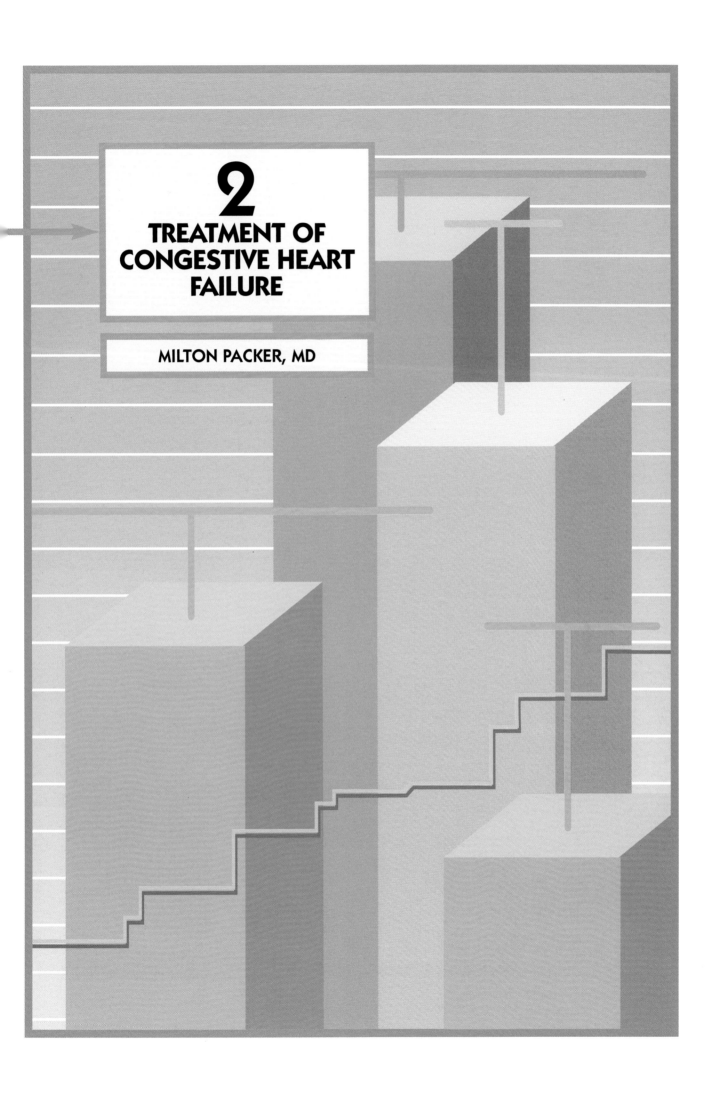

2

TREATMENT OF CONGESTIVE HEART FAILURE

MILTON PACKER, MD

Synopsis of Chapter Two

THE CLINICAL SYNDROME OF HEART FAILURE

During the last decade congestive heart failure has become one of the most important public health problems in cardiovascular medicine.[1] The disorder afflicts nearly four million people in the United States and over sixteen million people worldwide. Although the incidence of most cardiovascular disorders has decreased over the past 10 to 20 years, the incidence and prevalence of congestive heart failure has increased at a dramatic rate. Nearly 400,000 people in the United States develop congestive heart failure each year, and this number will rise further as patients who would normally die of an acute myocardial infarction survive, but with compromised ventricular function. The number of hospitalizations for congestive heart failure has increased more than threefold during the last 15 years. This disorder now represents the most common medical discharge diagnosis for patients over the age of 65. Over 200,000 patients die of heart failure annually.

DEFINITION OF HEART FAILURE

Congestive heart failure is a clinical syndrome characterized by a limitation of exercise tolerance due to dyspnea or fatigue, which is physiologically related to an identifiable abnormality of cardiac function. The limitation of exercise tolerance may be evident at rest or at varying levels of effort; the abnormality of cardiac function may be secondary to alterations in forward flow or in cardiac filling or both and may be associated with changes in systolic or diastolic performance. In most cases, these circulatory derangements become increasingly severe over time and are accompanied by:

- Worsening symptoms.
- Substantial disability despite aggressive therapy.
- The continuing need for hospitalization and emergency care.
- Death.

In addition to exercise intolerance and a high risk of premature death, patients with heart failure frequently, but not necessarily, manifest several associated physiologic abnormalities (Table 2.1):

- Sodium and water retention.
- Neurohormonal activation.
- Reduced peripheral blood flow and end-organ metabolic function.
- Impaired systolic or diastolic function of the heart.
- Reduced cardiac output or increased ventricular filling pressures at rest or during exercise.
- Atrial or ventricular arrhythmias.

Interestingly, there may be little relation between the severity of these associated physiologic abnormalities and degree of functional disability. For example, it is not unusual for patients with severe impairments of systolic function to have normal exercise capacity. Conversely, patients may be extremely disabled with a normal left ventricular ejection fraction[2] (Figure 2.1). Similarly, some severely ill patients have no evidence of fluid retention, whereas many patients with massive

● ● ● ● ● ● ● ● ● ● ● ● ● ● ●

TABLE 2.1 • PHYSIOLOGIC AND CLINICAL ABNORMALITIES IN HEART FAILURE

Exercise intolerance

Sodium and water retention

Neurohormonal activation

Reduced peripheral blood flow

Decreased end-organ metabolic function

Impaired systolic or diastolic function of the heart

Reduced cardiac output or increased pulmonary wedge pressure at rest or during exercise

Atrial and ventricular arrhythmias

Shortened survival

---

quantities of edema do not have congestive heart failure. The role played by these associated physiologic abnormalities in determining the functional capacity and mortality of patients with heart failure remains unknown.

CAUSES OF HEART FAILURE

The syndrome of heart failure may be produced by a variety of disease states (Table 2.2). These include:
- Ischemic heart disease (coronary artery disease).
- Dilated cardiomyopathy of unknown cause (idiopathic).
- Dilated cardiomyopathy of known cause (toxic, viral, parasitic, hypertensive, etc.).
- Valvular stenosis or regurgitation, with or without associated ventricular dysfunction.
- Hypertrophic or restrictive cardiomyopathy.
- Pericardial disease.
- Pulmonary hypertension.
- Congenital heart disease.
- High-output states.

These disorders produce either a loss of viable myocardium, mechanical stresses that increase loading conditions in the heart, impaired relaxation, or a combination of these mechanisms. It is important to elucidate the contribution of each of these factors to the development of the clinical syndrome, because each mechanism responds differently to therapeutic interventions.

ASSESSMENT OF SEVERITY

Since disability and mortality are the hallmarks of congestive heart failure, the severity of the disease is generally gauged by the degree of functional impairment and the risk of death.

The degree of functional disability can be estimated by either direct questioning or by formal exercise testing. These two approaches have resulted in two different classifications of disease severity. The first approach, initially developed by the New York Heart Association,[3] assigns a numerical value— Class I, II, III and IV—to the amount of effort required to provoke symptoms of dyspnea and fatigue (Table 2.3). The second approach, advocated by Weber et al.,[4] categorizes patients according to their maximum exercise capacity—Class A, B, C, D and E—which is evaluated by the direct measurement of oxygen consumption during a standardized bicycle or treadmill test (Table 2.4). The first approach permits physicians to determine how the symptoms of heart failure interfere with the lifestyle of the patient, but the assessment is highly subjective.

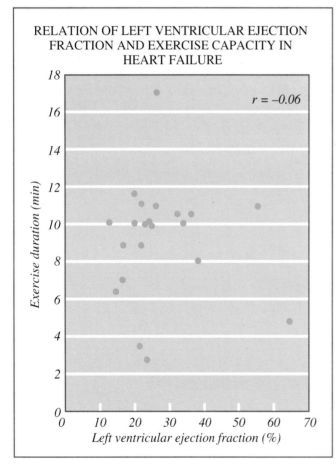

RELATION OF LEFT VENTRICULAR EJECTION FRACTION AND EXERCISE CAPACITY IN HEART FAILURE

$r = -0.06$

FIGURE 2.1 • Relation of left ventricular ejection fraction and exercise capacity in patients with heart failure. (Reproduced with permission. Franciosa JA, Park M, Levine TB: *Am J Cardiol* 1981;47:33.)

TABLE 2.2 • CAUSES OF HEART FAILURE
Coronary artery disease
Dilated cardiomyopathy of unknown cause
Dilated cardiomyopathy of known cause
• Hypertensive
• Toxic
• Viral
• Parasitic
Valvular stenosis or regurgitation
• With left ventricular dysfunction
• Without left ventricular dysfunction
Hypertrophic cardiomyopathy
Restrictive cardiomyopathy
Pericardial disease
Pulmonary hypertension
Congenital heart disease
High-output states

The second approach, although objective and reproducible, relies heavily on peak performance and thus fails to assess physical endurance—the capacity to perform prolonged activities at physiologically relevant submaximal workloads.

The severity of heart failure can also be assessed by estimating the risk of death. This goal is most commonly achieved in the clinical setting by quantifying the degree of patient's disability. When the cause of heart failure is left ventricular dysfunction, the annual mortality rate is 10% to 25% in patients with mild-to-moderate symptoms and 40% to 60% in patients with severe symptoms[5,6] (Figure 2.2). However, many other hemodynamic, functional, neurohormonal, and electrophysio-

TABLE 2.3 • NEW YORK HEART ASSOCIATION FUNCTIONAL CLASSIFICATION
Class I
No limitation of exercise tolerance
No symptoms during usual activities of daily living
Class II
Mild limitation of exercise tolerance
Symptoms are provoked by ordinary activity
Class III
Moderate limitation of exercise tolerance
Symptoms are provoked by less than ordinary activity
Class IV
Severe limitation of exercise tolerance
Symptoms are present at rest

TABLE 2.4 • WEBER CLASSIFICATION OF EXERCISE TOLERANCE
Class A
Maximum oxygen consumption > 20 mL/min/kg
Class B
Maximum oxygen consumption 16-20 mL/min/kg
Class C
Maximum oxygen consumption 10-15 mL/min/kig
Class D
Maximum oxygen consumption < 10 mL/min/kg

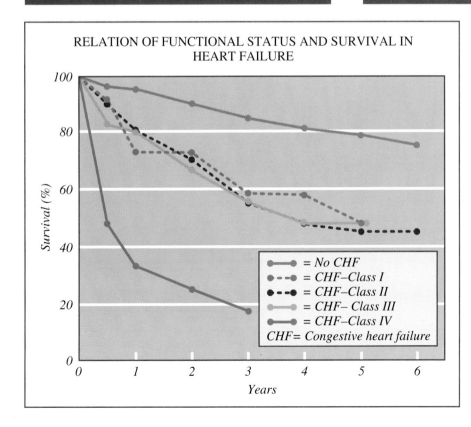

RELATION OF FUNCTIONAL STATUS AND SURVIVAL IN HEART FAILURE

- = No CHF
- = CHF–Class I
- = CHF–Class II
- = CHF– Class III
- = CHF–Class IV

CHF= Congestive heart failure

FIGURE 2.2 • Relation of functional status and survival in patients with congestive heart failure. (Reproduced with permission. Califf RM, Bounous P, Harrell FE, et al: The prognosis in the presence of coronary artery disease. In: Braunwald E, Mock MB, Watson JT, eds. *Congestive Heart Failure* New York, NY: Grune and Stratton; 1982:31.)

logic variables have been shown to have prognostic significance in patients with heart failure, and consequently, could be used to assess the severity of the disease. For example, patients with heart failure who have:

- Underlying coronary artery disease (Figure 2.3).
- Severe limitation of exercise tolerance (Figure 2.4).
- Markedly depressed right or left ventricular ejection fraction (Figure 2.5).

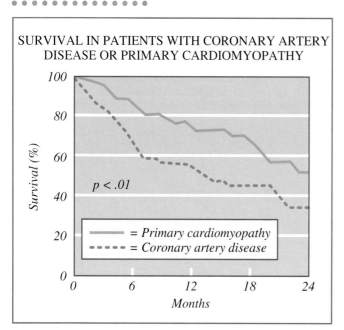

FIGURE 2.3 • Survival curves in patients with coronary artery disease or in primary cardiomyopathy. (Reproduced with permission. Franciosa, JA, Wilen M, Ziesche S, et al: *Am J Cardiol* 1983;51:831.)

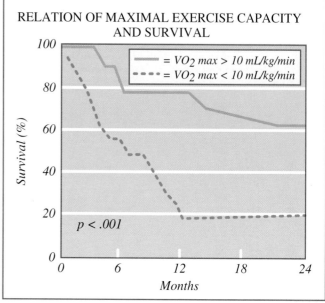

FIGURE 2.4 • Survival curves based on maximal exercise capacity, as measured by VO₂ max (maximal oxygen consumption). (Reproduced with permission. Szlachcic J, Massie BM, Kramer BL: *Am J Cardiol* 1985; 55:1037.)

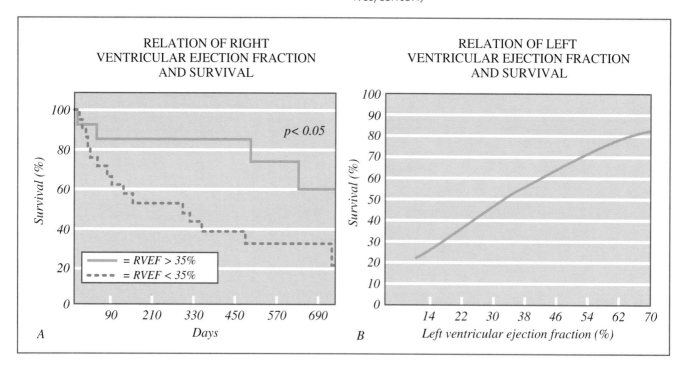

FIGURE 2.5 • Cumulative probability of survival for those patients with a right ventricular ejection fraction (RVEF) above or below 35% (A). (Reproduced with permission. Polack JF, Holman L, Wynne J, et al:*J Am Coll Cardiol* 1983;2:217.) Relation of left ventricular ejection fraction and survival in congestive heart failure (B). (Reproduced with permission. Califf RM, Bounous P, Harrel FE, et al: The prognosis in the presence of coronary artery disease. In: Braunwald E, Mock MB, Watson JT, eds. *Congestive Heart Failure* New York, NY: Grune and Stratton;1982:31.)

- Severely deranged central hemodynamic variables (Figure 2.6).
- Activation of the sympathetic nervous system and renin-angiotensin system (Figures 2.7, 2.8).

- Serious ventricular arrhythmias, especially nonsustained ventricular tachycardia, appear to have a particularly unfavorable long-term outcome[7] (Figure 2.9).

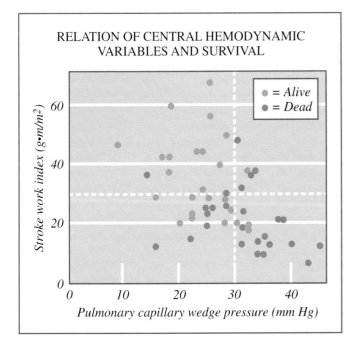

FIGURE 2.6 • Relation of central hemodynamic variables and survival in congestive heart failure. (Adapted with permission. Massie BM, T Ports, K Chatterjee, et al: *Circulation* 1981;63:2269 and the American Heart Association.)

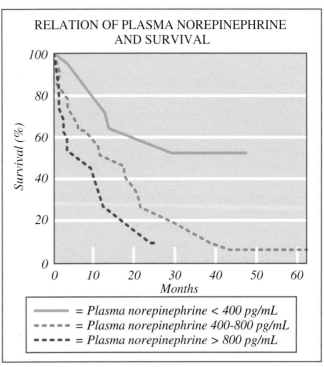

FIGURE 2.7 • Relation of plasma norepinephrine (PNE) and survival in congestive heart failure. (Reproduced with permission. Cohn JN, Levine TB, Olivari MT, et al: *N Engl J Med* 1984;31:819.)

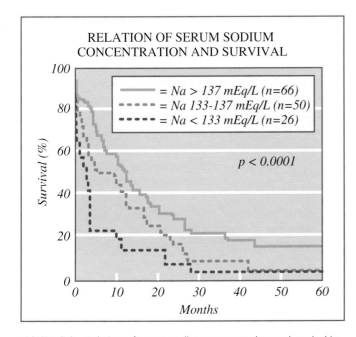

FIGURE 2.8 • Relation of serum sodium concentration and survival in congestive heart failure. (Adapted with permission. Lee WH, Packer M: *Circulation* 1986;73:257 and the American Heart Association.)

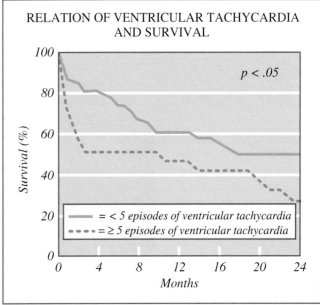

FIGURE 2.9 • Cumulative survival rates for patients with and without five or more episodes of ventricular tachycardia. (Reproduced with permission. Wilson JR, Schwartz JS, St. John Sutton M, et al: *J Am Coll Cardiol* 1983;2:403.)

Yet, the predictive value for each variable depends greatly on the patient cohort being evaluated. For example, although the left ventricular ejection fraction is a powerful prognostic indicator in patients with coronary artery disease,[8,9] its value in this setting derives primarily from the fact that comparisons are usually made between patients with normal and abnormal cardiac performance. In the setting of congestive heart failure, in which nearly all patients have an abnormal left ventricular ejection fraction, the measurement of ejection fraction may no longer be useful in predicting survival, especially in patients with refractory symptoms.[10,11] More important, changes in left ventricular ejection fraction, especially those produced by pharmacologic agents, have not been shown to predict changes in the risk of death. Similarly, in patients with mild-to-moderate heart failure in whom hyponatremia is uncommon, the measurement of serum sodium concentration is unlikely to provide useful information. However, in patients with severe heart failure in whom hyponatremia is a common occurrence, sodium serum concentration is a powerful predictor of long-term outcome.[11]

APPROACH TO THE PATIENT WITH HEART FAILURE

HISTORY AND PHYSICAL EXAMINATION

Since the syndrome of heart failure is defined as a reduction in exercise capacity that is related to an abnormality of heart function, it is essential to characterize the history of effort intolerance in the evaluation of each patient. Exercise tolerance in heart failure may be limited by dyspnea or fatigue. Elucidation of which symptom stops exertion is probably unimportant, since the precise sensation experienced by the patient may be a reflection of the type of exercise rather than the type of circulatory derangement.[12] Still, it is important to identify patients with heart failure who have exertional angina, since this symptom suggests that ventricular dysfunction may in part be related to myocardial ischemia.

History

A careful history not only confirms the symptoms of heart failure but allows the physician to assess its possible cause, both with respect to the nature of the underlying disease as well as the presence of any precipitating factors. The patient should be asked about a history of rheumatic fever, cardiac murmur, hypertension, diabetes and myocardial infarction. Present and past drug use and abuse should be evaluated, especially the use of alcohol, cocaine, cardiotoxic drugs such as adriamycin and cyclophosphamide, and cardiodepressant agents, for example disopyramide and verapamil.

Physicians should make every effort to identify factors that may have exacerbated symptoms (Table 2.5). Such events can be identified in up to 50% of heart failure episodes.[13] The most important precipitating causes include tachy- or brady-arrhythmias, myocardial ischemia, and changes in diet and therapy. Anemia, hyperthyroidism and hypothyroidism, worsening renal function and systemic infection may be important in selected patients.

Precipitating Causes of Heart Failure

Most of the cardiac arrhythmias that can worsen hemodynamic and clinical status of patients with heart failure are supraventricular in origin. These tachyarrhythmias reduce the time available for ventricular filling, an event that is particularly deleterious in patients with impaired ventricular relaxation.[14] Tachycardias may also increase myocardial oxygen consumption and decrease the time available for myocardial perfusion. These factors may act in concert to exacerbate myocardial ischemia.

The poor systolic function seen in many patients with heart failure may not only be the result of myocardial necrosis but may occur as a consequence of myocardial ischemia. Ischemia may manifest as episodes of typical angina, or it may occur without symptoms. An aggressive approach to the treatment of angina in patients with left ventricular dysfunction is warranted,[15,16] but the

TABLE 2.5 • PRECIPITATING CAUSES OF HEART FAILURE

Changes in diet
Tachy- and bradyarrhythmias
Myocardial ischemia
Failure to take prescribed drugs
Cardiodepressant drugs
Anemia
Hyper- and hypothyroidism
Metabolic deficiencies
Worsening renal function
Systemic infection

therapeutic implications of silent ischemia in patients with chronic heart failure remain unclear. In our experience, silent ischemia is a rare event in patients with chronic heart failure, even in patients with extensive coronary artery disease. Recurrent ischemic events, however, are likely to be an important cause of disease progression in patients with symptomatic ischemia, since coronary artery bypass surgery favorably modifies the long-term outcome of patients with multiple-vessel disease, left ventricular dysfunction and angina[15,16] (Figure 2.10).

Four types of commonly-used medications may exacerbate the symptoms of heart failure (Table 2.6). Anti-inflammatory drugs, such as corticosteroids and nonsteroidal agents, cause sodium retention, antagonize the compensatory actions of endogenous vasodilator systems and reduce the efficacy of diuretic drugs.[17,18]

Nearly all anti-arrhythmic drugs exert important cardiodepressant effects. Although the negative inotropic actions of disopyramide and flecainide are cited most commonly,[19,20]

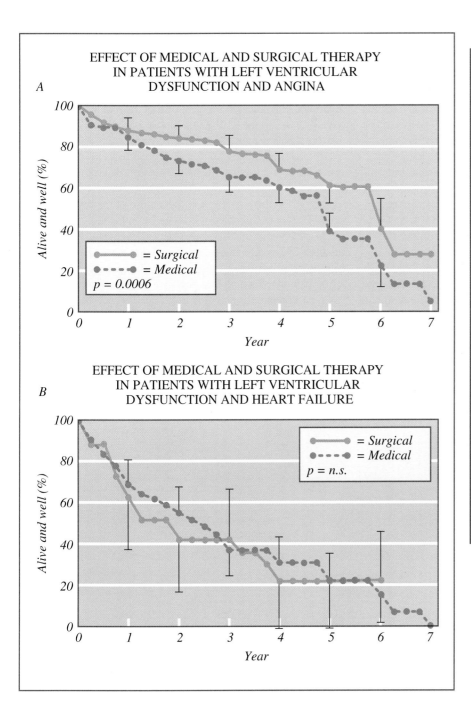

TABLE 2.6 • DRUGS THAT CAN WORSEN HEART FAILURE
Anti-inflammatory drugs
Corticosteroids
Nonsteroidal anti-inflammatory agents
Anti-arrhythmic agents
Disopyramide
Flecainide
Encainide
Mexiletine
Tocainide
Procainamide
Lidocaine
Calcium channel-blocking drugs
Verapamil
Diltiazem
Nifedipine
Nicardipine
ß-adrenergic blocking drugs

FIGURE 2.10 • Percentage of patients with left ventricular dysfunction with angina as the predominant symptom who are alive and free of moderate or severe limitation following medical or surgical therapy (A). Percentage of patients with left ventricular dysfunction with heart failure as the predominant symptom who are alive and free of moderate or severe limitation (B). (Reproduced with permission. Alderman EL, Fisher LD, Litwin P, et al: *Circulation* 1983;68:785 and the American Heart Association.)

cardiac performance may also deteriorate following the administration of encainide, mexilitene, tocainide, procainamide and lidocaine.[20–24]

Calcium-channel blocking drugs can depress cardiac contractility and thus can exacerbate the symptoms of heart failure and adversely affect long-term outcome.[25–27] Finally, β-blocking drugs can initially worsen the clinical condition of patients with heart failure, even though these drugs may exert favorable long-term effects in high-risk subsets when compared with calcium channel blocking drugs.[28]

Physical Examination

The physical examination should be directed towards both identifying the nature of the underlying heart disease—cardiac murmurs or chamber enlargement—and the severity of fluid retention. Aside from such information, however, the treating physician should not rely too heavily on the physical examination, because the presence or absence of specific physical findings cannot be used to predict specific hemodynamic abnormalities.[29] Since there is no reliable means of estimating left ventricular systolic or diastolic function by physical examination, patients with heart failure may not show any specific abnormality on examination of the heart. Similarly, since most patients with elevated pulmonary wedge pressures do not have pulmonary rales, it is nearly impossible to estimate the left ventricular filling pressure by examining the lungs.

Although signs of right heart failure—jugular venous distension and peripheral edema—provide the most reliable signs of fluid overload, fluid retention is not an invariable feature of heart failure, and thus, patients may have significant symptoms without any evidence of edema. Cheynes-Stokes respirations and cardiac cachexia are usually seen only in the late stages of the disease.[30,31]

LABORATORY EVALUATION

The chest roentgenogram is helpful in establishing the two cardinal radiographic features of the disease—cardiac dilatation and pulmonary congestion—but it is of limited value in clarifying the underlying cause or in defining the pathophysiology of the disease (Figures 2.11–2.13). Similarly, the electrocardiogram often demonstrates poor R wave progression, ST segment depression and T wave changes, whether or not coronary artery disease is the cause of heart failure.

The most useful laboratory test in evaluating patients with heart failure is the two-dimensional echocardiogram. This technique can detect and quantify the loss of functioning myocardium. Patients whose heart failure is the result of systolic dysfunction generally have a left ventricular ejection fraction of less than 35%. This noninvasive test, especially when combined with Doppler flow studies, can also be used to confirm the presence and estimate the severity of mechanical lesions that can cause heart failure—valvular stenosis and regurgitation, pericardial disease, pulmonary hypertension, and congenital heart defects (intracardiac shunts). If no mechanical lesion is discovered in a patient with preserved left ventricular systolic function, diastolic abnormalities of the heart should be suspected. If doubt persists about the nature of the cardiac abnormality, cardiac catheterization may be indicated.

Gas exchange measurements performed during the course of treadmill or bicycle exercise testing can provide an objective assessment of the presence and severity of exercise intolerance[4] (Figure 2.14). Such testing permits the evaluation of maximal oxygen consumption, exercise-induced hyperventilation and anaerobic threshold. The symptoms of heart failure are associated with:

- An excessive increase in blood lactate during low levels of exercise.

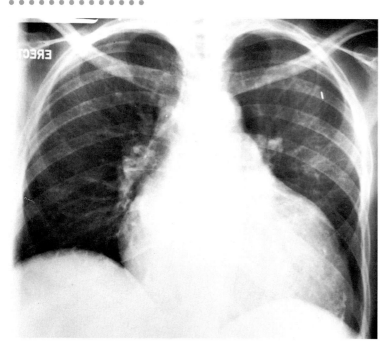

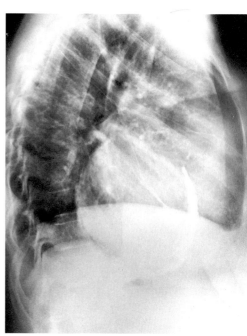

FIGURE 2.11 • Chest x-ray of patient with heart failure. (Reproduced with permission. Soto B, Kassner EG, Baxley WA: *Imaging of Cardiac Disorders. Volume 2* New York, NY: Gower Medical Publishing; 1992:126.)

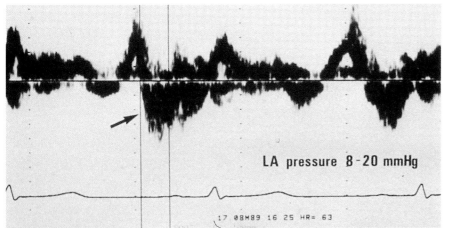

FIGURE 2.12 • Pulmonary venous flow profile from the left upper pulmonary vein in a patient with congestive heart failure and a left atrial pressure of 8-20 mm Hg. There is retrograde flow into the vein which starts early in diastole (arrow, first verticle line), before the onset of the P wave on the ECG (second verticle line). (Reproduced with permission. Tuccillo B, Fraser AG: Pulmonary venous flow. In: Sutherland GR, Roelandt JRTC, Fraser AG, et al: *Transesophageal Echocardiography in Clinical Practice* London, England: Gower Medical Publishing; 1991:5.14.)

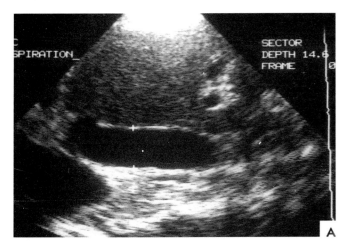

FIGURE 2.13 • Sagittal sonograms of the inferior vena cava at end inspiration (A) and end expiration (B) in a 52 year-old woman with right-sided congestive heart failure. The proximal inferior vena cava (arrow 1) is shown to be distended to 2.3 cm in caliber. As a rule of thumb, a caliber greater than 3.1 cm suggests venous engorgement secondary to right-sided congestive heart failure. Note the pleural effusion superiorly (arrow 2) (A). In expiration, no change in inferior vena cava (arrow 1) caliber is demonstrated. Right-sided congestive heart failure increases resistance to venous return to the heart, and the normal respiratory variation in the inferior vena cava caliber decreases in amplitude. (Reproduced with permission. Kassner EG: *Atlas of Radiologic Imaging* New York, NY: Gower Medical Publishing; 1989:5.38.)

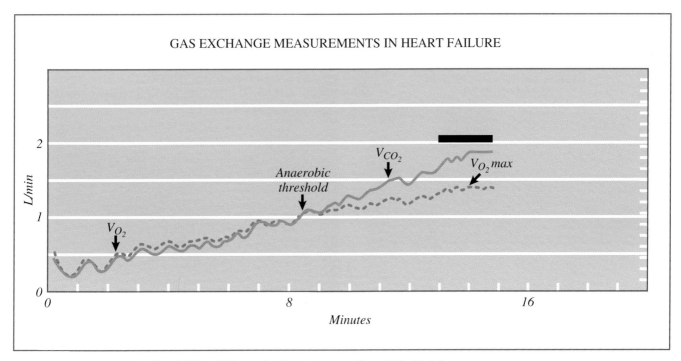

FIGURE 2.14 • The anaerobic threshold and VO_2 max in this patient were 12 and 17 mL/min/kg, respectively, and compatible with mild to moderately severe circulatory failure (Class B).

- A reduction in the quantity of oxygen consumed at peak effort.
- A disproportionate increase in the ventilatory equivalent for carbon dioxide.

Serial changes in these parameters may be used to evaluate the response to specific therapeutic interventions.

PATHOPHYSIOLOGIC ABNORMALITIES OF HEART FAILURE

Heart failure is characterized by complex changes in a variety of physiological systems. Some of these changes represent primary events that contribute directly to disease progression, while others reflect compensatory changes that permit the failing circulation to adapt to prolonged stress. An understanding of these abnormalities permits the formulation of rational therapeutic approaches to the management of patients with the disease (Table 2.7).

IMPAIRED CONTRACTILITY

Cardiac contractility is depressed in patients with heart failure, but the precise biochemical mechanisms that account for this mechanical deficiency—defective excitation-contraction coupling—have not been elucidated. In theory, a defect in contractility could be explained by (Table 2.8):

- A derangement in the sarcolemmal systems that bind calcium to the sarcoplasmic reticulum since a reduction in the calcium binding reduces the amount of calcium available to the myocardial cell at the time of the next contraction.

- A defect in the sarcolemmal systems that mediate the influx of calcium from the sarcoplasmic reticulum into the cardiac cell.
- A reduction in the activity of the myofibrillar, actomyosin and myosin ATPases that regulate contraction.
- A decrease in the responsiveness of the myofilaments to calcium.
- A reduced content of myofibrillar proteins.

Many of these abnormalities have emerged as potential targets for new pharmacologic agents.

Abnormalities in Intracellular Calcium Kinetics

The rate of calcium binding by the sarcoplasmic reticulum and thus, the amount of calcium bound to the sarcolemma is reduced in heart failure (Figure 2.15). The sarcoplasmic reticulum derived from the explanted hearts of patients with severe heart failure demonstrates slower rates of calcium accumulation and release than the reticulum derived from normal muscle.[32–34] In experimental models of heart failure, these abnormalities in calcium uptake precede the development of the clinical syndrome.[35] This finding suggests that defects in calcium uptake contribute directly to the disturbed excitation-contraction coupling of the failing heart.

Theoretically, changes in the intracellular level of cyclic adenosine monophosphate (AMP) could explain the abnormal intracellular calcium kinetics seen in heart failure.[36] By activating a variety of protein kinases, cyclic AMP increases the release of calcium from the sarcoplasmic reticulum, enhances the rate of dissociation of calcium from its binding sites on troponin C, and augments the rate of calcium uptake by the sarcoplasmic reticulum. Interestingly, the ability of physiologic stimuli (for example, catecholamines) to increase intracellular

● ● ● ● ● ● ● ● ● ● ● ● ● ● ● ● ●

TABLE 2.7 • MAJOR PATHOPHYSIOLOGIC ABNORMALITIES IN CHRONIC HEART FAILURE

Impaired myocardial contractility

Sodium retention

Enhanced impedance to left ventricular ejection

Neurohormonal activation

Electrophysiologic abnormalities

TABLE 2.8 • POTENTIAL BIOCHEMICAL MECHANISMS THAT COULD EXPLAIN IMPAIRED CONTRACTILITY IN HEART FAILURE

Reduced rate of calcium binding by sarcoplasmic reticulum

Decreased intracellular levels of cyclic adenosine monophosphate (cyclic AMP)
- Reduced ß-receptor density
- Impaired ß-receptor coupling

Decreased Na^+/Ca^{++} exchange

Reduced content of myofibrillar protein

Decreased activity of myofibrillar, actomyosin and myosin adenosine triphosphatase (ATPase)

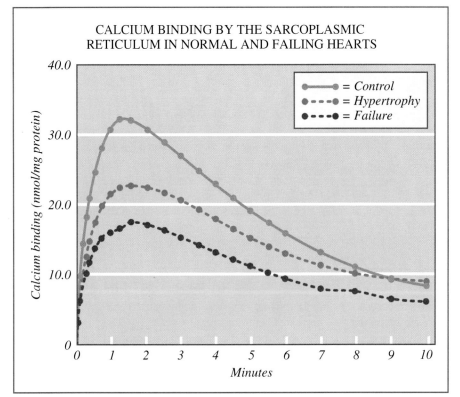

CALCIUM BINDING BY THE SARCOPLASMIC
RETICULUM IN NORMAL AND FAILING HEARTS

- = Control
- = Hypertrophy
- = Failure

FIGURE 2.15 • Calcium binding by fragments of the sarcoplasmic reticulum isolated from control, hypertrophied, and failing rabbit hearts. The reaction medium consisted of 0.1 M KCl, 10 mM $MgCl_2$, 20 mM Tris-maleate, 0.2 mM Murexide, 30 mM $CaCl_2$, and 0.2 mM ATP. The pH was 6.8 and the temperature was 30°C. (Reproduced with permission. Schwartz A, Sordahl LA, Entman ML, et al: Abnormal biochemistry in myocardial failure. In: Mason DT, ed. *Congestive Heart Failure* New York, NY: Yorke Medical Books; 1976:39.)

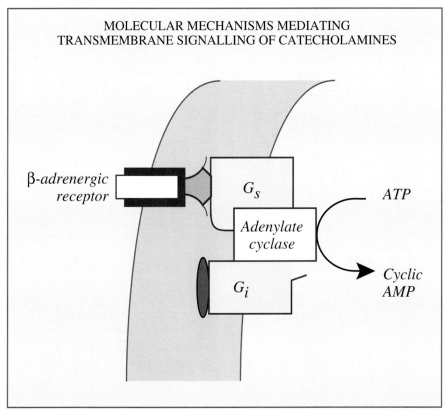

MOLECULAR MECHANISMS MEDIATING
TRANSMEMBRANE SIGNALLING OF CATECHOLAMINES

FIGURE 2.16 • Molecular mechanisms mediating transmembrane signalling of catecholamines. Interaction of ß-adrenergic receptor with adenylate cyclase is regulated by two guanine nucleotide binding proteins, G_s and G_i, which stimulate and inhibit, respectively, the interaction of the receptor and its effector enzyme.

levels of cyclic AMP is attenuated in chronic heart failure (Figures 2.16, 2.17), in part due to a decrease in the density of β-adrenergic receptors—primarily β_1 in idiopathic cardiomyopathy and both β_1 and β_2 in mitral valve disease[37,38]—and in part related to an uncoupling of these receptors from their effector enzyme, adenylate cyclase.[39] This uncoupling may be caused either by a decrease in the stimulatory or an increase in the inhibitory guanine nucleotide binding proteins that regulate the receptor-cyclase interaction.[39–42] The activity of adenylate cyclase itself appears to be normal in heart failure.

Other sarcolemmal systems—Na+/K+-ATPase activity and the Na+/Ca++ exchange mechanism—may also be defective in heart failure and may contribute to a reduction in the delivery of calcium to the myofilaments during systole.[43,44]

Alterations in Myofibrillar Content and Enzyme Activity

Force development and shortening by cardiac muscle occur as a result of the interaction between actin and myosin within the myofibrillar lattice. This interaction is not only dependent on the intracellular concentration of ionized calcium, but it is also controlled by the troponin-tropomyosin regulatory proteins that are situated along the actin filament. The amount of myofibrillar protein in the hearts of patients with heart failure is lower than that of normal hearts, the magnitude of the reduction being proportional to the severity of the disease.[45] Furthermore, the activities of myofibrillar, actomyosin and myosin ATPase are reduced in experimental heart failure,[46] and possibly, in human heart failure as well.[45,47] Previous work in experimental models of pressure overload has suggested that the reduction in ATPase activity may in part be related to a shift in the synthesis of cardiac myosin isozymes from the normal adult V_1 to the fetal V_3 isoform, which has reduced ATPase activity.[48] Such a shift, however, appears to occur only in the atria, but not in the ventricles, of patients with heart failure.[49]

The development of end-stage heart failure in man is not associated with changes in the sensitivity of the myofilaments to calcium under basal conditions, but heart failure may alter the myofibrillar responsiveness to calcium in the presence of pharmacologic agents.[50]

SODIUM RETENTION

Sodium retention in heart failure is the direct result of changes in intrarenal hemodynamic forces and tubular function that are triggered by the decline in cardiac performance[51,52] (Table 2.9). When cardiac output falls, enhanced neurohormonal activity leads to renal vasoconstriction, which occurs primarily at the level of the efferent arteriole. The resulting increase in filtration fraction increases the protein concentration in the peritubular

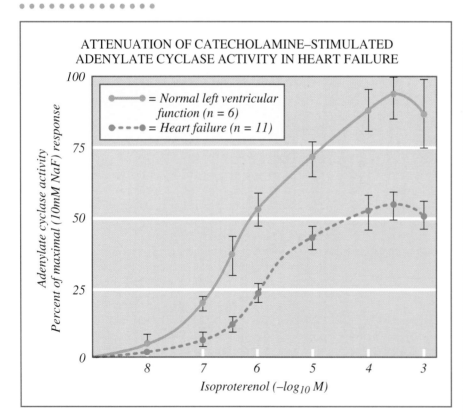

FIGURE 2.17 • L-Isoproterenol-stimulated adenylate cyclase activity in left ventricles in patients with normal left ventricular function and in patients suffering from heart failure. Activity is expressed as a percentage of the response to stimulation with 10 mM sodium fluoride (NaF). (Reproduced with permission. Bristow MR, Ginsburg R, Minobe W, et al: *N Engl J Med* 1982;307:208.)

TABLE 2.9 • FACTORS LEADING TO SODIUM RETENTION IN PATIENTS WITH HEART FAILURE
Intrarenal hemodynamic alterations resulting in enhanced proximal tubular sodium reabsorption
Redistribution of renal blood flow from cortical to juxtamedullary nephrons
Increased activity of renal sympathetic nerves
Enhanced formation of intrarenal angiotensin II, which directly increases tubular sodium reabsorption and exerts important intrarenal hemodynamic effects
Increased secretion of aldosterone by adrenal gland
Attenuated response to atrial natriuretic peptide

capillaries—thereby increasing the peritubular oncotic pressure—but decreases the postcapillary hydrostatic pressure. The interaction of these intrarenal hemodynamic events enhances the peritubular capillary uptake of proximal tubular fluid, thereby increasing the quantity of sodium reabsorbed by the proximal tubule. Furthermore, as renal perfusion declines, blood is redistributed from the cortical to the juxtamedullary nephrons, which have a greater capacity for sodium reabsorption. The net result of these intrarenal events is sodium retention.

In addition, most of the neurohormonal systems that are activated in heart failure can exert important effects on sodium balance, either by influencing the interplay of intrarenal hemodynamic factors or by exerting direct effects on the tubular reabsorption of sodium (Figure 2.18). On the one hand, enhanced renal sympathetic activity and activation of the intrarenal renin-angiotensin system can cause sodium retention by increasing the magnitude of efferent arteriolar vasoconstriction.[51–55] Angiotensin II may also augment the tubular reab-

sorption of sodium both by a direct tubular effect[55] and by its ability to stimulate the formation of aldosterone by the adrenal gland.[56] On the other hand, both atrial natriuretic peptide and intrarenal prostaglandins oppose the actions of angiotensin II within the kidney and act to enhance sodium excretion.[54,57,58]

ENHANCED IMPEDANCE TO SYSTOLIC EJECTION

The impaired ventricular function in most patients with heart failure is not merely the result of a depression of cardiac contractility but is related to an increase in the impedance that the failing ventricle must overcome in order to empty during systole. This impedance includes a resistance component that resides primarily in the small arteries and arterioles and a compliance component that resides in the larger arteries. The normal ventricle is able to adjust to large changes in impedance without any notable change in systolic function, in part because it can utilize an increase in loading conditions in the heart to en-

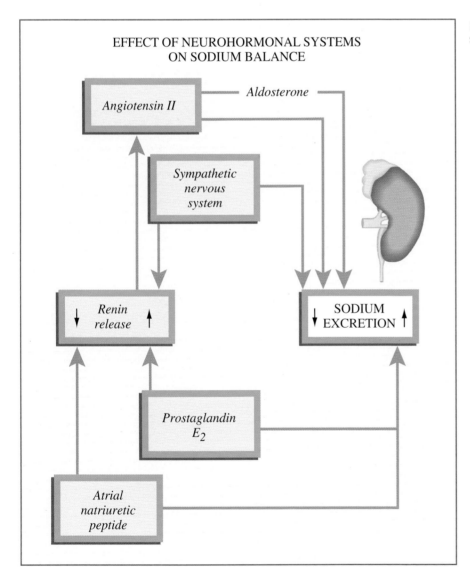

FIGURE 2.18 • Effect of neurohumoral systems on sodium balance.

hance ejection—Frank-Starling mechanism—and in part because the normal heart has an intrinsic ability to augment contractile force to overcome an increase in resistance[59] (Figure 2.19A). However, the failing ventricle loses both of these compensatory mechanisms. Increases in preload do not enhance systolic performance because the Frank-Starling curve is both depressed and flattened, and the abnormal myocardium cannot increase contractility in response to an increase in impedance[60] (Figure 2.19B). Consequently, the failing heart becomes exquisitely sensitive to small changes in its loading conditions. These may result either from sodium retention or from the constriction of peripheral arteries and veins. As a result, cardiac output remains depressed despite a marked increase in cardiac filling pressures.

Is the reduced cardiac output or the elevated cardiac filling pressures the most important hemodynamic abnormality in heart failure? For nearly 100 years, clinicians debated the relative merit of two seemingly conflicting hemodynamic theories

• • • • • • • • • • • • • • •

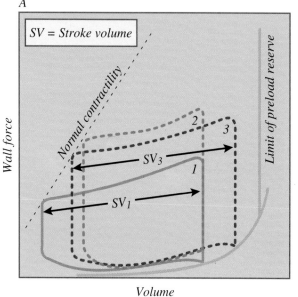

EFFECT OF CHANGES IN AFTERLOAD
IN THE NORMAL HEART

A

SV = Stroke volume

Wall force

Normal contractility

Limit of preload reserve

2

3

SV₃

1

SV₁

Volume

EFFECT OF CHANGES IN AFTERLOAD IN
THE FAILING VENTRICLE

B

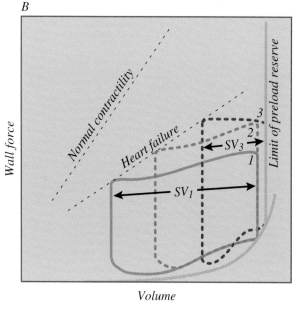

Wall force

Normal contractility

Heart failure

Limit of preload reserve

3

2

SV₃

1

SV₁

Volume

FIGURE 2.19 • Response of the normal heart to increases in ventricular afterload that occurs in the physiologic portion of the force-volume relationship (A). Loop 1, originating from a normal end-diastolic volume, ejects a normal quantity of blood (SV₁). With an increase in afterload, the initial result is loop 2, and a diminished stroke volume. However, through the redistribution of total load and a slight increase in end-systolic volume, the heart uses its preload reserve and moves to loop 3. This loop originates from a slightly larger end-diastolic volume and contracts with slightly less afterload than loop 2, but ejects the same or nearly the same quantity of blood as loop 1. This sequence of events describes the process of preload reserve and afterload matching that is within the capacity of the normal heart.

Result of increased afterload in a dilated, failing ventricle operating at a point in the wall force-volume plane that is very near the limit of preload reserve— loop 1 (B). With an increase in afterload, a significant reduction in stroke volume (SV) occurs. The heart attempts to compensate by using preload reserve, but quickly reaches the limit without a significant increment in diastolic volume. The small increment in diastolic volume, however, contributes further to the added afterload, loop 3, and produces a further decline in stroke volume. Thus, the failing heart, operating at the limit of preload reserve, is severely afterload dependent. Under these conditions, a very small reduction in ventricular afterload will produce a significant increase in stroke volume. (Reproduced with permission. Strobeck JE, Ross J Jr: *Heart Failure* 1985;1:84.)

pressure or volume seen in patients with heart failure will be transmitted to the left ventricle and cause an increase in left ventricular diastolic pressure without a change in left ventricular volume.[86]

Theoretically, changes in pulmonary wedge pressure produced by pharmacologic agents could be related to changes in left ventricular volume, to changes in the left ventricular pressure-volume relation or to changes in mitral regurgitant flow. Which is the primary mechanism by which vasodilator and inotropic drugs work? In most studies therapeutic interventions have produced changes in left ventricular filling pressure without changes in left ventricular volume. Indeed, a decrease in ventricular volume alone can never adequately explain the decline in left ventricular filling pressure seen during therapy.[87] To achieve the large decreases in left ventricular filling pressure seen during vasodilator therapy by a decrease in end-diastolic volume, the translocation of blood from the left ventricle would need to be so large that it would be mathematically impossible for the heart to maintain its stroke volume. As a result, changes in diastolic function or in mitral regurgitant flow must contribute greatly to the changes in pulmonary venous pressure seen in most patients with chronic heart failure.[67,88]

NEUROHORMONAL ACTIVATION

When cardiac output falls after an insult to the myocardium, several neurohormonal mechanisms are activated in an attempt to preserve circulatory homeostasis. These mechanisms include both endogenous vasoconstrictor systems—sympathetic nervous and renin-angiotensin systems—and endogenous vasodilator systems—atrial natriuretic peptide and prostaglandins[89] (Table 2.11).

Recent evidence also suggests that other endogenous humoral mechanisms may be altered in heart failure—arginine vasopressin,[90] neuropeptide Y,[91] enkephalin and opioid pathways,[92] endothelin,[93] endothelial-derived relaxing factor,[94] and tumor necrosis factor[95]—but their importance in the pathophysiology of heart failure has not been elucidated. As in the case of the biochemical and hemodynamic derangements outlined earlier, neurohormonal events provide an important target for pharmacologic interventions.

Sympathetic Nervous System

Plasma levels of norepinephrine are elevated in congestive heart failure in proportion to the clinical severity of the disease (Figure 2.22A). In patients with mild symptoms, plasma norepinephrine is normal at rest but rises to high levels on exertion.[96] As symptoms become more severe, plasma norepinephrine becomes elevated even at rest, and the magnitude of the elevation parallels the degree of the hemodynamic and functional impairment.[97,98] These observations may explain why plasma norepinephrine provides important prognostic information in these patients.[99] Interestingly, the increase in circulating norepinephrine appears to be related to both an increase in sympathetic outflow from the central nervous system, as demonstrated by intraneural recordings,[100] as well as a decrease in norepinephrine clearance.[101,102]

The cause of sympathetic activation in heart failure remains unclear, but recent studies suggest that abnormalities of barore-

---

TABLE 2.10 • FACTORS LEADING TO INCREASED PULMONARY CAPILLARY WEDGE PRESSURE IN HEART FAILURE

Increased ventricular volume
- Increased intravascular volume due to sodium retention
- Redistribution of blood to central circulation due to decreased venous capacitance
- Enhanced impedance to left ventricular ejection due to increased systemic arterial resistance

Increased mitral regurgitant flow

Impaired ventricular diastolic function

TABLE 2.11 • NEUROHORMONAL ACTIVATION IN HEART FAILURE

Vasoconstrictors	Vasodilators
Catecholamines	Atrial natriuretic peptide
Renin/angiotensin	Prostaglandins/kinins
Arginine vasopressin	Endothelial factors
Neuropeptide Y	• Endothelial-derived relaxing factor (EDRF)
Endothelin	Opioids/enkephalins
	Cytokines
	• Tumor necrosis factor (TNF)

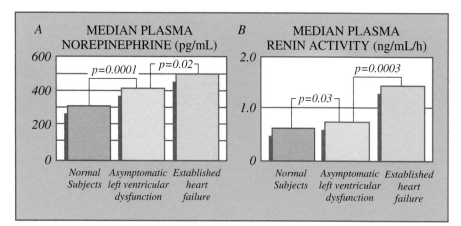

FIGURE 2.22 • Activation of sympathetic nervous and renin-angiotensin systems in patients with congestive heart failure. (Reproduced with permission. Francis GS, Benedict C, Johnstone, et al: *Circulation* 1990;82:1727.)

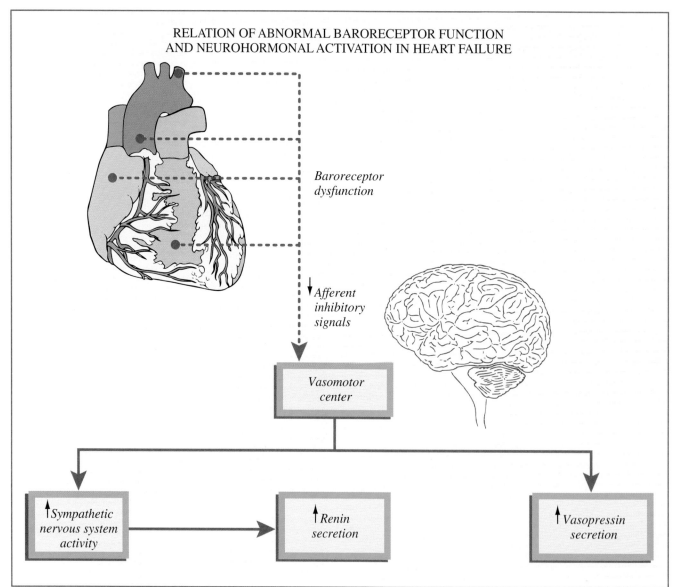

FIGURE 2.23 • Relationship of abnormal baroreceptor function to neurohormonal activation and regional blood flow in congestive heart failure. Increases in atrial and ventricular filling pressures and in mean arterial or pulse pressure normally stimulate cardiopulmonary and arterial baroreceptors. Baroreceptor activation sends inhibitory signals to the medullary vasomotor center, resulting in suppression of sympathetic efferent activity and increased vagal efferent activity (not shown). Baroreflex mechanisms are blunted in heart failure, resulting in activation of sympathetic and renin-angiotensin systems and increased neurohypophyseal release of vasopressin. (Adapted from Hirsch AT, Dzau VJ, Creager MA: *Circulation* 1986;74:815).

ceptor responsiveness play key roles.[81] These baroreflexes normally act as the primary mechanism that limits the magnitude of the adrenergic response to circulatory stress, but their modulating function is impaired in patients with heart failure. Consequently, pressure increases in the cardiac chambers and the great vessels no longer suppress, and may actually enhance, the outflow of sympathetic impulses from the central nervous system (Figure 2.23). The resulting activation of the sympathetic nervous system is accompanied by enhanced responsiveness of the peripheral vasculature, but reduced responsiveness of the myocardium, to adrenergic neurotransmitter activity.[37,103–106] The increased responsiveness of the peripheral vessels may be related to an enhanced vascular sensitivity to the vasoconstrictor actions of α-adrenergic agonists.[104] The decreased responsiveness of the myocardium is caused by both a reduction in the density and in the coupling of ß-adrenergic receptors to adenylate cyclase[36–42] (refer to the Biochemical Basis for Impaired Contractility section).

Activation of the sympathetic nervous system subserves both beneficial and deleterious roles in patients with chronic heart failure.[107] On the one hand, α-adrenergic impulses support systemic perfusion pressures, whereas β-adrenergic stimulation provides important inotropic and chronotropic support to the failing heart. On the other hand, prolonged α-adrenergically-mediated vasoconstriction adversely affects loading conditions in the heart, whereas β-adrenergic stimulation may provoke ventricular arrhythmias or exert a direct toxic effect on the myocardium.[108] Sympathetic activation is also a major stimulus to sodium retention by the kidney, both by virtue of its di-

rect effects on intrarenal hemodynamics as well as by its ability to activate the intrarenal renin-angiotensin system.[53,109]

Renin-Angiotensin System

As in the case of the sympathetic nervous system, the renin-angiotensin system is activated in patients with congestive heart failure in proportion to the severity of the disease[110] (Figure 2.22B). In patients with mild symptoms, plasma renin activity is normal at rest but rises to high levels on exertion.[111] As symptoms become progressively severe and renal perfusion pressure falls, plasma renin activity becomes elevated at rest, and the magnitude of the elevation parallels the degree of hemodynamic and functional impairment.[110] These observations may explain why plasma renin activity or its marker—serum sodium concentration—provides important prognostic information in these patients[11,112,113] (refer to Figure 2.8).

Several factors contribute to the activation of the renin-angiotensin system in chronic heart failure. In the early stages of the disease the increase in plasma renin activity is primarily due to stimulation of the renal sympathetic nerves and the use of diuretics[109,114,115] In the late stages of the disease the fall in renal perfusion pressure directly stimulates the release of renin from the kidneys[116] (Figure 2.24). Interestingly, renal hypoperfusion not only acts to release renin but also impairs the clearance of free water, leading to dilutional hyponatremia. The development of hyponatremia is further enhanced by an increased intake of water, which results from the direct stimulation of the cerebral thirst center by angiotensin II.[117] These interactions explain why an inverse relation exists between plasma renin activity

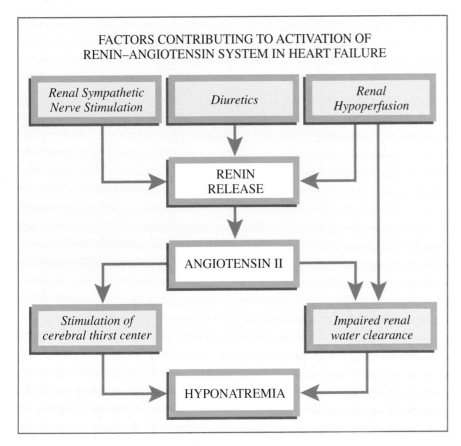

FIGURE 2.24 • Factors contributing to activation of renin-angiotensin system and the development of hyponatremia in heart failure.

and serum sodium concentration in chronic heart failure,[11,118] (Figure 2.25). It also explains why both hyponatremia and high levels of renin are markers of renal hypoperfusion.[116,119]

As in the case of the sympathetic nervous system, activation of the renin-angiotensin system subserves both beneficial and deleterious roles in patients with chronic heart failure.[54] Angiotensin II acts not only to support systemic perfusion pressures but also to preserve glomerular filtration rate during states of renal hypoperfusion.[120] Nevertheless, prolonged activation of the renin-angiotensin system may exert deleterious effects on ventricular function either by a direct toxic effect on the heart, by causing direct systemic vasoconstriction or by facilitating the vasoconstrictor actions of the sympathetic nervous system.[121,122] Furthermore, by stimulating the synthesis of aldosterone, angiotensin promotes the retention of salt and water by the kidneys (which may further exacerbate loading conditions in the failing heart) and the depletion of potassium and magnesium (which may increase the likelihood of complex ventricular arrhythmias).[123]

Endogenous Vasodilator Systems

Atrial Natriuretic Peptide • Under normal conditions, atrial natriuretic peptide exerts potent direct vasodilator and natriuretic effects and acts to inhibit the release and actions of the sympathetic nervous system, the renin-angiotensin system and arginine vasopressin.[89] These normal physiologic actions are preserved in acute heart failure,[124,125] but as the heart failure state becomes chronic, the ability of atrial distension to increase the release of natriuretic peptides is blunted,[126] and the ability of the released peptides to exert natriuretic effects and suppress neurohormonal activity is lost[127] (Table 2.12). This attenuation of the actions of atrial natriuretic factor may be related to a decline in the density of receptors for the peptide,[128,129] to a decline in renal blood flow,[130,131] or to the intrarenal antagonism of the peptide actions by the sympathetic nervous and the renin-angiotensin systems.[132] Regardless of the mechanism of attenuation, however, it is not clear that atrial natriuretic peptide functions as an important homeostatic hormone in most patients with chronic heart failure.

Prostaglandins • Renal hypoperfusion is a potent stimulus not only to renin release, but also the release of vasodilator prostaglandins from the kidneys. Consequently, patients with hyponatremic heart failure who have the most compromised renal perfusion[119] not only show the highest plasma renin activity but also the highest circulating levels of prostacyclin and prostaglandin E$_2$[17] (Figure 2.26). Both hormones are further released in response to diuretic therapy and to stimulation of the renal sympathetic nerves. Once formed within the kidney, both prostaglandins and angiotensin II stimulate the intrarenal release of one another.[133,134]

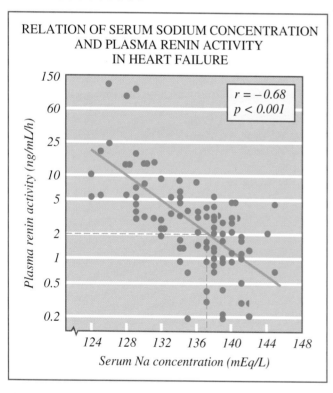

RELATION OF SERUM SODIUM CONCENTRATION AND PLASMA RENIN ACTIVITY IN HEART FAILURE

$r = -0.68$
$p < 0.001$

Plasma renin activity (ng/mL/h)

Serum Na concentration (mEq/L)

FIGURE 2.25 • Relationship between serum sodium concentration and plasma renin activity before vasodilator therapy in 96 patients with severe chronic heart failure. In the linear regression equation, the lower limit of normal for serum sodium concentration of 137 mEq/L corresponded to the lower limit of normal for plasma renin activity— 2 ng/mL/h). (Reproduced with permission. Lee WH, Packer M: *Circulation* 1986;73:261.)

TABLE 2.12 • ALTERATIONS IN ATRIAL NATRIURETIC PEPTIDE RELEASE AND ACTION IN HEART FAILURE

Ability of atrial distension to release atrial peptides is blunted

Ability of atrial peptides to suppress neurohormonal systems is reduced

Ability of atrial peptides to exert natriuretic effects is markedly attenuated because of:

- Decrease in receptors for the peptide
- Decline in renal blood flow
- Intrarenal antagonism by sympathetic nervous system
- Intrarenal antagonism by renin-angiotens in system

How do these hormones interact physiologically? Both prostaglandins and angiotensin II increase glomerular hydraulic filtration pressure and thus act to preserve glomerular filtration rate—the prostaglandins by a dilating action on the afferent arteriole and angiotensin II by a constricting effect on the efferent arteriole[54] (Figure 2.27). Yet, at nearly all other sites, the actions of renal prostaglandins oppose those of angiotensin II. Prostaglandins:

- Antagonize the actions of angiotensin II on systemic blood vessels and decrease loading conditions in the failing heart.[17]
- Directly inhibit sodium reabsorption in the renal tubules.[58]
- Antagonize the dipsogenic effects of angiotensin II[135]
- Oppose the actions of angiotensin II-mediated vasopressin release in the collecting duct.[136]

ELECTROPHYSIOLOGIC ABNORMALITIES

The progression of left ventricular dysfunction in heart failure is characterized by the parallel development of both mechanical and electrical abnormalities. Consequently, as left ventricular mechanical performance deteriorates, ventricular arrhythmias become more common. Nearly 80% to 90% of patients with Class III and IV heart failure have frequent and complex ventricular ectopic beats—40% to 60% have non-sustained ventricular tachycardia[137] (Table 2.13). As left ventricular dysfunction progresses, the risk of sudden death also increases. About 40% of patients with Class III-IV heart failure appear to die suddenly. The remaining deaths are attributed to progressive heart failure (50%) or recurrent ischemic events (10%).

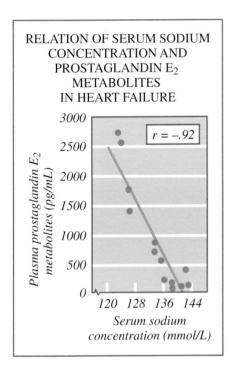

RELATION OF SERUM SODIUM CONCENTRATION AND PROSTAGLANDIN E₂ METABOLITES IN HEART FAILURE

$r = -.92$

FIGURE 2.26 • Relation between serum sodium concentration and levels of prostaglandin E_2 (PGE₂) metabolites in patients with severe heart failure. (Reproduced with permission. Dzau VJ, Packer M, Lilly JS, et al: *N Engl J Med* 1986;310:348.)

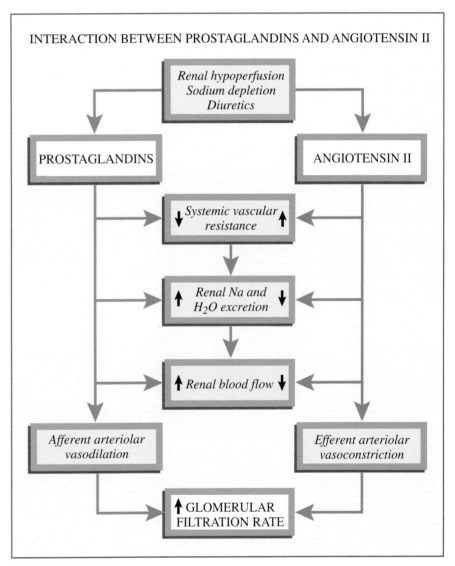

FIGURE 2.27 • Synergistic and counterregulatory interactions between two nephrogenic hormones—prostaglandins and angiotensin II—in patients with congestive heart failure. These two hormones exert qualitatively opposite effects on the systemic vasculature and on sodium and water excretion, but act in concert to preserve glomerular filtration rate during states of renal hypoperfusion or sodium depletion.

These observations have led physicians to expect that patients with the most frequent or serious arrhythmias would be at greatest risk of a fatal arrhythmia and thus, sudden death, but this does not seem to be the case. The finding of a malignant ventricular arrhythmia during ambulatory monitoring is a strong predictor of total mortality, but it does not presage which patients will die suddenly[7,137] (Table 2.13). Similarly, the results of ventricular stimulation during invasive electrophysiologic testing do not predict sudden death.[137-139] Hence, complex ventricular arrhythmias appear to be more a reflection of the severity of the patient's hemodynamic and functional abnormalities rather than a specific pathophysiologic event.[140] This concept may explain why antiarrhythmic drug therapy may suppress ventricular arrhythmias but not prolong life in these patients.[141-143] However, this issue remains unresolved.[113,144]

Why do ventricular arrhythmias fail to predict sudden death? Many sudden deaths in heart failure are due to bradyarrhythmias or electromechanical dissociation, not ventricular tachyarrhythmias[145]. Thus, although clinically sudden, such deaths appear to be related to mechanical, rather than electrical, events. This observation underscores the extreme difficulty encountered in attempting to classify the precise mode of death in a patient

· · · · · · · · · · · · · · · ·

TABLE 2.13 • VENTRICULAR ARRHYTHMIAS IN CONGESTIVE HEART FAILURE

Study[1]	Number of patients	Percent mortality	Percent of patients with ventricular tachycardia	Relation of ventricular tachycardia to total mortality	Relation of ventricular tachycardia to sudden death
Huang SK, et al, 1983[2]	35	11	60	No	No
von Olshausen K, et al, 1984[3]	60	12	42	Yes	No
Constanzo-Nordin MR, et al, 1985[4]	55	16	40	No	No
Meinertz T, et al, 1985[5]	42	17	36	Yes	No
Meinertz T, et al, 1984[6]	74	26	49	Yes	Yes
Unverferth DV, et al, 1984[7]	69	35	41	Yes	–
Chakko CS, et al, 1985[8]	43	37	48	Yes	No
Holmes J, et al, 1985[9]	31	45	39	Yes	No
Dargie HJ, et al, 1987[10]	84	58	61	Yes	–
Baim DS, et al, 1986[11]	100	63	59	Yes	No
Wilson JR, et al, 1983[12]	77	65	51	Yes	No
Maskin CS, et al, 1984[13]	35	71	71	–	–

[1] Studies listed in order of increasing severity of heart failure.

[2] Huang SK, Messer JV, Denes P: Significance of ventricular arrhythmias in idiopathic dilated cardiomyopathy: Observations in 35 patients. Am J Cardiol 1983;51:507.

[3] von Olshausen K, Schafer A, Mehmel HC, et al: Ventricular arrhythmias in idiopathic dilated cardiomyopathy. Br Heart J 1984;51:195.

[4] Constanzo-Nordin MR, O'Connell JB, Englemeier RS, et al: Dilated cardiomyopathy: Functional status, hemodynamics, arrhythmias, and prognosis. Cathet Cardiovasc Diagn 1985;11:445.

[5] Meinertz T, Tresse N, Kasper W, et al: Determinants of prognosis in idiopathic dilated cardiomyopathy as determined by programmed electrical stimulation. Am J Cardiol 1985;56:337.

[6] Meinertz T, Hofmann F, Kasper W, et al: Significance of ventricular arrhythmias in idiopathic dilated cardiomyopathy. Am J Cardiol 1984;53:902.

[7] Unverferth DV, Magorien DR, Moeschberger ML, et al: Factors influencing the one year mortality of dilated cardiomyopathy. Am J Cardiol 1984;54:147.

[8] Chakko CS, Gheorghiade M: Ventricular arrhythmias in severe heart failure: Incidence, significance, and effectiveness of antiarrhythmic therapy. Am Heart J 1985;109:497.

[9] Holmes J, Kubo SH, Cody RJ, et al: Arrhythmias in ischemic and nonischemic dilated cardiomyopathy: Prediction of mortality by ambulatory electrocardiography. Am J Cardiol 1985;55:146.

[10] Dargie HJ, Cleland JGF, Leckie BJ, et al: Relation of arrhythmias and electrolyte abnormalities to survival in patients with severe chronic heart failure. Circulation 1987;75(suppl IV):98.

[11] Baim DS, Colucci WS, Monrad ES, et al: Survival of patients with severe congestive heart failure treated with oral milrinone. J Am Coll Cardiol 1986;7:661.

[12] Wilson JR, Schwartz JS, St. John Sutton M, et al: Prognosis in severe heart failure: Relation to hemodynamic measurements and ventricular ectopic activity. J Am Coll Cardiol 1983;2:403.

[13] Maskin CS, Siskind SJ, LeJemtel TH: High prevalence of nonsustained ventricular tachycardia in severe congestive heart failure. Am Heart J 1984;107:896.

with heart failure. As patients with heart failure approach the time of death, they usually have both arrhythmias and severe symptoms, and it may be impossible to determine with confidence how these factors interact to lead to the patient's demise.[7,146] Even under close scrutiny, we cannot usually determine if a terminal arrhythmia played a primary or secondary role in the death of a particular patient. Consequently, the first goal of therapy in patients with heart failure is the reduction of total mortality. Claims that a specific treatment reduces the risk of a specific mode of death without reducing total mortality should be viewed with skepticism.

TREATMENT OF LEFT VENTRICULAR SYSTOLIC DYSFUNCTION

The most important pathophysiologic condition underlying the development of heart failure in the United States is left ventricular systolic dysfunction. Although this condition may be caused by a variety of disease states, its management is usually not directed towards the cause of heart failure, but instead, to its clinical manifestations. This approach is based on the fact that, regardless of its cause, left ventricular systolic dysfunction is generally irreversible and is not improved by surgical interventions, unless there is coexistent valvular disease or myocardial ischemia or unless cardiac transplantation is being considered. Efforts to identify the underlying cause are commonly futile[147] or lead to the use of interventions of unproven value: coronary artery bypass surgery for ischemic cardiomyopathy, chelation therapy for hemochromatosis, corticosteroids for sarcoidosis, immunosuppressive therapy for myocarditis and antiparasitic agents for Chagas' disease (Figures 2.28, 2.29). However, it is always important to remove potential toxins, such as alcohol, and to correct associated metabolic deficiencies (for example, beriberi or hypophosphatemia).

The therapeutic approach to the patient with heart failure due to left ventricular systolic dysfunction depends largely on the urgency of the clinical presentation. Chronic stable heart failure, even if severe, is generally managed with oral agents. Intravenous therapy is usually necessary for unstable patients during acute exacerbations of the disease, regardless of whether their heart failure symptoms are recent or long-standing.

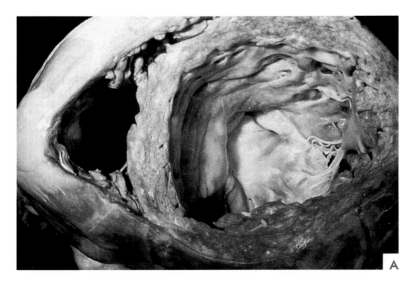

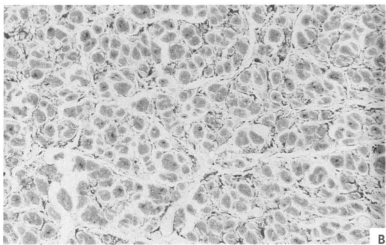

FIGURE 2.28 • In ischemic cardiomyopathy, the left ventricular cavity may be widely dilated with a hypertrophic wall (A). Histologically, there is extensive lace-like myocardial fibrosis. (Reproduced with permission. Hurst JW, Anderson RH, Becker AE, et al: *Atlas of the Heart* New York, NY: Gower Medical Publishing; 1988:6.41.)

PHARMACOLOGIC TREATMENT OF STABLE HEART FAILURE

Given the grave functional and prognostic consequences of heart failure, the primary goals of therapy in individuals with chronic stable symptoms are to make patients feel better and live longer. Therefore, physicians should strive to reduce:

- The symptoms of dyspnea and fatigue at rest or during exercise.
- The need for hospitalization and emergency care for worsening symptoms.
- Mortality.

Therapy is selected and adjusted to permit patients to carry out activities of daily living commensurate with their needs and desires, and the success of treatment is judged primarily by the relief of symptoms. Interventions that change the natural history of the disease and reduce mortality should be added to the therapeutic regimen—even in patients whose symptoms are well-controlled.

Several general measures are advisable for most patients with chronic heart failure (Table 2.14). Obese patients should lose weight, and concomitant cardiac conditions—hypertension and atrial arrhythmias—should be vigorously treated. Even if overt sodium retention can be controlled by the use of diuretics, moderate dietary sodium restriction is usually indicated to permit the effective use of lower, safer doses of diuretic drugs. Although patients should not participate in heavy labor or exhaustive sports, bed rest should not be encouraged—except during periods of acute decompensation—since the restriction of activity promotes physical deconditioning. Indeed, physical training alone may improve symptoms and exercise capacity in patients with mild-to-moderate heart failure.[148,149] Finally, since patients with marked ventricular dilatation and dysfunction are at risk for systemic and pulmonary emboli, physicians should consider the use of anticoagulants or antiplatelet agents, unless contraindications exist.

As stated earlier, there are four principal pathophysiologic abnormalities in heart failure:

- Impaired contractility.
- Sodium retention.
- Enhanced impedance to systolic ejection.
- Neurohormonal activation.

Since pharmacologic interventions have been developed to ameliorate each of these physiologic derangements, drugs for the treatment of heart failure can also be categorized into four groups:[150–152]

- Positive inotropic agents.
- Diuretic drugs.
- Direct-acting vasodilators.
- Neurohormonal antagonists.

POSITIVE INOTROPIC AGENTS

Two types of positive inotropic drugs have been identified: those that increase cardiac contractility by changing the activity of the sodium channel or sodium pump (for example, digitalis) and those that promote the synthesis or inhibit the degradation of cyclic AMP (for example, catecholamines and phosphodiesterase inhibitors). At present, only agents in the first category are available for oral use. Cyclic AMP-dependent agents are available solely for intravenous administration for the treatment of unstable heart failure.

Digoxin

It is commonly believed that the primary action of digitalis in heart failure is to increase cardiac contractility as a conse-

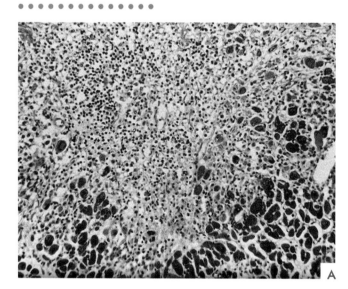

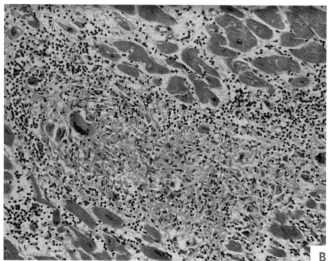

FIGURE 2.29 • In this case of viral myocarditis, extensive loss of monocytes is accompanied by massive infiltration of inflammatory cells, mainly lymphocytes (A). This histologic section of the myocardium shows a granulomatous inflammation with multinucleated giant cells in a case of tuberculous myocarditis (B). (Reproduced with permission. Becker AE, Anderson RH: *Cardiac Pathology* New York, NY: Gower Medical Publishing; 1983:3.37.)

quence of its inhibition of Na$^+$/K$^+$ ATPase.[153] However, there is little relation between the positive inotropic effects of digitalis and the clinical response to treatment with the drug.[154,155] Recent evidence suggests that the beneficial clinical effects of digitalis may be related to its ability to sensitize cardiac baroreceptors, thereby reducing the outflow of sympathetic impulses from the central nervous system[156,157] (Table 2.15 and Figure 2.30). In addition, as a consequence of its inhibitory action on Na$^+$/K$^+$ ATPase, digitalis inhibits the renal tubular reabsorption of sodium.[158] The resulting increase in the delivery of sodium to the distal tubules may contribute to the suppression of renin

secretion from the kidneys, and hence, plasma renin activity.[157] The most commonly used preparation of digitalis in the United States is digoxin.

Hemodynamic and Clinical Effects • Digoxin produces immediate and sustained increases in cardiac output and left ventricular ejection fraction and decreases in cardiac filling pressures and volumes in patients with chronic heart failure.[159–161] These favorable hemodynamic effects are accompanied by decreases in plasma norepinephrine and plasma renin activity.[157,162,163] Digoxin improves exercise tolerance and reduces the need for hospitalization and emergency care for

TABLE 2.14 • GENERAL MEASURES IN THE MANAGEMENT OF CHRONIC HEART FAILURE
Management of associated disorders
• Weight loss in obese patients
• Smoking cessation in persistent smokers
• Treatment of associated hypertension, myocardial ischemia and atrial arrhythmias
• Correction of anemia and metabolic disorders
Moderate dietary sodium restriction
Encourage mild-to-moderate exercise
Consider use of anticoagulants/antiplatelets agents

TABLE 2.15 • ACTIONS OF DIGITALIS GLYCOSIDES IN CHRONIC HEART FAILURE
Increase in cardiac contractility
Sensitization of baroreflex function, thereby suppressing outflow of sympathetic impulses from vasomotor center in the central nervous system
Inhibition of renal tubular reabsorption of sodium
Suppression of renin release by the kidney due to sympatholytic and renal tubular actions

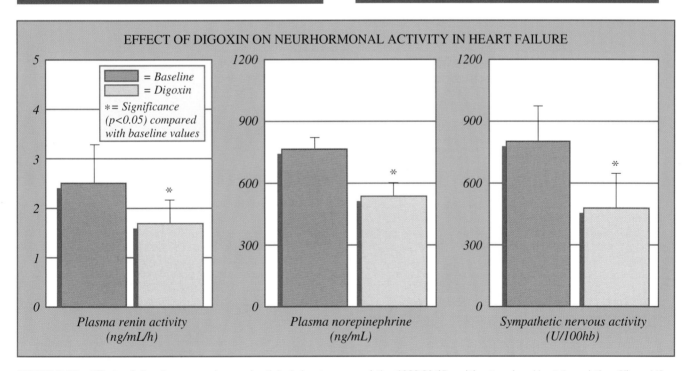

FIGURE 2.30 • Effects of digoxin on neurohumoral activity in heart failure. (Adapted from Ferguson DW, Berg WJ, Sanders JS, et al: *Circulation* 1989;80:65 and the American Heart Association; Ribner HS, Plucinski DA, Hsieh A-M: *Am J Cardiol* 1985;56:896.)

worsening heart failure.[159,161] When digoxin is withdrawn, the clinical status of patients deteriorates[154,164,165] (Table 2.16 and Figure 2.31).

The utility of long-term treatment with digoxin—0.125 to 0.50 mg once daily—in chronic heart failure has been demonstrated in six double-blind placebo-controlled trials.[154,159,161,164,166,167] Five trials enrolled only patients in normal sinus rhythm. These benefits have been observed in patients with mild, moderate and severe symptoms, but only if they had systolic dysfunction—as evidenced by a low ejection fraction, left ventricular dilatation or a third heart sound[159,161,164,167] (Table 2.17). In contrast, digoxin appears to be ineffective in patients with preserved systolic function or without cardiomegaly, regardless of the severity of symptoms.[166,168–170] In these patients, the syndrome of heart failure may be related to an abnormality of diastolic, rather than systolic function, which might not be expected to respond favorably to therapy with a positive inotropic agent. Digoxin is probably of little value in patients with constrictive pericarditis or mitral stenosis, unless there is coexistent atrial fibrillation or right ventricular failure, or hypertrophic cardiomyopathy. In the last case, digitalis may actually increase the severity of left ventricular outflow obstruction.

Adverse Effects • Toxic doses of digitalis can produce:
- Gastrointestinal symptoms—anorexia, nausea and vomiting.
- Neurologic complaints—visual disturbances, disorientation and confusion.
- Cardiac arrhythmias—ectopic and reentrant cardiac rhythms and heart block.

However, despite long-standing concerns about such side effects, recent reports indicate that therapeutic doses of digoxin are well tolerated by most patients with heart failure. In controlled trials, patients treated with digoxin experienced less toxicity than patients treated with placebo, primarily because placebo-treated patients deteriorated symptomatically and required increasing doses of diuretics.[159,164] In contrast to the converting-enzyme inhibitors, digoxin does not produce symptomatic hypotension or renal insufficiency.[159] In contrast to other positive inotropic agents, digoxin is associated with fewer episodes of palpitations and ventricular arrhythmia.[164] Adverse effects of digitalis seem to occur only when the drug is administered in large doses, but such large doses are not necessary to produce hemodynamic and symptomatic benefits. These observations suggest that the therapeutic-to-toxic ratio for digoxin may not be as narrow as has been previously feared.

Although retrospective analyses of trials of patients recovering from an acute myocardial infarction have identified digitalis therapy as a risk factor for enhanced mortality,[171] it is likely that this adverse association was related to the severity of heart failure in treated patients and not to drug therapy.[172] To the extent that digitalis contributes to clinical stability in chronic heart failure, we might even expect the drug to improve the long-term outcome of most patients. A formal trial to evaluate the impact of digitalis on survival is now being carried out by the National Heart, Lung, and Blood Institute.

Clinical Use • Digoxin is usually initiated and maintained at a dose of 0.25 mg daily. A lower dose of 0.125 mg every day

• • • • • • • • • • • • • • •

TABLE 2.16 • DIGITALIS GLYCOSIDES IN HEART FAILURE—RESULTS OF PLACEBO-CONTROLLED TRIALS

Improved symptoms
- Dobbs SM, Kenyon WL, Dobbs RJ, et al: Maintenance digoxin after an episode of heart failure: Placebo-controlled trial in outpatients. *Br Med J* 1977;2:749.
- Lee DC, Johnson RA, Bingham JB, et al: Heart failure in outpatients. A randomized trial in outpatients. *N Engl J Med* 1982;306:699.
- Guyatt GH, Sullivan MJ, Fallen EL, et al: A controlled trial of digoxin in congestive heart failure. *Am J Cardiol* 1988; 61:371.

Improved exercise tolerance
- Guyatt GH, Sullivan MJ, Fallen EL, et al: A controlled trial of digoxin in congestive heart failure. *Am J Cardiol* 1988;61:371.
- Captopril-Digoxin Multicenter Research Group: Comparative effects of captopril and digoxin in patients with mild to moderate heart failure. *JAMA* 1988;259:539.
- DiBianco R, Shabetai R, Kostuk W, et al: A comparison of oral milrinone, digoxin, and their combination in the treatment of patients with chronic heart failure. *N Engl J Med* 1989;320:677.

Reduction in cardiovascular morbidity
- Captopril-Digoxin Multicenter Research Group: Comparative effects of captopril and digoxin in patients with mild to moderate heart failure. *JAMA* 1988;259:539.
- DiBianco R, Shabetai R, Kostuk W, et al: A comparison of oral milrinone, digoxin, and their combination in the treatment of patients with chronic heart failure. *N Engl J Med* 1989;320:677

or every other day may be more appropriate if the patient is over 70 years old or has impaired renal function (Table 2.18). Although serum levels of digoxin have been advocated as a guide to the rational use of the drug, there is no relationship between serum digoxin concentration and the drug's therapeutic effects.[173,174] Large doses have not been shown to be more effective than small doses in the treatment of heart failure.[160]

Similarly, although some investigators have claimed that a relationship exists between serum levels of digoxin and the drug's adverse effects,[175] others have raised considerable doubts about the utility of digoxin levels in assessing the toxic patient,[176,177] since even low circulating levels of digoxin can be associated with toxicity if hypokalemia or hypomagnesemia coexist.[178,179] Quinidine, verapamil, spironolactone, flecainide, propafenone and amiodarone can increase the serum digoxin concentration.[180–185]

Cyclic AMP-Dependent Positive Inotropic Agents

These drugs can be classified into two groups:
- The β-adrenergic agonists
- The phosphodiesterase inhibitors (Table 2.19).

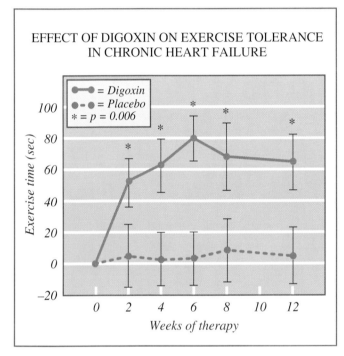

FIGURE 2.31 • Effect of digoxin on exercise tolerance in chronic heart failure. (Adapted from DiBianco R, Shabetai R, Kostuk W, et al: *N Engl J Med* 1989;320:677.)

TABLE 2.17 • DIGITALIS GLYCOSIDES— CONDITIONS MOST LIKELY TO RESPOND TO THERAPY

Systolic dysfunction	Hemodynamic abnormalities at rest
Left ventricular dilatation	Third heart sound

TABLE 2.18 • DIGITALIS GLYCOSIDES— APPROACH TO CLINICAL USE

Use of fixed doses of digoxin depending on patient's age and renal function

If age is less than 70 and normal serum Cr: Digoxin 0.25 mg once daily

If age is greater than 70 or elevated serum Cr: Digoxin 0.125 mg once daily

If age is greater than 70 and elevated serum Cr: Digoxin 0.125 mg every other day

---

TABLE 2.19 • CYCLIC AMP-DEPENDENT POSITIVE INOTROPIC AGENTS

ß-adrenergic agonists		Phosphodiesterase inhibitors	
ß₁-selective	ß₂-selective	Class I (no associated pharmacologic actions)	Class II (have pharmacologic properties in addition to PDE inhibition)
• Prenalterol	• Pirbuterol	• Amrinone	• Pimobendan
• Denopamine	• Salbutamol	• Milrinone	• Vesnarinone
• Xamoterol	• Terbutaline	• Enoximone	
		• Imazodan	
		• Indolidan	

Several cyclic AMP-dependent agents are available for intravenous use (refer to Treatment of Unstable Heart Failure section), and although none are available for oral use, many candidates are presently under active clinical investigation.

Investigational β-Adrenergic Agonists • Both β_1-selective (prenalterol, denopamine and xamoterol[186–188]) and β_2-selective agonists (pirbuterol and salbutamol[189,190]) produce short-term hemodynamic effects in chronic heart failure, but these initial favorable responses have not been translated into long-term clinical benefits. In most double-blind studies with these drugs, no difference has been seen in cardiac performance, symptoms or exercise tolerance between patients treated with active therapy and those treated with placebo.[191–194] This lack of benefit appears to be related to the development of pharmacologic tolerance during long-term treatment, probably due to the down-regulation of ß-adrenergic receptors that follows any prolonged exposure to catecholamines.[195] Concerns have also been raised that long-term treatment with these drugs may enhance the prevalence of ventricular arrhythmias and the risk of sudden death. Such fears have recently been confirmed by the results from two randomized, placebo-controlled trials—one with xamoterol (Figure 2.32) and one with intermittent intravenous dobutamine.[194,196]

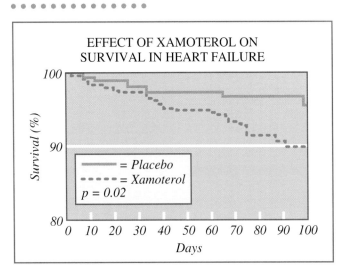

FIGURE 2.32 • Three-month survival during placebo and xamoterol therapy in patients with severe heart failure. (Reproduced with permission. The Xamoterol in Heart Failure Study Group. *Lancet* 1990;336:1.)

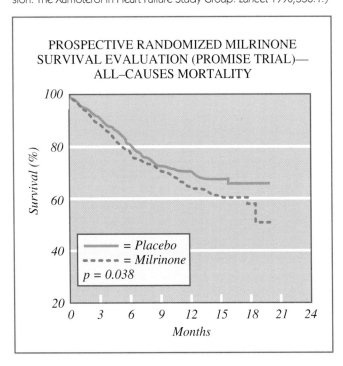

FIGURE 2.33 • Results of the Prospective Randomized Milrinone Survival Evaluation (PROMISE) trial. Milrinone increased the mortality of patients with severe heart failure by 28%. (Reproduced with permission. Packer M, Carver JR, Rodeheffer R, et al: *N Engl J Med* 1991;325:1468.)

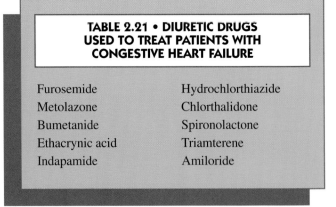

TABLE 2.20 • POTENTIAL ADVERSE EFFECTS OF CYCLIC AMP-DEPENDENT POSITIVE INOTROPIC DRUGS

Accelerated progression of underlying disease
Provocation of ventricular arrhythmias
Increased mortality

TABLE 2.21 • DIURETIC DRUGS USED TO TREAT PATIENTS WITH CONGESTIVE HEART FAILURE

Furosemide	Hydrochlorthiazide
Metolazone	Chlorthalidone
Bumetanide	Spironolactone
Ethacrynic acid	Triamterene
Indapamide	Amiloride

Treatment of Congestive Heart Failure

Investigational Phosphodiesterase Inhibitors • Like the β-adrenergic agonists, the phosphodiesterase inhibitors act by increasing intracellular cyclic AMP. Unlike the β-agonists, however, the primary hemodynamic effect of these drugs is probably peripheral vasodilation and not inotropic stimulation. All of the agents in this class—amrinone, milrinone, enoximone, piroximone, imazodan and indolidan—produce short-term hemodynamic effects,[197–201] but large-scale clinical trials have not yet been able to demonstrate the efficacy of these drugs in the treatment of heart failure.[164,202–207] Like the β-agonists, these agents have been reported to increase the frequency and complexity of ventricular arrhythmias,[164] and their long-term use has been accompanied by hemodynamic changes suggesting that these drugs accelerate progression of the underlying disease[208,209] (Table 2.20).

Three randomized, controlled studies have raised fears that phosphodiesterase inhibitors may increase mortality.[164,203,205] These fears have been confirmed by the results of a large-scale multicenter study—the Prospective Randomized Milrinone Survival Evaluation (PROMISE)—which showed that long-term treatment with oral milrinone, 40 mg daily, was associated with a 28% increase in the risk of death in patients with severe chronic heart failure treated with digitalis, diuretics, and angiotensin-converting enzyme inhibitors[206] (Figure 2.33).

DIURETICS

Diuretics have been used to treat heart failure for nearly 50 years (Table 2.21). These agents reduce sodium retention by inhibiting the reabsorption of sodium or chloride at specific sites in the renal tubules:

- Acetazolamide and mercurials at the proximal tubule
- Furosemide, ethacrynic acid, and bumetanide in the loop of Henle.
- Thiazides and metolazone in the distal tubule
- Potassium-sparing diuretics in the collecting duct (Figure 2.34).

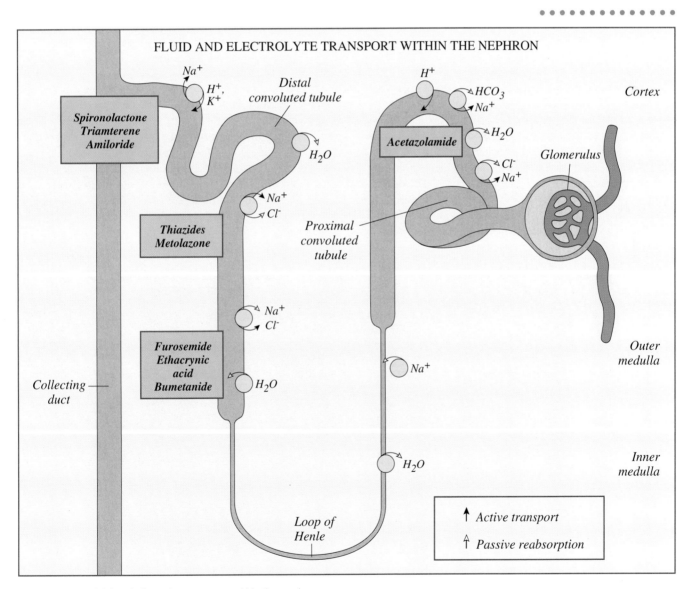

FIGURE 2.34 • Fluid and electrolyte transport within the nephron and the major sites of action of diuretics.

Furosemide, metolazone and spironolactone are the most often used diuretics in patients with chronic heart failure.

Pharmacologic Actions and Clinical Effects • All diuretics increase urine volume and sodium excretion, but these agents differ markedly in their pharmacologic properties[210] (Table 2.22). The loop diuretics:

- Increase sodium excretion up to 20% to 25% of the filtered load of sodium.
- Enhance the clearance of free water.
- Show reduced efficacy only when renal function is severely impaired—creatinine clearance less than 5 mL/min.

In contrast, the thiazides and the potassium-sparing diuretics:

- Increase the fractional excretion of sodium to only 5% to 10% of the filtered load.
- Tend to decrease free water clearance.
- Lose their effectiveness in patients with only moderately impaired renal function—creatinine clearance less than 30 mL/min).

Consequently, the loop diuretics—particularly furosemide—have emerged as the preferred diuretic agent for patients with chronic heart failure. When additional sodium excretion or potassium preservation, is desired, they are frequently combined with thiazide diuretics (particularly metolazone) and potassium-sparing diuretics (especially spironolactone).

Unlike thiazide and potassium-sparing diuretics, the loop diuretics exert hemodynamic and hormonal effects that are unrelated to their ability to increase sodium excretion. Furosemide enhances the renal release of prostaglandins, thereby increasing venous capacitance and renal blood flow.[211–213] The drug also promotes the renal release of renin, which causes arterial vasoconstriction.[214,215] Since both the prostaglandins and the renin-angiotensin system exert their own effects on sodium excretion, the simultaneous release of these hormones can modify the natriuretic response to furosemide, which is potentiated by converting-enyzme inhibition and attenuated by cyclo-oxygenase inhibition.[18,216] The activation of renal hormonal systems by furosemide also magnifies their importance in preserving the glomerular filtration rate in low-flow states. As a result, diuretics potentiate the risk of renal insufficiency seen during treatment with converting-enzyme inhibitors and nonsteroidal anti-inflammatory drugs.[217,218]

Adverse Reactions • The major side effects of diuretic therapy are electrolyte depletion and the activation of neurohormonal systems, both of which may predispose to serious cardiac arrhythmias[123] (Figure 2.35). In patients with a very low cardiac output, diuretic therapy may be complicated by increasing azotemia. Contrary to conventional wisdom, the development of prerenal azotemia is not necessarily the result of an excessive lowering of ventricular filling pressure but is a consequence of renal hypoperfusion.[219,220] Hence, the development of azotemia during diuretic therapy should not lead to a reduction in the dose of diuretics if the therapeutic endpoint—amelioration of peripheral edema—has not been reached (Table 2.23). Other adverse reactions of diuretics include hyperuricemia, carbohydrate intolerance and ototoxicity, especially with ethacrynic acid.

Diuretics enhance both the beneficial and deleterious effects of the converting-enzyme inhibitors. On the one hand, the hemodynamic effects of captopril, enalapril and lisinopril are attenuated in patients consuming a high-sodium diet, and conversely, the benefits of these drugs are potentiated by the use of diuretics.[221] On the other hand, furosemide increases the risk of hypotension and renal insufficiency during treatment with converting-enzyme inhibitors.[217] Concurrent therapy with potassium-sparing diuretics also increases the risk of hyperkalemia.[222]

· · · · · · · · · · · · · · · ·

TABLE 2.22 • PHARMACOLOGIC CHARACTERISTICS OF DIURETIC DRUGS

	Thiazide diuretics	Loop diuretics
Percent maximal fractional sodium excretion	5%-10%	20%-25%
Renal clearance of free water	Decrease	Increase
Actions reduced at glomerular filtration rate less than	25-30 mL/min	5 mL/min
Effect on renal blood flow	No effect	Increase
Release of renal prostaglandins	No	Yes
Systemic vasodilator effects	No	Yes

Clinical Use • Since one of the earliest pathophysiologic abnormalities of heart failure is the development of a sodium-avid state, the first goal of treatment is the restoration of sodium balance. This can generally be achieved by a combined approach in which dietary sodium is restricted and diuretic agents are administered to bring sodium excretion in line with a reduced salt load. Therapy is commonly initiated with furosemide, 20 to 40 mg daily, and the dose is increased until edema is controlled—even if prerenal azotemia develops (Table 2.23).

The response to furosemide is dependent on the concentration of the drug and time course of its entry into the urine[223] (Figure 2.36). As heart failure advances, the absorption of the drug may be delayed by bowel edema or intestinal hypoperfusion and the delivery of the drug may be delayed by the decline in renal perfusion and function.[224] Consequently, clinical progression is usually accompanied by the need for increasing doses of furosemide. Resistance to the drug can be overcome by:

• IV administration.
• The concomitant use of other diuretics, especially metolazone.
• Drugs that increase renal blood flow, such as dopamine and dobutamine.

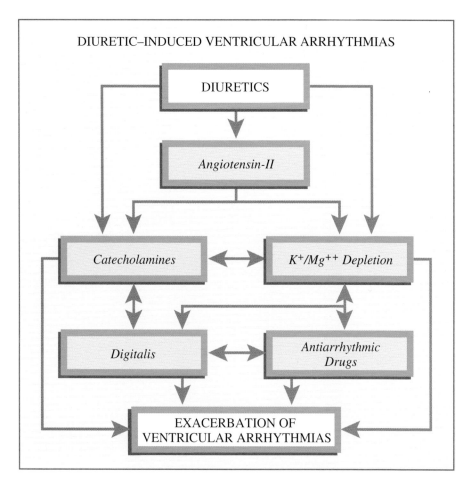

FIGURE 2.35 • Mechanisms of diuretic-induced ventricular arrhythmias in congestive heart failure.

TABLE 2.23 • DIURETIC DRUGS—APPROACH TO CLINICAL USE

Administration of incremental doses of diuretics until resolution of fluid retention (such as edema) regardless of asymptomatic changes in vital signs and renal function.	Converting-enzyme inhibitors potentiate the clinical benefits and antagonize the adverse metabolic and neurohormonal effects of diuretics, but increase the risk of hypotension and azotemia.

- The mechanical reduction of excess sodium—hemofiltration or peritoneal dialysis (Table 2.24)—but only as a last resort.

Diuretics produce symptomatic benefits more rapidly than any other drug. They can relieve dyspnea and edema within hours or days, whereas the effects of digitalis, angiotensin-converting enzyme inhibitors, or β-blockers may take weeks or months to become apparent. Nonetheless, even if symptoms and fluid retention are controlled, diuretics alone seem unable to maintain the clinical stability of patients with chronic heart failure for long periods of time. A high proportion of patients whose symptoms appear well-controlled deteriorate clinically during long-term follow-up when managed with diuretics alone.[159] The risk of clinical decompensation is reduced, however, when diuretics are combined with digoxin or an angiotensin-converting enzyme inhibitor.[159]

DIRECT-ACTING VASODILATORS

These agents have been traditionally classified according to their dominant site of action—arterial or venous or both—in the peripheral circulation. Several years ago, this classification achieved widespread popularity based on the belief that the site of drug action could guide the rational selection of a specific vasodilator for the individual patient. This approach assumed that increases in cardiac output and decreases in left ventricular filling pressure were invariably linked to dilation of the arterial resistance and venous capacitance vessels, respectively. Physicians were therefore advised to treat low cardiac output with an arterial vasodilator drug and high left ventricular filling pressure with a drug that dilated systemic veins. Although we now recognize that such a therapeutic approach is neither valid nor useful,[225] this classification of direct-acting vasodilators remains in common use.

Direct-acting vasodilators appear to exert beneficial effects in heart failure treatment primarily by reducing pulmonary venous pressures at rest and during exercise.[74] This effect may be achieved by:

- Decreasing left ventricular volumes as a consequence of venodilatation (nitrates).

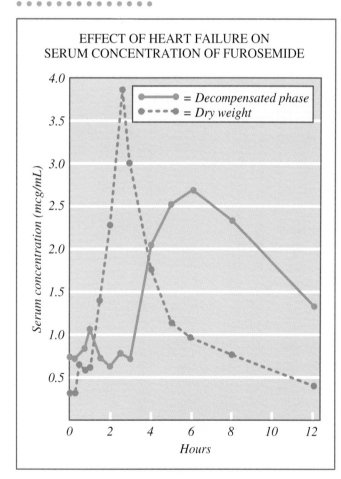

EFFECT OF HEART FAILURE ON SERUM CONCENTRATION OF FUROSEMIDE

= Decompensated phase
= Dry weight

FIGURE 2.36 • Serum concentrations of furosemide after oral administration of 160 mg of the drug. Furosemide was administered to patients in the decompensated phase of congestive heart failure and again after attaining dry weight. A higher and earlier peak concentration was noted when patients achieved dry weight. (Reproduced with permission Vasko MR, Brown-Cartwright D, Knochel JP, et al.: *Ann Intern Med* 1985;102:316.)

TABLE 2.24 • DIURETIC DRUGS—POSSIBLE APPROACHES TO THE REFRACTORY PATIENT
Increase in dose of diuretic drug
Change from oral to intravenous administration
Addition of a second/third diuretic (metolazone)
Addition of dopamine and dobutamine
Institution of hemofiltration/ peritoneal dialysis

- Improving left ventricular diastolic function through a reduction in right ventricular volume, thereby minimizing the pericardium's constraining effect on left ventricular filling (nitrates).
- Reducing the magnitude of mitral regurgitation (nitrates or hydralazine).[67,87,88]

Nitrates and Hydralazine

Nitrates such as nitroglycerin and isosorbide dinitrate exert their vasodilator action primarily on venous capacitance vessels by activating guanylate cyclase, thereby increasing cyclic GMP in vascular smooth muscle.[226] In contrast, hydralazine exerts its vasodilator effects primarily on arterial resistance vessels; its mechanism of action is unknown. A related vasodilator—minoxidil—acts as an agonist of the potassium channel in vascular smooth muscle.[227]

Hemodynamic Effects • The principal short-term hemodynamic effects of the organic nitrates in chronic heart failure is to lower right and left ventricular filling pressure at rest and during exercise[228] (Figure 2.37). Approximately 70% of patients experience immediate hemodynamic improvement after a single dose of oral isosorbide dinitrate, 20 to 40 mg. The remaining 30% show no initial response to the drug—nitrate resistance—perhaps related to a reduced ability of venous capacitance vessels to dilate in edematous states.[229,230] Nitrates produce only modest short-term increases in cardiac output in most patients with heart failure, unless mitral regurgitation is present.[231] Concerns have been raised that nitrates may actually lower cardiac output in patients who have low ventricular filling pressure before therapy (causing an excessive decline in cardiac preload),[232] but such an effect has never been shown to be clinically important.

Hydralazine and minoxidil primarily increase cardiac output and lower systemic vascular resistance in patients with chronic heart failure[233,234] (Figure 2.37). Although nearly all patients experience hemodynamic benefits after short-term treatment with these drugs, the doses required to achieve these effects are highly unpredictable, ranging from 150 to 3,000 mg daily for hydralazine and 5 to 20 mg daily for minoxidil.[234,235] Although neither hydralazine nor minoxidil exerts notable effect on venous capacitance vessels, they can decrease left ventricular filling pressure in patients who have severe mitral or aortic valvular regurgitation, in whom aortic impedance is an important determinant of the magnitude of regurgitant volume.[236,237]

Unfortunately, the short-term hemodynamic benefits of nitrates and hydralazine are not necessarily sustained during

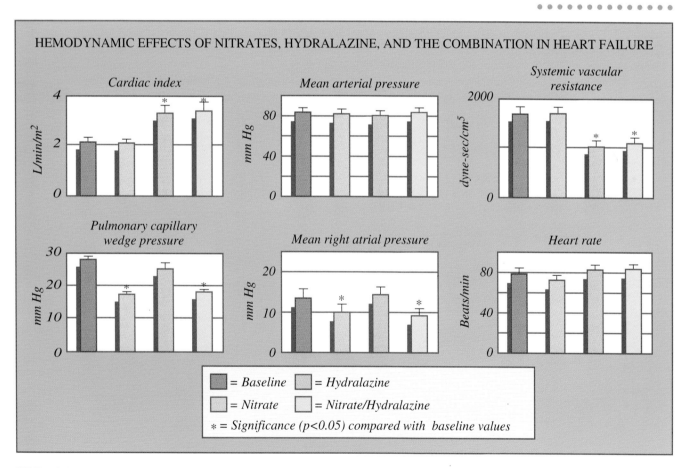

FIGURE 2.37 • Nitrates caused significant changes only in mean right atrial pressure and pulmonary capillary wedge pressure. Hydralazine primarily produced a marked increase in cardiac index and decrease in systemic vascular resistance. Combined therapy resulted in a decrease in both ventricular filling pressures along with an increase in cardiac index. Heart rate and mean arterial pressure were unaffected. (Reproduced with permission. Massie B, Chatterjee K, Werner J, et al: *Am J Cardiol* 1977;40:796.)

long-term treatment. Loss of pharmacologic activity (tolerance) is an important clinical problem with nitrates in chronic heart failure, the magnitude of tolerance development being proportional to the frequency of dosing. With continuous nitrate administration, as with intravenous and transdermal therapy, the initial effects of these drugs are nearly lost in most patients during long-term therapy[238,239] (Figure 2.38). This loss of efficacy, however, can be partially or totally circumvented by separating doses by at least 8 to 12 hrs.[238–241] Similarly, the initial hemodynamic improvement with hydralazine may not be sustained during long-term therapy. Tolerance may occur in up to 30% to 50% of treated patients[242] (Figure 2.39). Tolerance to nitrates and to hydralazine appears to be related to both a loss of the direct vasodilator effects of these drugs and to the activation of endogenous vasoconstrictor mechanisms that limit their circulatory actions.[239,242–244]

Clinical Effects • Five double-blind placebo-controlled clinical trials have investigated the utility of oral isosorbide dinitrate—40 mg four times daily—in patients with chronic heart failure[245–249] (Table 2.25). Although isosorbide dinitrate produced some favorable trends after 2 to 3 months of treatment in most of these studies, the increase in exercise capacity was not consistently greater than that seen with placebo and was not reliably accompanied by the relief of symptoms. Similarly, in five double-blind, placebo-controlled trials, hydralazine, 200 to 300 mg daily, failed to alleviate symptoms or improve effort tolerance.[75,249–252] In a single study with minoxidil, patients treated with the drug actually fared worse than those treated with placebo.[253] Even when hydralazine and isosorbide dinitrate were combined, the vasodilator combination failed to improve the clinical status or exercise capacity of treated patients after 2 to 6 months of therapy.[249]

Nevertheless, the Veterans Administration Vasodilator Heart Failure Trial (V-HeFT) showed that when used in combination with hydralazine and added to digitalis and diuretics, isosorbide dinitrate, 40 mg four times daily, could reduce mortality in patients with mild-to-moderate symptoms[254] (Figure 2.40). The magnitude of the effect was of borderline statistical significance, however, and the combination of both vasodilator drugs was poorly tolerated. During the period of follow-up, 38% of patients had to discontinue one or both of the vasodilators because of side effects. At the end of six months, only 55% of patients were taking full doses of both drugs. Because the side effects appeared to be more frequent with hydralazine than with isosorbide dinitrate and because nitrates used alone are associated with reduced mortality when administered after acute myocardial infarction,[255] many physicians have been tempted to use isosorbide dinitrate alone to prolong life in chronic heart failure. Unfortunately, such an approach cannot be supported by the available data. The reduction in mortality in V-HeFT was related to an increase in the left ventricular ejection fraction,[256] but such an increase is more likely to be seen with hydralazine than with isosorbide dinitrate.[257] In addition, the regression of cellular hypertrophy seen in patients with an idiopathic cardiomyopathy when both vasodilators are combined can be achieved with hydralazine alone but not with isosorbide dinitrate alone.[257] Consequently, the role of nitrate monotherapy in reducing mortality in chronic heart failure remains uncertain. Furthermore, according to the results of the recently completed V-HeFT II Trial, in which the effects of hydralazine plus isosorbide dinitrate on survival were compared to those of enalapril, angiotensin-converting enzyme inhibitors reduced mortality to a greater extent than the combination of the two direct-acting vasodilator drugs[258] (Figure 2.41).

• • • • • • • • • • • • • • • •

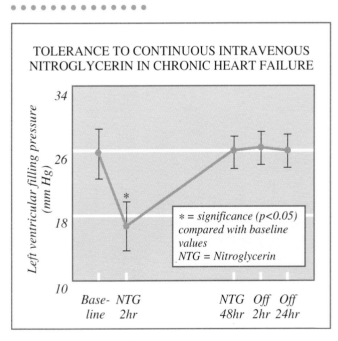

FIGURE 2.38 • Tolerance to continuous intravenous nitroglycerin in chronic heart failure. The initial fall in left ventricular filling pressure is no longer seen after 48 hours of continuous therapy. (Adapted with permission. Packer M, Lee WH, Kessler PD, et al: *N Engl J Med* 1987;317:799.)

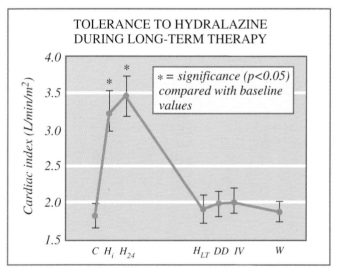

FIGURE 2.39 • Tolerance to hydralazine in patients with chronic heart failure. C is the control period; H_i is the initial dose of oral hydralazine (100 to 200 mg); H_{24} is after 24 hrs of hydralazine (100 to 200 mg every 8 hrs); H_{LT} is the time of hemodynamic reevaluation during long term therapy with oral hydralazine (100 to 200 mg); DD represents a double dose of oral hydralazine (200 to 400 mg); IV represents intravenous administration of 20 mg of hydralazine; and W is 24 to 72 hrs after withdrawal of the drug. (Reproduced with permission Packer M, Meller J, Medina N, et al: *N Engl J Med* 1982;306:57.)

Adverse Reactions • About 5% to 10% of patients with heart failure discontinue nitrates because of adverse reactions—primarily headaches, flushing and dizziness. Side effects are more frequent with hydralazine and minoxidil.[254] Headaches, palpitations, flushing and gastrointestinal distress occur in up to one third of treated patients.[77] Tachycardia and edema are potentially serious complications, especially with minoxidil.[253]

Clinical Use • Although the results of randomized clinical trials have been disappointing, many physicians believe that carefully selected patients can respond favorably to treatment with isosorbide dinitrate or hydralazine. However, because the angiotensin-converting enzyme inhibitors reduce mortality to a greater extent than the direct-acting vasodilators, most clinicians use nitrates and hydralazine only as adjuvant therapy together with other orally effective agents. Nitrates may be particularly

---

TABLE 2.25 • DIRECT-ACTING VASODILATORS— CONTROLLED CLINICAL TRIALS

- Franciosa JA, Nordstrom LA, Cohn JN: Nitrate therapy for congestive heart failure. *JAMA* 1978;240:443.
- Franciosa JA, Goldsmith SR, Cohn JN: Contrasting immediate and long-term effects of isosorbide dinitrate on exercise capacity in congestive heart failure. *Am J Med* 1980;69:559.
- Leier CV, Huss D, Magorien RD, et al: Improved exercise capacity and differing arterial and venous tolerance during chronic isosorbide dinitrate therapy for congestive heart failure. *Circulation* 1983;67:817.
- Aranda JM, Cintron G, Linares E, et al: Acute and long-term effects of Isordil Tembids capsules on cardiac and vascular hemodynamics in patients with congestive heart failure. *Clin Res* 1983;30:825A.

- Cohn JN, Archibald D, Johnson G, et al: Effects of vasodilator therapy on peak oxygen consumption in heart failure: V-HeFT. *Circulation* 1987;75:II-443.
- Franciosa JA, Weber KT, Levine TB, et al: Hydralazine in the long–term treatment of heart failure: Lack of difference from placebo. *Am Heart J* 1982;104:587.
- Conradson TB, Ryden L, Ahlmark G, et al: Clinical efficacy of oral hydralazine in chronic heart failure. One year double-blind placebo controlled study. *Am Heart J* 1984;108:1001.
- Reifart N, Bunge T, Kaltenbach M, et al: Acute effect and long-term treatment with dihydralazine at rest and during exercise in severe chronic heart failure. *Z Kardiol* 1982;71:75.

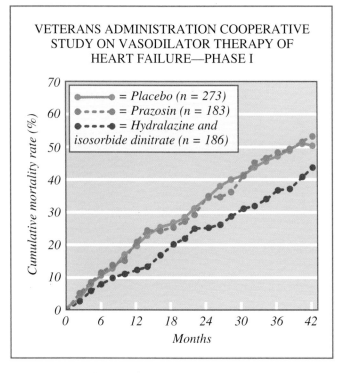

FIGURE 2.40 • Influence of direct-acting vasodilator drugs on mortality in congestive heart failure—The Veterans Administration Cooperative Study on Vasodilator Therapy of Heart Failure (V-HeFT). (Reproduced with permission Cohn JN, Archibald DG, Ziesche S, et al: *N Engl J Med* 1986;314:1547.)

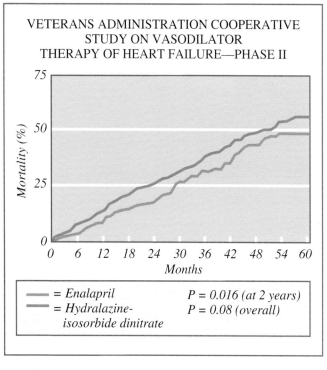

FIGURE 2.41 • Comparative effects of enalapril and the combination of hydralazine and isosorbide dinitrate on mortality in heart failure (V-HeFT II). (Reproduced with permission from Cohn JN, et al: *N Engl J Med* 1991;325:305.)

useful in patients with underlying coronary artery disease. Under such circumstances, intermittent therapy with oral isosorbide dinitrate, 20 to 40 mg twice or three times daily, is preferred over continuous therapy with transdermal nitroglycerin preparations. Hydralazine can be beneficial in patients with underlying severe mitral and aortic regurgitation.[236,237] Controlled trials suggest that the drug may exert long-term favorable effects on ventricular dimensions in such patients even when asymptomatic.[259] Minoxidil should not be used to treat chronic heart failure.

Flosequinan

A new vasodilator drug, flosequinan, exerts dilator effects on both arterial resistance and venous capacitance vessels, but unlike nitroprusside, the drug is effective when given orally and has a long duration of action, permitting once daily dosing[260] (Figures 2.42, 2.43). Short-term therapy with flosequinan, 75 to 100 mg once daily, produces increases in cardiac output and decreases in right and left ventricular filling pressures that are sustained during long-term treatment.[261] Like other vasodilators, flosequinan can activate endogenous neurohormonal systems, which can limit the efficacy of therapy.[262] However, such neurohormonal activation with flosequinan appears to be dose-related. If large doses of 150 mg daily are avoided, the drug can produce long-term hemodynamic and clinical benefits without notable increases in plasma renin activity.[261,262]

Four double-blind placebo-controlled trials have demonstrated that flosequinan, 75 to 100 mg once daily, can improve

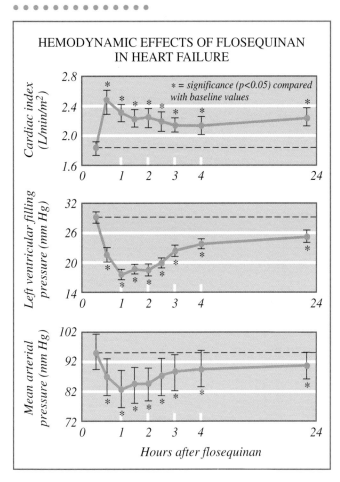

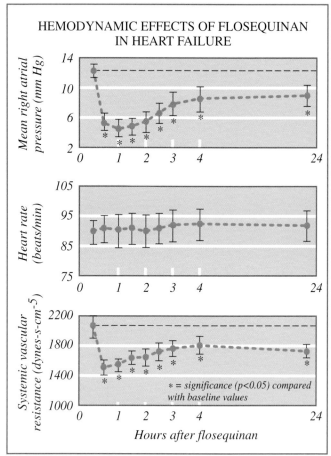

FIGURE 2.42 • Serial changes in cardiac index, left ventricular filling pressure, mean arterial pressure before and after the administration of flosequinan. (Reproduced with permission. Kessler PD, Packer M: *Am Heart J* 1987;113:137.)

FIGURE 2.43 • Mean right atrial pressure, heart rate, and systemic vascular resistance before and after the administration of flosequinan. Format as in Figure 2.42. (Reproduced with permission. Kessler PD, Packer M: *Am Heart J* 1987;113:137.)

exercise tolerance in patients with moderate to severe symptoms[263-266] (Figure 2.44), and the drug produces few side effects that limit long-term therapy. A large-scale trial—the Prospective Randomized Flosequinan Longevity Evaluation (PROFILE)—to evaluate the effect of flosequinan on survival is in progress.

Calcium Channel Blocking Drugs

All calcium channel blocking drugs—verapamil, nifedipine, diltiazem, and nicardipine—exert direct dilating effects on arterial resistance vessels and can increase cardiac output and lower systemic vascular resistance in patients with left ventricular dysfunction.[267,268] As in the case of other arterial vasodilators, however, these beneficial effects on cardiac performance have not been associated with symptomatic benefits or enhanced exercise tolerance in controlled clinical trials[76,269,270] (Table 2.26). In addition, short- and long-term treatment with these drugs can cause serious adverse cardiovascular reactions.[25,270-272] These limitations may be related either to the negative inotropic effects of these drugs or to their ability to activate neurohormonal systems.[273]

During short-term therapy, the cardiodepressant effects of the calcium channel blockers appear to be of primary impor-

tance. All calcium blocking drugs depress cardiac contractility.[26] This action is greatly exaggerated in patients with chronic heart failure who have a profound defect in the delivery of calcium to the contractile proteins[32-34] (refer to the Impaired Contractility section). Consequently, despite a marked reduction in systemic vascular resistance, cardiac performance may deteriorate rapidly following calcium channel blockade.[25] This acute hemodynamic deterioration may be accompanied by serious clinical reactions, including pulmonary edema and cardiogenic shock.

In contrast, during long-term therapy, the stimulatory action of the calcium channel blockers on neurohormonal systems may be more important than their negative inotropic effects.[273] Most calcium channel blockers increase the activity of both the sympathetic nervous system and the renin-angiotensin system.[271,274] Such neurohormonal activation may adversely affect both the clinical status and survival of patients with heart failure.[275] This effect may explain why calcium channel blocking drugs that enhance neurohormonal activity can exacerbate the clinical condition of many patients[270,271] (Figures 2.45, 2.46) and may increase the mortality of patients with congestive

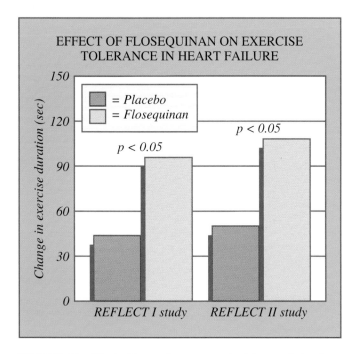

FIGURE 2.44 • Effect of flosequinan on exercise tolerance in heart failure. (Adapted from Packer M, Narahara KA, Elkayam U, et al: *Circulation* 1990;82(suppl II):II-323 and Pitt B, et al: *Circulation* 1991;84(suppl II):II-311.)

TABLE 2.26 • CONTROLLED TRIALS WITH CALCIUM CHANNEL-BLOCKERS IN PATIENTS WITH CHRONIC HEART FAILURE		
	Improved symptoms	Improved ETT
• Agostoni PG, et al, 1986[1]	No	No
• Figulla HR, et al, 1987[2]	No	No
• Tan LB, et al, 1987*	No	No
• Maisch AS, et al, 1988[3]	No	No
• Elkayam U, et al, 1990**	No	No

[1]Agostoni PG, DeCesare N, Doria E, Polese A, Tamborini G, Guazzi MD. Afterload reduciton: a comparison of captopril and nifedipine in dilated cardiomyopathy. *Br Heart J* 1986;55:391–399.

[2]Figulla HR, Luig H, Nieschlag F, Kreuzer H. Klinische und hämodynamische Wirkungen von Nisoldipin und Captopril bei der Herzinsuffinzienz: eine doppel blinde Vergleichsstudie der Kurz und Langzeitwirkungen. *Z Kardiol* 1987;76:167–174.

[3]Maisch B, Hofman J, Borst U, Drude L, Herzum M, Kochsiek K. Nisoldipine in dilated cardiomyopathy. *Circulation* 1988;87(suppl II):II-618.

*Reference 269.

**Reference 270.

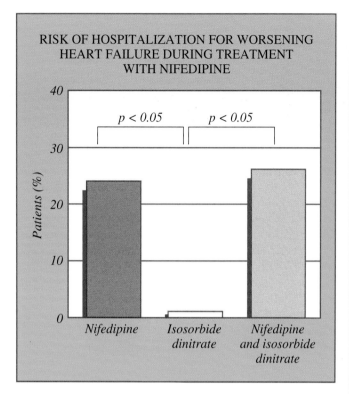

FIGURE 2.45 • Risk of hospitalization for worsening heart failure during treatment with nifedipine. (Adapted from Elkayam U, Amin J, Mehra A, et al: *Circulation* 1991;82:1954-1961.)

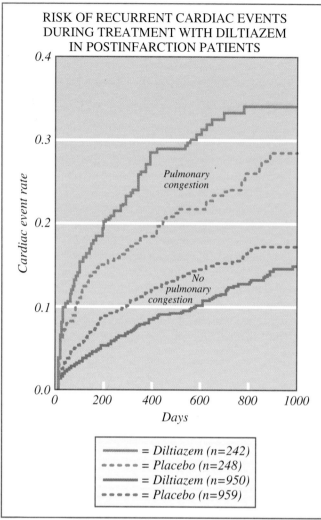

FIGURE 2.47 • Cumulative rate of first recurrent cardiac events in patients with and without pulmonary congestion following an acute myocardial infarction. Patients with pulmonary congestion treated with diltiazem had a higher rate of cardiac events than patients receiving placebo. (Reproduced with permission. Multicenter Diltiazem Postinfarction Research Group: *N Engl J Med* 1988;319:385.)

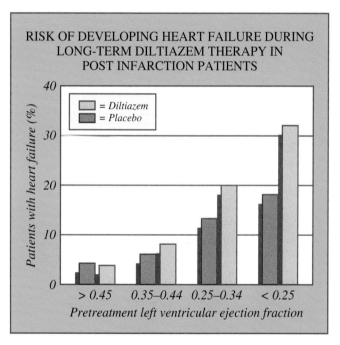

FIGURE 2.46 • Risk of developing heart failure during long-term diltiazem therapy in postinfarction patients. (Reproduced with permission.)

heart failure who have suffered a recent myocardial infarction[27] (Figure 2.47).

Because of ineffectiveness and concerns about safety, presently available calcium channel blocking drugs should not be used to treat chronic heart failure. However, newer calcium channel blockers—felodipine and amlodipine—that reduce neurohormonal activity by enhancing baroreceptor responsiveness, will soon be available. Preliminary results in controlled trials with these new agents suggest that they may prove to be effective agents[276,277] (Figure 2.48).

NEUROHORMONAL ANTAGONISTS

Although direct-acting vasodilator drugs can be used to antagonize the systemic vasoconstriction of chronic heart failure, such agents do not address one of the major causes of vasoconstriction—specifically, neurohormonal activation. Hence, there has been great interest in developing drugs that interfere with the formation or the action of endogenous vasoconstrictor hormones, primarily angiotensin and norepinephrine.

Angiotensin-Converting Enzyme Inhibitors

A large number of angiotensin-converting enzyme (ACE) inhibitors are now commercially available (Table 2.27), although only two agents—captopril and enalapril—have been specifically approved for use in heart failure by the US Food and Drug Administration.

Hemodynamic Effects • All angiotensin-converting enzyme (ACE) inhibitors produce sustained hemodynamic benefits in patients with chronic heart failure. The primary circulatory effect of these drugs is to reduce left ventricular filling pressure at rest and during exercise during long-term treatment.[278] Although these agents also decrease systemic vascular resistance, ACE inhibitors do not produce striking increases in cardiac output or left ventricular ejection fraction.[159,278] Tolerance may occasionally develop during long-term treatment with these drugs, but its occurrence is less common than with other vasodilators, perhaps because ACE inhibitors diminish rather than activate endogenous neurohormonal mechanisms. In fact, the long-term response to captopril, enalapril, and lisinopril in many patients may exceed that seen during initiation of treatment. Even the complete lack of any discernible short-term effect does not preclude long-term benefits in many patients.[278]

Clinical Effects • Angiotensin-converting enzyme inhibitors have produced long-term clinical improvement in a large number of clinical trials, and these responses are superior to the effects seen with other vasodilator drugs[76,159,279–289]

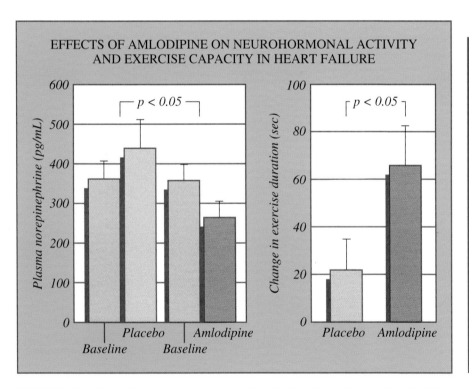

EFFECTS OF AMLODIPINE ON NEUROHORMONAL ACTIVITY AND EXERCISE CAPACITY IN HEART FAILURE

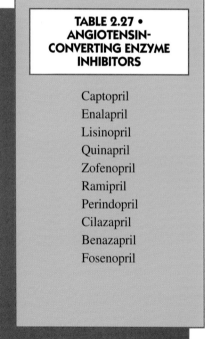

TABLE 2.27 •
ANGIOTENSIN-CONVERTING ENZYME INHIBITORS

Captopril
Enalapril
Lisinopril
Quinapril
Zofenopril
Ramipril
Perindopril
Cilazapril
Benazapril
Fosenopril

FIGURE 2.48 • Effects of amlodipine on neurohormonal activity and exercise capacity in heart failure. (Adapted from Packer M, Nicod P, Khandheria BR, et al: *J Am Coll Cardiol* 1991; 17:274A.)

(Table 2.28 and Figure 2.49). Dyspnea is relieved, exercise tolerance is prolonged (Figure 2.50), and the need for hospitalization and emergency care for worsening heart failure is reduced. This improvement is seen in patients with mild, moderate and severe symptoms, whether or not they are treated with digitalis.[159,279] However, captopril, enalapril and lisinopril should not be used before diuretics in patients with a history of fluid retention, since these drugs cannot control the tendency toward peripheral and pulmonary edema.[290] Nevertheless, the ACE inhibitors may reduce the need for diuretics and potassi-

TABLE 2.28 • ANGIOTENSIN-CONVERTING ENZYME INHIBITORS—CONTROLLED CLINICAL TRIALS

- Captopril Multicenter Research Group: A placebo-controlled trial of captopril in refractory chronic congestive heart failure. *J Am Coll Cardiol* 1983;2:755.
- Sharpe DN, Murphy J, Coxon R, et al: Enalapril in patients with chronic heart failure: A placebo-controlled, randomized, double-blind study. *Circulation* 1984;70:271.
- Chalmers JP, West MJ, Cyran J, et al: Placebo-controlled study of lisinopril in congestive heart failure: A multicenter study. *J Cardiovasc Pharmacol* 1987;9:S89.
- Riegger GAJ: Results of long-term therapy with angiotensin converting-enzyme inhibitor quinapril in patients with congestive heart failure. *Circulation* 1987;76:IV-178.
- Captopril-Digoxin Multicenter Research Group: Comparative effects of captopril and digoxin in patients with mild to moderate heart failure. *JAMA* 1988;259:539.
- Cleland JGF, Dargie HG, Hodsman GP, et al: Captopril in heart failure: A double-blind controlled trial. *Br Heart J* 1984;52:530.
- Cleland JGF, Dargie HG, Ball SG, et al: Effects of enalapril in heart failure: A double-blind study of effects on exercise performance, renal failure, hormones, and metabolic state. *Br Heart J* 1985;54:305.
- Cowley AJ, Rowley JM, Stainer KL, et al: Captopril therapy for heart failure. A placebo-controlled study. *Lancet* 1982;2:730.
- Creager MA, Massie BM, Faxon DP, et al: Acute and long-term effects of enalapril on the cardiovascular response to exercise and exercise tolerance in patients with congestive heart failure. *J Am Coll Cardiol* 1985;6:163.
- Drexler H, Banhardt U, Meinertz T, et al: Contrasting peripheral short-term and long-term effects of converting enzyme inhibition in patients with congestive heart failure. A double-blind, placebo-controlled trial. *Circulation* 1989;79:491.

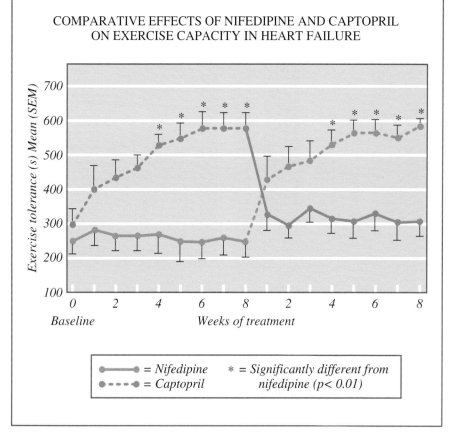

COMPARATIVE EFFECTS OF NIFEDIPINE AND CAPTOPRIL ON EXERCISE CAPACITY IN HEART FAILURE

= Nifedipine
= Captopril
* = Significantly different from nifedipine (p< 0.01)

FIGURE 2.49 • Comparative effects of nifedipine and captopril on exercise capacity in heart failure. (Reproduced with permission. Agostini PG, DeCeare N, Doria E, et al: *Br Heart J* 1986;55:394.)

um supplements,[159,217] may correct hyponatremia and hypokalemia,[117,284,285] and may decrease the frequency and complexity of ventricular arrhythmias[284,285] (Table 2.29). Most important, ACE inhibitors prolong life in patients with chronic heart failure.

In the Cooperative North Scandinavian Enalapril Survival Study (CONSENSUS), long-term treatment with enalapril markedly reduced the mortality of patients with severe (Class IV) symptoms[291] (Figure 2.51). Enalapril also reduced the mortality of patients with mild-to-moderate symptoms (Class II and III) and

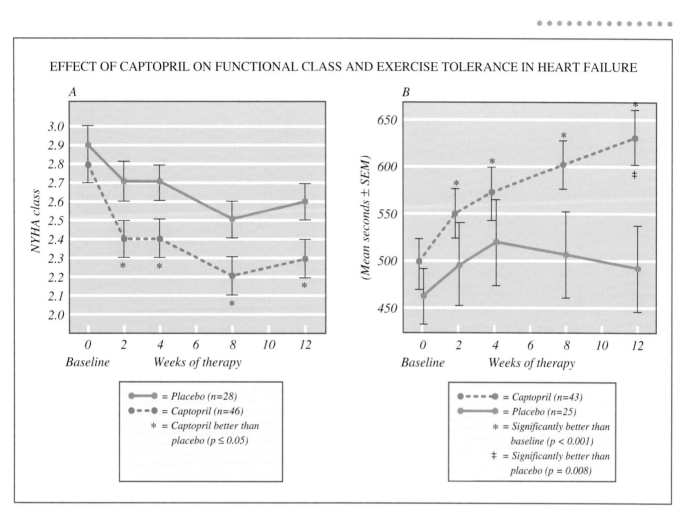

EFFECT OF CAPTOPRIL ON FUNCTIONAL CLASS AND EXERCISE TOLERANCE IN HEART FAILURE

A

= Placebo (n=28)
= Captopril (n=46)
* = Captopril better than placebo (p ≤ 0.05)

B

= Captopril (n=43)
= Placebo (n=25)
* = Significantly better than baseline (p < 0.001)
‡ = Significantly better than placebo (p = 0.008)

FIGURE 2.50 • Effect of captopril on New York Heart Association (NYHA) functional class (A) and exercise tolerance time (B) of patients with moderately severe heart failure. (Reproduced with permission. Captopril Multicenter Research Group: *J Am Coll Cardiol* 983;2:755.)

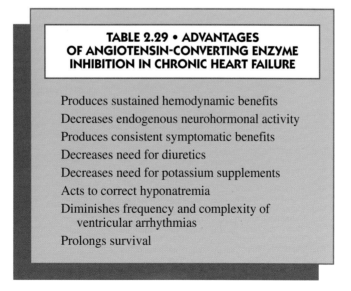

TABLE 2.29 • ADVANTAGES OF ANGIOTENSIN-CONVERTING ENZYME INHIBITION IN CHRONIC HEART FAILURE

Produces sustained hemodynamic benefits
Decreases endogenous neurohormonal activity
Produces consistent symptomatic benefits
Decreases need for diuretics
Decreases need for potassium supplements
Acts to correct hyponatremia
Diminishes frequency and complexity of ventricular arrhythmias
Prolongs survival

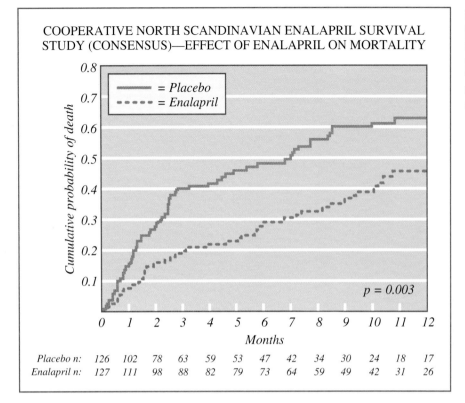

COOPERATIVE NORTH SCANDINAVIAN ENALAPRIL SURVIVAL
STUDY (CONSENSUS)—EFFECT OF ENALAPRIL ON MORTALITY

| Placebo n: | 126 | 102 | 78 | 63 | 59 | 53 | 47 | 42 | 34 | 30 | 24 | 18 | 17 |
| Enalapril n: | 127 | 111 | 98 | 88 | 82 | 79 | 73 | 64 | 59 | 49 | 42 | 31 | 26 |

FIGURE 2.51 • Influence of converting-enzyme inhibition with enalapril on mortality in severe chronic congestive heart failure—The Cooperative Northern Scandinavian Enalapril Survival Study (CONSENSUS) Trial (Reproduced with permission. The CONSENSUS Trial Study Group: *N Engl J Med* 1987;316:1429.)

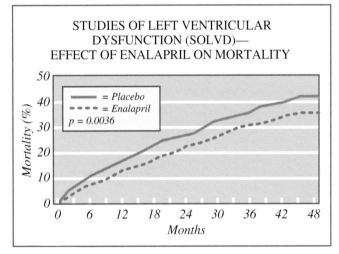

FIGURE 2.52 • Effect of enalapril on mortality in patients with mild-to-moderate heart failure. Results of the Studies of Left Ventricular Dysfunction (SOLVD) study. (Reproduced with permission. The SOLVD Investigators: *N Engl J Med* 1991;325:297.)

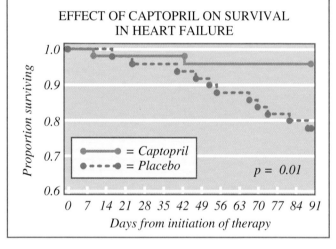

FIGURE 2.53 • Effect of captopril on survival in moderate-to-severe heart failure. (Reproduced with permission. Newman TJ, Maskin CS, Dennick LG, et al: *Am J Med* 1988;84:142.)

Treatment of Congestive Heart Failure

the risk of developing heart failure in patients with asymptomatic left ventricular dysfunction (Class I) in the recently completed Studies of Left Ventricular Dysfunction (SOLVD) trial[292] (Figure 2.52). Available data suggest that favorable effects on survival are seen with other ACE inhibitors, such as captopril[293] (Figure 2.53). Angiotensin-converting enzyme inhibitors may even retard the progression of left ventricular dysfunction in asymptomatic patients[294,295] (Figure 2.54).

Adverse Effects • The principal adverse effects of angiotensin-converting enzyme inhibition in heart failure are systemic hypotension, functional renal insufficiency and potassium retention[222] (Tables 2.30–2.32).

Hypotension • Blood pressure declines in nearly every patient who receives treatment with an ACE inhibitor, but these decreases, although occasionally quite marked, are usually asymptomatic. Hence, hypotension is a concern only if it is accompanied by dizziness, blurred vision or syncope. Such events

may occur at any time during the course of treatment but are seen most frequently during the first 24 hrs of therapy.[118]

Patients with extreme activation of the renin-angiotensin system are most likely to experience early hypotensive reactions. Such patients can be identified clinically by the presence of marked hyponatremia—serum sodium concentration less than 130 mmol/L—or by the recent occurrence of a profound diuresis.[118] In such individuals, converting-enzyme inhibitors should be initiated cautiously and in small doses—6.25 mg of captopril or 2.5 mg of enalapril or lisinopril). Attempts to decrease dependence of the patient on the renin-angiotensin system by withholding diuretics for 1 to 2 days may enhance the margin of safety. Should symptomatic hypotension occur with first doses, it may not recur with repeated administration of the same doses. However, it is prudent under such circumstances to reduce angiotensin dependence—by discontinuation of diuretics and/or liberalization of dietary salt—

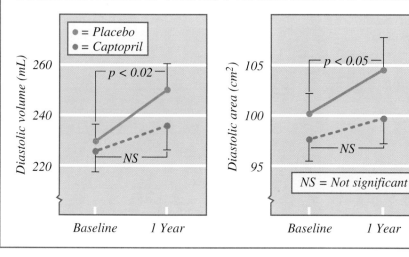

EFFECT OF CAPTOPRIL ON DIASTOLIC DIMENSIONS IN POST-INFARCTION PATIENTS WITH LEFT VENTRICULAR DYSFUNCTION

● = Placebo
● = Captopril

NS = Not significant

Baseline   1 Year

Baseline   1 Year

FIGURE 2.54 • Effect of captopril on diastolic dimensions in postinfarction patients with left ventricular dysfunction. Progressive dilatation of the left ventricle was seen only in the placebo group. (Reproduced with permission. Pfeffer MA, Lamas GA, Vaugh DE, et al: *N Engl J Med* 1986;319:83.)

TABLE 2.30 • ANGIOTENSIN CONVERTING ENZYME (ACE) INHIBITORS—CLASSIFICATION OF ADVERSE EFFECTS

Sodium-sensitive side effects
• Hypotension
• Functional renal insufficiency
• Potassium retention

Effects common to all ACE inhibitors
• Cough
• Angioneurotic edema

Effects of sulfhydryl-containing ACE inhibitors
• Rash
• Dysgeusia

TABLE 2.31 • ANGIOTENSIN CONVERTING ENZYME (ACE) INHIBITORS—RISK FACTORS FOR SODIUM-SENSITIVE SIDE EFFECTS

All risk factors are indicators of patients with marked activation of the renin-angiotensin system

• Sodium depletion
• High dose diuretic therapy

• Hyponatremia
• Advanced severity of symptoms

Class I	0%-10%
Class II	5%-20%
Class III	15%-30%
Class IV	30%-50%

Percentages indicate risk of sodium-sensitive side effects in patients with different functional classes.

before attempting to reinstitute treatment. Most patients who experience symptomatic hypotension remain excellent candidates for long-term angiotensin-converting enzyme inhibition, if appropriate measures are taken to minimize recurrent hypotensive reactions.

Functional Renal Insufficiency • Renal function may deteriorate during treatment with converting-enzyme inhibitors due to loss of angiotensin's vasoconstrictor effect on the efferent arteriole. The risk of functional renal insufficiency is increased by:

• The presence of hyponatremia.
• The use of high-dose diuretics.
• Diabetes mellitus.
• The use of long-acting ACE inhibitors.
• Advanced severity of symptoms.[296–299]

Functional renal insufficiency develops in 30% to 50% of patients with Class III and IV heart failure (in whom hyponatremia is common) but in only 5% to 20% of patients with Class II symptoms (in whom hyponatremia is rare).[298,299] As in the case of hypotension, azotemia can be ameliorated by reducing the dose of concomitantly administered diuretics, and thus, can generally be managed without withdrawing treatment.[217]

Potassium Retention • Hyperkalemia can occur during angiotensin-converting enzyme inhibition in patients with congestive heart failure and may be sufficient to cause cardiac conduction disturbances and heart block.[300,301] Such events usually occur, however, in patients who are taking potassium-sparing diuretics or large doses of oral potassium supplements.[222]

Noncirculatory adverse reactions may occur during treatment with ACE inhibitors. The most common reaction is cough—5% to 10%—which usually requires the withdrawal of therapy. The most serious reaction is angioneurotic edema. Both may be related to the accumulation of tissue kinins. Rash and dysgeusia may be seen during treatment with all ACE inhibitors, but are more frequent with captopril than with enalapril or lisinopril.

• • • • • • • • • • • • • • • •

TABLE 2.32 • ANGIOTENSIN-CONVERTING ENZYME (ACE) INHIBITORS—MANAGEMENT OF ADVERSE EFFECTS

Sodium-sensitive side effects
• Reduce dose of concomitant diuretic
• Reduce dose of ACE inhibitor
Effects common to all ACE inhibitors
• Discontinue ACE inhibitor
Effects characteristics of some ACE inhibitors
• Change to a nonsulfhydryl agent

TABLE 2.33 • ANGIOTENSIN-CONVERTING ENZYME (ACE) INHIBITORS—APPROACH TO CLINICAL USE

Initiate with low doses and then increase until dose is within therapeutic range. Lower doses used only if target doses (shown below) are not tolerated.
• Captopril 50 mg three times daily
• Enalapril 10 mg twice daily
• Lisinopril 20 mg once daily
Enhance tolerability of converting-enzyme inhibitors by reducing doses of concomitantly administered diuretic agents

---

TABLE 2.34 • FACTORS THAT DO NOT PREDICT THE LONG-TERM RESPONSE TO ANGIOTENSIN-CONVERTING ENZYME INHIBITIONS IN HEART FAILURE

Age
Sex
Cause of heart failure
Severity of heart failure
Left ventricular ejection fraction
Cardiac output and pulmonary wedge pressure
Initial hemodynamic response to the drug
Plasma renin activity

TABLE 2.35 • ANGIOTENSIN-CONVERTING ENZYME (ACE) INHIBITORS—PATIENTS LEAST LIKELY TO RESPOND TO THERAPY

Positive sodium balance attenuates response to ACE inhibitors. Thus,
• Patients with peripheral edema and those with markedly increased central venous pressures—mean right atrial pressures greater than 12 mm Hg—show reduced efficacy with these drugs.
Renal insufficiency impairs response to these drugs. Thus,
• Patients with serum creatinine > 3.0 mg/dL show reduced efficacy.

Clinical Use • Angiotensin-converting enzyme (ACE) inhibitors are generally initiated in small doses, which are then rapidly increased into the therapeutic range within 1 to 2 weeks (Table 2.33). The effective dose of an ACE inhibitor for most patients with heart failure remains unknown. Although some patients may respond favorably to low doses—for example 37.5 to 75 mg daily of captopril or 5 to 10 mg daily of enalapril or lisinopril—nearly all of the controlled trials that have shown that these agents can improve exercise tolerance or prolong life have employed large doses—150 to 300 mg daily of captopril, 20 to 40 mg daily of enalapril or 20 mg daily of lisinopril. Treatment should be continued for at least 3 to 4 weeks to determine if an individual patient will respond favorably to treatment. The full therapeutic effect may not become evident for 3 to 6 months.[279,302]

Although approximately 60% to 70% of patients with chronic heart failure improve symptomatically during long-term treatment with an ACE inhibitor, it is difficult to predict the response to these drugs short of a therapeutic trial. Neither the pretreatment hemodynamic state nor the plasma renin activity accurately presages the long-term effects of treatment[277,303] (Table 2.34). Among all of the variables that have been examined, only two pretreatment variables predict the clinical efficacy of converting-enzyme inhibitors—renal function and mean right atrial pressure.[304] Only 35% of patients who have both a mean right atrial pressure greater than 12 mm Hg and a serum creatinine concentration greater than 1.5 mg/dL will improve symptomatically, but if values for the two variables are low, nearly 85% will show sustained benefits (Table 2.35).

Antagonists of the Sympathetic Nervous System

α-Adrenergic Receptor Antagonists • The short-term administration of α-adrenergic antagonists, such as prazosin, produce marked hemodynamic effects in patients with chronic heart failure,[305] but double-blind placebo-controlled trials have shown that these drugs are no more effective than placebo in ameliorating symptoms, enhancing exercise tolerance or improving survival (refer to Figure 2.40).[254,306–308] The primary mechanism limiting the utility of α-adrenergic antagonists is the development of long-term tolerance to the pharmacologic actions of these drugs.[309,310]

ß-Adrenergic Receptor Antagonists • In contrast to other agents that have been used to treat chronic heart failure, the β-blocking drugs do not generally produce immediate hemodynamic benefits. In fact, cardiac function may deteriorate after the initiation of β-blockade due to interference with the positive inotropic actions of the sympathetic nervous system.[311] However, long-term therapy with some β-blockers—specifically, metoprolol 100 mg daily (Figure 2.55), bucindolol 200 mg daily (Figure 2.56), and carvedilol 50 mg daily—appears to improve cardiac performance, symptoms and perhaps exercise tolerance in some patients with an idiopathic dilated cardiomyopathy[312,313] by antagonizing the deleterious effects of prolonged adrenergic activation. Uncontrolled and controlled observations, both in patients with and without coronary artery disease, also suggest a favorable effect of β-blockers on the survival of patients with chronic heart failure[314,315] (Figure 2.57). Large-scale survival trials are now being planned.

However, little is known about how to select patients with chronic heart failure for treatment with β-adrenergic blocking drugs. The most marked hemodynamic and clinical improvement has been noted in patients without coronary artery disease[316] and those with the most advanced heart failure, as indicated by a very low left ventricular ejection fraction, a high resting heart rate and a high pretreatment plasma norepinephrine[312,313,317] (Table 2.36). However, these same pa-

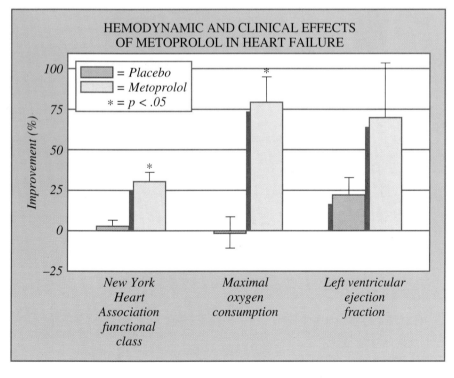

FIGURE 2.55 • Percent improvement in mean functional class, exercise capacity, and left ventricular ejection fraction during long-term metoprolol therapy in patients with an idiopathic dilated cardiomyopathy. (Reproduced with permission. Engelmeier RS, O'Connell JB, Walsh, et al: *Circulation* 1985;72:542 and the American Heart Association.)

tients—those with the most advanced cardiac dysfunction and highest plasma norepinephrine—are also most likely to experience clinical deterioration during initiation of treatment.[318,319] This pattern of response closely resembles that seen with the angiotensin-converting enzyme inhibitors, which also produce the highest frequency of adverse effects in patients most likely to benefit from treatment.[11,118] Fortunately, the early clinical instability seen with β-blockers is usually transient, and thus, as in the case of the converting-enzyme inhibitors, its occurrence is not necessarily a reason to withdraw treatment. Yet, because of the possibility of early deterioration, therapy with β-blockers is generally begun very cautiously with extremely low doses, (for example, 6.25 mg of metoprolol) followed by small increments achieved gradually over long periods of time. As with the angiotensin-converting enzyme inhibitors, a favorable clinical response to β-blockers in chronic heart failure may not become apparent for 2 to 6 months. This observation may explain why symptoms have not improved in trials that treated patients with β-blockers for only 1 month.[320,321]

Despite these early encouraging results, the use of β-blocking drugs in the management of chronic heart failure should be considered investigational at the present time. Experience with these drugs is limited. Rational selection of an appropriate dose

and appropriate patient population remains undefined and the long-term effects of these drugs have not been elucidated.

THERAPEUTIC APPROACH

As stated earlier, the goals of therapy in the management of chronic heart failure are:

- The amelioration of the symptoms of dyspnea and fatigue at rest or during exercise.
- The reduction of the need for hospitalization and emergency care for worsening symptoms.
- Prolongation of life.

These goals cannot be achieved with a single agent. Diuretics can control fluid retention, but when used alone they cannot maintain long-term clinical stability even in minimally symptomatic patients.[159] Digoxin improves the symptoms of heart failure and reduces long-term cardiovascular morbidity, but the effect of the drug on mortality is unknown. Angiotensin-converting enzyme (ACE) inhibitors improve symptoms and decrease both morbidity and mortality, but they cannot prevent fluid retention.[290] Hence, to achieve the goals of therapy in heart failure, the complementary actions of digoxin, diuretics, and ACE inhibitors need to be combined in an effort to improve symptoms, reduce the risk of clinical progression and to prolong

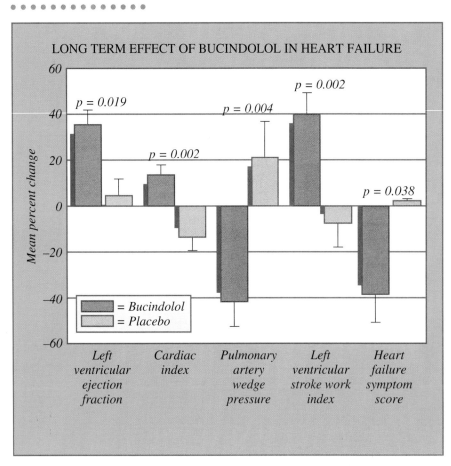

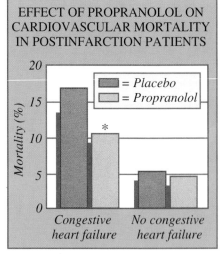

FIGURE 2.57 • Effect of propranolol on cardiovascular mortality in postinfarction patients with and without heart failure at the time of initial evaluation. Beta-blockade reduced cardiovascular mortality by 32% (p< 0.05) in patients with heart failure, but not significantly in patients without heart failure. (Reproduced with permission. Chadda K, Goldstein S, Byington R, et al: *Circulation* 1986;73:508 and the American Heart Association.)

FIGURE 2.56 • Effect of long-term bucindolol therapy on hemodynamic and clinical variables in patients with chronic heart failure. (Reproduced with permission. Gilbert EM, Anderson JL, Deitchman D, et al: *Am J Med* 1990;88:228.)

life. Even when minimally symptomatic, no patient with chronic heart failure should be treated with a single drug.[152]

Should all three first-line drugs be prescribed the first time the patient with chronic heart failure is seen by the physician? Therapy with diuretics should be used first to rapidly control symptoms of pulmonary congestion and to relieve edema. Additional therapy might be best withheld temporarily until this rapid diuretic phase has been completed. Premature institution of treatment with digitalis could increase the risk of digitalis toxicity if the diuresis has produced important potassium deficits. Similarly, premature institution of therapy with a converting-enzyme inhibitor could cause symptomatic hypotension if the diuresis has increased the circulation's dependency on angiotensin II. However, digoxin and an ACE inhibitor should be started once steady-state conditions have been achieved. This goal can generally be accomplished within 1 to 2 weeks after the acute symptoms of pulmonary and systemic congestion have subsided.

What is the role of direct-acting vasodilators and β-adrenergic blockers? Many patients with chronic heart failure remain symptomatic despite treatment with digitalis, diuretics and converting-enzyme inhibitors, and many of these individuals have responded favorably—in both controlled and uncontrolled reports—to treatment with a combination of hydralazine and isosorbide dinitrate, flosequinan, felodipine, amlodipine, or a β-blocker. Yet, little is known about which of these therapeutic interventions should be preferred or about the effect of these drugs on survival. Large-scale studies are in progress to investigate the effects of direct-acting vasodilators (flosequinan, felodipine and amlodipine) on mortality in chronic heart failure in patients who were treated with digoxin, diuretics and an ACE inhibitor. Should one of these drugs be shown to reduce mortality, it will become an indispensable part of heart failure treatment. and will join the first-line drugs that are already available. Conversely, should one of these drugs be shown to increase the risk of death, it will be discarded. Until such trials are completed, the choice of additional therapy in patients who remain symptomatic on conventional therapy will largely be guided by therapeutic trial and error.

PHARMACOLOGIC TREATMENT OF UNSTABLE HEART FAILURE

Patients with unstable heart failure have many of the pathophysiologic and clinical features of patients with chronic stable heart failure, except that the circulatory derangement is severe enough to be immediately life-threatening, unless treated aggressively. The clinical manifestations vary across a wide spectrum, from clinical states dominated by pulmonary congestion (pulmonary edema) to emergencies characterized by peripheral hypoperfusion (cardiogenic shock), or a combination of these features. The principal goals of treatment are immediate hemodynamic and clinical stabilization.

PULMONARY CONGESTION— ACUTE PULMONARY EDEMA

The cardinal symptom of pulmonary congestion is dyspnea at rest and the principal physical finding is pulmonary rales. The primary pathophysiologic feature is the massive transudation of fluid from the pulmonary capillaries into the alveolar space. Pulmonary congestion may develop in a patient without a previous history of heart failure or may complicate the course of a patient with long-standing disease. If severe, abrupt and accompanied by clinical evidence of sympathetic overactivity—tachycardia, diaphoresis and vasoconstriction—the syndrome is designated as acute pulmonary edema. Acute pulmonary edema is most commonly caused by cardiogenic disorders or direct injury to the alveolar-capillary membrane. Unusual causes of pulmonary edema include high-altitude stress, diseases of the central nervous system, narcotic overdose, pulmonary embolism and the delayed effects of cardiac procedures—cardioversion and cardiopulmonary bypass (Table 2.37).

Regardless of the cause, the syndrome of pulmonary edema is related to an imbalance in the factors that modulate the transport of fluid from the pulmonary microcirculation to the interstitial space of the lung. Under normal conditions, fluid is fil-

---

TABLE 2.36 • β-ADRENERGIC BLOCKERS— CONDITIONS MOST LIKELY TO RESPOND TO THERAPY

Idiopathic dilated cardiomyopathy

Elevated pretreatment heart rate

Elevated pretreatment plasma norepinephrine

Markedly decreased left ventricular ejection fraction

TABLE 2.37 • CAUSES OF ACUTE PULMONARY EDEMA

Congestive heart failure

Direct injury to alveolar-capillary membrane

High-altitude stress

Diseases of the central nervous system

Narcotic overdose

Pulmonary embolism

Complication of cardioversion

Complication of cardiopulmonary bypass

tered into the interstitial space and removed by the pulmonary lymphatic system. Pulmonary edema occurs when the rate of fluid transudation exceeds the drainage capacity of the lymphatics.[322] This may happen if the pulmonary capillary hydrostatic pressure exceeds the capillary colloid osmotic pressure (heart failure) or when the pulmonary alveolar membrane is injured, as is the case in patients with adult respiratory distress syndrome. When the cause of pulmonary edema is heart failure, the primary hemodynamic abnormality is a marked increase in pulmonary venous pressures. Consequently, the goal of all pharmacologic interventions for cardiogenic pulmonary edema is the rapid reduction of pulmonary venous pressures.

Several general measures are advisable for most patients with pulmonary congestion. Every effort should be made to identify an underlying precipitating factor, since its correction is often critical to the success of treatment. Bed rest should be enforced. Patients usually feel most comfortable in the upright position, since gravity enhances the peripheral pooling of blood. Special attention should be devoted to maintaining adequate oxygenation. This goal may be achieved simply by increasing the concentration of inspired oxygen or it may require endotracheal intubation and mechanical ventilation.

As in the treatment of stable heart failure, pharmacologic interventions that are useful in the treatment of pulmonary edema include:

- Neurohormonal antagonists (morphine).
- Diuretic drugs (furosemide).
- Direct-acting vasodilators (nitroglycerin and nitroprusside).
- Positive inotropic agents (dobutamine and amrinone).

Because of the need for rapid and reliable treatment, these interventions are generally administered intravenously.

Morphine

Morphine remains the most effective single agent for the treatment of cardiogenic pulmonary edema. The drug reduces pulmonary artery and pulmonary venous pressures and produces rapid symptomatic improvement, both in the experimental and

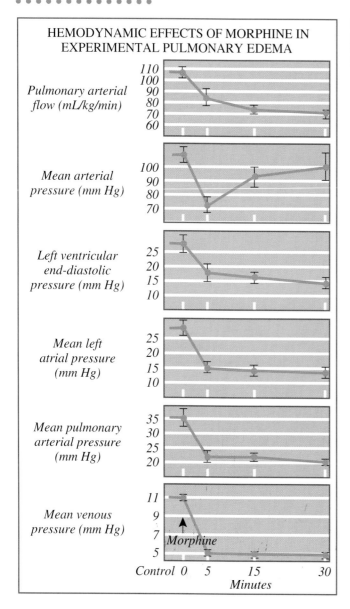

HEMODYNAMIC EFFECTS OF MORPHINE IN EXPERIMENTAL PULMONARY EDEMA

FIGURE 2.58 • Hemodynamic effects of morphine in dogs with experimental pulmonary edema induced by aortic or mitral regurgitation. (Reproduced with permission. Vasko JS, Henney RP, Oldman HN, et al: *Am J Cardiol* 1966;18:879.)

clinical settings[323,324] (Figure 2.58). Morphine achieves these hemodynamic and clinical benefits by causing arteriolar and venous dilatation through its ability to antagonize the peripheral vasoconstrictor effects of the sympathetic nervous system.[324–327] The drug not only attenuates peripheral adrenergic activity directly, but it also reduces the reflex arteriolar vasoconstriction that accompanies hypercapnia.[328] The precise site of the vasodilation produced by morphine is uncertain. The magnitude of venodilation in the limbs is insufficient to explain the hemodynamic actions of the drug.[324] Instead, morphine may act primarily to increase pooling in the splanchnic circulation as a result of arteriolar dilation and passive filling of previously unperfused mesenteric venous segments.[324,329] Regardless of its precise locus of action, however, morphine is not a direct-acting vasodilator.[330] Since it exerts beneficial hemodynamic effects only in hyperadrenergic states,[323,326] it acts principally as a neurohormonal antagonist. In addition, morphine blunts the chemoreceptor-mediated ventilatory reflexes that trigger the severe tachypnea characteristic of pulmonary edema; by doing so, the drug reduces the work of breathing and, consequently, oxygen demand.[331]

Morphine is administered in intermittent doses of 2 to 4 mg intravenously, until dyspnea is relieved and the diaphoresis subsides, or a dose of 10 to 15 mg is given. The patient should be monitored for respiratory depression, which can be reversed by narcotic antagonists.

Diuretics

Rapidly-acting intravenous loop diuretics can elicit a prompt diuresis in patients with pulmonary edema, and in doing so, these drugs can reduce pulmonary venous pressures by reducing total blood volume. However, loop diuretics may relieve pulmonary edema even before a diuresis has occurred (Figure 2.59). These immediate benefits are the direct result of the ability of these drugs to cause peripheral arterial and venous dilatation due to the release of prostaglandins from the kidney.[211,212] This direct vasodilator action is the primary advantage of loop diuretics over thiazide diuretics in the treatment of pulmonary edema. Although loop diuretics are more potent and have a faster onset of action than the thiazides, the rapidity of diuresis does not determine the clinical response to treatment in patients with acute pulmonary congestion.[332] Vasodilation, not diuresis, comprises the principal mechanism of symptom relief in pulmonary edema.

Furosemide is the most commonly used loop diuretic in the treatment of pulmonary edema. The dose of the drug is determined by the prior exposure of the patient to diuretic therapy. In patients who have never received loop diuretics, treatment is usually begun with low doses, 40 to 60 mg intravenously. Patients treated with diuretics chronically may require very large doses of the drug, 120 to 200 mg intravenously. Furosemide is usually well tolerated, although hypotension may occur when the drug is administered to patients with acute heart failure following an acute myocardial infarction. In these patients, pulmonary congestion may be related primarily to diastolic dysfunction and not volume overload.

Nitroprusside and Nitroglycerin

Although direct vasodilation can be achieved in patients with pulmonary edema through the use of sublingual nitroglycerin

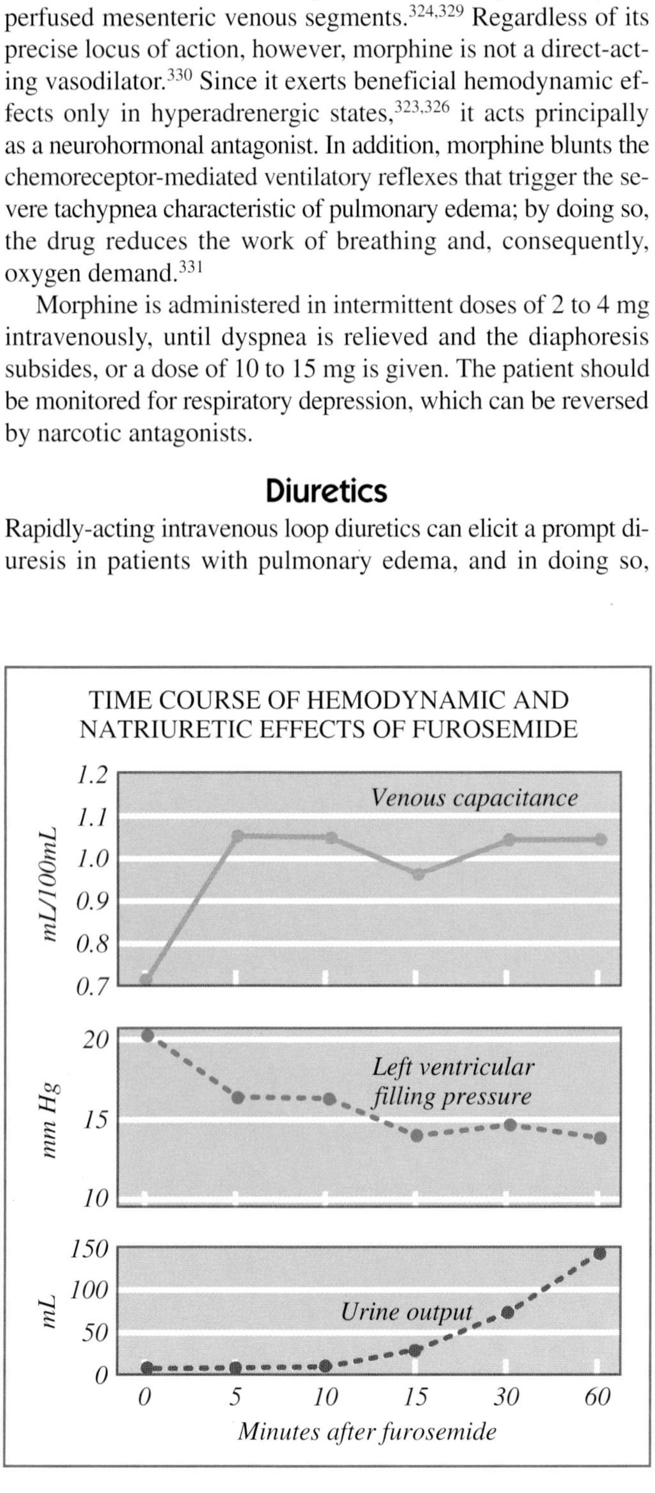

TIME COURSE OF HEMODYNAMIC AND NATRIURETIC EFFECTS OF FUROSEMIDE

FIGURE 2.59 • Temporal changes in mean left ventricular filling pressure, calf venous capacitance, and total urine output after intravenous furosemide. The decrease in left ventricular filling pressure within the first 15 mins is accompanied by a simultaneous increase in calf venous capacitance, during which there was an insignificant increase in urine output. Hence, the hemodynamic benefits of the drug were not solely related to its diuretic actions. (Reproduced with permission. Dikshit K, Vyden JK, Forrester JS, et al: *N Engl J Med* 288:1089.)

or oral isosorbide dinitrate, the intravenous infusion of either nitroprusside or nitroglycerin offers a more reliable and titratable therapeutic approach.

Hemodynamic Effects • By stimulating guanylate cyclase within the vascular smooth muscle cell, both nitroprusside and nitroglycerin exert dilating effects on arterial resistance and venous capacitance vessels.[226] The predominant site of action of both drugs usually depends on the dose being administered. When small doses are infused, both nitroprusside and nitroglycerin act principally on peripheral veins, and thus, reduce right and left ventricular filling pressures. When large doses are infused, both drugs exert dilating effects on arterial resistance vessels as well, and thus, act to enhance cardiac output.[333,334] The belief that nitroprusside exerts "balanced" peripheral effects but that nitroglycerin is only a venodilator stems largely from studies that have compared small doses of nitroglycerin to large doses of nitroprusside.[335]

Nevertheless, nitroprusside and nitroglycerin differ in important ways. Since the magnitude of arterial vasodilatation achieved with nitroprusside is greater than with nitroglycerin, nitroprusside has a greater potential to produce systemic hypotension. This hypotensive action may explain why nitro-

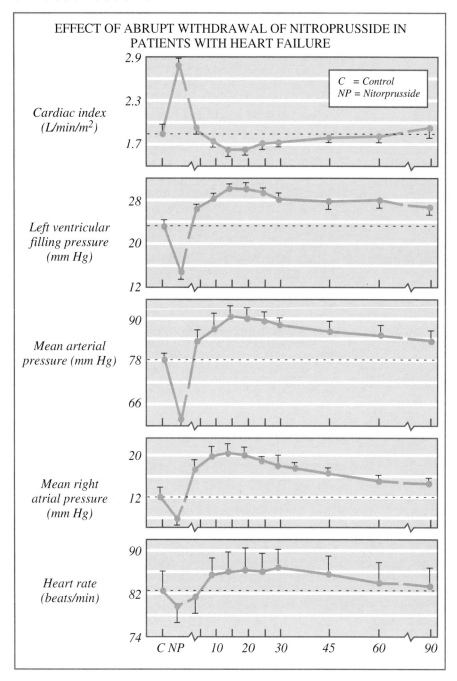

EFFECT OF ABRUPT WITHDRAWAL OF NITROPRUSSIDE IN
PATIENTS WITH HEART FAILURE

C = Control
NP = Nitorprusside

Cardiac index (L/min/m²)

Left ventricular filling pressure (mm Hg)

Mean arterial pressure (mm Hg)

Mean right atrial pressure (mm Hg)

Heart rate (beats/min)

C NP   10   20   30   45   60   90

FIGURE 2.60 • Changes in cardiac index, left ventricular filling pressure, mean arterial pressure, mean right atrial pressure, and heart rate before, during, and at 5-min intervals after discontinuation of nitroprusside administration. (Reproduced with permission. Packer M, Meller J, Medina N, et al: *N Engl J Med* 1979;301:1196.)

prusside, but not nitroglycerin, has been reported to reduce myocardial blood flow to ischemic cardiac tissue,[336,337] although this difference may be of little clinical relevance when the two drugs are titrated to achieve similar hemodynamic effects.[338] However, the greater arterial vasodilator effect of nitroprusside may also lead to more marked neurohormonal activation during infusion of the drug. This may explain why rebound hemodynamic effects following abrupt drug withdrawal occur more frequently with nitroprusside than with nitroglycerin[339] (Figure 2.60). The hemodynamic differences between nitroprusside and nitroglycerin become more marked during prolonged infusions of the drugs, since long-term exposure to nitroglycerin, but not nitroprusside, is predictably accompanied by the development of tolerance.[239,340]

Clinical Use • Therapy with both nitroprusside and nitroglycerin is usually initiated as a continuous low-dose intravenous infusion, the rate of which is increased to achieve specific hemodynamic or clinical goals. The initial infusion rate for both drugs is commonly 10 μg/min, and the rate may be increased to as much as 300 μg/min to achieve desired results.

Nitroglycerin is considered the agent of choice in patients with underlying ischemic heart disease. Nitroprusside is preferred for patients who have severe hypertension or valvular regurgitation.

Adverse Effects • Hypotension is the most common and most serious side effect of both nitroprusside and nitroglycerin. Thus, infusions of the drugs require close continuous monitoring of vital signs, frequently with the aid of a right heart catheter and indwelling arterial line (Table 2.38). Symptomatic hypotension is frequently associated with bradycardia, not tachycardia, particularly when nitroglycerin is used.[341] Both drugs can cause pulmonary vasodilatation, which can aggravate arterial hypoxemia in patients with ventilation-perfusion abnormalities.[342,343] Long-term (greater than 48 hrs) infusions of both drugs can lead to clinical difficulties, specifically, hemodynamic tolerance with nitroglycerin, and thiocyanate toxicity with nitroprusside.[239,340,344] High doses of nitroprusside can also cause cyanide toxicity.[345] Hence, these drugs should be used only for brief periods. If long-term therapy is needed, treatment with oral vasodilators should be initiated as soon as possible.

Intravenous Positive Inotropic Agents

All effective interventions in the treatment of pulmonary edema act to redistribute central blood volume from the pulmonary circulation to the systemic capacitance vessels. Many positive inotropic agents, such as dobutamine and amrinone, can achieve a similar therapeutic response not only by enhancing systolic function but by exerting a direct vasodilator effect on peripheral vascular systems. Digoxin should not be used to treat pulmonary edema—except in patients with rapid atrial fibrillation—because of its slow onset and prolonged duration of action.

Dobutamine • Dobutamine is a synthetic sympathomimetic agent that stimulates β_1-, β_2-, and α_1-adrenergic receptors. The drug is a racemic mixture—its α-adrenergic effects are primarily related to the l-enantiomer, the β-adrenergic effects to the d-enantiomer.[346] The drug increases cardiac contractility by virtue of its β_1 and α_1 effects, but because the α_1 effects in the peripheral circulation are generally offset by the drug's β_2 actions, there is generally no change in systemic blood pressure.[347] Yet, by virtue of its α_1-agonist effects, dobutamine exerts more positive inotropic, but fewer positive chronotropic effects than isoproterenol,[348] since any α_1-mediated vasoconstriction produced by dobutamine limits the magnitude of vasodilation and hence, the reflex tachycardia that would be expected with a pure β-agonist. The α_1-effects of dobutamine, however, are weaker than those of dopamine or norepinephrine. Furthermore, unlike dopamine, dobutamine does not release norepinephrine from adrenergic nerve terminals.[349]

Dobutamine markedly increases cardiac output but produces only modest decreases in pulmonary wedge pressures and virtually no increase in systemic blood pressure[350] (Figure 2.61). Heart rate generally increases only when doses greater than 10 μg/kg/min are used. Dobutamine produces smaller increases in heart rate than isoproterenol[348] and larger increases in cardiac output and decreases in pulmonary wedge pressures than dopamine.[350–352] However, compared with dobutamine,

---

TABLE 2.38 • ADVERSE EFFECTS OF NITROGLYCERIN AND NITROPRUSSIDE

Systemic hypotension

Aggravation of arterial hypoxemia in patients with ventilation-perfusion abnormalities

Cyanide toxicity (nitroprusside)

Long-term infusions lead to:
- Hemodynamic tolerance (nitroglycerin)
- Thiocyanate toxicity (nitroprusside)

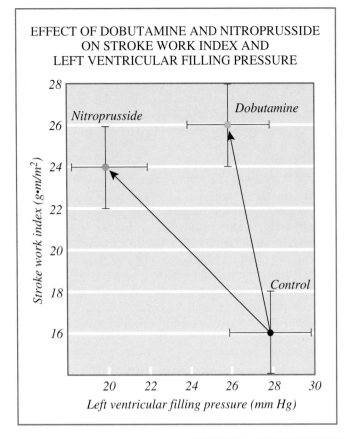

EFFECT OF DOBUTAMINE AND NITROPRUSSIDE
ON STROKE WORK INDEX AND
LEFT VENTRICULAR FILLING PRESSURE

FIGURE 2.61 • The effect of dobutamine and nitroprusside on stroke work index and left ventricular filling pressure in patients with advanced heart failure. (Adapted with permission. Berkowitz C, McKeever L, Croke RP, et al: *Circulation* 1977;56:918, American Heart Association.)

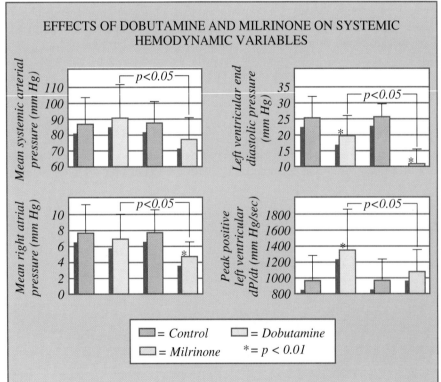

EFFECTS OF DOBUTAMINE AND MILRINONE ON SYSTEMIC
HEMODYNAMIC VARIABLES

FIGURE 2.62 • Comparative effects of intravenous dobutamine and milrinone on systemic hemodynamic variables. (Reproduced with permission. Grose RM, Strain JE, Greenberg MA, et al: *J Am Coll Cardiol* 1986;7:1110.)

dopamine is a better vasoconstrictor, and amrinone and milrinone are better vasodilators[350,353,354] (Figure 2.62). Dobutamine can be combined with nitroglycerin, nitroprusside, dopamine and amrinone to produce added hemodynamic benefits.[355–358]

The usual therapeutic dose of dobutamine is 2.5 to 15 µg/kg/min. Short-term infusions can be extremely effective in the treatment of unstable heart failure, especially when systemic blood pressures are relatively preserved. However, dobutamine can increase myocardial oxygen consumption[353] and can cause serious arrhythmias, either directly or by lowering the serum potassium concentration.[359,360] Long-term infusions should be avoided, since prolonged continuous administration of dobutamine is accompanied by the development of hemodynamic tolerance[354,361] (Figure 2.63). Although, as with nitroglycerin, intermittent therapy with dobutamine can circumvent the development of tolerance and produce sustained clinical effects, this approach may increase the mortality of patients with chronic heart failure.[196]

Amrinone and Milrinone • Amrinone is the only phosphodiesterase inhibitor that is presently available for intravenous use, although intravenous milrinone has also been approved by the Food and Drug Administration for the short-term treatment of heart failure. Both drugs produce dose-dependent increases in cardiac output and decreases in pulmonary wedge pressures as a result of the interaction of their direct positive inotropic, positive lusitropic and peripheral vasodilator actions[362–365] (Figure 2.64). The net result is a hemodynamic profile similar to a combination of dobutamine and nitroprusside.[366] Because of their peripheral vasodilator effects, amrinone and milrinone are less likely than dobutamine to increase heart rate and myocardial oxygen consumption[353,367]—although myocardial ischemia can occasionally be provoked.[208] Because of their positive inotropic effects, amrinone and milrinone may be less likely than nitroprusside to decrease systemic blood pressure—although marked hypotensive reactions have been observed.[368,369] These hypotensive events have led some investi-

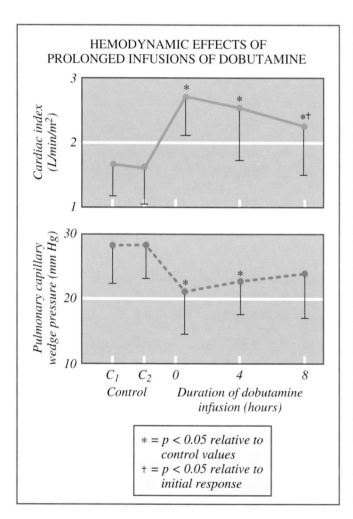

FIGURE 2.63 • The effects of dobutamine on cardiac index and pulmonary capillary wedge pressure. After a substantial increase in cardiac index and reduction in pulmonary capillary wedge pressure, these responses slowly return toward, but not completely to, the control values over a period of 8 hrs despite continued infusion of the drug. (Reproduced with permission. Klein NA, Siskind SJ, Frishman WH, et al: *Am J Cardiol* 1981;48:173.)

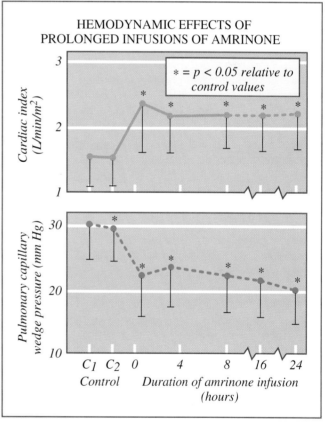

FIGURE 2.64 • Effects of amrinone on cardiac index and pulmonary capillary wedge pressure. The initial salutary effect on these variables is sustained over 24 hrs of drug infusion. (Reproduced with permission. Klein NA, Siskind SJ, Frishman WH, et al: *Am J Cardiol* 1981;48:173.)

gators to question the clinical relevance of the positive inotropic effects of these drugs,[370,371] since the inotropic actions of phosphodiesterase inhibitors are known to be attenuated in the failing heart.[36,370] However, direct intravenous and intracoronary infusion studies have demonstrated a positive inotropic effect of these drugs in the clinical setting.[368,372]

Therapy with amrinone is initiated as an initial bolus of 0.75 mg/kg, followed by an intravenous infusion of 5 to 20 μg/kg/min. The optimal dosing schedule for milrinone has not yet been elucidated. The major disadvantage of both drugs is their long duration of action. Hence, should adverse effects occur with amrinone and milrinone, they may persist for several hrs, whereas the hemodynamic actions of nitroglycerin, nitroprusside and dobutamine last for only minutes. Adverse circulatory effects include hypotension, worsening ventricular arrhythmias and acceleration of the ventricular response to atrial arrhythmias. Some noncardiac concerns associated with amrinone include gastrointestinal distress, abnormal liver function tests and thrombocytopenia.[369]

PERIPHERAL HYPOPERFUSION— CARDIOGENIC SHOCK

The cardinal symptoms of peripheral hypoperfusion are fatigue, altered mental status and oliguria. The principal physical finding is cutaneous vasoconstriction and the primary pathophysiologic feature is end-organ hypoperfusion and dysfunction. As in the case of pulmonary congestion, peripheral hypoperfusion may develop in patients without previous left ventricular dysfunction or may occur in patients with long-standing heart failure. If severe, abrupt, and accompanied by clinical evidence of sympathetic activity, the syndrome is designated as shock. Shock may be caused by cardiogenic disorders (usually acute myocardial infarction), hypovolemia or sepsis.

Regardless of its cause, peripheral hypoperfusion reduces effective blood flow to critical organs of the body. Although cardiac output is decreased in cardiogenic shock, it is increased in bacteremic states.[373] Hence, changes in cardiac output cannot be used to define the existence of shock. Similarly, although blood pressure is usually decreased in shock regardless of the cause, there is an imprecise relationship between blood pressure and perfusion. Some patients with severe hypotension—for example, patients with heart failure receiving angiotensin-converting enzyme inhibitors—maintain excellent end-organ perfusion and function and thus do not qualify as being in shock. Conversely, blood pressure may be inexplicably preserved in some patients with severe perfusion deficits. Hence, no central hemodynamic variable can be used to define shock. The definition is based solely on the presence of end-organ hypoperfusion.

The severity of shock is quantified in the clinical setting by the degree of hypoperfusion of the skin, skeletal muscle, and kidneys—the organs most likely to be impaired as blood flow is preferentially distributed to the brain and heart. Consequently, the cardinal manifestations of cardiogenic shock are:
- Cutaneous vasoconstriction—due to skin hypoperfusion.
- Lactic acidosis—due to skeletal muscle hypoperfusion.
- Oliguria—due to renal hypoperfusion.

The primary goal of treatment is the restoration of adequate perfusion to all organs of the body.

Several general measures are indicated in all patients in shock. Immediate hospitalization in a critical care unit is essential. Noninvasive measurements of ventricular function should be available to rapidly assess the magnitude of ventricular dysfunction and to allow the diagnosis of mechanical defects in the heart (for example, papillary muscle rupture, ventricular septal defect, and prosthetic valve thrombosis). Invasive hemodynamic monitoring may be extremely helpful in characterizing the hemodynamic derangement and guiding the use of pharmacologic agents. Serial measurements of urine output, arterial blood gases and blood lactate are important in monitoring the adequacy of oxygen delivery to peripheral tissues.

The most important therapeutic measures in the treatment of cardiogenic shock are:
- Fluid management.
- The intravenous administration of pressor agents—dopamine and levarterenol.
- Intraaortic balloon counterpulsation.

Fluid Management

Fluid management represents a direct means of altering loading conditions in the heart without changing cardiac contractility or peripheral vascular resistance. Since the therapeutic administration of fluids increases the pressure and volume in the cardiac chambers during both systole and diastole, the infusion of fluids acts to enhance cardiac preload and afterload. Interestingly, the performance of the normal left ventricle is extremely responsive to changes in cardiac preload but is resistant to changes in cardiac afterload.[59] Hence, the administration of fluids is generally beneficial in treating shock patients who have normal left ventricular function (for example, hypovolemia, bacteremic shock and right ventricular infarction). In contrast, the performance of the impaired left ventricle is resistant to changes in cardiac preload, but it is exquisitely sensitive to changes in cardiac afterload.[60] The administration of fluids, therefore, may exacerbate the hemodynamic abnormalities of cardiogenic shock. Consequently, physicians should attempt to reduce intravascular volume in overloaded patients by administering diuretics. If used judiciously, diuretics may improve cardiac function by reducing wall stress and reducing the magnitude of secondary volume-dependent mitral regurgitation.[374]

The measurement of left ventricular filling pressure—pulmonary wedge pressure—by means of a right-heart balloon-floatation catheter is an essential tool in monitoring the volume status of patients with shock (Figure 2.65). However, physicians should recognize that this pressure is not an estimate of intravascular volume, since changes in cardiac contractility, diastolic function, mitral valve function and peripheral circulation can also affect intracardiac pressures. Instead, the measurement of the pulmonary wedge pressure indicates how likely it is that increases in intravascular volume will be beneficial (by enhancing the pumping function of the left ventricle) or detrimental (by jeopardizing the oxygen exchange function of the lungs). If the pulmonary wedge pressure is less than 14 mm Hg, volume expansion is likely to increase the cardiac output with minimal risk of pulmonary edema. If the pulmonary wedge pressure is markedly elevated—greater than 20 mm Hg—volume expansion is likely to produce little improvement and may be dangerous. If the pulmonary wedge pressure is between 12 and 20 mm Hg, the effects of changes in intravascular volume are unpredictable. In such patients, the response to a cautious volume expansion using a specific volume of fluid infused over a defined interval may be very helpful.[375] If volume expansion leads to an increase in cardiac output—preferably, with increased urine output but minimal change in pulmonary wedge pressure— additional volume repletion is likely to be beneficial. Nevertheless, if volume expansion leads to a rapid rise in pulmonary wedge pressure without beneficial effects on peripheral perfusion, additional volume challenges should be avoided.

Intravenous Pressor Agents

A variety of catecholamines that act to support systemic blood pressure are commercially available for the treatment of shock, based on the concept that an increase in perfusion pressure will lead to a restoration of peripheral blood flow. The most popular agents are the two endogenous neurotransmitters, dopamine and norepinephrine (levarterenol).

Dopamine • Dopamine is an endogenous catecholamine that interacts with the following receptors in the heart and peripheral circulation:

- Dopamine receptors—both DA_1 and DA_2 subtypes.
- β_1-adrenergic receptors, but not β_2.
- α-adrenergic receptors—both α_1 and α_2 subtypes.

As a result of these receptor interactions, the drug:

- Causes vasodilation due to its agonist effects on DA_1 receptors.
- Stimulates cardiac contractility due to its agonist effects on β_1 receptors and its ability to release norepinephrine from sympathetic nerve terminals.
- Causes constriction of peripheral arterial and venous vessels due to its agonist effects on α_1 receptors, and perhaps, serotonergic receptors.[376–378]

The hemodynamic effects of dopamine depend largely on dose of the drug administered.[379,380] Low doses of less than 2 µg/kg/min, which stimulate DA_1- and DA_2- receptors, act to dilate the renal and splanchnic circulations. Moderate doses between 2 to 5 µg/kg/min, which activate β_1-receptors, increase cardiac output but produce little change in pulmonary wedge pressure, heart rate, or systemic vascular resistance. High dos-

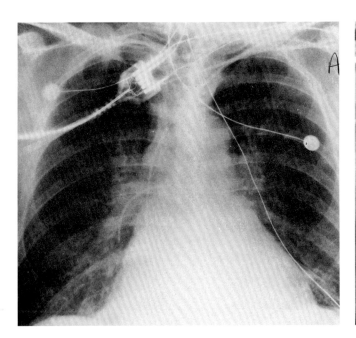 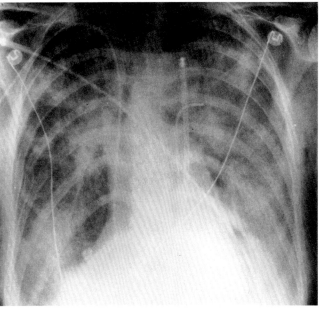

FIGURE 2.65 • Placement of a Swan-Ganz catheter in patients with unstable heart failure. (Reproduced with permission. Soto B, Kassner EG, Baxley WA: *Imaging of Cardiac Disorders. Volume 2* New York, NY: Gower Medical Publishing; 1992:132.)

es (greater than 5 µg/kg/min, which stimulate α_1-receptors) increase pulmonary wedge pressure, blood pressure and heart rate, and may reduce renal blood flow (Figure 2.66).

Dopamine may be useful in the treatment of both the pulmonary congestion and the peripheral hypoperfusion of unstable heart failure. In normotensive patients with pulmonary congestion, low doses of dopamine increase renal blood flow and are used to potentiate the diuretic actions of furosemide.[381–383] Should a diuresis fail to occur, two other options should be considered:

• Low doses of dopamine may be combined with dobutamine.[357,384] In this combination, the enhanced cardiac output produced by dobutamine is preferentially directed to the kidneys.

• Moderate doses of dopamine may be combined with nitroprusside or nitroglycerin[385,386] (Figure 2.67).

Dopamine acts to minimize the hypotensive effects of the vasodilators, whereas the vasodilators act to reduce the venoconstrictor effects of dopamine. In hypotensive patients with peripheral hypoperfusion, large doses of dopamine are utilized to support systemic blood pressure, either alone or in combination with norepinephrine.[380,387,388]

Levarterenol • This commercial preparation of the endogenous catecholamine (norepinephrine) preferentially stimulates intrasynaptic receptors—α_1 and β_1—when administered in therapeutic doses. Due to its lack of β_2-agonist effects, levarterenol produces less vasodilation and tachycardia than epinephrine or isoproterenol.[389,390] Due to its lack of DA_1-agonist effects, norepinephrine increases systemic vascular resistance and blood pressure more than dopamine.[388] Systemic vasoconstriction may be intense enough to reduce renal blood flow and to limit any increase in cardiac output that might be expected to result from β_1-adrenergic stimulation.[391,392] Consequently, levarterenol is used only in patients with shock when blood pressure cannot be supported adequately with dopamine. Levarterenol is generally infused in doses ranging from 0.03 to 0.12 µg/kg/min.

Other Catecholamines and Sympathomimetic Amines • Isoproterenol and epinephrine exert potent agonist effects on β_1- and β_2-adrenergic receptors. This combination of activities not only causes marked positive inotropic effects, but also marked vasodilation and tachycardia due to the β_2-actions of these drugs.[389,393] Consequently, isoproterenol and low doses of epinephrine may lower systemic blood pressures and reduce urine output in patients with cardiogenic shock.[389,392,394,395] Thus, neither drug is useful in the management of this condi-

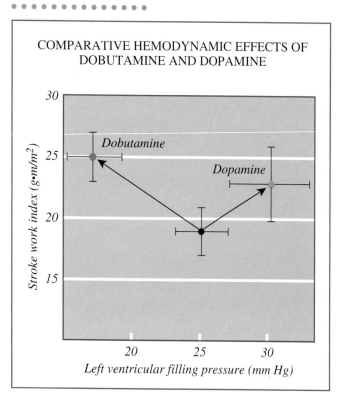

FIGURE 2.66 • The effect of dobutamine and high-dose dopamine on stroke work index and left ventricular filling pressure in patients with advanced heart failure. (Adapted with permission. Loeb HS, Bredakis J, Gunnar RM: *Circulation* 1977;55:375 and the American Heart Association.)

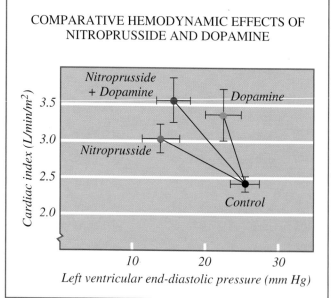

FIGURE 2.67 • The effect of nitroprusside and dopamine, alone and in combination, on left ventricular end-diastolic pressure and cardiac index in patients with advanced heart failure. (Adapted with permission. Miller RR, Awan NA, Joye JE: *Circulation* 1977;55:881 and American Heart Association.)

tion. Although large doses of epinephrine, unlike isoproterenol, can stimulate peripheral α_1-receptors and raise blood pressure, such large doses frequently produce excessive degrees of tachycardia and serious arrhythmias.[90]

Phenylephrine, methoxamine, mephentermine and metarminol act primarily as α_1-adrenergic receptor agonists by causing peripheral vasoconstriction. All four drugs can be used to support systemic blood pressure.[395–398] Unlike phenylephrine and methoxamine, mephentermine and metarminol also promote the release of norepinephrine from sympathetic nerve terminals, and thus, exert modest positive inotropic effects.[399–403] Because of this additional property, mephentermine and metarminol were the preferred α-adrenergic agonists for the treatment of shock for many years, whereas phenylephrine and methoxamine were primarily utilized for the management of supraventricular tachycardia. Compared with dopamine and levarterenol, however, these agents exert fewer beneficial effects on cardiac performance and may occasionally decrease cardiac output.[391,395] Hence, they are now rarely used.

All catecholamines have the potential for causing serious adverse cardiovascular effects. Drugs with potent α-agonist effects can reduce peripheral perfusion, especially renal blood flow, and if extravasated during infusion, can cause local tissue necrosis.[404] Drugs with potent β-agonist effects can produce serious atrial and ventricular arrhythmias and may exacerbate myocardial ischemia.[405] In addition, unlike other catecholamines, dopamine may cause nausea and vomiting—presumably due to its DA_1-agonist effects.[380]

Intraaortic Balloon Counterpulsation

The cyclical inflation during diastole of a balloon positioned in the descending aorta can produce beneficial hemodynamic effects in patients with cardiogenic shock who are resistant to fluid and pressor therapy.[406] Like vasodilators, this intervention reduces ventricular loading conditions in the failing heart during systole. Like vasoconstrictors, the inflation of the balloon acts to improve coronary perfusion during diastole. Pharmacologic interventions cannot accomplish these cycle-specific goals, since the simultaneous administration of vasodilators and vasoconstrictors neutralizes each other's circulatory effects. Yet, both hemodynamic goals can be achieved with the use of intraaortic balloon counterpulsation. This technique is useful in managing cardiogenic shock that is caused by an acute myocardial infarction, particularly when there is a coexistent mechanical defect, ventricular septal defect or papillary muscle rupture,[407] or when there is ongoing myocardial ischemia.[408]

THERAPEUTIC APPROACH TO UNSTABLE HEART FAILURE

The approach to management of unstable heart failure depends largely on the severity of the condition and the relative contributions of pulmonary congestion and peripheral hypoperfusion to the clinical presentation of the patient.

Pulmonary Congestion

Patients who present with acute pulmonary edema generally respond favorably to interventions that reduce the constriction of the peripheral arterial and venous circulations. Such patients should receive bolus injections of morphine and furosemide followed by intravenous infusion of nitroglycerin. Tourniquets are rarely used now. Nitroprusside is preferred over nitroglycerin if the patient is severely hypertensive or has severe mitral or aortic valvular regurgitation. If dyspnea, diaphoresis and peripheral vasoconstriction persist, dobutamine should be added. If additional inotropy and vasodilation is desired, amrinone may be tried. If the syndrome becomes immediately life-threatening, phlebotomy is essential. All of these interventions are well tolerated as long as hypotension does not develop.

Patients who present with chronic pulmonary congestion and massive peripheral edema respond favorably to interventions that enhance the excretion of sodium by the kidneys. Therapy should be initiated with IV furosemide, the dose of which should be increased up to 120 to 200 mg per dose until a diuresis is achieved. If urine output is not adequately enhanced, metolazone should be added. This diuretic combination predictably elicits a marked diuresis, but this is frequently complicated by the development of hypokalemia. If the diuretic response remains insufficient, dobutamine alone or combined with low doses of dopamine should be used to potentiate the response to furosemide and metolazone. Vasodilators may reduce renal perfusion pressure and attenuate the effects of furosemide and should be used cautiously. If the edema proves to be refractory to these interventions, hemofiltration or peritoneal dialysis may be needed.[409,410] Fortunately, these are generally required only in patients with impaired renal function.

Peripheral Hypoperfusion

Patients who present with acute circulatory shock should be treated with intravenous pressors until systemic blood pressure rises to the low-normal range—blood pressure of 85 to 90 mm Hg systolic). The agent of first choice is dopamine. Levarterenol may be added if the pressor response to dopamine is inadequate. If pulmonary rales are not heard, fluids should be infused cautiously until a balloon-floatation catheter can be inserted to measure pulmonary wedge pressure. If pulmonary rales are present, diuretics or vasodilators can be used once the blood pressure has been supported by intravenous pressors. Unfortunately, once treatment is initiated, there may be little relation between the presence of pulmonary rales and the level of the left ventricular filling pressure. Rales may persist for long periods after the pulmonary wedge pressure has decreased to low values. If there are doubts about fluid therapy, hemodynamic monitoring is essential. Ventilatory support may be needed to maintain adequate oxygenation.

If the patient fails to respond favorably to fluids and pharmacologic agents, intra-aortic balloon counterpulsation may be helpful, especially when there is a coexistent mechanical defect—ventricular septal defect or papillary muscle rupture—or when there is continuing myocardial ischemia. Other mechanical options include temporary or permanent ventricular assist devices and the total artificial heart—usually as a bridge to transplantation.[411,412]

TREATMENT OF HEART FAILURE WITH PRESERVED SYSTOLIC FUNCTION

Some patients who present with the clinical syndrome of heart failure show little impairment of left ventricular systolic function. The hemodynamic and clinical features in these patients are related to an abnormality of diastolic function—ventricular filling—or to a prolonged increase in loading conditions in the heart—valvular stenosis or regurgitation.

DISORDERS OF LEFT VENTRICULAR DIASTOLIC FUNCTION

Diastolic dysfunction not only leads to an increase in left ventricular filling pressures as a consequence of the altered pressure-volume relations in the left ventricle, but it may impair cardiac output, since the left ventricle can eject only a limited ventricular volume. Surveys suggest that 15% to 25% of patients with the clinical syndrome of heart failure have diastolic rather than systolic dysfunction as their primary cardiac abnormality.[413,414] Three types of cardiac disorders can cause heart failure by adversely affecting diastolic function:
- Hypertrophic cardiomyopathy.
- Restrictive cardiomyopathy.
- Constrictive pericarditis.

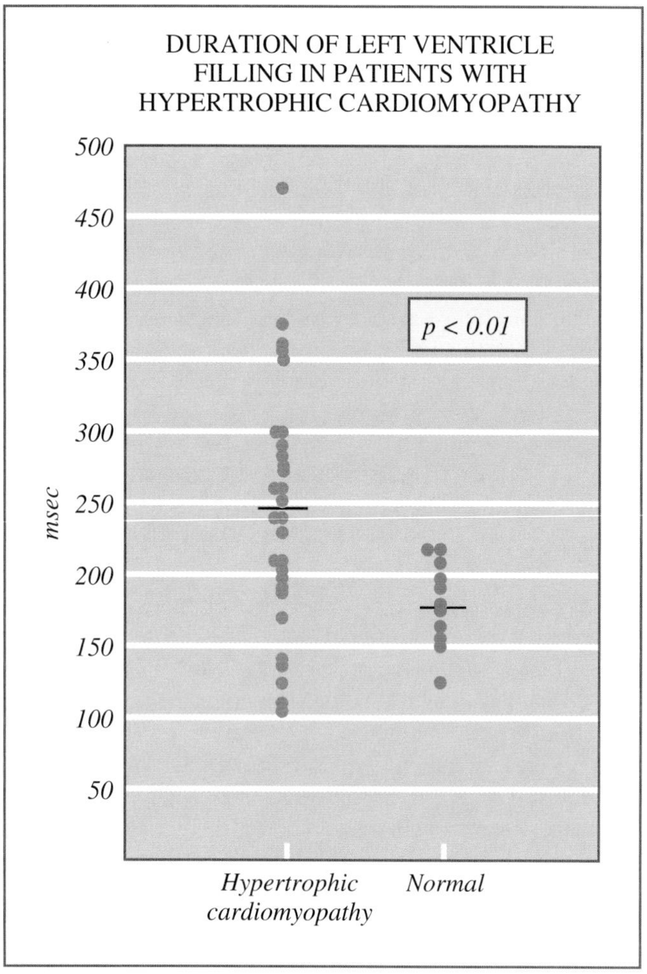

DURATION OF LEFT VENTRICLE FILLING IN PATIENTS WITH HYPERTROPHIC CARDIOMYOPATHY

$p < 0.01$

(y-axis label: *msec*, with values 50, 100, 150, 200, 250, 300, 350, 400, 450, 500)

(x-axis labels: *Hypertrophic cardiomyopathy*, *Normal*)

FIGURE 2.68 • Although there is wide variation in left ventricular filling period in patients with hypertrophic cardiomyopathy compared with the normal, mean value is significantly greater than normal. (Reproduced with permission. St. John Sutton MG, Tajik AJ, Gibson DG, et al: *Circulation* 1978;57:515.)

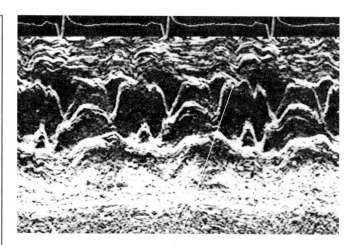

systolic anterior
displacement of mitral valve

A

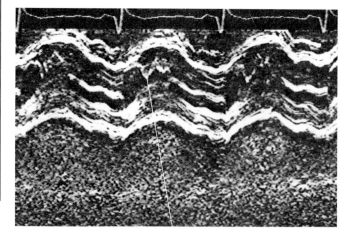

early systolic closure
of aortic valve

B

FIGURE 2.69 • M-mode echocardiogram of a middle-aged female with hypertrophic cardiomyopathy and left ventricular outflow tract obstruction. There is abnormal systolic anterior motion of the mitral valve (A) and early systolic closure of the aortic valve (B). (Reproduced with permission. Hurst JW, Anderson RH, Becker AE, et al: *Atlas of the Heart* New York, NY: Gower Medical Publishing; 1988:5.14.)

Hypertrophic Cardiomyopathy

This hereditary disorder is characterized by myocardial hypertrophy that is out of proportion to and cannot be explained by an increase in ventricular wall stress. The primary symptoms are dyspnea, angina and syncope; the clinical course is variable, but in most cases the symptoms progress slowly over a period of many years. The most feared complication is sudden death, which may occur in symptomatic or asymptomatic patients.[415]

Pathophysiology • The most important pathophysiologic abnormality is an impairment of diastolic relaxation. Patients show an abnormal prolongation of relaxation, often associated with a reduced increase in left ventricular dimension during a shortened rapid filling phase[416] (Figure 2.68). Many patients also have a functional subvalvular obstruction to left ventricular outflow that results from rapid, early emptying of the hyperdynamic left ventricle acting in concert with a narrowing of the outflow tract. The constricted outflow tract is produced by systolic anterior motion of the mitral valve against the hypertrophic septum[417] (Figures 2.69, 2.70).

The clinical significance of the outflow tract obstruction remains controversial. Many patients do not have a subvalvular gradient at rest or during provocative maneuvers, and the reproducibility of the gradient from day to day is poor.[418] Furthermore, a reduced ventricular emptying during the late phases of systole may be more closely related to an excessive emptying of the ventricle during the early phases of systole rather than the development of an outflow obstruction;[419] a similar gradient may be produced in normal hearts made hyperdynamic by the infusion of isoproterenol or severe hypovolemia.[420,421] These observations may explain why the magnitude of the outflow gradient fails to predict either symptoms or prognosis in these patients.[422,423] In contrast, symptoms are closely related to the magnitude of diastolic dysfunction.[424]

Medical Management • Although the clinical features of hypertrophic cardiomyopathy are primarily related to abnormalities of diastolic function, therapy has been primarily directed towards alleviating the functional outflow obstruction of the left ventricle. Based on this logic, physicians traditionally employed interventions that decreased cardiac contractility or increased ventricular volume, since positive inotropic agents and hypovolemia can produce an outflow gradient even in a normal heart.[420,421] Consequently, the treatment of hypertrophic cardiomyopathy has largely relied on the use of β-adrenergic blockers and calcium channel blockers. Digitalis has generally been avoided, unless there is associated atrial fibrillation. Diuretics have usually been proscribed, unless there is associated right heart failure related to pulmonary hypertension. However, since doubts have been raised about the clinical significance of the outflow gradient, presently accepted therapeutic approaches lack strong physiologic support. This may explain why traditional treatments have not changed the natural history of the disease. It is possible that therapy directed at the primary abnormality (for example, diastolic dysfunction) may prove to be more useful.

Aside from pharmacologic interventions, patients with hypertrophic cardiomyopathy should not engage in vigorous exercise, since this has been linked to sudden death.[415] All efforts, including cardioversion, should be made to treat atrial arrhythmias. Atrial fibrillation is poorly tolerated primarily because it reduces the time for ventricular filling. Some patients may also deteriorate because of the loss of the atrial contribution to ventricular filling.

β–Adrenergic Blocking Drugs • Beta-blockers have become an accepted mode of therapy for hypertrophic cardiomyopathy, although controlled clinical trials to support their use are lacking. The most experience has been gained with pro-

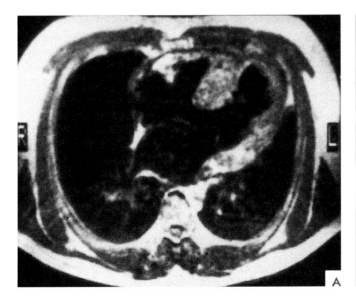 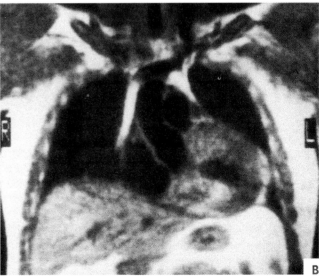

FIGURE 2.70 • MRI of a 31-year-old male with hypertrophic cardiomyopathy who experienced two episodes of syncope. The transverse sections were made during end diastole (A). An image in the coronal plane was also made during mid-systole (B). Left ventricular hypertrophy is evident and systolic anterior motion of the mitral valve is seen in all of the systolic images. (Reproduced with permission. Hurst JW, Anderson RH, Becker AE, et al: *Atlas of the Heart* New York, NY: Gower Medical Publishing; 1988:5.16.)

pranolol, usually 160 to 320 mg daily. The mechanism underlying the efficacy of β-blockers remains controversial. Physicians traditionally believed that β-blockers work by reducing the outflow tract gradient. However, β-blockers only inhibit the increase in outflow gradient that occurs during exercise, but do not affect the gradient at rest.[425,426] Therefore, it is possible that the effect of β-blockers on diastolic filling is more important than their effect on systolic obstruction. Specifically, β-blockers reduce the heart rate response to exercise and thus favorably prolong the time available for ventricular filling.[427,428] Despite these physiologic benefits, β-blockers are effective in only about 50% of patients with the disease. Angina and syncope appears to be alleviated more effectively than dyspnea. Some patients with very high left ventricular end-diastolic pressures may even experience more dyspnea following treatment with β-blockers.[429,430]

Calcium Channel Blocking Drugs • Calcium channel blocking drugs, particularly verapamil, have been used with increasing success. Like β-blockers, these drugs reduce the inotropic state of the heart and blunt its response to exercise, but they also reduce the basal and provoked outflow gradients[403] by improving diastolic relaxation[431,432] (Figure 2.71). Even patients who show no immediate effect on the gradient may experience a decrease in the magnitude of obstruction during long-term use.[434] In addition to its hemodynamic advantages, verapamil possesses many clinical advantages over β-blockers.

Verapamil, 360 to 480 mg daily, improves symptoms and exercise tolerance in approximately two thirds of treated patients[435,436] (Figure 2.72). Verapamil produces greater relief of angina but less fatigue and depression than β-blockers. There-

fore, some patients who remain symptomatic despite maximal β-blockade may show significant improvement when their medication is changed to verapamil.[434] During long-term use, verapamil may reduce left ventricular hypertrophy more than β-blockers.[434,437] Nevertheless, verapamil, like β-blockers, can exacerbate dyspnea and even cause pulmonary edema in patients with a very high left ventricular end-diastolic pressure before treatment.[438]

Verapamil is the preferred calcium channel blocker for patients with hypertrophic cardiomyopathy. Although both nifedipine and diltiazem may also favorably affect diastolic function in these patients, the potent vasodilator effects of nifedipine can increase the outflow tract gradient,[439] and clinical experience with diltiazem is limited.

Other Interventions • Disopyramide improves the hemodynamic and clinical status of some patients with hypertrophic cardiomyopathy.[440] Amiodarone can abolish the frequent atrial and ventricular arrhythmias and may prevent sudden death; some patients experience hemodynamic and clinical benefits following the institution of amiodarone therapy.[441] If symptoms persist despite maximal medical therapy, surgical approaches—septal myotomy-myectomy—should be considered.

Restrictive Cardiomyopathy and Constrictive Pericarditis

Patients with restrictive cardiomyopathy or constrictive pericarditis present with signs and symptoms of heart failure, but left ventricular systolic function is preserved. As in patients with hypertrophic cardiomyopathy, the primary hemodynamic abnormality is an impairment in ventricular filling (Figure 2.73).

• • • • • • • • • • • • • • •

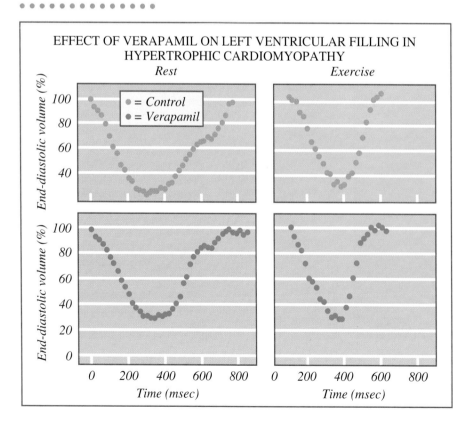

EFFECT OF VERAPAMIL ON LEFT VENTRICULAR FILLING IN HYPERTROPHIC CARDIOMYOPATHY

FIGURE 2.71 • Left ventricular time activity curves obtained in one patient at rest and during exercise before and after verapamil. Despite increases in cardiac cycle length, verapamil increases peak filling rate both at rest—from 2.5 to 4.0 EDV/sec—and during exercise—from 5.7 to 7.1 EDV/sec. There is a decrease in time to peak filling rate at rest—from 184 to 149 msec—and exercise—from 123 to 75 msec. Verapamil augmented exercise tolerance in this patient from 3.0 to 5.6 min. (Reproduced with permission. Bonow RO, Dilisizian V, Rosing DR, et al: *Circulation* 1985;72:857 and the American Heart Association.)

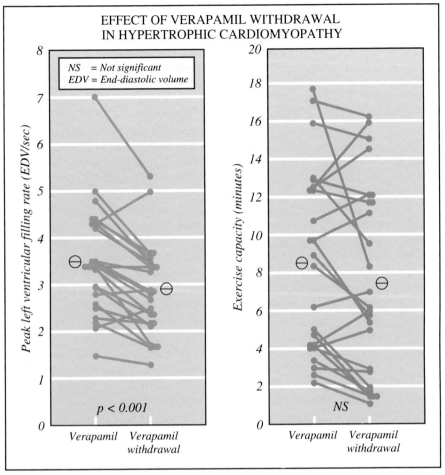

EFFECT OF VERAPAMIL WITHDRAWAL
IN HYPERTROPHIC CARDIOMYOPATHY

NS = Not significant
EDV = End-diastolic volume

Peak left ventricular filling rate (EDV/sec)

$p < 0.001$

Verapamil   Verapamil
withdrawal

Exercise capacity (minutes)

NS

Verapamil   Verapamil
withdrawal

FIGURE 2.72. • Effects of withdrawal after long-term verapamil therapy on peak left ventricular filling rate at rest and on exercise capacity. (Reproduced with permission. Bonow RO, Dilisizian V, Rosing DR, et al: *Circulation* 1985;72:861 and the American Heart Association.)

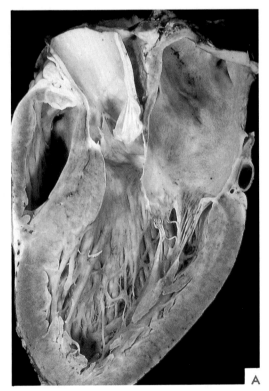

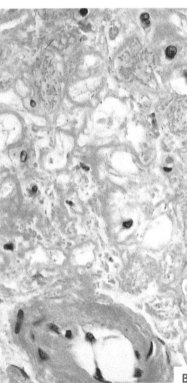

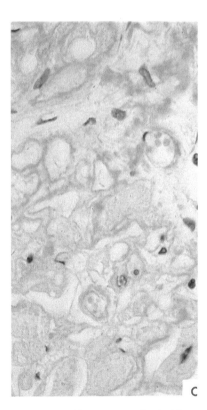

FIGURE 2.73 • Long axis section through a heart with amyloid disease demonstrates the sandy appearance of the left atrial endocardium (A). Histologic section shows myocardial cell degeneration and extensive extracellular deposition of amorphous material enclosing the cells (B). The amyloid stains positive with a Congo red stain (C). (Reproduced with permission. Hurst JW, Anderson RH, Becker AE, et al: *Atlas of the Heart* New York, NY: Gower Medical Publishing; 1988:5.18.)

Restrictive Cardiomyopathy

A variety of systemic disorders can cause myocardial fibrosis, hypertrophy and infiltration, thereby producing restrictive cardiomyopathy. These include amyloidosis, hemachromatosis, glycogen storage disorders, sarcoidosis, endomyocardial fibrosis, fibroelastosis, hypereosinophilic syndromes, and pseudoxanthoma elasticum. Occasionally, infiltrative disorders of the heart may be related to neoplasia. Infiltrative fibrosis may also be of unknown cause.

The clinical features of patients with restrictive cardiomyopathy are typical of heart failure—exertional dyspnea and peripheral edema. Yet, the left ventricular ejection fraction is usually greater than 40%. Cardiac catheterization reveals marked increases in right and left ventricular filling pressures, and typically, a deep and rapid early decline in the ventricular pressure tracing at the onset of diastole followed by a rapid rise to a plateau in early diastole—"square root sign."[442] These hemodynamic and clinical features, however, are also typical of patients with constrictive pericarditis. Three hemodynamic findings favor the diagnosis of restrictive cardiomyopathy:

- Left ventricular diastolic pressure that is 5 mm Hg or greater than the right ventricular diastolic pressure—a difference which becomes accentuated during exercise
- Pulmonary artery systolic pressure greater than 45 mmHg
- Right ventricular diastolic pressure plateau that is less than 30% of the peak right ventricular systolic pressure.[442]

The presence of atrioventricular block and conduction disturbances favors the diagnosis of restrictive cardiomyopathy. When doubt persists, endocardial biopsy, CT, and MRI may be helpful in distinguishing between pericardial and myocardial thickening. Exploratory thoracotomy is rarely necessary.

Treatment • There is no controlled evidence that therapy targeted at the underlying disease improves the outlook of patients with known causes of restrictive cardiomyopathy. Nevertheless, reports of success have been published with the use of iron-chelating agents and phlebotomy in hemachromatosis,[443,444] corticosteroids in sarcoidosis,[445] and steroids and hydroxyurea in eosinophilic syndromes.[446] Surgical excision of fibrotic endocardium may offer significant hemodynamic and symptomatic benefits in patients with Loeffler's endocarditis and endomyocardial fibrosis.[447,448]

There is no specific treatment for restrictive cardiomyopathy, and most drugs used in the management of heart failure due to systolic dysfunction produce unsatisfactory, and occasionally deleterious, results. Digitalis is of limited value and may be deleterious in patients with amyloidosis, possibly because of the selective binding of digoxin to amyloid fibrils in the myocardium.[449] Diuretics may be used to control peripheral edema, but should be employed cautiously, if at all, to treat exertional dyspnea, since the elevation of left ventricular filling pressure in patients with restrictive cardiomyopathy is not related to volume expansion. Even mild volume depletion may compromise critical levels of cardiac preload and produce excessive degrees of hypotension. For similar reasons, most vasodilators are both hemodynamically and symptomatically ineffective in this disorder and are likely to produce severe decreases in blood pressure. Although calcium channel blockers may have beneficial effects on diastolic function in patients with hypertrophic cardiomyopathy, there is no evidence that such benefits extend to patients with restrictive disease. Indeed, any improvement in ventricular relaxation following the administration of nifedipine is likely to be related to reflex activation of the sympathetic nervous system, since calcium channel blockers act directly to impair diastolic performance.[450]

The only drugs that can directly improve the diastolic properties of the left ventricle are agents that increase intracellular levels of cyclic AMP.[451] Both β-agonists and phosphodiesterase inhibitors enhance ventricular relaxation,[85,452] but there is little experience with these drugs in the treatment of restrictive cardiomyopathy. Some patients with coronary artery disease present with exertional dyspnea and manifest hemodynamic abnormalities similar to those with restrictive heart

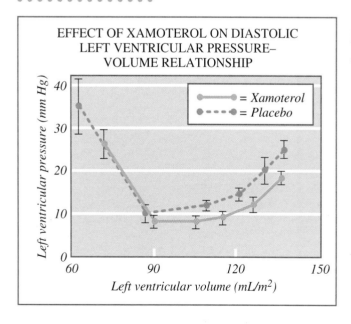

EFFECT OF XAMOTEROL ON DIASTOLIC LEFT VENTRICULAR PRESSURE–VOLUME RELATIONSHIP

FIGURE 2.74 • Effect of xamoterol on left ventricular diastolic pressure-volume relationship in patients with ischemic heart disease. Therapy with xamoterol was administered for 3 months. (Reproduced with permission. Pouleur H, van Eyll C, Hanet C, et al: *Circulation* 1988;77:1081.)

disease. Exercise intolerance in such individuals appears to be directly related to diastolic dysfunction of the left ventricle.[453] Of note, both the diastolic abnormality and the symptoms of the patients have improved following treatment with the partial β-agonist, xamoterol[453—455] (Figure 2.74). Whether xamoterol exerts beneficial hemodynamic and clinical effects in other disorders characterized primarily by diastolic dysfunction remains unknown.

Constrictive Pericarditis

Constrictive pericarditis is characterized by the presence of a fibrotic, thickened and adherent pericardium that restricts ventricular filling during diastole. Most cases are of unknown etiology. Known causes of constrictive pericarditis include: tuberculosis, chronic renal failure treated with hemodialysis, connective tissue disorders, neoplastic infiltration, mediastinal radiation. Constrictive pericarditis may also be one of the long-term complications of hemopericardium (Figure 2.75).

Patients present with signs and symptoms of heart failure, but systolic function is usually preserved. The diagnosis must be distinguished from restrictive cardiomyopathy. Both disorders may show atrial fibrillation and diffuse low QRS voltage. On a chest roentgenograph restrictive disorders are more likely to show conduction system disturbances, and constrictive disorders to show pericardial calcification, but an accurate differential diagnosis requires cardiac catheterization (refer to the Restrictive Cardiomyopathy section). Computed tomography and MRI may be helpful in distinguishing between pericardial and myocardial thickening. The definitive treatment of constrictive pericarditis is complete resection of the pericardium.

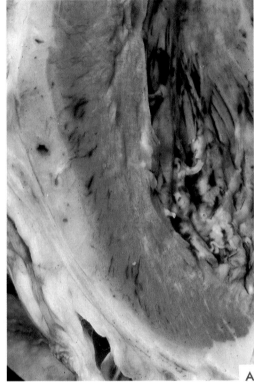

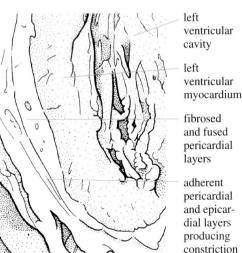

left ventricular cavity

left ventricular myocardium

fibrosed and fused pericardial layers

adherent pericardial and epicardial layers producing constriction

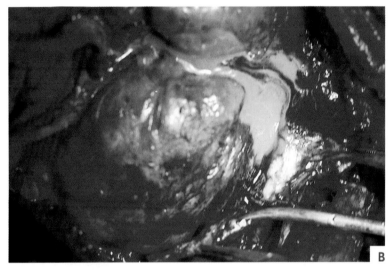

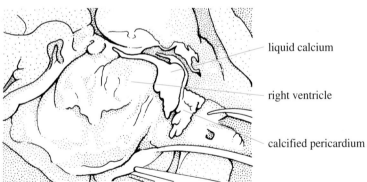

liquid calcium

right ventricle

calcified pericardium

FIGURE 2.75 • Fibrosed pericardial layers encapsulating the heart characterizes constrictive pericarditis (A). The creamy fluid on this patient's heart contains calcium crystals. There was more extensive calcification seen on radiographic examination (B). (Reproduced with permission. Hurst JW, Anderson RH, Becker AE, et al: *Atlas of the Heart* New York, NY: Gower Medical Publishing; 1988:7.10.)

VALVULAR HEART DISEASE

Heart failure may occur in patients with normal systolic function if the effective ejection of blood from the heart is impaired either as a consequence of valvular stenosis or valvular regurgitation. The most frequent valvular lesions are mitral stenosis and insufficiency and aortic stenosis and insufficiency.

MITRAL STENOSIS

Mitral stenosis implies an obstruction to the flow of blood from the left atrium to the left ventricle during diastole (Figure 2.76). As a result, at any given level of exercise, cardiac output is lower and pulmonary artery pressures are higher than in normal individuals (Figure 2.77). The most common cause is rheumatic fever. The severity of the disease is determined by:

- The quantity of blood crossing the valve per unit time.
- The duration of diastole—the amount of time available for transmitral transport.
- The severity of the obstruction to flow.

The medical management of mitral stenosis is focussed on modifying the first two factors. Surgery is directed at altering the third.

Pharmacologic Considerations

In patients with mitral stenosis and normal sinus rhythm, the symptoms of heart failure generally respond favorably to drugs that reduce the quantity of blood crossing the mitral valve per unit time, or that prolong the duration of diastole. The first goal can be achieved by diuretics and the second by the use of β-blockers[456] (Figure 2.78). Digitalis does not produce beneficial hemodynamic effects in patients with mitral stenosis who are in sinus rhythm.[457]

Patients in atrial fibrillation also respond favorably to diuretics and β-blockers, but digitalis is also of value in slowing the ventricular response and producing notable clinical benefits. Once the ventricular rate is controlled, consideration should be given to the restoration of normal sinus rhythm. This option should be strongly considered in patients with new onset atrial fibrillation or in those without marked left atrial enlargement. Cardioversion should generally be preceded by 2 to

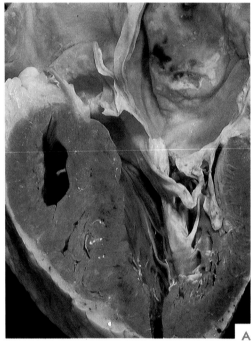

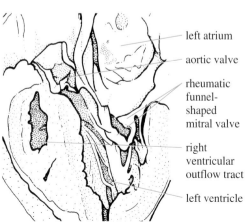

left atrium

aortic valve

rheumatic funnel-shaped mitral valve

right ventricular outflow tract

left ventricle

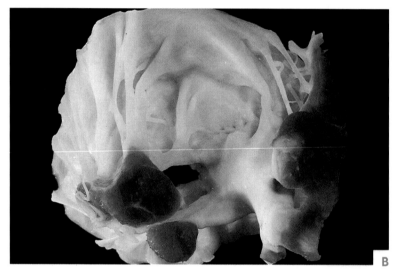

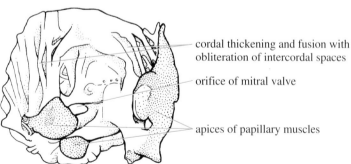

cordal thickening and fusion with obliteration of intercordal spaces

orifice of mitral valve

apices of papillary muscles

FIGURE 2.76 • Long axis cross section through a heart with a rheumatic valve shows a funnel-like stenosis (A). A resected rheumatic mitral valve shows extensive obliteration of intercordal space and leaflet fibrosis (B). These are the features of mitral stenosis. (Reproduced with permission. Hurst JW, Anderson RH, Becker AE, et al: *Atlas of the Heart* New York, NY: Gower Medical Publishing; 1988:4.25.)

3 weeks of anticoagulation and, if successful, should be followed by long-term treatment with quinidine or procainamide to reduce the risk of recurrent fibrillation.

Anticoagulant therapy is mandatory for all patients with mitral stenosis who are in atrial fibrillation or who have previously experienced an embolic event, and it is recommended for all patients with mitral stenosis who have symptoms of heart failure. Anticoagulant therapy should also be considered for patients without heart failure, especially if the left atrium is enlarged.

Surgical Considerations

Surgery should be performed in all patients with severe mitral stenosis who have Classes III and IV symptoms. Surgery should be considered for patients with mild symptoms (functional Class II) if a mitral commisurotomy, rather than mitral valve prosthetic replacement, can be performed, or if severe pulmonary hypertension is present. Asymptomatic patients with mitral stenosis are not candidates for mitral valve surgery. Physicians should consider the fact that many patients with mitral stenosis have a remarkable ability to adapt to the lim-

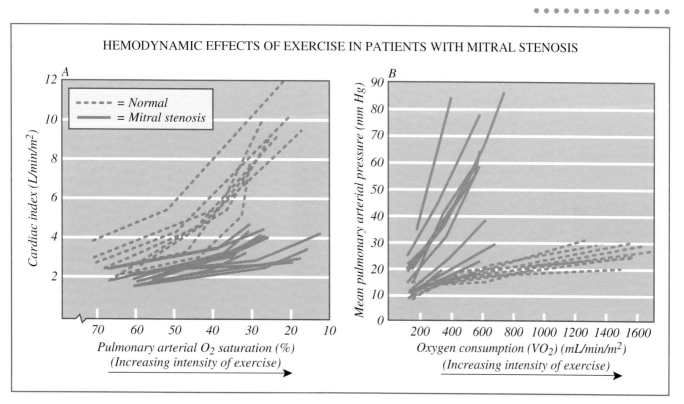

FIGURE 2.77 • Changes in cardiac index (A) and mean pulmonary arterial pressure (B) during submaximal and maximal levels of exercise in normal subjects and patients with mitral stenosis. (Reproduced with permission. Beiser GDS, Epstein SE, Stampfer M, et al: *N Engl J Med* 1968;278:133.)

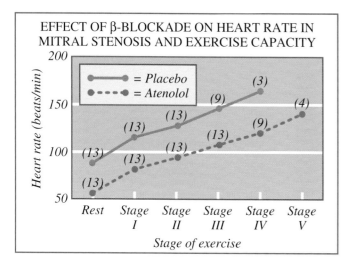

FIGURE 2.78 • Effect of atenolol on heart rate and exercise capacity in mitral stenosis. Beta-blockade reduced the heart rate response to submaximal exercise, but prolonged maximal exercise capacity. (Reproduced with permission. Klein HO, Sareli P, Schamroth CL, et al: *Am J Cardiol* 1985;56:599.)

itations of the disease over long periods of time, and thus, the patient's history of disability may be misleading.

MITRAL REGURGITATION

Mitral regurgitation can occur as a result of abnormalities of the mitral valve leaflets (rheumatic fever), the mitral annulus (left ventricular dilatation), the chordae tendineae (infective endocarditis) and the papillary muscles (myocardial ischemia) (Figure 2.79). The hemodynamic severity of the disease is determined by:

• The size of the regurgitant orifice.
• The pressure gradient between the left ventricle and left atrium during systole.

Both are dynamic processes that can be altered by a variety of physiologic and pharmacologic interventions. The size of the regurgitant orifice is enhanced by increases in preload and afterload and is diminished by increases in

contractility.[458,459] In mitral regurgitation, left ventricular systolic ejection begins earlier and occurs more rapidly than in normal individuals. Almost half of the regurgitant volume is ejected into the left atrium before the aortic valve opens.[460] By permitting earlier opening of the aortic valve, a reduction in afterload favors the flow of ejected blood towards the aorta, and away from the left atrium.

Pharmacologic Considerations

Symptomatic patients with mitral regurgitation should be treated with agents that act to reduce the size of the regurgitant orifice area. This can be achieved with the use of drugs that increase contractility—digitalis—and reduce ventricular preload and afterload—diuretics and vasodilators. Digitalis and diuretics are accepted therapeutic approaches in the management of patients with chronic mitral regurgitation, but the use of vasodilators remains controversial. Beneficial hemodynamic effects have been reported with the use of hydralazine,[236] but no

• • • • • • • • • • • • • •

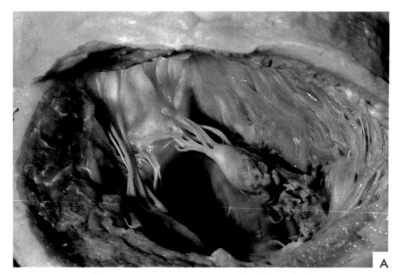

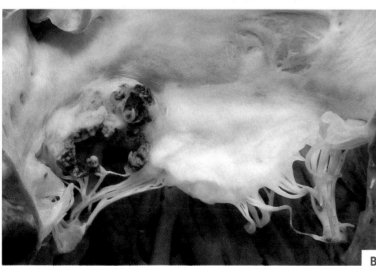

FIGURE 2.79 • Acute mitral regurgitation may result from a ruptured papillary muscle as a complication of acute myocardial infarction (A). Infective endocarditis of the mitral valve, localized in the area of the anterolateral commissure, may also result in mitral regurgitation (B). (Reproduced with permission. Hurst JW, Anderson RH, Becker AE, et al: *Atlas of the Heart* New York, NY: Gower Medical Publishing; 1988:4.39.)

studies have evaluated the long-term effects of this drug. Since corrective surgery is generally recommended in symptomatic patients, there may be little opportunity or need for the long-term use of vasodilator drugs in this cohort. In asymptomatic patients in whom corrective surgery is not recommended, it is not known if the long-term administration of vasodilators can reduce the rate of disease progression or delay the need for valve replacement.

In contrast, vasodilators have an established role in the management of severely ill patients with acute mitral regurgitation. Nitroprusside produces dramatic hemodynamic and clinical benefits in this setting and is the agent of first choice[461,462]. Vasodilators should be used to stabilize the patient prior to valve replacement surgery. Intra-aortic balloon counterpulsation may be particularly helpful if nitroprusside proves to be insufficient.[407]

Surgical Considerations

Patients with severe mitral regurgitation who remain symptomatic despite medical therapy should be considered for surgical repair or replacement of the mitral valve. Surgery is recommended in patients with:
- Recent-onset of severe mitral regurgitation.
- Class III or IV symptoms.
- Class II symptoms with evidence of progressive cardiac dilatation.

In evaluating the minimally symptomatic patient, end-systolic wall stress parameters are useful in the early detection of ventricular dysfunction.[463]

AORTIC STENOSIS

Aortic stenosis in the adult may result from rheumatic fever or calcific degeneration of a congenitally bicuspid or normal tricuspid valve (Figures 2.80, 2.81). The hemodynamic severity of the disease is determined by:
- The size of the stenotic orifice.
- The adequacy of left ventricular hypertrophy, which is required to normalize wall stress and preserve ventricular function.
- The preservation of atrial transport, which is required to maintain adequate filling of the hypertrophic, noncompliant left ventricle.

Pharmacologic Considerations

Most pharmacologic interventions that are used in the treatment of chronic heart failure are inappropriate for the patient with aortic stenosis. Digitalis provides little benefit when the ejection fraction is normal. Diuretics may excessively lower left ventricular filling pressures. Vasodilators are associated with an unacceptable risk of hypotension, since aortic stenosis impedes the ability of the heart to respond to a fall in systemic vascular resistance.

Patients with aortic stenosis should be advised against vigorous activity. Atrial arrhythmias should be treated aggressively in order to avoid the loss of atrial transport function.

Surgical Considerations

Surgery is recommended for symptomatic patients with severe aortic stenosis. Valve replacement may be extremely helpful even in patients with severe left ventricular dysfunction and

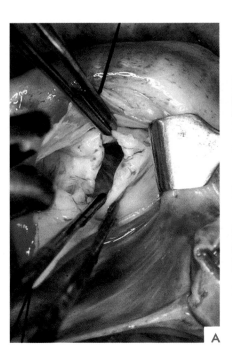 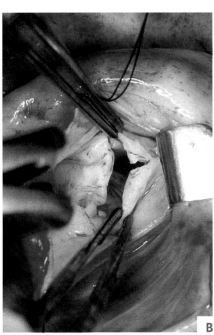

FIGURE 2.80 • In this operative view of aortic valve stenosis in an infant (A), the fused commissure is opened (B). (Reproduced with permission. Hurst JW, Anderson RH, Becker AE, et al: *Atlas of the Heart* New York, NY: Gower Medical Publishing; 1988:4.9.)

advanced symptoms of heart failure.[464] The role of surgery for asymptomatic patients with preserved left ventricular function remains controversial.

AORTIC REGURGITATION

Aortic regurgitation can occur as a result of abnormalities of the aortic valve leaflets—rheumatic fever, congenital bicuspid valve and infective endocarditis—or of the aortic root—syphilis and Marfan's syndrome (Figure 2.82). The hemodynamic severity of the disease is determined by:

- The size of the regurgitant orifice.
- The pressure gradient between the aorta and the left ventricle during diastole.
- The relation between pressure and volume in the left ventricle.

In chronic aortic regurgitation, the left ventricle becomes enormously compliant and is able to accept large regurgitant volumes without notable increases in end-diastolic pressure. In acute aortic regurgitation, however, these adaptive changes have not had time to develop. Consequently, the regurgitant flow leads a marked increase in left ventricular diastolic pressure; the pressure rise in the ventricle can be severe enough to cause premature closure of the mitral valve.

Pharmacologic Considerations

Symptomatic patients with severe aortic regurgitation should be treated with digitalis, diuretics and vasodilators until their condition improves enough to permit valve replacement surgery. Vasodilator drugs play an indispensable role in this process. Hydralazine,[237] nifedipine,[465] and nitroprusside[466] have been shown to produce short-term hemodynamic benefits in these patients. Sustained therapy with hydralazine—for weeks and months—can lead to an improvement in left ventricular systolic function and a reduction in left ventricular dilatation.[467]

The role of vasodilators in asymptomatic patients with severe aortic regurgitation remains controversial. Two controlled studies with hydralazine[258,468] showed modest increases in left ventricular ejection fraction and decreases in left ventricular dimensions and wall stress after 6 to 24 months of therapy (Figure 2.83), but the drug was poorly tolerated. A single controlled study with nifedipine[78] for 12 months showed more impressive hemodynamic benefits, but the placebo-treated group in this study unexpectedly exhibited an inexplicably large deterioration in left ventricular function during the course of follow-up. Although some favorable effects of vasodilators were noted in all three studies, it is not clear that these drugs can retard the rate of disease progression or delay the need for valve replacement surgery.

Surgical Considerations

Surgery is generally recommended for symptomatic patients with severe aortic regurgitation, but the timing of valve replacement in asymptomatic patients is uncertain. Asymptomatic patients with normal ventricular function and exercise tolerance should be observed closely with serial monitoring of ventricular function. During follow-up, some patients will develop irreversible changes in systolic performance before symptoms become apparent, but in most cases symptoms develop in parallel to any decline in left ventricular function. Surgery should be considered for the preservation of ventricular function when serial studies reveal a progressive decline in left ventricular ejection fraction to less than 40% or a progressive increase in left ventricular dimension—end-diastolic diameter greater than 70 mm or end-systolic diameter greater than 50 mm.[469,470]

• • • • • • • • • • • • • • • •

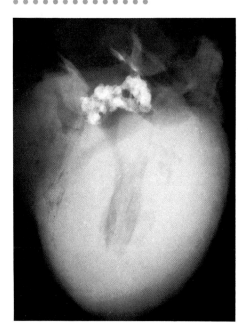

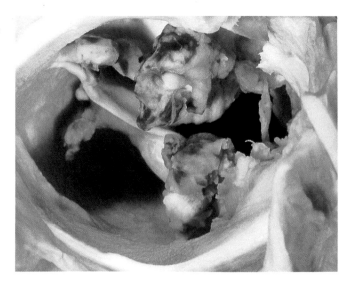

FIGURE 2.81 • Postmortum x-ray of the heart reveals isolated calcified aortic stenosis. (Reproduced with permission. Hurst JW, Anderson RH, Becker AE, et al: *Atlas of the Heart* New York, NY: Gower Medical Publishing; 1988:4.3.)

FIGURE 2.82 • Infective endocarditis of the aortic valve with extensive destruction of leaflet tissue leading to acute regurgitation. (Reproduced with permission. Hurst JW, Anderson RH, Becker AE, et al: *Atlas of the Heart* New York, NY: Gower Medical Publishing; 1988:4.18.)

PRIMARY PULMONARY HYPERTENSION

Primary pulmonary hypertension represents a heterogenous group of disorders in which pulmonary artery pressure and pulmonary vascular resistance are markedly elevated in the absence of known causes (Figure 2.84). Three distinct pathologic subtypes of primary pulmonary hypertension are recognized by the World Health Organization[471]—plexogenic arteriopathy, microthromboembolism, and pulmonary veno-occlusive disease, but it is not clear whether these categories represent distinct etiologies with a common clinical picture or different pathologic manifestations of the same disease.

Regardless of the diversity of the underlying pathologic changes, the clinical picture is strikingly similar among afflicted patients, since the symptoms and signs of patients with primary pulmonary hypertension reflect the hemodynamic abnormalities and not the pathologic or etiologic causes of the disease. The obstructive pulmonary vascular disease acts to limit transpulmonary blood flow, which leads in turn to an increase in pulmonary artery pressures, and eventually, right ventricular hypertrophy, dilatation, dysfunction and failure. The accompanying dyspnea, fatigue, angina, and syncope are directly attributed to the limitation of transpulmonary blood flow. The disorder carries an extremely poor prognosis. Nearly 50% of patients with primary pulmonary hypertension die within 3 to 5 years of initial diagnosis (Figure 2.85).

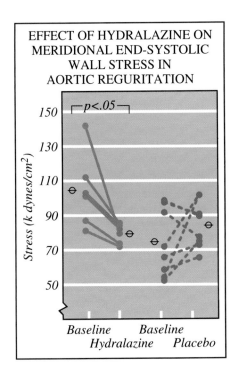

FIGURE 2.83 • M-mode echo-derived meridional end-systolic wall stress in hydralazine and placebo patients before and after a 6-month treatment period. End systolic stress was greater in the hydralazine group at intake and decreased significantly at 6 months. End systolic stress was unchanged in the placebo group. (Reproduced with permission. Kleaveland JP, Reichek N, McCarthy DM, et al: *Am J Cardiol* 1986;57:1114.)

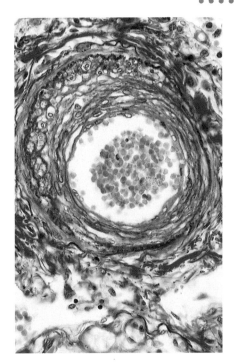

FIGURE 2.84 • Histologic section of a pulmonary arteriole depicts eccentric intimal thickening due to a proliferation of longitudinally oriented smooth muscle cells—often seen in hypoxic pulmonary hypertension. (Reproduced with permission. Hurst JW, Anderson RH, Becker AE, et al: *Atlas of the Heart* New York, NY: Gower Medical Publishing; 1988:8.3.)

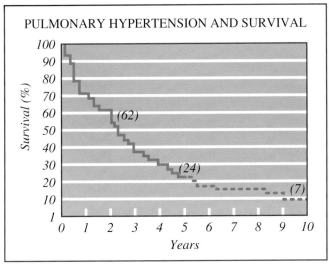

FIGURE 2.85 • Survival of patients with primary pulmonary hypertension. (Reproduced with permission. Fuster V, Steele PM, Edwards WD, et al: *Circulation* 1984;70:582.)

TREATMENT OF PRIMARY PULMONARY HYPERTENSION

No therapy has been shown to consistently improve the hemodynamic abnormalities and clinical manifestations of primary pulmonary hypertension or modify progression of the disease, but a variety of therapeutic approaches have been tried with limited success.

General Measures

Several general measures can be recommended in the management of patients with primary pulmonary hypertension. Exercise elevates pulmonary artery pressures in these patients and could theoretically accelerate the progress of right ventricular hypertrophy. On the other hand, therapeutic restriction of exercise may lead to a state of progressive physical deconditioning, which could exacerbate the exercise intolerance. Hence, exercise should be neither restricted nor encouraged. Patients should be specifically questioned about the use of appetite suppressants and oral contraceptives, both of which have been implicated in reported cases.[472,473]

Nonsteroidal anti-inflammatory agents, such as indomethacin, and histamine H_2 antagonists, such as cimetidine, have been reported to aggravate the severity of pulmonary hypertension in experimental models of the disease and should be avoided, if possible.[474,475] Patients should be advised to stop smoking, since nicotine's inhibitory effects on prostacyclin production could act to further elevate pulmonary vascular resistance.[476]

General Anesthesia and Pregnancy

Because of the inability of the pulmonary vasculature to respond adequately to changes in circulatory dynamics, patients with primary pulmonary hypertension are particularly susceptible to rapid decreases in intravascular volume. Such volume shifts are more likely to produce marked hypotension in these patients than in normal individuals. This may explain why patients with primary pulmonary hypertension have an increased risk with general anesthesia and surgical procedures.[477] Many of these adverse reactions result from abnormal cardiopulmonary reflexes elicited by the disease, which may account for the fatalities reported during pulmonary arterial catheterization.[478,479]

Pregnancy and fetal delivery can induce sudden changes in intravascular volume similar to those seen during the induction of general anesthesia, and thus, gestation places the patient with primary pulmonary hypertension at considerable risk.[480] Pregnancy should be avoided, and strict birth control measures—other than oral contraceptives—should be followed by all women of child-bearing potential. Should pregnancy occur, termination should be strongly considered, since pregnancy may accelerate the pulmonary hypertensive state and reduce responsiveness to therapeutic interventions. Nearly one fifth of patients who first present to the physician with signs and symptoms of pulmonary hypertension do so shortly after the birth of a child.[481]

General Pharmacologic Interventions

Several pharmacologic approaches commonly used in the management of patients with left ventricular failure are considered for the patient with primary pulmonary hypertension, but their efficacy has not been established.

Oxygen • Oxygen is frequently administered to patients with primary pulmonary hypertension and other obliterative pulmonary vascular disorders for diagnostic and therapeutic purposes. Such patients receive oxygen during cardiac catheter-

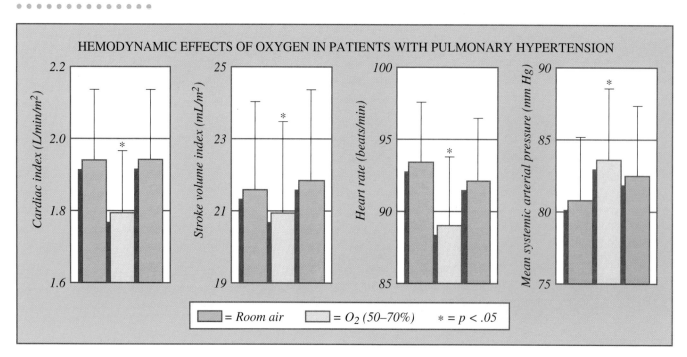

FIGURE 2.86 • Cardiac index, stroke volume index, heart rate and mean systemic arterial pressure while breathing room air, during the administration of 50% to 70% oxygen and after its withdrawal.

(Reproduced with permission. Packer M, Lee WH, Medina N, et al: *Am J Cardiol* 1986;57:853.)

ization to gauge the reversibility of the pulmonary hypertensive state and to evaluate the potential responsiveness of the pulmonary vessels to vasodilator agents.[482] It is unclear whether such testing is logical, however, because the hemodynamic response to oxygen administration does not predict the response to vasodilator therapy.[482] Oxygen is prescribed to relieve dyspnea in primary pulmonary hypertension, but these patients do not generally have hypoxia-mediated pulmonary vasoconstriction and rarely show hemodynamic or symptomatic improvement after oxygen inhalation.[483]

Unfortunately, the administration of oxygen is not entirely without hazards. Oxygen therapy may produce systemic vasoconstriction in patients with primary pulmonary hypertension (Figure 2.86), and this may be severe enough to lower cardiac output, compromise renal function, and limit the natriuretic responses to concomitantly administered treatment.[484,485]

Digitalis and Diuretics • Some investigators have proposed that digitalis be utilized early in the course of primary pulmonary hypertension,[486] based on observations that digitalis can retard the progression of right ventricular dysfunction and hypertrophy that is caused by experimentally-induced right ventricular pressure overload.[487] However, there is little clinical evidence to support this concept, and the risk of digitalis toxicity is likely to be heightened by the hemodynamic abnormalities present in these patients and by the metabolic abnormalities induced by attempts to treat the disease.

Similarly, some investigators have suggested that diuretics be routinely administered to patients with primary pulmonary hypertension, even in the absence of right heart failure.[486] This approach is based on the concept that, despite low pulmonary venous pressures, the actual closing pressures of the pulmonary vascular bed may be markedly elevated,[488] and this may lead to an increase in pulmonary lung water that contributes to the sensation of dyspnea. There is little evidence, however, that diuretics improve the lifestyle and exercise tolerance of patients with the disease. Furthermore, their administration to patients with very low left ventricular filling pressures may further deplete intravascular volume and predispose patients to catastrophic hypotensive events, particularly after the administration of systemic vasodilator drugs.

Anti-Inflammatory Drugs • The frequent association of primary pulmonary hypertension and collagen vascular disease[489–493] suggests that the pulmonary vessels may be the target of an autoimmune process, and that anti-inflammatory measures may be useful in the management of the disorder. However, vasculitic changes in the pulmonary arterial system are a rare finding in patients with primary pulmonary hypertension, even when associated with a systemic collagen vascular disorder. Furthermore, neither corticosteroids nor azothiaprine have produced any beneficial hemodynamic and clinical effects.[494]

Anticoagulants • Several authors have postulated that numerous, small, clinically silent pulmonary emboli might be an important cause of many cases of primary pulmonary hypertension.[481] Based on this hypothesis, oral anticoagulants have been recommended as a routine measure for all patients with this disorder.[495–497] In the absence of clinical contraindications, such an approach would seem reasonable, particularly since the presence of vascular microthrombi cannot be distinguished clinically from plexogenic pulmonary hypertension and since patients with pulmonary hypertension are unlikely to tolerate even a small pulmonary embolus without serious circulatory compromise. Nevertheless, there remains no definitive evidence that such an approach has improved the clinical status or prognosis of these patients. Although one retrospective study has suggested a beneficial effect of anticoagulants on survival[481] (Figure 2.87), others have not been able to document any improvement from this treatment in patients with the disease.[495–497]

Vasodilator Therapy • Although several lines of evidence support the hypothesis that reversible pulmonary vasoconstriction plays an important role in the pathogenesis of primary pulmonary hypertension, the administration of pulmonary

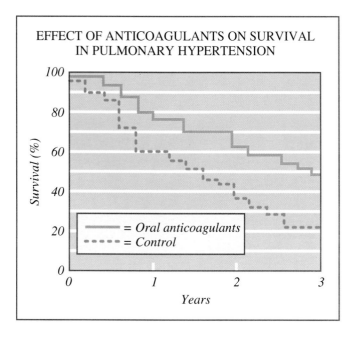

EFFECT OF ANTICOAGULANTS ON SURVIVAL IN PULMONARY HYPERTENSION

FIGURE 2.87 • Observed survival with and without anticoagulant treatment in patients with primary pulmonary hypertension. Survival rate was better among 78 patients who received oral anticoagulants than among the 37 who did not. (Reproduced with permission. Fuster V, Steele PM, Edwards WD, et al: *Circulation* 1984;70:583.)

vasodilator drugs have not proved to be consistently useful for most patients with the disease.

The principal goal of vasodilator therapy is to selectively dilate the pulmonary vasculature without producing important systemic vasodilator effects.[498] Active pulmonary vasodilation can be presumed to have occurred if the magnitude of the decrease in pulmonary resistance exceeds the decline in systemic resistance.[499] If pulmonary vasoconstriction is playing an essential role in the pathogenesis of primary pulmonary hypertension, this hemodynamic goal should be easy to achieve, since the heightened tone of the pulmonary vasculature should make it especially sensitive to the actions of pharmacologic vasodilators. Ironically, the pulmonary vasculature of patients with primary pulmonary hypertension appear to be abnormally hyporesponsive to vasodilator stimuli, possibly because the pulmonary vascular endothelium—essential to the actions of many vasodilator drugs—is destroyed by the underlying disease process,[500] or because the elevated pulmonary resistance in these patients is the result of structural obliteration of the pulmonary vascular bed and not active vasoconstriction.[501] Paradoxically, the systemic vasculature of patients with primary pulmonary hypertension appears to be exquisitely hypersensitive to vasodilator stimuli. The veins constrict in an attempt to support systemic blood pressure, as cardiac output is limited by the obliterative changes in the pulmonary vasculature.[499]

The administration of vasodilator drugs to such patients neutralizes this compensatory systemic vasoconstriction without exerting notable dilatory effects on the diseased pulmonary vessels. Hence, vasodilator therapy is likely to result in marked systemic vasodilation without producing pulmonary vasodilator effects. This lack of pulmonary vasodilator selectivity leads to the predictable development of four important adverse circulatory reactions during the administration of vasodilator drugs.[498]

Systemic Hypotension • If systemic vasodilation is produced without similar degrees of pulmonary vasodilation, the obliterative changes in the pulmonary vasculature act to limit any increase in cardiac output that is needed to prevent a substantial fall in systemic blood pressure.[502] The resultant hypotension is initially accompanied by reflex tachycardia, but if the decrease in systemic pressure persists and progresses, perfusion of the right ventricle may become severely compromised, and secondary ischemic right ventricular dysfunction leads to bradycardia, refractory hypotension, and death.[482]

Exacerbation of Pulmonary Hypertension • Even if the decrease in resistance in the systemic circulation greatly exceeds that in the pulmonary circuit, marked declines in systemic blood pressure may be avoided if cardiac output increases as a result of reflex activation of the sympathetic nervous system.[503] Such adrenergic stimulation can augment right ventricular output directly by increasing heart rate and contractility, and indirectly by enhancing venous return to the right heart consequent to venoconstriction. Unfortunately, any increase in cardiac output directed into an unresponsive pulmonary circulation will cause a further elevation of pulmonary artery pressures. This may be great enough to produce chest pain and dyspnea.[504]

Worsening of Right Ventricular Failure • Vasodilator therapy may exacerbate right ventricular dysfunction by several mechanisms. Systemic hypotension may cause hypoperfusion of the right ventricle and provoke ischemic right ventricular failure.[482] The exacerbation of pulmonary hypertension following sympathetic activation may, if persistent, lead to progressive right ventricular overload and failure, especially if vasodilator therapy is accompanied by notable fluid retention.[503] Moreover, some pulmonary vasodilator drugs—particularly calcium chan-

TABLE 2.39 • HEMODYNAMIC EFFECT OF VASODILATOR DRUGS IN PULMONARY HYPERTENSION

	Cardiac output	Heart rate	Pulmonary artery pressure	Right atrial pressure	Systemic vascular resistance	Pulmonary vascular resistance	Systemic blood pressure
Acetylcholine	0-↑	0	↓↓	0	0	↑	0
Tolazoline	↑	↑	0-↓	?	0-↑	0-↓	0-↓
Phentolamine	↑	↑	0-↓	?	0-↓	0-↓	0-↓
Isoproterenol	↑↑	↑↑	0-↑	?	↓↓	0-↓	0-↓
Diazoxide	↑	↑	0	0	↓↓	↓	↓
Hydralazine	↑	↑	0	0	↓↓	↓	↓
Verapamil	0-↓	0	↓↓	↑	↓	0-↓	↓↓
Nifedipine	0-↑	0-↑	↓↓	↑	↓↓	↓	↓↓
Nitroglycerin	0-↑	0	↓↓	↓	0-↓	↓	↓
Captopril	0	0	0	0	↓↓	0-↓	↓
Prostaglandins	↑	0-↑	↓	?	↓↓	↓	↓

(Reproduced with permission. Packer M: *Ann Intern Med* 1985;103:262.)

nel blocking agents—may exert direct negative inotropic effects on the right ventricle that may exacerbate the fall in systemic pressures during acute drug testing and worsen clinical heart failure during long-term therapy.[505,506]

Systemic Arterial Oxygen Desaturation • Even if selective pulmonary vasodilation is achieved, it may occur not in the diseased arterioles, but rather in the adjacent normal pulmonary vessels that are responsible for the maintenance of normal ventilation-perfusion relationships.[507,508] This type of pulmonary vasodilation redistributes blood flow to alveoli with low ventilation-perfusion ratios, and hence, leads to systemic arterial hypoxemia. If cardiac output fails to increase to maintain oxygen transport to the tissues, systemic arterial hypoxemia can result.[502,506]

Results with Specific Vasodilator Drugs • Isolated case reports have noted short-term hemodynamic improvement following the administration directly into the pulmonary artery of agents that interact with the autonomic nervous system—acetylcholine,[509] tolazoline,[510] phentolamine,[511] and isoproterenol[512] (Table 2.39). Unfortunately, the pulmonary vasculature in most patients has proved to be unresponsive to such interventions,[494,513] and the need for parenteral administration has been an important limitation. Even if hemodynamic improvement were observed, attempts to sustain the benefit with long-term oral or sublingual drug administration have been generally ineffective, impractical or associated with disabling gastrointestinal reactions. The use of other types of neurohormonal antagonists (for example, angiotensin-converting enzyme inhibitors) has met with equally disappointing results.[514]

Direct-Acting Vasodilator Drugs • Nitrates, hydralazine, and diazoxide have produced short-term hemodynamic benefits in some patients with primary pulmonary hypertension.[515–519] In a few cases, these effects have been sustained during long-term use and have been accompanied by an amelioration of symptoms.[515,516,519] In one patient, oral diazoxide was reported to induce hemodynamic and clinical remission of the disease.[520] Unfortunately, most experience with these drugs has not been favorable. Only a minority of patients have responded well to treatment, and many have experienced potentially serious adverse effects. Specifically, nitrates may lower cardiac output and cause oxygen desaturation.[521] Hydralazine may produce marked hypotension and provoke severe angina and dyspnea.[502,503] Diazoxide has been associated with circulatory collapse, nausea and vomiting, fluid retention, glucose intolerance, and hirsutism.[522–524]

Calcium Channel Blocking Drugs • Nifedipine has produced beneficial short- and long-term hemodynamic and clinical effects in some patients with primary pulmonary hypertension.[525-528] High doses of nifedipine have been used successfully by one group of investigators to produce marked hemodynamic and symptomatic improvement that was sustained for one year and associated with regression of right ventricular hypertrophy.[529] Isolated case reports have showed similar long-term benefit with diltiazem and felodipine.[530,531] Unfortunately, these benefits are seen in a minority of patients, and many patients experience adverse reactions. Amongst the most serious is the potential of these drugs to depress right ventricular function, which can result in cardiogenic shock during short-term therapy and worsening right heart failure during long-term therapy.[505,506]

Prostaglandin Infusions • The infusion of prostaglandin E$_1$ and prostacyclin has produced marked short-term hemodynamic benefits in patients with primary pulmonary hypertension.[532,533] The drug has been used to determine the reactivity of the pulmonary circulation to vasodilator stimuli and to predict the response to subsequently administered orally active agents.[534,535] Prolonged ambulatory infusion of the drug has been reported to produce dramatic clinical benefits.[536] Unfortunately, these dramatic effects could not be confirmed in a recent randomized controlled trial of ambulatory IV prostacyclin, which observed only a trend towards hemodynamic and clinical improvement in the treated group.[537] Furthermore, infusion of the drug is frequently associated with adverse reactions, including hypotension, flushing, headaches, nausea, vomiting, epigastric pain and bradycardia.[538,539]

Therapeutic Recommendations

At present, the administration of vasodilator drugs cannot be considered an established approach to the treatment of patients with primary pulmonary hypertension. The benefits of vasodilator therapy have never been demonstrated in a controlled clinical trial.[540] Even the most optimistic advocates suggest that favorable hemodynamic responses are uncommon (25%), probably because pulmonary vasoconstriction does not play an important role in most symptomatic patients with this disorder. Whether the detection and treatment of asymptomatic patients will produce more positive results remains to be determined.

In considering the use of vasodilator drugs in a specific patient with primary pulmonary hypertension, physicians should keep certain concepts in mind. The principal hemodynamic goal of vasodilator therapy is the selective reduction of pulmonary vascular resistance. However, because changes in pulmonary vascular resistance are unpredictable and cannot be assessed clinically and because drugs may produce serious adverse circulatory reactions, hemodynamic monitoring is mandatory to evaluate the efficacy and ensure the safety of any therapeutic intervention. Because the hemodynamic response to a specific vasodilator drug cannot be predicted before drug administration, the efficacy of any given agent can only be assessed by a process of trial and error. It is prudent to evaluate several drugs while the patient is being hemodynamically monitored, since agents that appear promising during acute invasive testing may produce intolerable adverse effects during sustained treatment.

Heart-Lung Transplantation

The definitive treatment for primary pulmonary hypertension is heart-lung transplantation. The operation produces marked clinical improvement and normalizes exercise tolerance.[541,542] Importantly, there has been no recurrence of pulmonary hypertension in patients studied by cardiac catheterization one to two years after surgery.

REFERENCES

1. Packer M: Prolonging life in patients with congestive heart failure: The next frontier. *Circulation* 1987;75(suppl IV):1.

2. Franciosa JA, Park M, Levine TB: Lack of correlation between exercise capacity and indexes of resting left ventricular performance in heart failure. *Am J Cardiol* 1981;47:33.

3. Criteria Committee, New York Heart Association, Inc In: *Diseases of the Heart and Blood Vessels. Nomenclature and Criteria for Diagnosis* 6th ed. Boston, Mass: Little, Brown and Co; 1985.

4. Weber KT, Janicki JS, McElroy PA: Determination of aerobic capacity and the severity of chronic cardiac and circulatory failure. *Circulation* 1987;76(suppl VI):40.

5. Califf RM, Bounous P, Harrell FE, et al: The prognosis in the presence of coronary artery disease. In: Braunwald E, Mock MB, Watson JT, eds. *Congestive Heart Failure* New York, NY: Grune and Stratton; 1982:31.

6. McKee PA, Castelli WP, McNamara PM: Role of blood pressure in the development of congestive heart failure: The Framingham Study. *N Engl J Med* 1972;287:781.

7. Packer M: Survival in patients with chronic congestive heart failure and its potential modification by drug therapy. In: Cohn JN, ed. *Drug Treatment of Heart Failure* Secaucus, NJ: Advanced Therapeutics Communications International; 1988:261.

8. Brushke AVG, Proudfit WL, Sones FM Jr: Progress study of 590 consecutive nonsurgical cases of coronary artery disease followed 5-9 years: II. Ventriculographic and other correlations. *Circulation* 1973;47:1154.

9. Taylor GJ, Humphries JO, Mellits ED, et al: Predictors of clinical course, coronary anatomy and left ventricular function after recovery from acute myocardial infarction. *Circulation* 1980;62:960.

10. Wilson JR, Schwartz JS, St. John Sutton M, et al: Prognosis in severe heart failure: Relation to hemodynamic measurements and ventricular ectopic activity. *J Am Coll Cardiol* 1983;2:403.

11. Lee WH, Packer M: Prognostic importance of serum sodium concentration and its modification by converting-enzyme inhibition in patients with severe chronic heart failure. *Circulation* 1986;73:257.

12. Lipkin DP, Canepa-Anson R, Stephens MR, et al: Factors determining symptoms in heart failure: comparison of fast and slow exercise tests. *Br Heart J* 1986;55:439.

13. Sodeman WA, Burch GE: The precipitating causes of congestive heart failure. *Am Heart J* 1938;15:22.

14. Ng KS, Gibson DG: Impairment of diastolic function by shortened filling period in severe left ventricular disease. *Br Heart J* 1989;62:246.

15. Luchi RJ, Scott SM, Deupree RH, et al: Comparison of medical and surgical treatment for unstable angina pectoris. Results of a Veterans Administration Cooperative Study. *N Engl J Med* 1987;316:977.

16. Alderman EL, Fisher LD, Litwin P, et al: Results of coronary artery surgery in patients with poor left ventricular function CASS. *Circulation* 1983;68:785.

17. Dzau VJ, Packer M, Lilly JS, et al: Prostaglandins in heart failure: Relation to activation of the renin-angiotensin system and hyponatremia. *N Engl J Med* 1984;310:347.

18. Oliw E, Kover G, Larsson C, et al: Reduction by indomethacin of furosemide effects in the rabbit. *Eur J Pharmacol* 1976;38:95.

19. Jackson N, Verna SP, Frais MA, et al: Hemodynamic dose-response effects of flecainide in acute myocardial infarction with and without left ventricular decompensation. *Clin Pharmacol Ther* 1985;37:619.

20. Silke B, Frais MA, Verna SP, et al: Comparative hemodynamic effects of intravenous lignocaine, disopyramide and flecainide in uncomplicated acute myocardial infarction. *Br J Clin Pharmacol* 1986;22:707.

21. Gottlieb SS, Kukin ML, Medina N, et al: Cardiodepressant effects of encainide in patients with severe left ventricular dysfunction. *Ann Intern Med* 1989;110:505.

22. Gottlieb SS, Packer M: Deleterious hemodynamic effect of lidocaine in congestive heart failure. *Am Heart J* 1989;118:611.

23. Gottlieb SS, Kukin ML, Medina N, et al: Comparative hemodynamic effects of procainamide, tocainide and encainide in chronic heart failure. *Circulation* 1990;81:860.

24. Gottlieb SS, Weinberg M: Cardiodepressant effects of mexiletine in patients with severe left ventricular dysfunction: Relation to plasma concentrations. *Circulation* 1990;80(suppl II):II-429. Abstract.

25. Packer M, Lee WH, Medina N, et al: Prognostic importance of the immediate hemodynamic response to nifedipine in patients with severe left ventricular dysfunction. *J Am Coll Cardiol* 1987;10:1303.

26. Packer M, Kessler PD, Lee WH: Calcium channel blockade in the management of severe chronic congestive heart failure: A bridge too far. *Circulation* 1987;75(suppl V):56.

27. Multicenter Diltiazem Post-Infarction Research Group: The effect of diltiazem on mortality and reinfarction after myocardial infarction. *N Engl J Med* 1988;319:385.

28. Chadda K, Goldstein S, Byington R, et al: Effect of propranolol after acute myocardial infarction in patients with congestive heart failure. *Circulation* 1986;73:503.

29. Stevenson LW, Perloff JK: The limited reliability of physical signs for estimating hemodynamics in chronic heart failure. *JAMA* 1989;10:884.

30. Gottlieb SS, Kessler P, Lee WH, et al: What is the significance of Cheynes-Stokes respiration in severe chronic heart failure? Hemodynamic and clinical correlates in 167 patients. *J Am Coll Cardiol* 1986;7:43A.

31. Carr JG, Stevenson LW, Walden JA, et al: Prevalence and hemodynamic correlates of malnutrition in severe congestive heart failure secondary to ischemic or idiopathic dilated cardiomyopathy. *Am J Cardiol* 1989;63:709.

32. Harigaya S, Schwartz A: Rate of calcium binding and uptake in normal animal and failing human cardiac muscle. *Circ Res* 1969;25:781.

33. Lindemayer GE, Sordahl LA, Harigaya S, et al: Some biochemical studies on subcellular systems isolated from fresh recipient human cardiac tissue obtained during transplantation. *An J Cardiol* 1971;27:277.

34. Gwathmey JK, Copelas L, MacKinnon R, et al: Abnormal intracellular calcium handling in myocardium from patients with end-stage heart failure. *Circ Res* 1987;61:70.

35. Ito Y, Suko J, Chidsey CA: Intracellular calcium and myocardial contractility. Calcium uptake of sarcoplasmic reticulum reticulum fractions in hypertrophied and failing rabbit hearts. *J Mol Cell Cardiol* 1974;6:237.

36. Feldman MD, Copelas L, Gwanthmey JK, et al: Deficient production of cyclic AMP: Pharmacologic evidence of an important cause of contractile dysfunction in patients with end-stage heart failure. *Circulation* 1987;75:331.

37. Bristow MR, Ginsburg R, Umans V, et al: β_1- and β_2-adrenergic-receptor subpopulations in nonfailing and failing human ventricular myocardium: Coupling of both receptor subtypes to muscle contraction and selective β_1-receptor down-regulation in heart failure. *Circ Res* 1986;59:297.

38. Brodde OE, Zerkowski HR, Doetsch N, et al: Myocardial beta-adrenoceptor changes in heart failure: Concomitant reduction in beta 1- and beta 2-adrenoceptor function related to the degree of heart failure in patients with mitral valve disease. *J Am Coll Cardiol* 1989;14:323.

39. Longabaugh JP, Vatner DE, Vatner SF, et al: Decreased stimulatory guanosine triphosphate binding protein in dogs with pressure-overload left ventricular failure. *J Clin Invest* 1988;81:420.

40. Horn EM, Corwin SJ, Steinberg SF, et al: Reduced lymphocyte stimulatory guanine nucleotide regulatory protein and beta-adrenergic receptors in congestive heart failure and reversal with angiotensin converting enzyme inhibitor therapy. *Circulation* 1988;78:1373.

41. Feldman AM, Cates AE, Veazey WB, et al: Increase of the 40,000 mol wt. pertussis toxin substrate G-protein in the failing human heart. *J Clin Invest* 1988;82:189.

42. Neumann J, Schmitz W, Scholz H, et al: Increase in myocardial Gi-proteins in heart failure. *Lancet* 1988;2:936.

43. Norgaard A, Bagger JP, Bjerregaard P, et al: Relation of left ventricular function and Na,K pump concentration in suspected idiopathic dilated cardiomyopathy. *Am J Cardiol* 1988;61:1312.

44. Gwanthmey JK, Slawsky MT, Briggs GM, et al: The role of intracellular sodium in the regulation of calcium and contractility. Effects of DPI 201-106 on excitation-contraction coupling in human ventricular myocardium. *J Clin Invest* 1988;82:1592.

45. Pagani ED, Alousi AA, Grant AM, et al: Changes in myofibrillar content and Mg-ATPase activity in ventricular tissues from patients with heart failure caused by coronary artery disease, cardiomyopathy, or mitral valve insufficiency. *Circ Res* 1988;63:380.

46. Chandler BM, Sonnenblick EH, Spann JR Jr, et al: Association of depressed myofibrillar adenosine triphosphate and reduced contractility in experimental heart failure. *Circ Res* 1967;21:717.

47. Unverferth DV, Lee SW, Wallick ET: Human myocardial adenosine triphosphate activities in health and heart failure. *Am Heart J* 1988;115:139.

48. Lompre A-M, Schwartz K, d'Albis A, et al: Myosin isoenzyme redistribution in chronic heart overload. *Nature* 1979;282:105.

49. Gorza L, Mercadier JJ, Schwartz K, et al: Myosin types in the human heart: An immunofluorescence study of normal and hypertrophied atrial and ventricular myocardium. *Circ Res* 1984;54:694.

50. Hajjar RJ, Gwathmey JK, Briggs GM, et al: Differential effect of DPI 201-106 in the sensitivity and myofilaments to Ca++ in intact and skinned trabeculae from control and myopathic human hearts. *J Clin Invest* 1988;82:1578.

51. Skorecki KL, Brenner BM: Body fluid homeostasis in congestive heart failure and cirrhosis with ascites. *Am J Med* 1982;72:323.

52. Hostetter TH, Pfeffer JM, Pfeffer MA, et al: Cardiorenal hemodynamics and sodium excretion in rats with myocardial infarction. *Am J Physiol* 1983;245:H98.

53. DiBona GF, Herman PJ, Sawin LL: Neural control of renal function in edema-forming states. *Am J Physiol* 1988;254:R101.

54. Packer M: Interaction of prostaglandins and angiotensin II in the modulation of renal function in congestive heart failure. *Circulation* 1988;77(suppl I):64.

55. Hall JE: Control of sodium excretion by angiotensin II: Intrarenal mechanisms and blood pressure regulation. *Am J Physiol* 1986;250:R960.

56. Fredlund P, Saltman S, Catt K: Aldosterone production by isolated adrenal glomerulosa cells: Stimulation by physiological concentrations of angiotensin II. *Endocrinology* 1975;97:1577.

57. Laragh JH: Atrial natriuretic hormone, the renin-angiotensin axis, and blood pressure-electrolyte homeostasis. *N Engl J Med* 1985;313:1330.

58. Stokes JB, Kokko JP: Inhibition of sodium transport by prostaglandin E2 across the isolated perfused rabbit collecting tubule. *J Clin Invest* 1977;59:1099.

59. Sarnoff SJ, Mitchell JH, Gilmore JP, et al: Homeometric autoregulation of the heart. *Circ Res* 1960;8:1077.

60. Cohn JN: Vasodilator therapy for heart failure: The influence of impedance on left ventricular performance. *Circulation* 1973;48:5.

61. Mackenzie J: *Diseases of the Heart* 3rd ed. London, England: Oxford University Press; 1913.

62. Hope JA: *Treatise on the Diseases of the Heart and Great Vessels* London, England: Williams-Kidd; 1832.

63. Mancini DM, Maskin CS, Licido D, et al: Failure to augment maximal limb blood flow in response to one-leg versus two-leg exercise in patients with severe heart failure. *Circulation* 1986;74:245.

64. Cowley AJ, Stainer K, Rowley JM, et al: Abnormalities of the peripheral circulation and respiratory function in patients with severe heart failure. *Br Heart J* 1986;55:75.

65. Fink LI, Wilson JR, Ferraro N: Exercise ventilation and pulmonary artery wedge pressure in chronic stable congestive heart failure. *Am J Cardiol* 1986;57:249.

66. Szlachcic J, Massie BM, Kramer BL, et al: Correlates and prognostic implication of exercise capacity in chronic congestive heart failure. *Am J Cardiol* 1985;55:1037.

67. Packer M: Abnormalities of diastolic function as a potential cause of exercise intolerance in chronic heart failure. *Circulation* 1990;81(suppl III):78.

68. Weiner D, Fink LI, Maris J, et al: Abnormal skeletal muscle bioenergetics during exercise in patients with heart failure: Role of reduced muscle blood flow. *Circulation* 1986;73:1127.

69. Massie B, Conway M, Yonge R, et al: Skeletal muscle metabolism in patients with congestive heart failure: Relation to clinical severity and blood flow. *Circulation* 1987;76:1009.

70. Franciosa JA, Baker BJ, Seth L: Pulmonary versus systemic hemodynamics in determining exercise capacity of patients with chronic left ventricular failure. *Am Heart J* 1985;110:807.

71. Baker BJ, Wilen MM, Boyd LM, et al: Relation of right ventricular ejection fraction to exercise capacity in chronic left ventricular failure. *Am J Cardiol* 1984;54:596.

72. Konstam MA, Weiland DS, Conlon TP, et al: Hemodynamic correlates of left ventricular versus right ventricular radionuclide volumetric responses to vasodilator therapy in congestive heart failure secondary to ischemic or dilated cardiomyopathy. *Am J Cardiol* 1987;59:1131.

73. Baker BJ, Wilen MM, Boyd CM, et al: Right ventricular ejection fraction as a predictor of changes in exercise capacity in heart failure. *Circulation* 1984;70(suppl II):II-156.

74. Packer M: How should we judge the efficacy of drug therapy in patients with chronic congestive heart failure? The insights of six blind men. *J Am Coll Cardiol* 1987;9:433.

75. Franciosa JA, Weber KT, Levine TB, et al: Hydralazine in the long-term treatment of chronic heart failure: Lack of difference from placebo. *Am Heart J* 1982;104:587.

76. Agostoni PG, DeCesare N, Doria E, et al: Afterload reduction: a comparison of captopril and nifedipine in dilated cardiomyopathy. *Br Heart J* 1986;55:391.

77. Packer M, Meller J, Medina N, et al: Importance of left ventricular chamber size in determining the response to hydralazine in severe chronic heart failure. *N Engl J Med* 1980;303:250.

78. Scognamiglio R, Fasoli G, Ponchia A, et al: Long-term nifedipine unloading therapy in asymptomatic patients with chronic severe aortic regurgitation. *J Am Coll Cardiol* 1990;16:424.

79. Franciosa JA, Jordan RA, Wilen MM, et al: Minoxidil in patients with left heart failure: contrasting hemodynamic and clinical effects in a controlled trial. *Circulation* 1984;70:63.

80. Zucker IH, Earle AM, Gilmore JP: The mechanism of adaptation of left atrial stretch receptors in dogs with chronic congestive heart failure. *J Clin Invest* 1977;60:323.

81. Hirsch AT, Dzau VJ, Creager MA: Baroreceptor function in congestive heart failure: Effect on neurohormonal activation and regional vascular resistance. *Circulation* 1987;75(suppl IV):36.

82. Carroll JD, Lang RM, Neumann AL, et al: The differential effects of positive inotropic and vasodilator therapy on diastolic properties in patients with congestive cardiomyopathy. *Circulation* 1986;74:815.

83. Grossman W, McLaurin LP, Rolett EL: Alterations in left ventricular relaxation and diastolic compliance in congestive cardiomyopathy. *Cardiovasc Res* 1979;13:514.

84. Katz AM: Role of the basic sciences in the practice of cardiology. *J Mol Cell Cardiol* 1987;19:3.

85. Little WC, Rassi A, Freeman GL: Comparison of effects of dobutamine and ouabain on left ventricular contraction and relaxation in closed-chest dogs. *J Clin Invest* 1987;80: 613.

86. Juneman M, Smiseth DA, Refsum H, et al: Quantification of effect of pericardium on left ventricular diastolic pressure-volume relation in dogs. *Am J Physiol* 1987;252:H963.

87. Smith ER, Smiseth OA, Kingma I, et al: Mechanism of action of nitrates. Role of changes in venous capacitance and in the left ventricular diastolic pressure-volume relation. *Am J Med* 1984;76 3A.:14.

88. Keren G, Katz S, Strom J, et al: Dynamic mitral regurgitation. An important determinant of the hemodynamic response to load alterations and inotropic therapy in severe heart failure. *Circulation* 1989;80:306.

89. Packer M: Neurohormonal interactions and adaptations in congestive heart failure. *Circulation* 1988;77:721.

90. Goldsmith SR, Francis GS, Cowley AW, et al: Increased plasma arginine vasopressin levels in patients with congestive heart failure. *J Am Coll Cardiol* 1983;1:1385.

91. Maisel AS, Scott NA, Motulsky HJ, et al: Elevation of plasma neuropeptide Y levels in congestive heart failure. *Am J Med* 1989;86:430.

92. Kawashima S, Fukutake N, Nishian K, et al: Elevation of plasma levels of beta-endorphin in patients with congestive heart failure. *Circulation* 1989;80(suppl II):II-672. Abstract.

93. Robertson RM, Susawa T, Sugiura M, et al: Circulatory endothelin levels: Modulation by heart failure in man. *Clin Res* 1990;38:414A. Abstract.

94. Kaiser L, Spickard RC, Olivier NB: Heart failure depresses endothelium-dependent responses in canine femoral artery. *Am J Physiol* 1989;256:H962.

95. Levine B, Kalman J, Mayer L, et al: Elevated circulating levels of tumor necrosis factor in congestive heart failure. *N Engl J Med* 1990;323:236.

96. Chidsey CA, Harrison DC, Braunwald E: Augmentation of the plasma norepinephrine response to exercise in patients with congestive heart failure. *N Engl J Med* 1962;267:650.

97. Thomas JA, Marks BH: Plasma norepinephrine in congestive heart failure. *Am J Cardiol* 1978;41:233.

98. Francis GS, Goldsmith SR, Cohn JN: Relationship of exercise capacity to resting left ventricular performance and basal plasma norepinephrine levels in patients with congestive heart failure. *Am Heart J* 1982;104:725.

99. Cohn JN, Levine TB, Olivari MT, et al: Plasma norepinephrine as a guide to prognosis in patients with chronic congestive heart failure. *N Engl J Med* 1984;311:819.

100. Leimbach WN Jr, Wallin BG, Victor RG, et al: Direct evidence from intraneural recordings for increased central sympathetic outflow in patients with heart failure. *Circulation* 1986;73:913.

101. Hasking GJ, Esler MD, Jennings GL, et al: Norepinephrine spillover to plasma during steady-state supine bicycle exercise. Comparison of patients with congestive heart failure and normal subjects. *Circulation* 1988;78:516.

102. Davis D, Baily R, Zelis R: Abnormalities in systemic norepinephrine kinetics in human congestive heart failure. *Am J Physiol* 1988;254:E760.

103. Kramer RS, Mason DT, Braunwald E: Augmented sympathetic neurotransmitter activity in the peripheral vascular bed of patients with congestive heart failure and cardiac norepinephrine depletion. *Circulation* 1968;38:629.

104. Forster C, Carter SL, Armstrong PW: Alpha 1-adrenoceptor activity in arterial smooth muscle following congestive heart failure. *Can J Physiol Pharmacol* 1989;67:110.

105. Covell JW, Chidsey CA, Braunwald E: Reduction in the cardiac response to postganglionic sympathetic nerve stimulation in experimental heart failure. *Circ Res* 1966;19:51.

106. Colucci WS, Ribeiro JP, Rocco MB, et al: Impaired chronotropic response to exercise in patients with congestive heart failure. Role of postsynaptic beta-adrenergic desensitization. *Circulation* 1989;80:314.

107. Packer M: Role of the sympathetic nervous system in chronic heart failure. A historical and philosophical perspective. *Circulation* 1990;82(suppl I):1.

108. Tanaka M, Tsuchihashi Y, Katsumi H, et al: Comparison of cardiac lesions induced in rats by isoproterenol and by repeated stress of restraints and water immersion with special reference to etiology of cardiomyopathy. *Jpn Circ J* 1980;44:971.

109. Dibner-Dunlap ME, Thames MD: Baroreflex control of renal sympathetic nerve activity is preserved in heart failure despite reduced arterial baroreceptor sensitivity. *Circ Res* 1989;65:1526.

110. Dzau VJ, Colucci WS, Hollenberg NK, et al: Relation of renin-angiotensin-aldosterone system to clinical state in congestive heart failure. *Circulation* 1981;63:645.

111. Kirlin PC, Grekin R, Das S, et al: Neurohumoral activation during exercise in congestive heart failure. *Am J Med* 1986;81:623.

112. Rockman HA, Juneau C, Chatterjee K, et al: Long-term predictors of sudden and low output death in chronic congestive heart failure secondary to coronary artery disease. *Am J Cardiol* 1989;64:1344.

113. Dargie HJ, Cleland JGF, Leckie BJ, et al: Relation of arrhythmias and electrolyte abnormalities to survival in patients with severe chronic heart failure. *Circulation* 1987;75(suppl IV):98.

114. Francis GS, Siegel RM, Goldsmith SR, et al: Acute vasoconstrictor response to intravenous furosemide in patients with chronic congestive heart failure. *Ann Intern Med* 1985;103:1.

115. Kubo SH, Clark M, Laragh JH, et al: Identification of normal neurohormonal activity in mild congestive heart failure and stimulating effect of upright posture and diuretics. *Am J Cardiol* 1987;60:1322.

116. Goldenberg IF, Levine TB, Olivari MT, et al: Markers of reduced renal blood flow in patients with congestive heart failure. *Circulation* 1985;72(suppl III):III-284. Abstract.

117. Packer M, Medina M, Yushak M: Correction of dilutional hyponatremia in patients with severe chronic heart failure by converting-enzyme inhibition. *Ann Intern Med* 1984;100:782.

118. Packer M, Medina N, Yushak M: Relationship between serum sodium concentration and the hemodynamic and clinical responses to converting-enzyme inhibition with captopril in severe heart failure. *J Am Coll Cardiol* 1984;3:1035.

119. Lilly LS, Dzau VJ, Williams GH, et al: Hyponatremia in congestive heart failure: Implications for neurohormonal activation and response to orthostasis. *J Clin Endocrinol Metab* 1984;59:924.

120. Packer M, Lee WH, Kessler PD: Preservation of glomerular filtration rate in human heart failure by activation of the renin-angiotensin system. *Circulation* 1986;74:766.

121. Tan LB, Jalil JE, Janicki JS, et al: Cardiotoxic effects of angiotensin II. *J Am Coll Cardiol* 1989;13:2A. Abstract.

122. Francis GS, Goldsmith SR, Olivari MT, et al: The neurohormonal axis in congestive heart failure. *Ann Intern Med* 1984;1091:370.

123. Packer M, Gottlieb SS, Kessler PD, et al: Hormone-electrolyte interactions in the pathogenesis of lethal cardiac arrhythmias in patients with congestive heart failure. The basis of a new physiologic approach to control of arrhythmia. *Am J Med* 1986;80:23.

124. Lee ME, Miller WL, Edwards BS, et al: Role of endogenous atrial natriuretic factor in acute congestive heart failure. *J Clin Invest* 1989;84:1962.

125. Villarreal D, Freeman RH, Davis JO, et al: Atrial natriuretic factor secretion in dogs with experimental high-output heart failure. *Am J Physiol* 1987;252:H692.

126. Redfield MM, Edwards BS, McGoon MD, et al: Failure of atrial natriuretic factor to increase with volume expansion in acute and chronic congestive heart failure in the dog. *Circulation* 1989;80:651.

127. Cody RJ, Atlas SA, Laragh JH, et al: Atrial natriuretic factor in normal subjects and heart failure patients: Plasma levels and renal, hormonal, and hemodynamic responses to peptide infusion. *J Clin Invest* 1986;78:1362.

128. Schiffrin EL: Decreased density of binding sites for atrial natriuretic peptide on platelets of patients with severe congestive heart failure. *Clin Sci* 1988;74:213.

129. Tsunoda K, Mendelsohn FA, Sexton PM, et al: Decreased atrial natriuretic peptide binding in renal medulla in rats with chronic heart failure. *Circ Res* 1988;62:155.

130. Sosa RE, Volpe M, Marion DN, et al: Relationship between renal hemodynamic and natriuretic effects of atrial natriuretic factor. *Am J Physiol* 1986;250:F520.

131. Redfield MM, Edwards BS, Heublein DM, et al: Restoration of renal response to atrial natriuretic factor in experimental low-output heart failure. *Am J Physiol* 1989;257:R917.

132. Petersson A, Hedner J, Hedner T: Renal interaction between sympathetic activity and ANP in rats with chronic ischaemic heart failure. *Acta Physiol Scand* 1989;135:487.

133. Katayama S, Attallah AA, Stahl RAK, et al: Mechanism of furosemide-induced natriuresis by direct stimulation of renal prostaglandin E2. *Am J Physiol* 1984;247:F555.

134. DeForrest JH, Davis JO, Freeman RH, et al: Effects of indomethacin and meclofenamate in renin release and renal hemodynamic function during chronic sodium depletion in conscious dogs. *Circ Res* 1980;47:99.

135. Guaita DP, Chiaravigilio E: Effect of prostaglandin E1 and its biosynthesis inhibitor indomethacin on drinking in the rat. *Pharmacol Biochem Behav* 1980;13:787.

136. Anderson RJ, Berl T, McDonald KM, et al: Evidence for an in vivo antagonism between vasopressin and prostaglandin in the mammalian kidney. *J Clin Invest* 1975;56:420.

137. Packer M: Sudden unexpected death in patients with congestive heart failure: a second frontier. *Circulation* 1985;72:681.

138. Meinertz T, Tresse N, Kasper W, et al: Determinants of prognosis in idiopathic dilated cardiomyopathy as determined by programmed electrical stimulation. *Am J Cardiol* 1985;56:337.

139. Stevenson WG, Stevenson LW, Weiss J, et al: Inducible ventricular arrhythmias and sudden death during vasodilator therapy of severe heart failure. *Am Heart J* 1988;116:1447.

140. Surawicz B: Prognosis of ventricular arrhythmias in relation to sudden cardiac death: Therapeutic implications. *J Am Coll Cardiol* 1987;10:435.

141. Chakko CS, Gheorghiade M: Ventricular arrhythmias in severe heart failure: Incidence, significance and effectiveness of antiarrhythmic therapy. *Am Heart J* 1985;109:497.

142. Neri R, Mestroni L, Salvi A, et al: Ventricular arrhythmias in dilated cardiomyopathy: Efficacy of amiodarone. *Am Heart J* 1987;113:707.

143. Wilson JR: Use of antiarrhythmic drugs in patients with heart failure: clinical efficacy, hemodynamic results, and relation to survival. *Circulation* 1987;75(suppl IV):64.

144. Simonton CA, Daly PA, Kereiakes D, et al: Survival in severe left ventricular failure treated with the new nonglycosidic, nonsympathomimetic oral inotropic agents. *Chest* 1987;92:118.

145. Luu M, Stevenson WG, Stevenson LW, et al: Diverse mechanisms of unexpected cardiac arrest in advanced heart failure. *Circulation* 1989;80:1675.

146. Bigger JT Jr: Why patients with congestive heart failure die: arrhythmias and sudden cardiac death. *Circulation* 1987;75(suppl IV):28.

147. Chow LC, Dittrich HC, Shabetai R: Endomyocardial biopsy in patients with unexplained congestive heart failure. *Ann Intern Med* 1988;109:535.

148. Sullivan MJ, Higginbotham MB, Cobb FR: Exercise training in patients with chronic heart failure delays ventilatory anaerobic threshold and improves submaximal exercise performance. *Circulation* 1989;79:324.

149. Shabetai R: Beneficial effects of exercise training in compensated heart failure. *Circulation* 1988;78:775.

150. Packer M: Vasodilator and inotropic therapy for severe chronic heart failure: Passion and skepticism. *J Am Coll Cardiol* 1983;2:841.

151. Packer M: Vasodilator and inotropic drugs for chronic heart failure: Distinguishing hype from hope. *J Am Coll Cardiol* 1988;12:1299.

152. Packer M: Therapeutic options in the management of chronic heart failure: Is there a drug of first choice? *Circulation* 1989;79:198.

153. Akera T, Baskin SI, Tobin T, et al: Ouabain: temporal relationship between inotropic effect and the in vitro binding to, and dissociation from, Na+, K+.-activated ATPase. *Naunyn Schmiedebergs Arch Pharmacol* 1973;277:151.

154. Pugh SE, White NJ, Aronson JK, et al: Clinical, haemodynamic, and pharmacologic effects of withdrawal and reintroduction of digoxin in patients with heart failure in sinus rhythm after long-term treatment. *Br Heart J* 1989;61:529.

155. Taggart AJ, Johnston GD, McDevitt DG: Digoxin withdrawal after cardiac failure in patients with sinus rhythm. *J Cardiovasc Pharmacol* 1983;5:229.

156. Ferguson DW, Berg WJ, Sanders JS, et al: Sympathoinhibitory responses to digitalis glycosides in heart failure patients. Direct evidence from sympathetic neural recordings. *Circulation* 1989;80:65.

157. Covit AB, Schaer GL, Sealey JE, et al: Suppression of the renin-angiotensin system by intravenous digoxin in chronic congestive heart failure. *Am J Med* 1983;75:445.

158. Torretti J, Hendler E, Weinstein E, et al: Functional significance of Na-K ATPase in the kidney: Effect of ouabain inhibition. *Am J Physiol* 1972;222:1398.

159. The Captopril-Digoxin Multicenter Research Group: Comparative effects of captopril and digoxin in patients with mild to moderate heart failure. *JAMA* 1988;259:539.

160. Arnold SB, Byrd RC, Meister W, et al: Long-term digitalis therapy improves left ventricular function in heart failure. *N Engl J Med* 1980;303:1443.

161. Guyatt GH, Sullivan MJJ, Fallen EL, et al: A controlled trial of digoxin in congestive heart failure. *Am J Cardiol* 1988;61:371.

162. Gheorghiade M, Hall V, Lakier JB, et al: Comparative hemodynamic and neurohormonal effects of intravenous captopril and digoxin and their combinations in patients with severe heart failure. *J Am Coll Cardiol* 1989;13:134.

163. Ribner HS, Plucinski DA, Hsieh A-M, et al: Acute effects of digoxin on total systemic vascular resistance in congestive heart failure due to dilated cardiomyopathy: A hemodynamic-hormonal study. *Am J Cardiol* 1985;56:896.

164. DiBianco R, Shabetai R, Kostuk W, et al: A comparison of oral milrinone, digoxin, and their combination in the treatment of patients with chronic heart failure. *N Engl J Med* 1989;320:677.

165. Jaeschke R, Oxman AD, Guyatt GH: To what extent do congestive heart failure patients in sinus rhythm benefit from digoxin therapy? A systematic overview and meta-analysis. *Am J Med* 1990;88:279.

166. Lee DC, Johnson RA, Bingham JB, et al: Heart failure in outpatients. A randomized trial of digoxin versus placebo. *N Engl J Med* 1982;306:699.

167. Dobbs SM, Kenyon WL, Dobbs RJ: Maintenance digoxin after an episode of heart failure: placebo-controlled trial in outpatients. *Br Med J* 1977;1:749.

168. The German and Austrian Xamoterol Study Group: Double-blind placebo-controlled comparison of digoxin and xamoterol in chronic heart failure. *Lancet* 1988;1:489.

169. Fleg JL, Gottlieb SH, Lakatta EG: Is digoxin really important in treatment of compensated heart failure? A placebo-controlled crossover trial in patients with sinus rhythm. *Am J Med* 1982;73:244.

170. Gheorghiade M, Beller GA: Effects of discontinuating maintenance digoxin therapy in patients with ischemic heart disease and congestive heart failure in sinus rhythm. *Am J Cardiol* 1983;51:1243.

171. Bigger JT, Fleiss KR, Rolnitsky LM, et al: Effect of digitalis treatment on survival after acute myocardial infarction. *Am J Cardiol* 1985;55:623.

172. Yusuf S, Wittes J, Bailey K, et al: Digitalis—a new controversy regarding an old drug. The pitfalls of inappropriate methods. *Circulation* 1986;73:14.

173. Goldstein S, Pitt B, Packer M, et al: The relationship of digoxin dose, serum concentration and left ventricular ejection fraction in mild to moderate heart failure. *1st International Symposium on Heart Failure* 233.

174. Ware JA, Snow E, Luchi JM, et al: Effect of digoxin on ejection fraction in elderly patients with congestive heart failure. *J Am Geriatric Soc* 1984;32:631.

175. Beller GA, Smith TW, Abelman WH, et al: Digitalis intoxication. A prospective clinical study with serum level correlations. *N Engl J Med* 1971;284:989.

176. Fogelman AM, LaMont JT, Finkelstein S, et al: Fallibility of plasma digoxin in differentiating toxic from non-toxic patients. *Lancet* 1971;2:727.

177. Ingelfinger JA, Goldman P: The serum digitalis concentration—Does it diagnose digitalis toxicity. *N Engl J Med* 1976;294:867.

178. Steiness E, Olesen KH: Cardiac arrhythmias induced by potassium loss during maintenance digoxin therapy. *Br Heart J* 1976;38:167.

179. Ghani MF, Smith JR: The effectiveness of magnesium chloride in the treatment of ventricular tachyarrhythmias due to digitalis intoxication. *Am Heart J* 1974;88:621.

180. Hager WD, Fenster PE, Mayersohn M, et al: Digoxin-quinidine interaction. *N Engl J Med* 1979;300:1238.

181. Klein HO, Lang R, Weiss E, et al: The influence of verapamil on serum digoxin concentration. *Circulation* 1982;65:998.

182. Paladino JA, Davidson KH, McCall B: Influence of spironolactone on serum digoxin concentration. *JAMA* 1984;251:470.

183. Lewis GP, Holtzxman JL: Interaction of flecainide with digoxin and propranolol. *Am J Cardiol* 1984;53:52B.

184. Belz GG, Matthews J, Doering WE, et al: Digoxin-antiarrhythmics: Pharmacodynamic and pharmacokinetic studies with quinidine, propafenone, and verapamil. *Clin Pharrmacol Ther* 1982;31:202.

185. Moysey JO, Jaggarao NSV, Grundy EN, et al: Amiodarone increase plasma digoxin concentrations. *Br Med J* 1981;282:272.

186. Awan NA, Needham KE, Eevenson MK, et al: Hemodynamic actions of prenalterol in severe congestive heart failure due to chronic coronary disease. *Am Heart J* 1981;101:158.

187. Bito K, Kiroshita M, Mashiro I, et al: Clinicopharmacological studies of a newly synthesized cardiotonic agent TA-064 in patients with congestive heart failure. *Clin Cardiol* 1988;11:334.

188. Rousseau MF, Pouleur H, Vincent MF: Effects of a cardioselective beta 1-partial agonist Corwin on left ventricular function and myocardial metabolism in patients with previous myocardial infarction. *Am J Cardiol* 1983;51:1267.

189. Awan NA, Evenson MK, Needham KE, et al: Hemodynamic effects of oral pirbuterol in chronic severe congestive heart failure. *Circulation* 1981;63:96.

190. Sharma B, Goodwin JF: Beneficial effect of salbutamol on cardiac function of severe congestive cardiomyopathy. *Circulation* 1978;58:449.

191. Lambertz H, Meyer J, Erbel R: Long-term effects of prenalterol in patients with severe congestive heart failure. *Circulation* 1984;69:298.

192. Roubin GS, Choong CY, Devenish-Meares S, et al: Beta-adrenergic stimulation of the failing left ventricle: A double-blind, randomized trial of sustained oral therapy with prenalterol. *Circulation* 1984;69:955.

193. Weber KT, Andrews V, Janicki JS, et al: Pirbuterol, an oral beta-adrenergic receptor agonist, in the treatment of chronic cardiac failure. *Circulation* 1982;66:1262.

194. Xamoterol in Severe Heart Failure Study Group: Xamoterol in severe heart failure. *Lancet* 1990;336:1.

195. Colucci WS, ALexander RW, Williams GH, et al: Decreased lymphocyte beta-adrenergic receptot density in patients with heart failure and tolerance to the beta-adrenergic agonist pirbuterol. *N Engl J Med* 1981;305:185.

196. Dies F, Krell MJ, Whitlow P, et al: Intermittent dobutamine in ambulatory outpatients with chronic cardiac failure. *Circulation* 1986;74 (suppl II):II-138. Abstract.

197. Le Jemtel TH, Keung M, Ribner HS, et al: Sustained beneficial effects of oral amrinone on cardiac and renal function in patients with severe congestive heart failure. *Am J Cardiol* 1980;45:122.

198. Simonton CA, Chatterjee K, Cody RJ, et al: Milrinone in congestive heart failure: Acute and chronic hemodynamic and clinical evaluation. *J Am Coll Cardiol* 1985;6:453.

199. Uretsky BT, Generalovich T, Veralis JG, et al: MDL 17,043 therapy in severe congestive heart failure: Characterization of the early and late hemodynamic pharmacokinetic, hormonal and clinical response. *J Am Coll Cardiol* 1985;5:1414.

200. Jafri SM, Burlew BS, Goldberg AD, et al: Hemodynamic effects of a new type III phosphodiesterase inhibitor CI-914 for congestive heart failure. *Am J Cardiol* 1986;57:254.

201. Weber KT, Janicki JS, Jain MC: Piroximone MDL 19,205. in the treatment of unstable and stable chronic cardiac failure. *Am Heart J* 1987;114:805.

202. DiBianco R, Shabetai R, Silverman BD, et al: Oral amrinone for the treatment of chronic congestive heart failure: Results of a multicenter randomized double-blind and placebo-controlled withdrawal study. *J Am Coll Cardiol* 1984;4:855.

203. Uretsky BF, Jessup M, Konstam MA, et al: Multicenter trial of oral enoximone in patients with moderately severe congestive heart failure: Lack of benefit compared to placebo. *Circulation* 1989;80(suppl II):II-174. Abstract.

204. Narahara KA and the Western Enoximone Study Group: Enoximone Versus Placebo: A Double-Blind Trial in Chronic Congestive Heart Failure. *Circulation* 1989;80(suppl II):II-175. Abstract.

205. Goldberg AD, Goldstein S, Nicklaus J, for the Imazodan Study Group. Multicenter trial of imazodan in patients with chronic congestive heart failure. *Circulation* 1990;82(suppl III):III-673. Abstract.

206. Packer M, Carver JR, Rodenheffer R, et al: Effect of oral milrinone on mortality in severe chronic heart failure. *N Engl J Med* 1991;325:1468.

207. Dies F, McNay JL, Andrejasich CM, et al: Indolidan a new phosphodiesterase inhibitor in chronic heart failure. *Circulation* 1989;80(suppl II):II-175. Abstract.

208. Packer M, Medina N, Yushak M: Hemodynamic and clinical limitation of long-term inotropic therapy with amrinone in patients with severe chronic heart failure. *Circulation* 1984;70:1038.

209. Chesebro JH, Browne KF, Fenster PE, et al: The hemodynamic effects of chronic oral milrinone therapy: A multicenter controlled trial. *J Am Coll Cardiol* 1988;11:144A. Abstract.

210. Doherty JE: Use of digitalis and diuretics in the treatment of heart failure. In: Cohn JN, ed. *Drug Treatment of Heart Failure* Secaucus, NJ: Advanced Therapeutics Communications International; 1988:147.

211. Dikshit K, Vyden JK, Forrester JS, et al: Renal and extrarenal hemodynamic effects of furosemide in congestive heart failure after acute myocardial infarction. *N Engl J Med* 1973;288:1087.

212. Johnston GD, Hiatt WR, Nies AS, et al: Factors modifying the early nondiuretic vascular effects of furosemide in man: The possible role of renal prostaglandins. *Circ Res* 1983;53:630.

213. Nies AS, Gal S, Fadul S, et al: Indomethacin-furosemide interaction: The importance of renal blood flow. *J Pharmacol Exp Ther* 1983;226:27.

214. Francis GS, Siegel RM, Goldsmith SR, et al: Acute vasoconstrictor response to intravenous furosemide in patients with chronic congestive heart failure. *Ann Intern Med* 1985;103:1.

215. Goldsmith SR, Francis G, Cohn JN: Attenuation of the pressor response to intravenous furosemide by angiotensin converting enzyme inhibition in congestive heart failure. *Am J Cardiol* 1989;64:1382.

216. Dzau VJ, Hollenberg NK: Renal response to captopril in severe heart failure: Role of furosemide in natriuresis and reversal of hyponatremia. *Ann Intern Med* 1984;100:777.

217. Packer M, Lee WH, Kessler PD: Functional renal insufficiency during long-term therapy with captopril and enalapril in severe chronic heart failure. *Ann Intern Med* 1987;106:346.

218. Walshe JJ, Venturo RC: Acute oliguric renal failure induced by indomethacin: Possible mechanisms. *Ann Intern Med* 1979;91:47.

219. Kessler P, Lee WH, Packer M: What causes prerenal azotemia in patients with congestive heart failure? A hemodynamic-hormonal correlative study in 231 consecutive patients. *Circulation* 1985;72(suppl III):III-284. Abstract.

220. Goldenberg IF, Levine TB, Olivari MT: Markers of reduced renal blood flow in patients with congestive heart failure. *Circulation* 1985;72(suppl III):III-284. Abstract.

221. Cody RJ, Covit AB, Schaer GL, et al: Sodium and water balance in chronic congestive heart failure. *J Clin Invest* 1986;77:1441.

222. Packer M, Kessler PD, Gottlieb SS: Adverse effects of converting-enzyme inhibition in patients with severe congestive heart failure: Pathophysiology and management. *Postgrad Med J* 1986;62(suppl I):179.

223. Brater DC: Resistance to loop diuretics: Why it happens and what to do about it. *Drugs* 1985;30:427.

224. Vasko MR, Brown-Cartwright D, Knochel JP, et al: Furosemide absorption altered in decompensated congestive heart failure. *Ann Intern Med* 1985;102:314.

225. Packer M: Conceptual dilemmas in the classification of vasodilator drugs for severe heart failure. Advocacy of a pragmatic approach to the selection of a therapeutic agent. *Am J Med* 1984;76:3.

226. Edwards JC, Ignarro LJ, Hyman AL, et al: Relaxation of intrapulmonary artery and vein by nitrogen-oxide-containing vasodilators and cyclic GMP. *J Pharmacol Exp Ther* 1984;228:33.

227. Meisheri KD, Cipkus LA, Taylor CJ: Mechanism of action of minoxidil sulfate-induced vasodilation: A role of increased K+ permeability. *J Pharmacol Exp Ther* 1988;245:751.

228. Gray R, Chatterjee K, Vyden JK, et al: Hemodynamic and metabolic effects of isosorbide dinitrate in chronic congestive heart failure. *Am Heart J* 1975;90:346.

229. Kulick D, Roth A, McIntosh N, et al: Resistance to isosorbide dinitrate in patients with severe chronic heart failure: Incidence and attempt at hemodynamic prediction. *J Am Coll Cardiol* 1988;12:1023.

230. Magrini F, Niarchos AP: Ineffectiveness of sublingual nitroglycerin in acute left ventricular failure in the presence of massive peripheral edema. *Am J Cardiol* 1980;45:841.

231. Sniderman AD, Marpole DGF, Palmer WH, et al: Response of the left ventricle to nitroglycerin in patients with and without mitral regurgitation. *Br Heart J* 1974;36:357.

232. Bussman WD, Lohner J, Kaltenbach M: Orally administered isosorbide in patients with and without left ventricular failure due to acute myocardial infarction. *Am J Cardiol* 1977;39:84.

233. Chatterjee K, Parmley WW, Massie B, et al: Oral hydralazine therapy for chronic refractory heart failure. *Circulation* 1976;54:879.

234. Franciosa JA, Cohn JN: Effects of minoxidil on hemodynamics in patients with congestive heart failure. *Circulation* 1981;63:652.

235. Packer M, Meller J, Medina N, et al: Dose requirements of hydralazine in patients with severe chronic congestive heart failure. *Am J Cardiol* 1980;45:655.

236. Greenberg BH, Massie BM, Brundage BH, et al: Beneficial effects of hydralazine in severe mitral regurgitation. *Circulation* 1978;58:273.

237. Greenberg BH, DeMots H, Murphy E, et al: Beneficial effects of hydralazine on rest and exercise hemodynamics on patients with chronic severe aortic regurgitation. *Circulation* 1980;62:49.

238. Sharpe N, Coxon R, Webster M, et al: Hemodynamic effects of intermittent transdermal nitroglycerin in chronic congestive heart failure. *Am J Cardiol* 1987;59:895.

239. Packer M, Gottlieb SS, Kessler PD, et al: Prevention and reversal of nitrate tolerance in patients with congestive heart failure. *N Engl J Med* 1987;317:799.

240. Packer M, Gottlieb SS, Kessler PD, et al: What drug-free interval is required to prevent the development of nitrate tolerance in heart failure? *Circulation* 1987;76(suppl IV):IV-255. Abstract.

241. Elkayam U, Kulick D, Roth A, et al: Early tolerance to oral nitrate therapy in patients with chronic heart failure: Effect of dosing intervals. *Circulation* 1987;76(suppl IV):IV-256. Abstract.

242. Packer M, Meller J, Medina N, et al: Hemodynamic characterization of tolerance to long-term hydralazine therapy in severe chronic heart failure. *N Engl J Med* 1982;306:57.

243. Reifart N, Kaltenbach M, Bussman WD: Loss of effectiveness of dihydralazine in the long-term treatment of chronic heart failure. *Eur Heart J* 1983;5:568.

244. Ueda K, Sakai M, Matsushita S, et al: Effect of orally administered hydralazine therapy on neurohumoral factors and hemodynamic response in aged patients with chronic congestive heart failure. *Jpn Heart J* 1983;24:711.

245. Franciosa JA, Nordstrom LA, Cohn JN: Nitrate therapy for congestive heart failure. *JAMA* 1978;240:443.

246. Leier CV, Huss P, Magorien RD, et al: Improved exercise capacity and differing arterial and venous tolerance during chronic isosorbide dinitrate therapy for congestive heart failure. *Circulation* 1983;67:817.

247. Franciosa JA, Goldsmith SR, Cohn JN: Contrasting immediate and long-term effects of isosorbide dinitrate on exercise capacity in congestive heart failure. *Am J Med* 1980;69:559.

248. Aranda JM, Cintron G, Linares E, et al: Acute and long term effects of Isordil Tembids capsules on cardiac and vascular hemodynamics in patients with congestive heart failure. *Clin Res* 1983;30:825A. Abstract.

249. Cohn JN, Archibald DG, Johnson G: Effects of vasodilator therapy on peak exercise oxygen consumption in heart failure: V-HeFT. *Circulation* 1987;75(suppl II):II-443. Abstract.

250. Magorien RD, Unverferth DV, Leier CV: Hydralazine therapy in chronic congestive heart failure. Sustained central and regional hemodynamic responses. *Am J Med* 1984;77:267.

251. Conradson TB, Ryden L, Ahlmark G, et al: Clinical efficacy of oral hydralazine in chronic heart failure. One year double-blind placebo controlled study. *Am Heart J* 1984;108:1001.

252. Reifart N, Bunge T, Kaltenbach M, et al: Acute effect and long-term treatment with dihydralazine at rest and during exercise in severe chronic heart failure. *Z Kardiol* 1982;71:75.

253. Franciosa JA, Jordan RA, Wilen MM, et al: Minoxidil in patients with left heart failure: Contrasting hemodynamic and clinical effects in a controlled trial. *Circulation* 1984;70:63.

254. Cohn JN, Archibald DG, Ziesche S, et al: Effect of vasodilator therapy on mortality in chronic congestive heart failure. Results of a Veterans Administration Cooperative Study. *N Engl J Med* 1986;314:1547.

255. Yusuf S, Collins R, MacMahon S, et al: Effect of intravenous nitrates on mortality in acute myocardial infarction: An overview of the randomized trials. *Lancet* 1988;1:1088.

256. Archibald DG, Cohn JN: A treatment-associated increase in ejection fraction predicts long-term survival in congestive heart failure: The V-HeFT study. *Circulation* 1987;75(suppl II):II-309. Abstract.

257. Unverferth DV, Mehegan JP, Magorien RD, et al: Regression of myocardial cellular hypertrophy with vasodilator therapy in chronic congestive heart failure associated with idiopathic cardiomyopathy. *Am J Cardiol* 1983;51:1392.

258. Cohn JN, Johnson G, Ziesche S, et al: A comparison of enalapril with hydralizine-isosorbide dinitrate in the treatment of congestive heart failure. *N Engl J Med* 1991;325:303.

259. Greenberg B, Massie B, Bristow JD, et al: Long-term vasodilator therapy of chronic aortic insufficiency. A randomized double-blinded, placebo-controlled clinical trial. *Circulation* 1988;78:92.

260. Kessler PD, Packer M: Hemodynamic effects of BTS 49465, a new long-acting systemic vasodilator drug, in patients with severe congestive heart failure. *Am Heart J* 1987;113:137.

261. Kessler P, Packer M, Medina N, et al: Long-term hemodynamic and clinical responses to flosequinan, a new once-daily balanced direct-acting vasodilator, in severe heart failure. *Circulation* 1986;74(suppl II):II-509. Abstract.

262. Kessler PD, Packer M, Medina N, et al: Activation of the renin-angiotensin system limits the long-term hemodynamic and clinical responses to the direct-acting vasodilator, flosequinan, in heart failure. *J Am Coll Cardiol* 1987;9:120A. Abstract.

263. Cowley AJ, Wynne RD, Stainer K, et al: Flosequinan in heart failure: acute hemodynamic and longer term symptomatic effects. *Br Med J* 1988;297:169.

264. Elborn JS, Stanford CF, Nicholls DP: Effect of flosequinan on exercise capacity and symptoms in severe heart failure. *Br Heart J* 1989;61:331.

265. Packer M, Narahara KA, Elkayam U, et al: Randomized, multicenter, double-blind, placebo-controlled study of the efficacy of flosequinan, a new, long-acting vasodilator drug, in patients with chronic heart failure. *Circulation* 1990;82(suppl III):III-323. Abstract.

266. Pitt B, The REFLECT II Study Group: A randomized, multicenter, double-blind placebo-controlled study of the efficacy of flosequinan on patients with chronic heart failure. *Circulation* 1991;84(suppl II):II-311. Abstract.

267. Ryman KS, Kubo SH, Lystash J, et al: Effect of nicardipine on rest and exercise hemodynamics in chronic congestive heart failure. *Am J Cardiol* 1986;58:583.

268. Walsh RW, Porter CB, Starling MR, et al: Beneficial hemodynamic effects of intravenous and oral diltiazem in severe congestive heart failure. *J Am Coll Cardiol* 1984;4:1044.

269. Tan LB, Murray RG, Littler WA: Felodipine in patients with chronic heart failure: Discrepant hemodynamic and clinical effects. *Br Heart J* 1987;58:122.

270. Elkayam U, Amin J, Mehra A, et al: A prospective, randomized, double-blind, crossover study to compare the efficacy and safety of chronic nifedipine therapy to isosorbide dinitrate and their combination in the treatment of chronic congestive heart failure. *Circulation* 1992. In press.

271. Barjon JN, Rouleau JL, Bichet D, et al: Chronic renal and neurohumoral effects of the calcium entry blocker nisoldipine in patients with congestive heart failure. *J Am Coll Cardiol* 1987;9:622.

272. Packer M, Lee WH, Medina N, et al: Comparative negative inotropic effects of nifedipine and diltiazem in patients with severe left ventricular dysfuntion. *Circulation* 1985;72(suppl III):III-275. Abstract.

273. Packer M: Second generation calcium channel blockers in the treatment of chronic heart failure: Are they any better than their predecessors? *J Am Coll Cardiol* 1989;14:1339.

274. Elkayam U, Roth A, Hsueh W, et al: Neurohumoral consequences of vasodilator therapy with hydralazine and nifedipine in severe congestive heart failure. *Am Heart J* 1986;111:1130.

275. Packer M, Lee WH, Kessler PD, et al: Role of neurohormonal mechanisms in determining the survival of patients with severe chronic heart failure. *Circulation* 1987;75(suppl IV):80.

276. Kassis E, Amtorp O: Cardiovascular and neurohumoral postural responses and baroreflex abnormalities during a course of adjunctive vasodilator therapy with felodipine for congestive heart failure. *Circulation* 1987;75:1204.

277. Packer M, Nicod P, Khandheria BR, et al: Randomized, multicenter, double-blind, placebo-controlled evaluation of amlodipine in patients with mild-to-moderate heart failure. *J Am Coll Cardiol* 1991;17:274 A. Abstract.

278. Packer M, Medina N, Yushak M, et al: Hemodynamic patterns of response during long-term captopril therapy for severe chronic heart failure. *Circulation* 1983;68:803.

279. Captopril Multicenter Research Group: A placebo-controlled trial of captopril in refractory chronic congestive heart failure. *J Am Coll Cardiol* 1983;2:755.

280. Massie BM, Kramer BL, Topic N: Lack of relationship between short-term hemodynamic effects of captopril and subsequent clinical responses. *Circulation* 1984;69:1135.

281. Sharpe DN, Murphy J, Coxon R, et al: Enalapril in patients with chronic heart failure: A placebo-controlled, randomized, double-blind study. *Circulation* 1984;70:271.

282. Creager MA, Massie BM, Faxon DP, et al: Acute and long-term effects of enalapril on the cardiovascular response to exercise and exercise tolerance in patients with congestive heart failure. *J Am Coll Cardiol* 1985;6:163.

283. Chalmers JP, West MJ, Cyran J, et al: Placebo-controlled study of lisinopril in congestive heart failure: A multicenter study. *J Cardiovasc Pharmacol* 1987;9(suppl III):S89.

284. Cleland JGF, Dargie HG, Hodsman GP, et al: Captopril in heart failure: A double-blind controlled trial. *Br Heart J* 1984;52:530.

285. Cleland JGF, Dargie HG, Ball SG, et al: Effects of enalapril in heart failure: A double-blind study of effects on exercise performance, renal function, hormones, and metabolic state. *Br Heart J* 1985;54:305.

286. Cowley AJ, Rowley JM, Stainer KL, et al: Captopril therapy for heart failure. A placebo-controlled study. *Lancet* 1982;2:730.

287. Drexler H, Banhardt U, Meinertz T, et al: Contrasting peripheral short-term and long-term effects of converting enzyme inhibition in patients with congestive heart failure. A double-blind, placebo-controlled trial. *Circulation* 1989;79:491.

288. Bayliss J, Noreel MS, Canepa-Anson R, et al: Clinical importance of the renin-angiotensin system in chronic heart failure: double-blind comparison of captopril and prazosin. *Br Med J* 1985;290:1861.

289. Mettauer B, Rouleau JL, Bichet D, et al: Differential long-term intra-renal and neurohormonal effects of captopril and prazosin in patients with chronic congestive heart failure: Importance of initial plasma renin activity. *Circulation* 1986;73:492.

290. Richardson A, Bayliss J, Scriven A, et al: Double-blind comparison of captopril alone against frusemide plus amiloride in mild heart failure. *Lancet* 1987;2:709.

291. The CONSENSUS Trial Study Group: Effects of enalapril on mortality in severe congestive heart failure. Results of the Cooperative North Scandinavian Enalapril Survival Study (CONSENSUS). *N Engl J Med* 1987;316:1429.

292. The SOLVD Investigators: Effect of enalapril on survival in patients with reduced left ventricular ejection fractions and congestive heart failure. *N Engl J Med* 1991;325:293.

293. Newman TJ, Maskin CS, Dennick LG, et al: Effects of captopril on survival in patients with heart failure. *Am J Med* 1988;84:140.

294. Sharpe N, Murphy J, Smith H, et al: Treatment of patients with symptomless left ventricular dysfuntion after myocardial infarction. *Lancet* 1988;1:255.

295. Pfeffer MA, Lamas GA, Vaughn DE, et al; Effect of captopril on progressive ventricular dilatation after anterior myocardial infarction. *N Engl J Med* 1988;319:80.

296. Packer M, Lee WH, Kessler PD, et al: Identification of hyponatremia as a risk factor for the development of functional renal insufficiency during converting-enzyme inhibition in severe chronic heart failure. *J Am Coll Cardiol* 1987;10:837.

297. Packer M, Lee WH, Medina N, et al: Influence of diabetes mellitus on changes in left ventricular performance and renal function produced by converting-enzyme inhibition in patients with severe chronic heart failure. *Am J Med* 1987;82:1119.

298. Packer M, Lee WH, Yushak M, et al: Comparison of captopril and enalapril in patients with severe chronic heart failure. *N Engl J Med* 1986;315:847.

299. Powers ER, Chiaramida A, DeMaria AN, et al: A double-blind comparison of lisinopril with captopril in patients with symptomatic congestive heart failure. *J Cardiovasc Pharmacol* 1987;9(suppl III):S82.

300. Packer M, Lee WH, Medina N, et al: Identification of patients with heart failure at risk of potassium retention during converting-enzyme inhibition. *Circulation* 1987;76(suppl IV):IV-273. Abstract.

301. Packer M, Lee WH: Provocation of hyper- and hypokalemic sudden death during treatment with and withdrawal of converting-enzyme inhibition in patients with severe chronic heart failure. *Am J Cardiol* 1986;57:347.

302. Massie BM, Kramer BL, Topic N: Long-term captopril therapy for chronic congestive heart failure. *Am J Cardiol* 1984;53:1316.

303. Packer M, Medina N, Yushak M, et al: Usefulness of plasma renin activity in predicting hemodynamic and clinical responses and survival during long-term converting-enzyme inhibition in severe chronic heart failure. Experience in 100 consecutive patients. *Br Heart J* 1985;54:298.

304. Packer M, Lee WH, Medina N, et al: Identification of patients with severe heart failure most likely to fail long-term therapy with converting-enzyme inhibitors. *J Am Coll Cardiol* 1986;7:181A. Abstract.

305. Miller RR, Awan NA, Maxwell KS, et al: Sustained reduction of cardiac impedance and preload in congestive heart failure with the antihypertensive vasodilator prazosin. *N Engl J Med* 1977;297:303.

306. Markham RV, Corbett JR, Gilmore A, et al: Efficacy of prazosin in the management of chronic congestive heart failure: A 6-month randomized, double-blind, placebo-controlled study. *Am J Cardiol* 1983;51:1346.

307. Reifart N, Schmidt-Moritz AD, Nadj M, et al: Absence of symptomatic and haemodynamic long-term effects of prazosin in chronic heart failure. *Z Kardiol* 1985;74:205.

308. Kirlin PC, Das S, Pitt B: Chronic alpha-adrenoceptor blockade with trimazosin in congestive heart failure. *Int J Cardiol* 1985;8:89.

309. Packer M, Meller J, Gorlin R, et al: Clinical and hemodynamic tachyphylaxis to prazosin mediated afterload reduction in severe congestive heart failure. *Circulation* 1979;59:531.

310. Packer M, Medina N, Yushak M: Role of the renin-angiotensin system in the development of hemodynamic and clinical tolerance to long-term prazosin therapy in patients with severe chronic heart failure. *J Am Coll Cardiol* 1986;7:671.

311. Ikram H, Chan W, Bennett SI, et al: Hemodynamic effects of acute beta adrenergic receptor blockade in congestive cardiomyopathy. *Br Heart J* 1979;42:311.

312. Englemeier RS, O'Connell JB, Walsh R, et al: Improvement in symptoms and exercise tolerance by metoprolol in patients with dilated cardiomyopathy: A double-blind, randomized, placebo-controlled trial. *Circulation* 1985;72:536.

313. Gilbert EM, Anderson JL, Deitchman D, et al: Long-term ß-blocker vasodilator therapy improves cardiac function in idiopathic dilated cardiomyopathy: A double-blind, randomized study of bucindolol versus placebo. *Am J Med* 1990;88:223.

314. Swedberg K, Jhalmarson A, Waagstein F, et al: Prolongation of survival in congestive cardiomyopathy by beta-receptor blockade. *Lancet* 1979;1:1374.

315. Chadda K, Goldstein S, Byington R, et al: Effect of propranolol after acute myocardial infarction in patients with congestive heart failure. *Circulation* 1986;73:503.

316. Woodley SL, Gilbert EM, Anderson JL, et al: Differing effect of chronic ß-blockade with bucindolol on cardiac function in patients with idiopathic vs ischemic cardiomyopathy. *Circulation* 1989;80(suppl II):II-118. Abstract.

317. Gilbert EM, Mestroni L, Anderson JL, et al: Can response to ß-blocker therapy in idiopathic dilated cardiomyopathy be predicted by baseline parameters? *Circulation* 1989;80(suppl II):II-428. Abstract.

318. Binkley PF, Lewe R, Lima JJ, et al: Hemodynamic-inotropic response to beta-blocker with intrinsic sympathomimetic activity in patients with congestive cardiomyopathy. *Circulation* 1986;74:1390.

319. Valentine HA, Billingham ME, Heilbrunn SM, et al: Response to beta-blockers in dilated cardiomyopathy predicted by myocardial biopsy. *Circulation* 1986;72(suppl II):II-309. Abstract.

320. Currie PJ, Kelly MJ, McKenzie A, et al: Oral beta-adrenergic blockade with metoprolol in chronic severe dilated cardiomyopathy. *J Am Coll Cardiol* 1984;3:203.

321. Ikram H, Fitzpatrick D: Double-blind trial of chronic oral beta blockade in congestive cardiomyopathy. *Lancet* 1981;2:490.

322. Robin ED, Cross CE, Zelis R: Pulmonary edema. *N Engl J Med* 1973;288:239.

323. Vasko JS, Henney RP, Oldham HN, et al: Mechanism of action of morphine in the treatment of experimental pulmonary edema. *Am J Cardiol* 1966;18:876.

324. Vismara LA, Leaman DM, Zelis R: Effect of morphine on venous tone in patients with acute pulmonary edema. *Circulation* 1976;54:335.

325. Henney HN, Vasko JS, Brawley RK, et al: The effects of morphine on the resistance and capacitance vessels of the peripheral circulation. *Am Heart J* 1966;72:242.

326. Ward JM, McGrath RL, Weil JV: Effects of morphine on the peripheral vascular response to sympathetic stimulation. *Am J Cardiol* 1972;29:659.

327. Flaim SF, Zelis R, Eisele JH: Differential effects of morphine on forearm blood flow: Attenuation of sympathetic control of the cutaneous circulation. *Clin Pharmacol Ther* 1978;23:542.

328. Zelis R, Flaim SF, Eisele JH: The effects of morphine on reflex arteriolar vasoconstriction induced in man by hypercapnia. *Clin Pharmacol Ther* 1977;22:172.

329. Brooksby GA, Donald DE: Release of blood from the splachnic circulation in dogs. *Circ Res* 1972;31:105.

330. Zelis R, Mansour EJ, Capone RJ, et al: The cardiovascular effects of morphine: The peripheral capacitance and resistance vessels in human subjects. *J Clin Invest* 1974;54:1247.

331. Zelis R, Kinney EL, Flaim SF, et al: Morphine: Its use in pulmonary edema. *Cardiovasc Rev Rep* 1981;2:257.

332. Lesch M, Caranasos GJ, Mulholland JH, et al: Controlled study comparing ethacrynic acid to mercaptomerin in the treatment of acute pulmonary edema. *N Engl J Med* 1968;279:115.

333. Packer M, Meller J, Medina N, et al: Comparative hemodynamic effects of low dose and high dose nitroprusside in patients with refractory congestive heart failure. *Clin Res* 1979;27:192A. Abstract.

334. Packer M, Meller J, Medina N, et al: Dose dependence of the hemodynamic responses to nitrate therapy in patients with refractory congestive heart failure. *Clin Res* 1979;27:192A. Abstract.

335. Miller RR, Vismara LA, Williams DO, et al: Pharmacologic mechanisms for left ventricular unloading in clinical congestive heart failure. Differential effects of nitroprusside, phentolamine and nitroglycerin on cardiac function and peripheral circulation. *Circ Res* 1976;39:127.

336. Chiariello M, Gold HK, Leinbach RC, et al: Comparison between the effects of nitroprusside and nitroglycerin on ischemic injury during acute myocardial infarction. *Circulation* 1976;54:766.

337. Mann T, Cohn PF, Holman BL, et al: Effect of nitroprusside on regional myocardial blood flow in coronary disease: Results in 25 patients and comparison with nitroglycerin. *Circulation* 1978;57:732.

338. Breisblatt WM, Navratil DL, Burns MJ, et al: Comparable effects of intravenous nitroglycerin and intravenous nitroprusside in acute ischemia. *Am Heart J* 1988;116:465.

339. Packer M, Meller J, Medina N, et al: Rebound hemodynamic events after the abrupt withdrawal of nitroprusside in patients with severe chronic heart failure. *N Engl J Med* 1979;301:1193.

340. Elkayam U, Kulick D, McIntosh N, et al: Incidence of early tolerance to hemodynamic effects of continuous infusion of nitroglycerin in patients with coronary artery disease and heart failure. *Circulation* 1987;76:577.

341. Come P, Pitt B: Nitroglycerin-induced severe hypotension and bradycardia in patients with acute myocardial infarction. *Circulation* 1976;54:624.

342. Hales CA, Westphal D: Hypoxemia following the administration of sublingual nitroglycerin. *Am J Med* 1978;65:911.

343. Mookherjee S, Keighly JFH, Warner RA, et al: Hemodynamic, ventilatory and blood gas changes during infusion of sodium nitroprusside: studies in patients with congestive heart failure. *Cest* 1977;72:273.

344. Palmer RF, Lasseter KC: Drug therapy: Sodium nitroprusside. *N Engl J Med* 1975;300:294.

345. Davies DW, Kadar D, Steward DJ, et al: A sudden death associated with the use of sodium nitroprusside for induction of hypotension during anesthesia. *Can Anaesth Soc J* 1975;22:547.

346. Ruffulo RR, Spradlin TA, Pollack GD, et al: Alpha- and beta-adrenergic effects of the stereoisomers of dobutamine. *J Pharmacol Exp Ther* 1981;219:447.

347. Ruffulo RR, Messick K: Systemic hemodynamic effects of dopamine, dobutamine and the enantiomers of dobutamine in anesthestized normotensive rates. *Eur J Pharmacol* 1985;109:173.

348. Loeb HS, Khan M, Saudaye A, et al: Acute hemodynamic effects of dobutamine and isoproterenol in patients with low output cardiac failure. *Circ Shock* 1976;3:55.

349. Kawashima S, Combes J, Liang CS, et al: Contrasting effects of dopamine and dobutamine on myocardial release of norepinephrine during acute myocardial infarction. *Jpn Heart J* 1985;26:975.

350. Leier CV, Heban P, Huss P, et al: Comparative systemic and regional hemodynamic effects of dopamine and dobutamine in patients with cardiomyopathic heart failure. *Circulation* 1978;58:466.

351. Loeb HS, Bredakis J, Gunnar RM: Superiority of dobutamine over dopamine for augmentation of cardiac output in patients with chronic low output cardiac failure. *Circulation* 1977;55:375.

352. Robie NW, Goldberg LI: Comparative systemic and regional hemodynamic effects of dopamine and dobutamine. *Am Heart J* 1975;90:340.

353. Grose RM, Strain JE, Greenberg MA, et al: Systemic and coronary effects of intravenous milrinone and dobutamine in congestive heart failure. *J Am Coll Cardiol* 1986;7:1107.

354. Klein NA, Siskind SJ, Frishman WH, et al: Hemodynamic comparison of intravenous amrinone and dobutamine in patients with chronic congestive heart failure. *Am J Cardiol* 1981;48:170.

355. Awan NA, Evenson MK, Needham KE, et al: Effects of combined nitroglycerin and dobutamine infusion in left ventricular dysfunction. *Am Heart J* 1983;106:35.

356. Mikulic E, Cohn JN, Franciosa JA: Comparative hemodynamic effects of inotropic and vasodilator drugs in severe heart failure. *Circulation* 1977;56:528.

357. Richard C, Ricome JL, Rimailho JA, et al: Combined hemodynamic effects of dopamine and dobutamine in cardiogenic shock. *Circulation* 1983;67:620.

358. Gage J, Rutman H, Lucido D, et al: Additive effects of dobutamine and amrinone in myocardial contractility and ventricular performance in patients with severe heart failure. *Circulation* 1986;74:367.

359. David D, Zaks JM: Arrhythmias associated with intermittent outpatient dobutamine infusion. *Angiology* 1986;37:86.

360. Goldenberg IF, Olivari MT, Levine TB, et al: Effect of dobutamine on plasma potassium in congestive heart failure secondary to idiopathic or ischemic cardiomyopathy. *Am J Cardiol* 1989;63:843.

361. Unverferth DV, Blaunford H, Kates RE, et al: Tolerance to dobutamine after a 72-hour continuous infusion. *Am J Med* 1980;69:262.

362. Benotti JR, Grossman W, Brauwald E, et al: Hemodynamic assessment of amrinone—a new inotropic agent. *N Engl J Med* 1978;299:1373.

363. LeJemtel TH, Keung E, Sonnenblick EH, et al: Amrinone: a new non-glycosidic, non-adrenergic cardiotonic agent effective in the treatment of intractable myocardial failure in man. *Circulation* 1979;59:1098.

364. Baim DS, McDowell AV, Cherniles J, et al: Evaluation of a new bipyridine inotropic agent—milrinone—in patients with severe congestive heart failure. *N Engl J Med* 1983;309:748.

365. Monrad ES, McKay RG, Maim DS, et al: Improvement in the indices of diastolic performance in patients with congestive heart failure with milrinone. *Circulation* 1984;70:1030.

366. Colucci WS, Wright RF, Jaski BE, et al: Milrinone and dobutamine in severe heart failure: differing hemodynamic effects and individual patient responsiveness. *Circulation* 1986;73 (suppl III):175.

367. Biddle TL, Benotti JR, Creager MA, et al: Comparison of intravenous milrinone and dobutamine for congestive heart failure secondary to either ischemic or dilated cardiomyopathy. *Am J Cardiol* 1987;59:1345.

368. Konstam MA, Cohen SR, Weiland DS, et al: Relative contributions to inotropic and vasodilation effects to amrinone-induced hemodynamic improvement in congestive heart failure. *Am J Cardiol* 1986;54:242.

369. Wilmhurst PT, Webb-Peploe MM: Side effects of amrinone therapy. *Br Heart J* 1983;49:447.

370. Wilmhurst PT, Walker JM, Fry CH, et al: Inotropic and vasodilator effects of amrinone on isolated human tissue. *Cardiovasc Res* 1984;18:302.

371. Firth BG, Ratner AV, Grassman ED, et al: Assessment of the inotropic and vasodilation effects of amrinone versus isoproterenol. *Am J Cardiol* 1984;54:1331.

372. Ludmer PL, Wright RF, Arnold JMO, et al: Separation of the direct myocardial and vasodilator actions of milrinone administered by an intra-coronary infusion technique. *Circulation* 1986;73:130.

373. Weil MH, Shubin H, Biddle M: Shock caused by gram-negative microorganisms. Analysis of 169 cases. *Ann Intern Med* 1964;60:384.

374. Wilson JR, Reichek N, Dunkman WB, et al: Effect of diuresis on the performance of the failing left ventricle in man. *Am J Med* 1981;70:234.

375. Weil MH, Henning RJ: New concepts in the diagnosis and fluid treatment of circulatory shock. *Anesth Analg* 1979;58:124.

376. Goldberg LI: Cardiovascular and renal actions of dopamine. Potential clinical applications. *Pharmacol Rev* 1972;24:1.

377. Yeh BK, McNay JL, Goldberg LI: Attenuation of dopamine renal and mesenteric vasodilatation by haloperidol. Evidence for a specific receptor. *J Pharmacol Exp Ther* 1969;168:303.

378. Gilbert JC, Goldberg LI: Characterization by cyproheptadine of the dopamine-induced contraction in canine isolated arteries. *J Pharmacol Exp Ther* 1975;193:435.

379. Beregovich J, Bianchi C, Rubler S, et al: Dose-related hemodynamic and renal effects of dopamine in congestive heart failure. *Am Heart J* 1974;87:550.

380. Goldberg LI, Talley RC, McNay JL: The potential role of dopamine in the treatment of shock. *Progr Cardiovasc Dis* 1969;12:40.

381. Henderson IS, Beattie TJ, Kennedy AC: Dopamine hydrochloride in oliguric states. *Lancet* 1980;2:827.

382. Lindner A: Synergism of dopamine and furosemide in diuretic-resistant, oliguric acute renal failure. *Nephron* 1983;33:121.

383. Goldberg LI, McDonald RH Jr, Zimmerman AM: Sodium diuresis produced by dopmaine in patients with congestive heart failure. *N Engl J Med* 1963;269:1060.

384. Pederson JE, Mortensen SA: Hemodynamic steady state via combined infusion of dobutamine and dopamine in the pretransplant phase. *Acta Cardiol* 1987;42:295.

385. Miller RR, Awan NA, Joye JA, et al: Combined dopamine and nitroprusside therapy in congestive heart failure. *Circulation* 1977;55:881.

386. Loeb HS, Ostenga JP, Gaul W, et al: Beneficial effects of dopamine combined with intravenous nitroglycerin on hemodynamics in patients with severe left ventricular failure. *Circulation* 1983;68:813.

387. Schaer GL, Fink MP, Parillo JE: Norepinephrine alone versus norepinephrine plus low-dose dopamine: Enhanced renal blood flow with combination pressor therapy. *Crit Care Med* 1985;13:492.

388. Loeb HS, Winslow EBJ, Rahimtoola SH, et al: Acute hemodynamic effects of dopamine in patients with shock. *Circulation* 1971;44:163.

389. Gunnar RM, Loeb HS, Pietras RJ, et al: Ineffectiveness of isoproterenol in shock due to acute myocardial infarction. *JAMA* 1967;202:1124.

390. Goldenberg M, Pines KL, Baldwin E, et al: The hemodynamic response of man to nor-epinephrine and epinephrine and its relation to the problem of hypertension. *Am J Med* 1948;5:792.

391. Smulyan H, Cuddy RP, Eich RH: Hemodynamic effects of pressor agents in septic and myocardial infarction shock. *JAMA* 1964;190:188.

392. Nickel JF, Smythe CM, Paper EM, et al: A study of the mode of action of adrenal medullary hormones on sodium, potassium and water excretion in man. *J Clin Invest* 1954;33:1687.

393. Dodge HJ, Lord JD, Sandler H: Cardiovascular effects of isoproterol in normal subjects and subjects with congestive heart failure. *Am Heart J* 1960;60:94.

394. Talley RC, Goldberg LI, Johnson CE, et al: A hemodynamic comparison of dopamine and isoproterenol in patients with shock. *Circulation* 1969;39:361.

395. Smith HJ, Oriol A, Morich J, et al: Hemodynamic studies in cardiogenic shock. Treatment with isoproterenol and metarminol. *Circulation* 1967;35:1084.

396. Brofman BL, Heelerstein HK, Caskey WH: Mephentermine—an effective pressor amine. *Am Heart J* 1952;44:396.

397. Smith NT, Whitcher C: Acute hemodynamic effects of methoxamine in man. *Anesthesiology* 1967;28:735.

398. Horvath SM, Knapp DW: Hemodynamic effects of Neo-Synephrine. *Am J Physiol* 1954;178:387.

399. Swaine CR, Perlmutter JF, Ellis S: The release of catecholamines from the isolated heart by mephentermine. *Naunyn-Schmiedebergs Arch Pharmacol Exp Pathol* 1964;248:331.

400. Shore PA, Brisfield D, Aplers HS: Binding and release of metarminol: mechanism of norepinephrine depletion by a-methyl-M-tyrosine and related agents. *J Pharmacol Exp Ther* 1964;146:194.

401. Eger EI, Hamilton WK: The effect of reserpine on the action of various vasopressors. *Anesthesiology* 1959;20:641.

402. Goldberg LI, Bloodwell RD, Braunwald E, et al: The direct effects of morepinephrine, epinephrine and methoxamine on myocardial contractile force in man. *Circulation* 1960;22:1125.

403. Gazes PC, Goldberg LI, Darby TD: Heart force effects of sympathomimetic amines as a basis for their use in shock accompanying myocardial infarction. *Circulation* 1953;8:883.

404. Pelner L, Waldman S, Rhoades MG: The problem of levarterenol Levophed. extravasation: An experimental study. *Am J Med Sci* 1958;236:755.

405. Loeb HS, Khan M, Klodnycky ML, et al: Hemodynamic effects of dobutamine on man. *Circ Shock* 1975;2:29.

406. Bregman D: Assessment of intra-aortic balloon counterpulsation in cardiogenic shock. *Crit Care Med* 1975;3:90.

407. Gold HK, Leimbach RC, Sanders CA, et al: Intraaortic balloon pumping for ventricular septal defect or mitral regurgitation complicating acute myocardial infarction. *Circulation* 1973;47:1191.

408. Gold HK, Leinbach RC, Mundth ED, et al: Reversal of myocardial ischemia complicating acute myocardial infarction by intra-aorta balloon pumping. *Circulation* 1972;45,46(suppl II):22.

409. Cairns KB, Porter GA, Kloster FE, et al: Clinical and hemodynamic results of peritoneal dialysis for severe cardiac failure. *Am Heart J* 1968;76:227.

410. Rimondini A, Cipolla CM, Della Bella P, et al: Hemofiltration as short-term treatment for refractory congestive heart failure. *Am J Med* 1987;83:43.

411. Richenbacher WE, Pennock JL, Pae WE Jr, et al: Artificial heart implantation for end-stage cardiac disease. *J Cardiac Surgery* 1986;1:3.

412. Griffith BP, Hardesty RL, Kormos RL, et al: Temporary use of the Jarvik-7 total artificial heart before transplantation. *N Engl J Med* 1987;316:130.

413. Soufer R, Wohlgelertner D, Vita NA, et al: Intact systolic left ventricular function in clinical congestive heart failure. *Am J Cardiol* 1985;55:1032.

414. Dougherty AH, Naccarelli GV, Gray EL, et al: Congestive heart failure with normal systolic function. *Am J Cardiol* 1984;54:778.

415. Baron BJ, Roberts WC, Epstein SE: Sudden death in hypertrophic cardiomyopathy: A profile of 78 patients. *Circulation* 1982;65:1388.

416. Sanderson JE, Traill TA, St John Sutton MG, et al: Left ventricular relaxation and filling in hypertrophic cardiomyopathy: An echocardiographic study. *Br Heart J* 1978;40:596.

417. Maron BJ, Gottdiener JS, Arce J, et al: Dynamic subaortic obstruction in hypertrophic cardiomyopathy: Analysis by pulsed Doppler echocardiography. *J Am Coll Cardiol* 1985;6:1.

418. Whalen RE, Cohen AI, Sumner RG, et al: Demonstration of the dynamic nature of idiopathic hypertrophic subaortic stenosis. *Am J Cardiol* 1963;11:8.

419. Murgo JP, Alter BR, Dorethy JF, et al: Dynamics of left ventricular ejection in obstructive and nonobstructive hypertrophic cardiomyopathy. *J Clin Invest* 1980;66:1369.

420. Criley JM, Lewis KB, White RI Jr, et al: Pressure gradients without obstruction: A new concept of "hypertrophic subaortic stenosis". *Circulation* 1965;32:881.

421. Martin AM, Hackel DB, Sieker HO: Intraventricular pressure changes in dogs during hemorrhagic shock. *Fed Proc* 1963;22:252. Abstract.

422. Shah PM, Adelman AG, Wigle ED, et al: The natural and unnatural. history of hypertrophic obstructive cardiomyopathy: A multicenter study. *Circ Res* 1974;35(suppl II):179.

423. Frank S, Braunwald E: Idiopathic hypertrophic subaortic stenosis: Clinical analysis and 126 patients with emphasis on the natural history. *Circulation* 1968;37:759.

424. St. John Sutton MG, Tajik AJ, Gibson DG, et al: Echocardiographic assessment of left ventricular filling and septal and posterior wall dynamics in idiopathic hypertrophic subaortic stenosis. *Circulation* 1978;57:512.

425. Adelman AG, Shah PM, Gramiak R, et al: Long-term propranolol therapy in muscular subaortic stenosis. *Br Heart J* 1970;32:804.

426. Flamm MD, Harrison DC, Hancock EW: Muscular subaortic stenosis: Prevention of outflow obstruction with propranolol. *Circulation* 1968;38:846.

427. Bourmayan C, Razavi A, Fournier C, et al: Effect of propranolol on left ventricular relaxation in hypertrophic cardiomyopathy: An echocardiographic study. *Am Heart J* 1985;109:1311.

428. Alvares RF, Goodwin JF: Noninvasive assessment of diastolic function in hypertrophic cardiomyopathy on and off beta adrenergic blocking drugs. *Br Heart J* 1982;48:204.

429. Swan DA, Bell B, Oakley CM, et al: Analysis of symptomatic course and prognosis and treatment of hypertrophic obstructive cardiomyopathy. *Br Heart J* 1971;33:671.

430. Sloman G: Propranolol in the management of muscular subaortic stenosis. *Br Heart J* 1967;29:783.

431. Hanrath P, Mathey DG, Kremer P, et al: Effect of verapamil on left ventricular isovolumic relaxation time and regional left ventricular filling in hypertrophic cardiomyopathy. *Am J Cardiol* 1980;45:1258.

432. Bonow RO, Dilsizian V, Rosing DR, et al: Verapamil-induced improvement in left ventricular diastolic filling and increased exercise tolerance in patients with hypertrophic cardiomyopathy: short- and long-term effects. *Circulation* 1985;72:853.

433. Rosing DR, Kent KM, Borer JS, et al: Verapamil therapy: A new approach to the pharmacologic treatment of hypertrophic cardiomyopathy. I. Hemodynamic effects. *Circulation* 1979;60:1201.

434. Kaltenbach M, Hopf R, Kober G, et al: Treatment of hypertrophic cardiomyopathy with verapamil. *Br Heart J* 1979;42:35.

435. Rosing DR, Kent KM, Maron BJ, et al: Verapamil therapy: A new approach to the pharmacologic treatment of hypertrophic cardiomyopathy. II. Effects on exercise capacity and symptomatic status. *Circulation* 1979;60:1208.

436. Rosing DR, Condit JR, Maron BJ, et al: Verapamil therapy: A new approach to the pharmacologic treatment of hypertrophic cardiomyopathy. III. Effects of long-term administration. *Am J Cardiol* 1981;48:545.

437. Cherian G, Brockington IF, Shah PM, et al: Beta-adrenergic blockade in hypertrophic obstructive cardiomyopathy. *Br Med J* 1966;1:895.

438. Epstein SE, Rosing DR: Verapamil: Its potential for causing serious complications in patients with hypertrophic cardiomyopathy. *Circulation* 1981;64:437.

439. Fedor JM, Stack RS, Pryor DB, et al: Adverse effects of nifedipine therapy in hypertrophic cardiomyopathy. *Chest* 1983;83:704.

440. Pollick C: Muscular subaortic stenosis. Hemodynamic and clinical improvements after disopyramide. *N Engl J Med* 1982;307:997.

441. McKenna WJ, Harris L, Rowland E, et al: Amiodarone for long-term management of patients with hypertrophic cardiomyopathy. *Am J Cardiol* 1984;54:802.

442. Shabetai R: Profiles in constrictive pericarditis, cardiac tamponade and restrictive cardiomyopathy. In: Grossman W, ed. *Cardiac Catheterization and Angiography* Philadelphia, PA: Lea and Febiger; 1974:304.

443. Cutler DJ, Isaner JM, Bracey AW, et al: Hemochromatosis heart disease: an unemphasized cause of potentially reversible restrictive cardiomyopathy. *Am J Med* 1980;69:923.

444. Short EM, Winkle RA, Billingham ME: Myocardial involvement in idiopathic hemochromatosis. Morphologic and clinical improvement following venesection. *Am J Med* 1981;70:1275.

445. Ishikawa T, Kondoh H, Nakagawa S, et al: Steroid therapy in cardiac sarcoidosis: increased left ventricular contractility comcomitant with electrocardiographic improvement after prednisolone. *Chest* 1984;85:445.

446. Fauci AS, Karley JB, Roberts WC, et al: NIH conference. The idiopathic eosinophilic syndrome. Clinical, pathophysiologic and therapeutic considerations. *Ann Intern Med* 1982;97:78.

447. Fournial G, Schlanger R, Berthoumieu F, et al: Surgery for cardiac complications caused by endocardial mural fibrin deposits in a hypereosinophilic syndrome. *Circulation* 1982;65:1010.

448. Bertrand E, Chauvet J, Assamoi MO, et al: Results, indications and contraindications of surgery in restrictive endomyocardial fibrosis. *East Afr Med JH* 1985;62:151.

449. Rubinow A, Skinner M, Cohen AS: Digoxin sensitivity in amyloid cardiomyopathy. *Circulation* 1981;63:1285.

450. Walsh RA, O'Rourke RA: Direct and indirect effects of calcium entry blocking agents on isovolumtetric relaxation in conscious dogs. *J Clin Invest* 1985;75:1426.

451. Katz AM: Interplay between inotropic and lusitropic effects of cyclic adenosine monophosphate on the myocardial cell. *Circulation* 1990;82(suppl I):7.

452. Piscione F, Jaski BE, Wenting GJ, et al: Effect of a single oral dose of milrinone on left ventricular diastolic performance in the failing human heart. *J Am Coll Cardiol* 1987;10:1294.

453. Pouleau H, Hanet C, Rousseau MF, et al: Relation of diastolic function and exercise capacity in ischemic left ventricular dysfunction. Role of B-agonists and B-antagonists. *Circulation* 1990;82 suppl I.:89.

454. Pouleur H, van Eyll C, Cheron P, et al: Changes in left ventricular filling dynamics after long-term xamoterol therapy in sichemic left ventricular dysfunction. *Heart Failure* 1986;2:176.

455. Pouleur H, van Eyll C, Hanet C, et al: Long-term effects of xamoterol on left ventricular diastolic function and late remodeling: a study in patients with anterior myocardial infarction and single-vessel disease. *Circulation* 1988;77:1081.

456. Klein HO, Sareli P, Schamroth CL, et al: Effects of atenolol on exercise capacity in patients with mitral stenosis with sinus rhythm. *Am J Cardiol* 1985;56:598.

457. Beiser GDS, Epstein SE, Stampfer M, et al: Studies on digitalis. Effects of ouabain on the hemodynamic response to exercise in patients with mitral stenosis in normal sinus rhythm. *N Engl J Med* 1968;278:131.

458. Yellin EL, Yoran C, Sonnenblick EH, et al: Dynamic changes in the canine mitral regurgitant orifice area during ventricular ejection. *Circ Res* 1979;45:677.

459. Yoran C, Yellin EL, Becker RM, et al: Dynamic aspects of acute miral regurgitation: effects of ventricular volume, pressure and contractility on the effective regurgitant orifice area. *Circulation* 1979;60:170.

460. Eckberg DL, Gault JH, Bouchard RL, et al: Mechanics of left ventricular contraction in chronic severe mitral regurgitation. *Circulation* 1973;47:1252.

461. Harshaw C, Grossman W, Munro A, et al: Reduced systemic vascular resistance as therapy for severe mitral regurgitation of valvular origin. *Ann Intern Med* 1975;83:312.

462. Chatterjee K, Parmley WW, Swan HJC, et al: Beneficial effects of vasodilator agents in severe mitral regurgitation due to dysfunction of subvalvular apparatus. *Circulation* 1973;48:884.

463. Carabello BA, Nolan SP, McGuire LD: Assessment of preoperative left ventricular function in patients with mitral regurgitation: Value of end-systolic wall stress/end-systolic volume ratio. *Circulation* 1986;64:1212.

464. Smith N, McAnulty JH, Rahimtoola SH: Severe aortic stenosis with impaired left ventricular function and clinical heart failure: Results of valve replacement. *Circulation* 1978;58:255.

465. Fioretti P, Bennusi B, Sacrdi S, et al: Afterload reduction with nifedipine in aortic insufficiency. *Am J Cardiol* 1982;49:1728.

466. Miller RR, Vismara LA, DeMaria AN, et al: Afterload reduction with nitroprusside in severe aortic regurgitation: Improved cardiac performance and reduced regurgitant volume. *Am J Cardiol* 1976;38:564.

467. Greenberg BH, Rahimtoola SH: Long-term vasodilator therapy in aortic insufficiency: evdience for regression of left ventricular dilatation and hypertrophy and improvement in systolic pump function. *Ann Intern Med* 1980;93:440.

468. Kleaveland JP, Reichek N, McCarthy DM, et al: Effects of six-month afterload reduction therapy with hydralazine in chronic aortic regurgitation. *Am J Cardiol* 1986;57:1109.

469. Borow KM, Green LH, Mann T, et al: End-systolic volume as a predictor of postoperative left ventricular performance in volume overload from valvular regurgitation. *Am J Med* 1980;65:655.

470. Bonow RO, Rosing DR, Kent KM, et al: Timing of operation for chronic aortic regurgitation. *Am J Cardiol* 1982;50:325.

471. World Health Organization: Primary pulmonary hypertension: Report of a WHO meeting. 1975.

472. Gurtner HP: Pulmonary hypertension, plexogenic pulmonary arteriopathy and appetite depressant drug aminorex: Post or propter? *Bull Eur Physiopath Resp* 1979;15:897.

473. Kleiger RE, Boxer M, Ingham RE, et al: Pulmonary hypertension in patients using oral contraceptives. *Chest* 1976;69:143.

474. Weir EK, McMurtry IF, Tucker A, et al: Prostaglandin synthetase inhibitors do not decrease hypoxic pulmonary vasoconstriction. *J Appl Physiol* 1976;41:714.

475. Tucker A, Weir EK, Reeves JT, et al: Failure of histamine antagonists to prevent hypoxic pulmonary vasocosntriction in dogs. *J Appl Physiol* 1976;40:496.

476. Wennmalm A: Interaction of nicotine and prostaglandins in the cardiovascular system. *Prostaglandins* 1982;23:139.

477. Inkley SR, Gillespie L, Funkhouser RK: Two cases of primary pulmonary hypertension with sudden death associated with the administration of barbiturates. *Ann Intern Med* 1955;43:396.

478. Caldini P, Gensini GC, Hoffman MS: Primary pulmonary hypertension in a child: Response to pharmacologic agents. *Circulation* 1969;40:583.

479. Keane JF, Fyler DC, Nadas AS: Hazards of cardiac catheterization in children with primary pulmonary vascular obstruction. *Am Heart J* 1978;96:556.

480. Jewett JF, Ober WB: Primary pulmonary hypertension as a cause of maternal death. *Am J Obstet Gynec* 1956;71:1335.

481. Fuster V, Steele PM, Edwards WD, et al: Primary pulmonary hypertension: Natural history and the importance of thrombosis. *Circulation* 1984;70:580.

482. Hermiller JB, Bambach D, Thompson MJ, et al: Vasodilators and prostaglandin inhibitors in primary pulmonary hypertension. *Ann Intern Med* 1982;97:480.

483. Nagasaka Y, Akutsu H, Lee YS, et al: Long-term favorable effect of oxygen administration in a patient with primary pulmonary hypertension. *Chest* 1978;74:299.

484. Packer M, Lee WH, Medina N, et al: Systemic vasoconstrictor effects of oxygen administration in obliterative pulmonary vascular disorders. *Am J Cardiol* 1986;57:853.

485. Aber GM, Harris AM, Bishop JM: The effect of acute changes in inspired oxygen concentration on cardiac, respiratory and renal function in patients with chronic obstructive airways disease. *Clin Sci* 1964;26:133.

486. Rich S: Primary pulmonary hypertension: Recent advances. *Herz* 1986;11:197.

487. Coulson RL, Rubio E, Bove AA, et al: Digoxin prophylaxis for prevention of contractile defect produced by pressure preload. *Clin Res* 1975;23:177.

488. McGregor M, Sniderman A: On pulmonary vascular resistance: the need for more precise definition. *Am J Cardiol* 1985;55:217.

489. Walcott G, Burchell HB, Brown AL: Primary pulmonary hypertension. *Am J Med* 1979;49:70.

490. Nair SS, Askari AD, Popelka CG, et al: Pulmonary hypertension and systemic lupus erythematosus. *Arch Intern Med* 1980;140:109.

491. Young RH, Mark G: Pulmonary vascular changes in scleroderma. *Am J Med* 1978;64:998.

492. Caldwell IW, Aitchison JD: Pulmonary hypertension in dermatomyositis. *Br Heart J* 1956;18:273.

493. Bunch TW, Tancredi RG, Lie JT: Pulmonary hypertension in polymyositis. *Chest* 1981;79:105.

494. Daoud FS, Reeves JT, Kelly DB: Isoproterenol as a potential pulmonary vasodilator in primary pulmonary hypertension. *Am J Cardiol* 1978;42:817.

495. Storstein O, Efskind L, Muller C, et al: Primary pulmonary hypetension with emphasis on its etiology and treatment. *Acta Med Scand* 1966;79:197.

496. Goodwin JF, Harrison CV, Wilcken DE: Obliterative pulmonary hypertension and thromboembolism. *Br Med J* 1963;1:777.

497. Sleeper JC, Orgain ES, McIntosh HD: Primary pulmonary hypertension. *Circulation* 1962;26:1358.

498. Packer M: Vasodilator therapy for primary pulmonary hypertension: Limitations and hazards. *Ann Intern Med* 1985;103:258.

499. Packer M: Does pulmonary vasoconstriction play an important role in patients with primary pulmonary hypertension? A skeptic's view of vasodilator therapy. *Chest* 1985;88:265S.

500. Furchgott RF, Zawadzki JV: The obligatory role of endothelial cells in relaxation of arterial smooth muscle by acetylcholine. *Nature* 1980;288:373.

501. Yu PN: Primary pulmonary hypertension: report of six cases and review of literature. *Ann Intern Med* 1958;49:1138.

502. Packer M, Greenberg B, Massie B, et al: Deleterious effects of hydralazine in patients with pulmonary hypertension. *N Engl J Med* 1982;306:1326.

503. Kronzon I, Cohen M, Winer HE: Adverse effect of hydralazine in patients with primary pulmonary hypertension. *JAMA* 1982;247:3112.

504. Elkayam U, Frishman WH, Yoran C, et al: Unfavorable hemodynamic and clinical effets of isoproterenol in primary pulmonary hypertension. *Cardiovasc Med* 1978;3:1177.

505. Packer M, Medina N, Yushak M, et al: Detrimental effects of verapamil in patients with primary pulmonary hypertension. *Br Heart J* 1984;52:106.

506. Packer M, Medina N, Yushak M: Adverse hemodynamic and clinical effects of calcium channel blockade in pulmonary hypertension secondary to obliterative pulmonary vascular disease. *J Am Coll Cardiol* 1984;4:890.

507. Dantzker DR, Bower JS: Mechanisms of gas exchange abnormality in patients with chronic obliterative pulmonary vascular disease. *J Clin Invest* 1979;64:1050.

508. Dantzker DR, Bower JS: Pulmonary vascular tone improves VA/Q matching in oblierative pulmonary hypertension. *J Appl Physiol* 1981;51:607.

509. Wood P: Pulmonary hypertension with special reference to the vasoconstrictor factor. *Br Heart J* 1958;20:557.

510. Dresdale DT, Michtom RJ, Schultz M: Recent studies in primary pulmonary hypertension including pharmacodynamic observations on pulmonary vascular resistance. *Bull NY Acad Med* 1954;30:195.

511. Ruskin JN, Hutter AM Jr: Primary pulmonary hypertension treated with oral phentolamine. *Ann Intern Med* 1979;90:772.

512. Shettigar UR, Hultgren HN, Specter M, et al: Primary pulmonary hypertension: Favorable effect of isoproterenol. *N Engl J Med* 1976;295:1414.

513. Lee TD Jr, Roveti GC, Ross RS: The hemodynamic effects of isoproterenol on pulmonary hypertension in man. *Am Heart J* 1963;65:361.

514. Leier CV, Bambach D, Nelson S, et al: Captopril in primary pulmonary hypertension. *Circulation* 1983;67:155.

515. Pearl RG, Rosenthal MH, Schroeder JS, et al: Acute hemodynamic effects of nitroglycerin in pulmonary hypertension. *Ann Intern Med* 1983;99:9.

516. Rubin LJ, Peter RH: Oral hydralazine therapy for primary pulmonary hypertension. *N Engl J Med* 1980;302:69.

517. Lupi-Herrera E, Sandoval J, Seaone M, et al: The role of hydralazine therapy for pulmonary arterial hypertension of unknown cause. *Circulation* 1982;65:645.

518. Wang SW, Pohl JE, Rowlands DJ, et al: Diazoxide in treatment of primary pulmonary hypertension. *Br Heart J* 1978;40:572.

519. Klinke WP, Gilbert JA: Diazoxide in primary pulmonary hypertension. *N Engl J Med* 1980;302:91.

520. Hall DR, Petch MC: Remission of primary pulmonary hypertension during treatment with diazoxide. *Br Med J* 1981;282:1118.

521. Chick TW, Kochukoshy KN, Matsumoto S, et al: The effect of nitroglycerin on gas exchange, hemodynamics, and oxygen transport in patients iwht chronic obstructive pulmonary disease. *Am J Med* Sci 1978;276:105.

522. Rubino JM, Schroeder JS: Diazoxide in treatment of primary pulmonary hypertension. *Br Heart J* 1979;42:362.

523. Buch J, Wennevold A: Hazards of diazoxide in pulmonary hypertension. *Br Heart J* 1981;46:401.

524. Honey M, Cotter L, Davies N, et al: Clinical and hemodynamic effects of diazoxide in primary pulmonary hypertension. *Thorax* 1980;35:269.

525. Camerini F, Alberti E, Klugmann S, et al: Primary pulmonary hypertension: effects of nifedipine. *Br Heart J* 1980;44:352.

526. Saito D, Haraoka S, Yoshida H, et al: Primary pulmonary hypertension improved by long-term oral administration of nifedipine. *Am Heart J* 1983;105:1041.

527. Wise JR: Nifedipine in the treatment of primary pulmonary hypertension. *Am Heart J* 1983;105:693.

528. De Feyter PJ, Kerkkamp HJJ, de Jong JP: Sustained beneficial effect of nifedipine in primary pulmonary hypertension. *Am Heart J* 1983;105:333.

529. Rich S, Brundage BH: High-dose calcium channel-blocking therapy for primary pulmonary hypertension: Evidence for long-term reduction in pulmonary arterial pressure and regression of right ventricular hypertrophy. *Circulation* 1987;76:135.

530. Kambara H, Fujimoto K, Wakabayashi A, et al: Primary pulmonary hypertension: beneficial therapy with diltiazem. *Am Heart J* 1981;101:230.

531. Arnman K, Ryden L, Smedgard P, et al: Felodipine in primary pulmonary hypertension: Report of two cases. *Acta Med Scand* 1984;215:275.

532. Watkins WD, Peterson MB, Crone RK, et al: Prostacyclin and prostaglandin E_1 for severe idiopathic pulmonary artery hypertension. *Lancet* 1980;1:1083.

533. Jones R, Higenbottam T, Wallwork J: Pulmonary vasodilation with prostacyclin in primary and secondary pulmonary hypertension. *Chest* 19879;96:784.

534. Rozhovec A, Minty K, Stradling J, et al: Value of acute vasodilator studies in the management of primary pulmonary hypertension. *Circulation* 1982;66(suppl II):II-49.

535. Groves BH, Rubin LJ, Reeves JT, et al: Comparable hemodynamic effects of prostacyclin and hydralazine in primary pulmonary hyperension. *Circulation* 1980;64(suppl IV):IV-297. Abstract.

536. Higenbottam T, Wheeldon D, Wells F, et al: Long-term treatment of primary pulmonary hypertension with continuous intravenous epoprostenol prostacyclin. *Lancet* 1984;1:1046.

537. Rubin LJ, Mendoza J, Hood M, et al: Treatment of primary pulmonary hypertension with continuous intravenous prostacyclin epoprostenol: Results of a randomized trial. *Ann Intern Med* 1990;112:489.

538. Rubin LJ, Groves BM, Reeves JT, et al: Prostacyclin-induced acute pulmonary vasodilation in primary pulmonary hypertension. *Circulation* 1982;66:334.

539. Guadagni DN, Ikram H, Maslowski AH: Hemodynamic effects of prostacyclin PGI2. in pulmonary hypertension. *Br Heart J* 1981;45:385.

540. Packer M: Is it ethical to administer vasodilator drugs to patients with primary pulmonary hypertension? *Chest* 1989;95:1173.

541. Reitz BA, Wallwork JL, Hunt SA, et al: Heart-lung transplantation: Successful therapy for patients with pulmonary vascular disease. *N Engl J Med* 1982;306:557.

542. Dwakins KD, Hunt SA, Jamieson SW, et al: Heart-lung transplantation for pulmonary vascular disease: Follow-up hemodynamic data. *J Am Coll Cardiol* 1984;3:596.

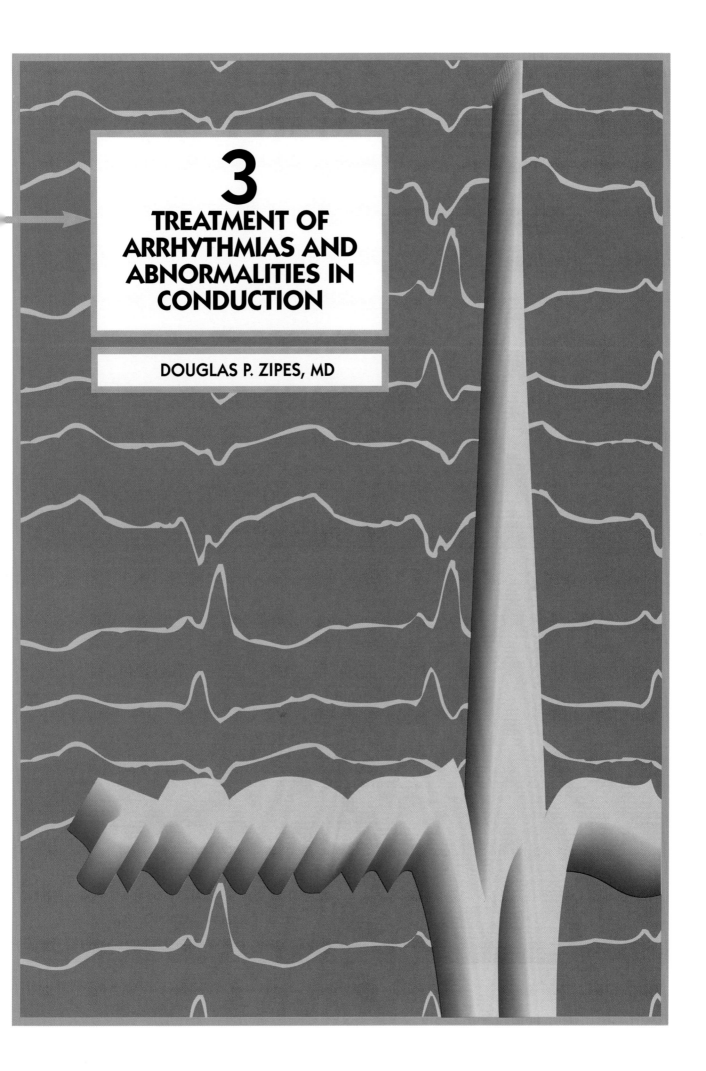

3

TREATMENT OF ARRHYTHMIAS AND ABNORMALITIES IN CONDUCTION

DOUGLAS P. ZIPES, MD

Synopsis of Chapter Three

HISTORY

The discovery of the impulse-forming and impulse-conducting system of the heart took place over many years. In 1845, Purkinje described the cells in the subendocardium of the pig and lamb heart that bear his name. In 1893, His described a connecting bundle of modified muscle fibers as the only path linking atria and ventricles. Thirteen years later, Tawara demonstrated that the bundle described by His was part of a larger conducting muscular pathway with a "node" at its beginning and the bundle branches at its end. Thus, the atrioventricular (AV) conduction system became fully known. Keith and Flack identified the sinus node in 1907. Bachmann described a muscular connection between the right and left atria in 1916.

Conceptions about cardiac arrhythmias probably began with the art of feeling the pulse as practiced in ancient China as early as 500 B.C. It was believed that pulse reading would lead to the diagnosis of all diseases. In the second century A.D., Galen taught that an intermittent pulse, depending upon the degree, had an ominous significance. Such feelings held sway for many hundreds of years. The first human electrocardiograms were recorded by Waller in 1889, with the greatest contribution—that of the string galvanometer—introduced in 1901 by Einthoven. A series of observations on arrhythmias by MacKenzie and Lewis in London, and Wenckebach and Rothberger in Vienna, followed quickly. Pick, Langendorf and Katz in Chicago, using the standard electrocardiograph machine, made some of the most important contributions to modern day understanding of cardiac arrhythmias.

ANATOMY

The sinus node is a spindle-shaped structure near the epicardial surface of the right atrium at its junction with the superior vena cava (Figure 3.1). No single cell in the sinus node serves as the underlying pacemaker; the cells function as electrically coupled oscillators discharging synchronously. Postganglionic adrenergic and cholinergic nerve fibers richly innervate the sinus node and help modulate its discharge rate. Vagal stimulation slows sinus nodal discharge rate, by releasing acetylcholine, while adrenergic stimulation releases norepinephrine and speeds the discharge rate. The impulse spreads radially from the sinus node and most evidence does not support the presence of specialized internodal tracks resembling the bundle branches. More rapid conduction occurs in some parts of the atrium due to fiber orientation, size, geometry or other factors rather than to discrete, histologically identifiable tracks of tissue between the nodes.

The atrioventricular (AV) node lies just beneath the right atrial endocardium, anterior to the ostium of the coronary sinus, and directly above the insertion of the septal leaflet of the tricuspid valve. The distal portion of the AV node becomes the penetrating portion of the His bundle at the point where it enters the central fibrous body. It then penetrates the membranous septum, continuing on as the bundle branches, with cells of the left bundle branch cascading downward as a continuous sheet onto the septum beneath the noncoronary aortic cusp. In some hearts, an anterosuperior and posteroinferior branch of the left bundle branch may arise, providing two fascicles of the left bundle branch. The right bundle branch continues as an unbranched extension of the AV bundle down the right side of the intraventricular septum. The bundle branches terminate in Purkinje fibers that form interweaving networks on the endocardial surface of both ventricles, transmitting the cardiac impulse almost simultaneously to the entire right and left ventricular endocardium[1,2] (Figure 3.2).

CARDIAC ELECTROPHYSIOLOGY

The cell membrane constitutes a bilayer boundary of phospholipid molecules that provide a high resistance insulated wrapping around the cell. The sarcolemma exhibits selective permeability to ions and creates an electrical potential across the cell membrane. At rest, the resistance to ion flow is greater across the cell membrane than in the cytoplasm of the cell interior. The cell membrane has openings called channels that serve as conduits through which ions move. Gates, influenced by the electric field and by time, control ion movement through the channels. In addition to the channels, protein molecules may help regulate ionic fluxes.

The cell membranes of some types of adjacent cells form close margins called intercalated discs. The nexus, also called a tight or gap junction, is a region in the intercalated disc where cells are in functional contact with each other. Nexuses provide low resistance electrical coupling between adjacent cells, reducing cell-to-cell resistance.

Depolarization of a typical cardiac cell causes the transmembrane potential to move through five phases that are the result of passive ion fluxes (Figure 3.3). Ions move down electrochemical gradients established by active ion pumps and exchange mechanisms. Each ion moves primarily through its own ion specific channel.

During **phase 4**, or **resting membrane potential**, the cell membrane is permeable to potassium and relatively impermeable to sodium. Intracellular potassium concentration remains high while intracellular sodium concentration remains low. A stimulus delivered to the cell that reduces membrane potential to a threshold value in the range of –70 mV for normal Purkinje fibers causes a sudden increase in membrane conductance to sodium, producing the upstroke of the cardiac action potential, **phase 0**. In normal atrial and ventricular muscle and in fibers of the His-Purkinje system, action potentials have very rapid upstrokes due to sodium rushing inward through ion specific channels and are called fast responses. Action potentials in the normal sinus and atrioventricular nodes have very slow upstrokes caused by the ingress of the slow inward current—predominately calcium rather than sodium—and are called slow responses.

Following phase 0, the membrane repolarizes rapidly and transiently to **phase 1**, and then enters the plateau phase, **phase 2**,

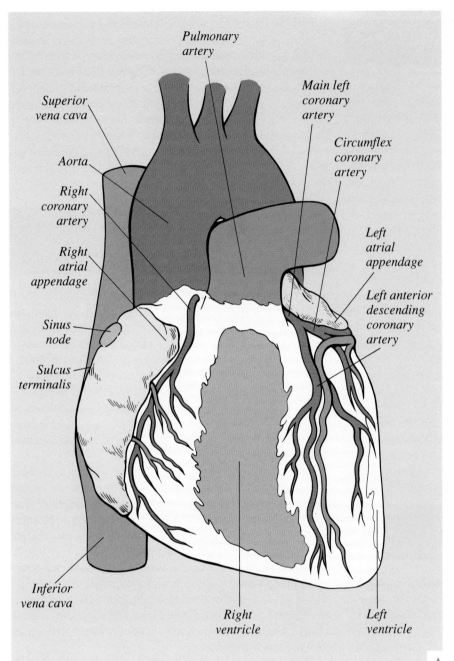

FIGURE 3.1 • The site of the sinus node (A). Operative views of the terminal sulcus, site of the sinus node (B) and the safe incision into the right atrium (C). (Figures 3.1B,C reproduced with permission. Wilcox BR, Anderson RH: *Surgical Anatomy of the Heart* New York, NY: Gower Medical Publishing/Raven Press;1985:2.4.)

Pulmonary artery

Superior vena cava

Aorta

Right coronary artery

Right atrial appendage

Sinus node

Sulcus terminalis

Inferior vena cava

Right ventricle

Main left coronary artery

Circumflex coronary artery

Left atrial appendage

Left anterior descending coronary artery

Left ventricle

A

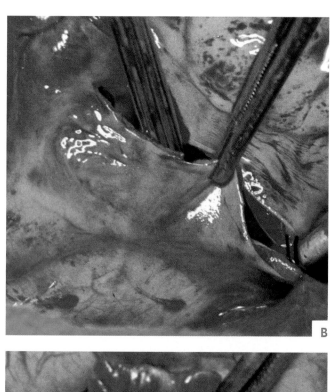

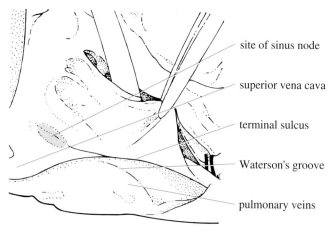

site of sinus node

superior vena cava

terminal sulcus

Waterson's groove

pulmonary veins

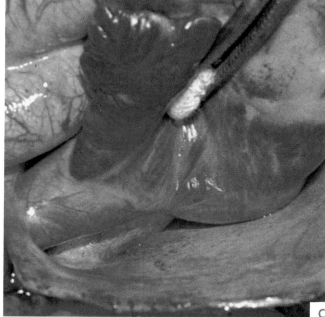

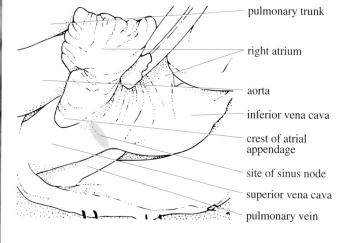

pulmonary trunk

right atrium

aorta

inferior vena cava

crest of atrial appendage

site of sinus node

superior vena cava

pulmonary vein

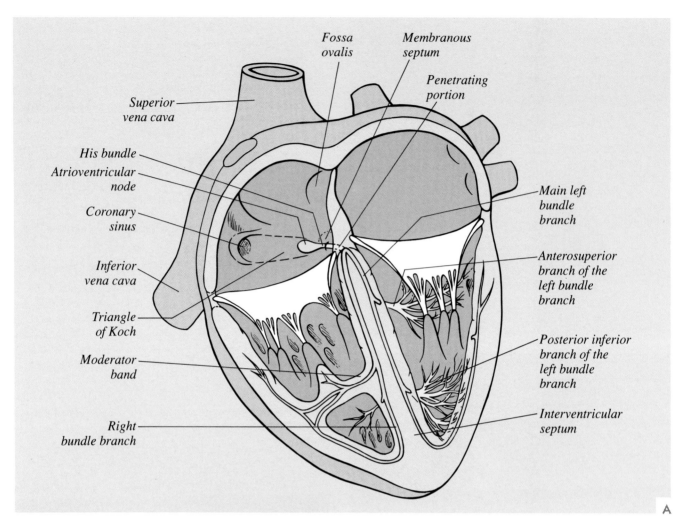

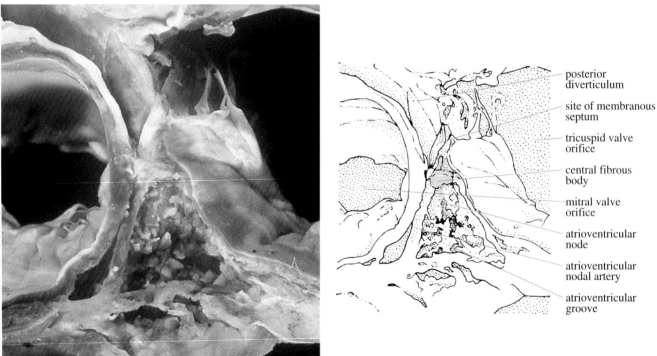

FIGURE 3.2 • The site of the atrioventricular node, His bundle, and bundle branches (A). Coronary sinus floor showing the course of the atrioventricular nodal artery through an epicardial tissue plate (B). Note that the site of the atrioventricular node is superimposed. (Figure 3.2B reproduced with permission. Wilcox BR, Anderson RH: *Surgical Anatomy of the Heart* New York, NY: Gower Medical Publishing/Raven Press; 1985.)

Treatment of Arrhythmias and Abnormalities in Conduction

during which membrane conductance to all ions falls to rather low values. The termination of phase 2, final rapid repolarization or **phase 3**, results in extrusion of potassium and restoration of the intracellular negative voltage. Sodium and potassium concentrations then return to diastolic levels during **phase 4**. Some cells, such as the sinus node, have the property of automaticity during which a net gain in intracellular positive charges occurs during diastole. When threshold potential is reached, the cell spontaneously discharges[2] (Figure 3.4).

MECHANISMS OF ARRHYTHMOGENESIS

The causes of cardiac arrhythmias are generally divided into categories of disorders of impulse formation, disorders of impulse conduction, or combinations of both. Disorders of impulse formation include inappropriate spontaneous discharge of a cell or group of cells that takes control of the cardiac rhythm. Automaticity probably causes parasystole, independently discharging pacemaker focus. Another cause is called triggered activity. It is not an automatic, self-generating mechanism since it requires prior stimulation to produce afterdepolarizations. These afterdepolarizations can occur before full repolarization and are termed early afterdepolarizations. When occuring after completion of full repolarization, they are called delayed afterdepolarizations. Early afterdepolarizations appear to be important in the long QT syndrome and associated torsades de pointes. Delayed afterdepolarizations may be important in some digitalis-induced arrhythmias.

Disorders of impulse conduction result from conduction delay or block. When the propagating impulse is blocked and followed by asystole, a bradyarrhythmia results. If the delay or block causes reentrant excitation, a tachyarrhythmia may transpire. Reentry occurs when a group of fibers—not activated because of unidirectional block during the initial wave of depolarization—recovers excitability in time to be discharged before the impulse dies out. These fibers serve as a link to reexcite areas that were just discharged and have now recovered from the initial depolarization. For reentry to occur, there must exist an area of unidirectional block, conduction sufficiently slowed in an alternate route to allow previously activated tissue to recover excitability, and recirculation of the impulse to its point of origin (Figure 3.5). Reentry occurs in several forms (refer to Fig-

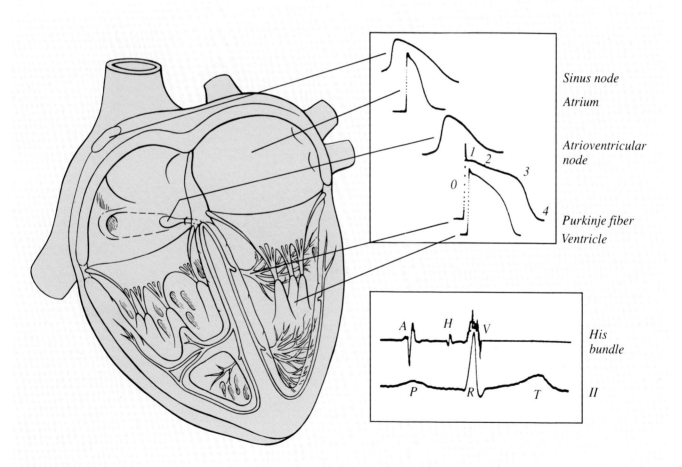

FIGURE 3.3 • Transmembrane potentials from different cell types. These are portrayed in order of depolarization with a superimposed His bundle recording and scalar ECG. 0, 1, 2, 3, and 4 indicate the five phases of the cardiac action potential which are labeled for the Purkinje fiber.

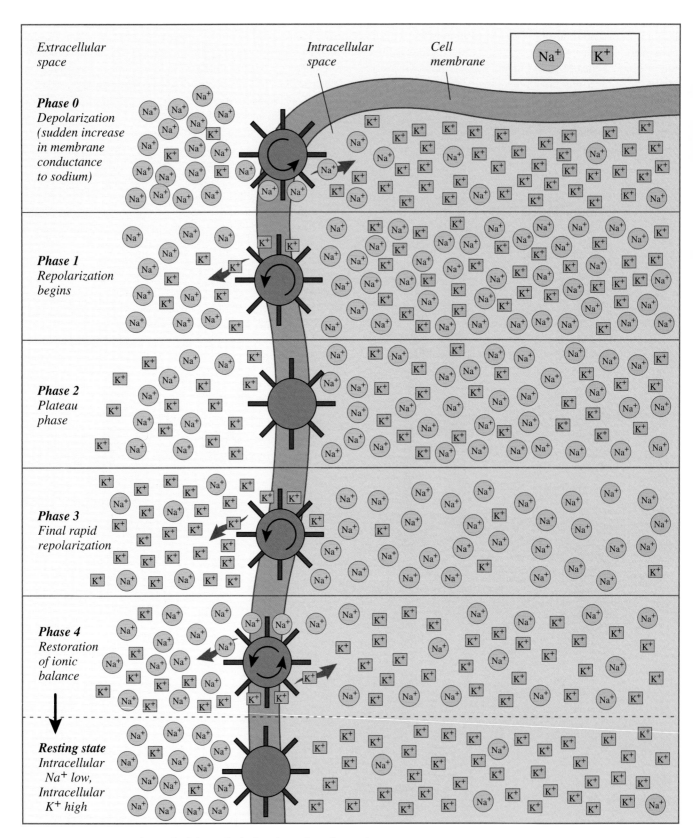

FIGURE 3.4A • Cardiac electrophysiology—ionic flow from phase 0 to resting state

ure 3.5) and is probably the cause of many tachyarrhythmias such as atrial flutter, some atrial tachycardias, sinus node reentry, AV nodal reentrant tachycardia and AV reciprocating tachycardia associated with Wolff-Parkinson-White syndrome. In AV nodal reentry, the reentrant loop is confined in or very near the AV node, while in AV reentrant tachycardia, the reentrant loop is comprised of the AV node in one direction (usually anterograde) and the accessory pathway in the other direction (usually retrograde). Ventricular tachycardia is often due to reentry, particularly in patients with ischemic heart disease. Reentry over the bundle branches can cause ventricular tachycardia in patients with dilated cardiomyopathy. Multiple wavelets of reentry are probably responsible for atrial and ventricular fibrillation.[2]

APPROACH TO THE DIAGNOSIS OF CARDIAC ARRHYTHMIAS

Critical to therapy is the concept that the physician evaluates a patient who has a rhythm disturbance and does not evaluate a rhythm disturbance in isolation. With that in mind, it is important to stress that some arrhythmias, such as rapid ventricular tachycardias, can be hazardous to the patient regardless of the clinical setting, while others, such as AV nodal reentry, can be hazardous because of the clinical setting. Patients with cardiac rhythm disturbances commonly present with symptoms such as palpitations, syncope, near syncope, or congestive heart failure. Individual patient perception of regular or irregular rhythms varies greatly. Some patients perceive slight variations in their heart rhythms with exquisite accuracy, while others are oblivious even to sustained episodes of ventricular tachycardia. Still others complain of palpitations when they actually have regular sinus rhythm.

Evaluation should proceed from the simplest to the most complex test, from the least invasive and safest to the most invasive and potentially dangerous, and from out-of-hospital studies to those that require hospitalization and sophisticated, costly procedures. Depending on the clinical circumstances, one may need to proceed directly to a high-risk, expensive procedure, such as an electrophysiological study, prior to obtaining a safe, noninvasive test, such as a 24-hr ECG recording. Exercise testing, long-term electrocardiographic recordings, invasive electrophysiologic studies, signal averaged ECG and tilt testing are some of the tests that can be used for evaluation.

Three major avenues available for treatment of patients with cardiac arrhythmias include pharmacologic, surgical and electrical approaches.

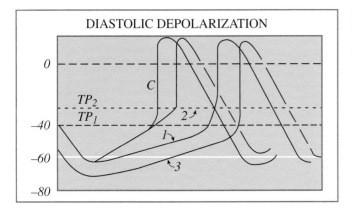

DIASTOLIC DEPOLARIZATION

FIGURE 3.4B • Diastolic depolarization. The sinus node is undergoing diastolic depolarization.
• (1) Depression of phase 4 diastolic depolarization.
• (2) Elevation in threshold potential (from TP_1 to TP_2).
• (3) Hyperpolarization of the membrane demonstrates mechanism responsible for the change in the normal rate.

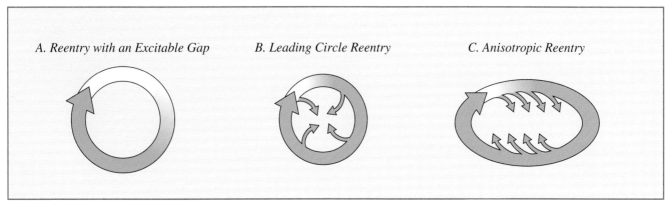

A. Reentry with an Excitable Gap

B. Leading Circle Reentry

C. Anisotropic Reentry

FIGURE 3.5 • Reentry. Three types of reentry are demonstrated. Reentry with an excitable gap (pale area), occurring commonly in tachycardias such as AV reentrant tachycardia (refer to preexcitation syndrome) (A). Leading circle reentry which has no excitable gap and has been shown in experimental atrial preparations (B). Anisotropic reentry due to anatomical features of cell-to-cell alignment has been demonstrated experimentally in ventricular tachycardia models (C).

PHARMACOLOGIC THERAPY

The primary objective of pharmacologic treatment of a patient with a cardiac arrhythmia is to to reach an effective and well-tolerated plasma drug concentration as rapidly as possible and to maintain this concentration for as long as required without producing adverse effects. In many, but not all situations and not with all drugs, serum concentration after equilibration correlates with the antiar-rhythmic and adverse effects of the drug. The therapeutic plasma concentration for an individual patient is the amount of drug required for that patient to suppress or terminate the cardiac arrhythmia without producing adverse effects, and can vary greatly.[3]

Antiarrhythmic agents have narrow toxic therapeutic relationships and important complications of therapy can result from amounts of drug that only slightly exceed the amount necessary to produce beneficial effects. Lesser concentrations are often subtherapeutic. It is obvious that careful dosing with

TABLE 3.1 • DOSAGE AND THERAPEUTIC SERUM CONCENTRATIONS FOR ANTIARRHYTHMIC AGENTS

| | Usual dose ranges | | | |
| | Intravenous (mg) | | Oral (mg) | |
Drug	Loading	Maintenance	Loading	Maintenance
Quinidine	6 - 10 mg/kg at 0.3 - 0.5 mg/kg/min		600 - 1,000	300 - 600 q6h
Procainamide	6 - 13 mg/kg at 0.2 - 0.5 mg/kg/min	2 - 6 mg/min	500 - 1,000	350 - 1000 q3–6h
Disopyramide	1 - 2 mg/kg over 45 min[1]	1 mg/kg/hr[1]		100 - 400 q6–8h
Lidocaine	1 - 3 mg/kg at 20 - 50 mg/min	1 - 4 mg/min	N/A	N/A
Mexiletine[1]	500 mg	0.5 - 1.0 g/24 hr	400 - 600	150 - 300 q6–8h
Tocainide[1]	750 mg		400 - 600	400 - 600 q8–12h
Phenytoin	100 mg q5min for ≤ 1,000 mg		1000	100 - 400 q12–24h
Moricizine			300	100 - 400 q8h
Flecainide[1]	2 mg/kg			100 - 200 q12h
Encainide[2]	0.6 - 0.9 mg/kg			25 - 75 q6–8h
Propafenone	1 - 2 mg/kg		600 - 900	150 - 300 q8–12h
Propranolol	0.25 - 0.5 mg, q5min for ≤ 0.15 - 0.20 mg/kg			10 - 200 q6–8h
Bretylium	5 - 10 mg/kg at 1 - 2 mg/kg/min	1/2 - 2 mg/min	N/A	4 mg/kg/d[1]
Amiodarone[1]	5 - 10 mg/kg over 20–30 min then 1 gm/24 hr		800 - 1,600 QD for 1 to 3 weeks	200 - 400 QD
Verapamil	10 mg over 1 - 2 min	0.005 mg/kg/min		80 - 120 q6–8h
Adenosine	6–12 mg (rapidly)		NA	NA

[1]IV administration; investigational only.
[2]Removed from the market.
Results presented may vary according to doses, disease state, and IV or oral administration.

(Reproduced with permission. Zipes DP: Management of cardiac arrhythmias. In: Braunwald E, ed. *Heart Disease. A Textbook of Cardiovascular Medicine* Philadelphia, Pa: WB Saunders; 1992.)

these agents is essential to maintain adequate but nontoxic amounts of drug in the body (Table 3.1).

CLASSIFICATION

Although the usefulness of drug classifications is limited, the available antiarrhythmic drugs (Figure 3.6) can be divided into those that exert blocking actions predominantly on sodium, potassium or calcium channels and those that block ß-adrenoceptors[4] (Tables 3.2, 3.3).

Class 1 Drugs that block the sodium channel
- Class 1A: Drugs that reduce the rapid upstroke and prolong action potential duration—quinidine, procainamide, disopyramide.
- Class 1B: Drugs that do not reduce the rapid upstroke and shorten action potential duration—lidocaine, mexiletine, tocainide, phenytoin, moricizine.
- Class 1C: Drugs that significantly reduce the rapid upstroke, primarily slow conduction, and prolong refractoriness minimally—flecainide, encainide, propafenone.

Drug	Time to peak plasma concentration (oral) (hr)	Effective serum or plasma concentration (µg/mL)	Elimination half-life (hr)	Bioavail-ability (%)	Major route of elimination
Quinidine	1.5 - 3.0	3 - 6	5 - 9	60 - 80	Liver
Procainamide	1	4 - 10	3 - 5	70 - 85	Kidneys
Disopyramide	1 - 2	2 - 5	8 - 9	80 - 90	Kidneys
Lidocaine	N/A	1 - 5	1 - 2	N/A	Liver
Mexiletine	2 - 4	0.75 - 2	10 - 17	90	Liver
Tocainide	0.5 - 2	4 - 10	11	90	Liver
Phenytoin	8 - 12	10 - 20	18 - 36	50 - 70	Liver
Moricizine		0.1			
Flecainide	3 - 4	0.2 - 1.0	20	95	Liver
Encainide	1 - 2	0.5 - 1.0	3 - 4	40	Liver
Propafenone	1 - 3	0.2 - 3.0	5 - 8	25 - 75	Liver
Propranolol	2 - 4	0.04 - 0.90	3 - 6	20 - 50	Liver
Bretylium		0.5 - 1.5	8 - 14	25	Kidneys
Amiodarone	4	1 - 2.5	50 days	35 - 65	Liver
Verapamil	1 - 2	0.10 - 0.15	3 - 8	10 - 35	Liver
Adenosine	NA	NA	1 - 6 sec	NA	See text

TABLE 3.1 • DOSAGE AND THERAPEUTIC SERUM CONCENTRATIONS FOR ANTIARRHYTHMIC AGENTS (Cont'd)

Results presented may vary according to doses, disease state, and IV or oral administration.

(Reproduced with permission. Zipes DP: Management of cardiac arrhythmias. In: Braunwald E, ed. *Heart Disease. A Textbook of Cardiovascular Medicine* Philadelphia, Pa: WB Saunders; 1992.)

Class 2 Drugs that block ß-adrenoceptors—propranolol, timolol, and others.

Class 3 Drugs that block potassium channels and prolong repolarization—bretylium, amiodarone.

Class 4 Drugs that block the slow calcium channel—verapamil, diltiazem, nifedipine.

Other drugs—adenosine.

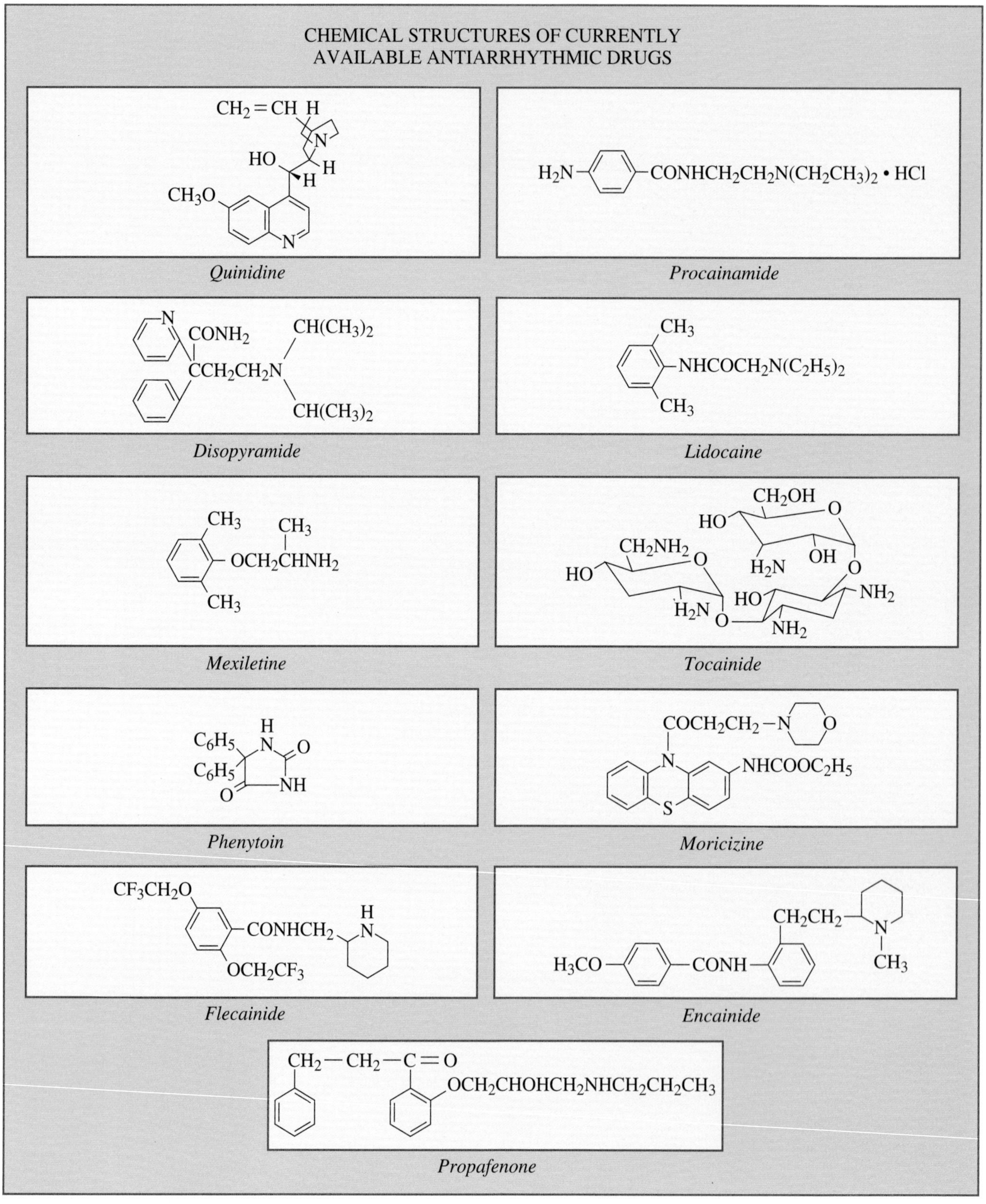

• • • • • • • • • • • • • • •

CHEMICAL STRUCTURES OF CURRENTLY AVAILABLE ANTIARRHYTHMIC DRUGS

Quinidine

Procainamide

Disopyramide

Lidocaine

Mexiletine

Tocainide

Phenytoin

Moricizine

Flecainide

Encainide

Propafenone

FIGURE 3.6 • Chemical structures of currently available drugs to treat arrhythmias.

A recently proposed model suggests that antiarrhythmic drugs cross the cell membrane and interact with receptors in the membrane channels when the latter are in the rested, activated, or inactivated states and that each of these interactions is characterized by different association and dissociation rate constants. Such interactions are voltage- and time-dependent. When the drug is bound to a receptor site or is very close to the ionic channel, the latter cannot conduct, resulting in a degree of

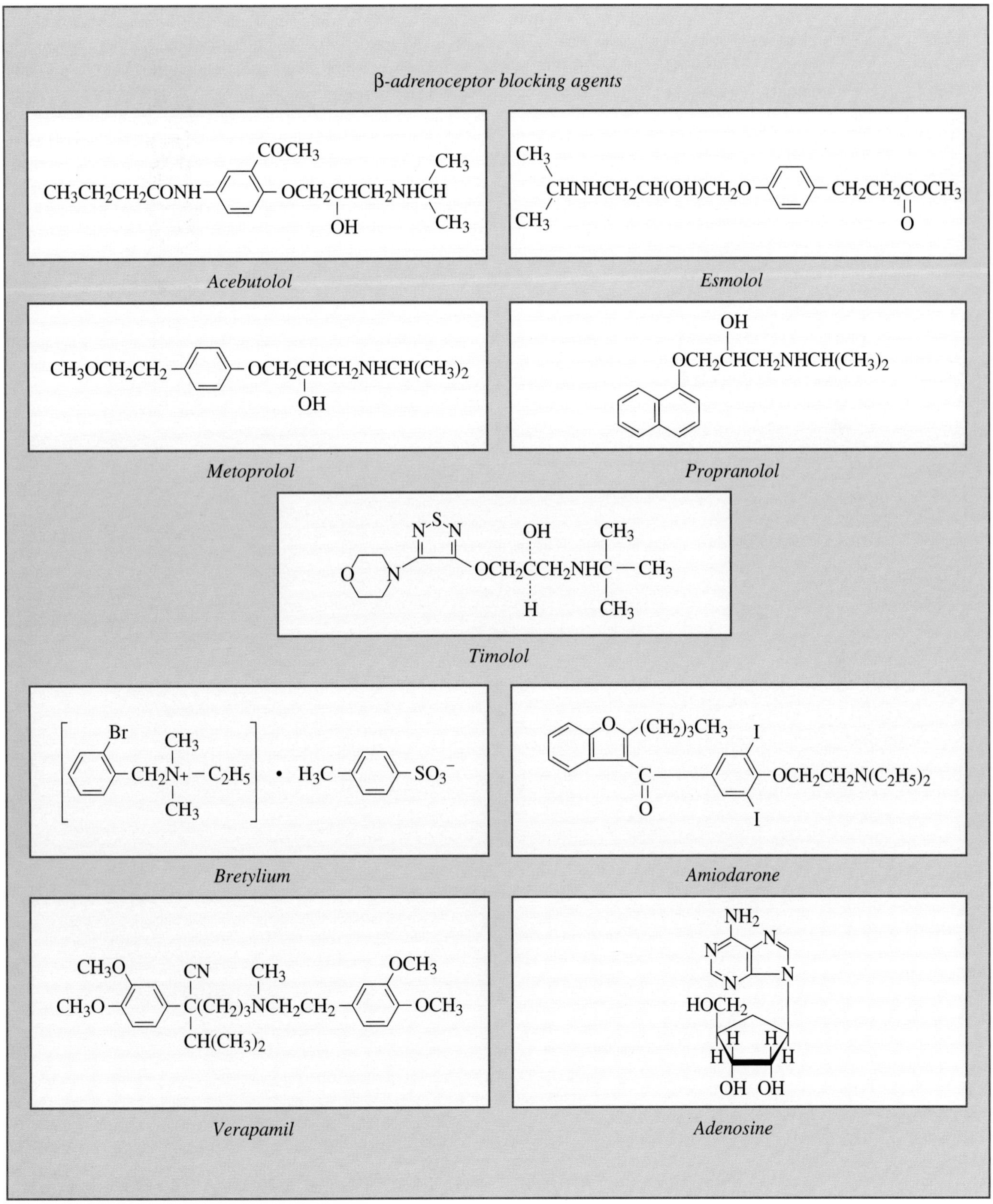

β-adrenoceptor blocking agents

Acebutolol

Esmolol

Metoprolol

Propranolol

Timolol

Bretylium

Amiodarone

Verapamil

Adenosine

ionic blockade. While 1B agents bind and dissociate quickly from the receptors, 1C agents have slow binding and dissociation kinetics and 1A drugs are intermediate.[5]

Some drugs exert greater inhibitory effects on the upstroke of the action potential at rapid rates or after longer periods of stimulation, a characteristic called "use dependence." With an increased time spent in diastole—slower rate—a greater proportion of receptors become drug free and the drug effect is less.

Antiarrhythmic agents can eliminate arrhythmias by depressing the automaticity of arrhythmogenic foci or by eliminating reentry. The latter can occur if a drug depresses conduction, transforming the unidirectional block to bidirectional block, or improves conduction to eliminate the unidirectional block. Further, it can allow a reentrant waveform to return too quickly and encroach on refractory fibers. Drugs can also suppress triggers that initiate the arrhythmia, such as premature complexes, or interact with blood flow, the autonom-

ic nervous system and electrolyte concentrations and other modulating influences.

ANTIARRHYTHMIC DRUGS
Class 1A

Quinidine • Quinidine has little effect on automaticity of the normal sinus node, but suppresses automaticity in ectopic pacemakers. Quinidine lengthens the duration of action potential and refractoriness of atrial and ventricular muscle and Purkinje fibers.[6] It prolongs conduction time in atria, ventricles and the His-Purkinje system. It exerts a significant anticholinergic action and causes reflex sympathetic stimulation resulting from alpha adrenergic blockade and peripheral vasodilation. These responses can increase sinus nodal discharge rate and improve atrioventricular (AV) nodal conduction, while direct effects can prolong AV nodal and His-Purkinje conduction times. No significant direct negative inotropic action occurs. Quinidine can be given intravenously if it is infused slowly. Approxi-

· · · · · · · · · · · · · · ·

TABLE 3.2 IN VIVO ELECTROPHYSIOLOGIC CHARACTERISTICS OF ANTIARRHYTHMIC DRUGS

Drug	Electrocardiographic intervals						Electrophysiologic intervals				
	Sinus rate	P-R	QRS	Q-T	A-H	H-V	ERP[1] AVN	ERP[1] HPS	ERP[1] A	ERP[1] V	ERP[1] AP
Quinidine	0↑	↓0↑	↑	↑	0↑	↑	0↑	↑	↑	↑	↑
Procainamide	0	0↑	↑	↑	0↑	↑	0↑	↑	↑	↑	↑
Disopyramide	0↑	0	↑	↑	0	↑	0↓	↑	↑	↑	↑
Lidocaine	0	0	0	0↓	0↓	0↑	0↓	0↑	0	0	0
Mexiletine	0	0	0	0	0↑	0↑	0↑	0↑	0	0	0
Tocainide	0↓	0	0	0↓	0	0	0	0	0	0	0
Phenytoin	0	0	0	0↓	0↓	0	0↓	↓	0	0	0
Moricizine	0↓	0↑	0↑	0	↑	↑	0	0	0↑	0↑	↑
Flecainide	0↓	↑	↑	0↑	↑	↑	↑	↑	↑	↑	↑
Encainide[2]	0↓	↑	↑	0↑	↑	↑	↑	↑	↑	↑	↑
Propafenone	0↓	↑	↑	0↑	↑	↑	0↑	0↑	0↑	↑	↑
Propranolol	↓	0↑	0	0↓	0↑	0	↑	0	0	0	0↑
Bretylium	0↓	0	0	0↑			0	↑	↑	↑	0
Amiodarone	↓	0↑	↑	↑	↑	↑	↑	↑	↑	↑	↑
Verapamil	0↓	↑	0	0	↑	0	↑	0	0	0	0↑
Adenosine	↓ then ↑	↑	0	0	↑	0	↑	0	↓	0	0↓

ERP = Effective refractory period
AVN = Atrioventricular node
HPS = His-Purkinje system
A = Atrium
V = Ventricle
AP = Accessory pathway (Wolff-Parkinson-White)

↑ = increase
↓ = decrease
0 = no change
0↑ or 0↓ = slight inconsistent increase or decrease

Results presented may vary according to tissue type, experimental conditions, and drug concentration.
[1]Longest S$_1$-S$_2$ interval at which S$_2$ fails to produce a response.
[2]Removed from the market.
(Reproduced with permission. Zipes DP: Management of cardiac arrhythmias. In: Braunwald E, ed. *Heart Disease. A Textbook of Cardiovascular Medicine* Philadelphia, Pa: WB Saunders; 1992.)

TABLE 3.3 • IN VITRO ELECTROPHYSIOLOGIC CHARACTERISTICS OF ANTIARRHYTHMIC DRUGS ON CANINE PURKINJE FIBERS

Drug	APA	APD	dV/dt	MDP	ERP	Conduction velocity	Sinus nodal automaticity	Purkinje fiber phase 4
Quinidine	↓	↑	↓	0	↑	↓	0	↓
Procainamide	↓	↑	↓	0	↑	↓	0	↓
Disopyramide	↓	↑	↓	0	↑	↓	↑0↓	↓
Lidocaine	0↓	↓	0↓	0	↓	0↓	0	↓
Mexiletine	0	↓	0↓	0	↓	0	0	↓
Tocainide	0	↓	0↓	0	↓	0	0	↓
Phenytoin	0	↓	↑0↓	0	↓	0	0	↓
Moricizine	↓	↓	↓	0	↓	↓	0	0
Flecainide	↓	0↑	↓	0	↑	↓↓	0	↓
Encainide	↓	0↑	↓	0	↑	↓↓	0	↓
Propafenone	↓	0↑	↓	0	↑	↓↓	↓	↓
Propranolol	0↓	0↓	0↓	0	↓	0	↓	↓[1]
Bretylium	0	↑	0	0	↑	0	0↓	0↓[1]
Amiodarone	0	↑	0↓	0	↑	↓	↓	↓
Verapamil	0	↓	0	0	0	0↓	↓	↓[1]
Adenosine	0	0	0	0	0	0	↓	0

Drug	Membrane responsiveness	ET	VFT	Contractility	Slow inward current	Autonomic nervous system	Local anesthetic effect
Quinidine	↓	↑	↑	0	0	Antivagal; α-blocker	Yes
Procainamide	↓	↑	↑	0	0	Slight antivagal	Yes
Disopyramide	↓	↑	↑	↓	0	Central: antivagal, antisympathetic	Yes
Lidocaine	0↓	0↑	↑	0	0	0	Yes
Mexiletine	↓	↑	↑	↓	0	0	Yes
Tocainide	↓	↑	↑	0	0	0	Yes
Phenytoin	0↑	0			0	0	No
Moricizine	↓	↑	0		0	0	Yes
Flecainide	↓	↑		↓	0	0	Yes
Encainide	↓	↑		↓	0	0	Yes
Propafenone	↓	↑	↑	↓	May inhibit	Antisympathetic	Yes
Propranolol	0↑	0	0↑	↓	0	Antisympathetic	Yes
Bretylium	0	0	↑	0↑	0	Antisympathetic	Yes
Amiodarone	↓			↓	0↓	Antisympathetic	No
Verapamil	0	0	0	↓	Inhibit	? Block α-receptors; enhance vagal	Yes
Adenosine	0	0	0	0	May inhibit	Vagomimetic	No

APA = Action potential amplitude
APD = Action potential duration
dV/dt = Rate of rise of action potential
MDP = Maximum diastolic potential
ERP = Effective refractory period
ET = Excitability threshold
VFT = Ventricular fibrillation threshold

[1]With a background of sympathetic activity.

(Reproduced with permission. Zipes DP: Management of cardiac arrhythmias. In: Braunwald E, ed. *Heart Disease. A Textbook of Cardiovascular Medicine* Philadelphia, Pa: WB Saunders; 1992.)

mately 80% of plasma quinidine is protein bound and removal occurs both by the liver and kidneys, with hepatic metabolism being more important. Approximately 20% is excreted unchanged in the urine. Elimination half-life is eight hours after oral administration.

The usual oral dose of quinidine sulfate for an adult is 300 to 600 mg four times daily. Quinidine is a versatile antiarrhythmic agent useful for treating premature supraventricular and ventricular complexes and sustained tachyarrhythmias. It can prevent AV nodal reentrant tachycardia by prolonging atrial and ventricular refractoriness and depressing conduction in the retrograde fast pathway. Prior to administering quinidine to patients with atrial flutter or fibrillation, the ventricular response should be slowed sufficiently with digitalis, propranolol or verapamil, since quinidine-induced slowing of the atrial flutter rate, and its vagolytic effect on AV nodal conduction, can increase the ventricular response. In patients with Wolff-Parkinson-White syndrome, quinidine increases the effective refractory period of the accessory pathway to prevent AV reciprocating tachycardia and to slow ventricular response from conduction over the accessory pathway during atrial flutter or fibrillation.

The most common adverse effects of chronic oral quinidine therapy are gastrointestinal, including nausea, vomiting, diarrhea, abdominal pain and anorexia. Central nervous system toxicity includes tinnitus, hearing loss, visual disturbances, confusion, delirium and psychosis. Allergic reactions can be manifested as rash, fever, immune-mediated thrombocytopenia, hemolytic anemia and, rarely, anaphylaxis. Quinidine can produce syncope, most often as the result of prolonged QT interval and torsades de pointes.[7] Conduction block can also result.

Procainamide • The electrophysiologic actions of procainamide on automaticity, refractoriness and conduction resemble those of quinidine. Procainamide exerts minimal anticholinergic effects compared with quinidine but produces more potent local anesthetic effects. Procainamide has a major metabolite, n-acetylprocainamide (NAPA) that prolongs action potential duration of ventricular muscle and Purkinje fibers more than does the parent compound. Procainamide can depress myocardial contractility in high doses. It does not produce α-blockade, but can result in peripheral vasodilation via a mild ganglionic blocking action.

Approximately 80% of oral procainamide is bioavailable, with 20% bound to serum proteins. Elimination half-life is 3 to 5 hrs, with 50% to 60% of the drug eliminated by the kidneys and 10% to 30% eliminated by hepatic metabolism. A prolonged release form of procainamide can be given every 6 hrs. The drug is acetylated to NAPA, which is excreted almost exclusively by the kidneys. In patients with decreased renal function or heart failure, procainamide serum concentration, particularly the NAPA metabolite, increases and maintenance doses must be reduced.

Procainamide can be given orally and intravenously to achieve plasma concentrations in the range of 4 to 10 μg/mL. The prolonged release procainamide is administered every six

hours in doses of 750 to 1000 mg. Given intravenously, maximum infusion rates of 0.5 mg/kg/min have been used, with a range of 25 to 50 mg/min until the arrhythmia is controlled, hypotension results or the QRS complexes are prolonged by 50%. Procainamide is used to treat both supraventricular and ventricular arrhythmias and has a spectrum of application comparable to that of quinidine.[8]

Multiple adverse noncardiac effects have been reported, including skin rashes, myalgia, digital vaculitis and Raynaud's phenomenon. Gastrointestinal side effects are less frequent than with quinidine. Adverse central nervous system side effects are less common than with lidocaine. Tachyarrhythmias and AV block can result, as with quinidine. Fever and agranulocytosis can be due to hypersensitivity reactions and blood counts should be performed at regular intervals. Arthralgia, fever, pleuropericarditis, hepatomegaly and hemorrhagic pericardial effusion with tamponade have been described in a systemic lupus erythematosus-like syndrome. Approximately 60% to 70% of patients who receive procainamide on a chronic basis develop antinuclear antibodies, with clinical symptoms in 20% to 30% that are reversible when the procainamide is discontinued.

Disopyramide • Although structurally different from quinidine and procainamide, disopyramide produces similar cardiac electrophysiologic effects. The positive isomer of the clinically used racemic mixture has important vagolytic actions, exceeding those of quinidine, that can speed sinus nodal discharge rate and shorten AV nodal conduction time and refractoriness. Disopyramide can also slow sinus nodal discharge rate by direct effects, especially in patients with sinus node dysfunction. Disopyramide's negative inotropic action can produce profound hemodynamic deterioration in patients who have abnormal ventricular function because they tolerate the negative inotropic effects of disopyramide poorly. In these patients, the drug should be used with extreme caution or not at all.

Disopyramide has a mean elimination half-life of 8 to 10 hrs, prolonged by renal insufficiency. Approximately one half an oral dose is recovered unchanged in the urine with about 30% as the mono n-dealkylated metabolite. Doses are generally 100 to 200 mg orally every 6 hrs with a range of 400 to 1200 mg/d. A sustained-release preparation may be given every 12 hrs. Disopyramide is comparable to quinidine and procainamide in overall efficacy and indications.

Adverse effects comprise three categories:
• Potent parasympatholytic response causing urinary hesitancy or retention, constipation, blurred vision, closed angle glaucoma, and dry mouth. Symptoms can be minimized by concomitant administration of pyridostigmine.
• Disopyramide can produce ventricular tachyarrhythmias that are commonly associated with QT prolongation and torsades de pointes.
• Disopyramide can reduce contractility of the normal ventricle, but the depression of ventricular function is much more pronounced in patients with pre-existing ventricular failure. The agent should be used cautiously or not at all in these patients.

Class 1B

Lidocaine • Lidocaine does not affect normal sinus nodal automaticity, but it depresses both normal and abnormal forms of automaticity in Purkinje fibers *in vitro*. Lidocaine also suppresses early and late afterdepolarizations, but it has minimal effect on normal conduction. However, faster rates of stimulation, reduced pH, increased extracellular potassium concentration and reduced membrane potential—all changes that can result from ischemia—increase the ability of lidocaine to block the fast sodium channels. Lidocaine can increase refractoriness in partially depolarized fibers, but generally decreases it. Lidocaine, except in very high concentrations, does not affect slow channel-dependent action potentials. It significantly reduces action potential duration and the effective refractory period of Purkinje fibers and ventricular muscle due to blocking of tetrodotoxin-sensitive sodium channels and decreasing entry of sodium into the cell. It has little effect on atrial fibers and does not affect conduction in accessory pathways. Clinically significant adverse hemodynamic effects are rarely noted at usual drug concentrations, unless left ventricular function is severely impaired.

Lidocaine is used only parenterally because oral administration results in extensive first pass hepatic metabolism and unpredictable low plasma levels with excessive metabolites that can produce toxicity. Hepatic metabolism of lidocaine depends greatly on hepatic blood flow, thus severe hepatic disease, heart failure or shock can markedly decrease the rate of lidocaine metabolism. Its elimination half-life averages about 1 to 2 hrs in normal subjects, more than four hours in patients after relatively uncomplicated myocardial infarction, more than 10 hrs in patients after myocardial infarction complicated by cardiac failure and even longer in the presence of cardiogenic shock. Maintenance doses should be reduced by one third to one half in patients with low cardiac output.

Although lidocaine can be given intramuscularly, the IV route is most commonly used. Intramuscular lidocaine is given in doses of 4 to 5 mg/kg (250 to 350 mg), resulting in effective serum levels in about 15 mins and lasting for approximately 90 mins. Intravenously, lidocaine is given as initial bolus of 1 to 2 mg/kg body weight at a rate of approximately 20 to 50 mg/min, with a second injection of one half the initial dose 20 to 40 mins later. Patients treated with an initial bolus followed by a maintenance infusion can experience transient subtherapeutic plasma concentrations at 30 to 120 mins after initiation of therapy. The second bolus of about 25 mg/kg, without increasing the maintenance infusion rate, reestablishes therapeutic serum concentrations. If recurrence of arrhythmia appears after a steady state has been achieved, a similar bolus should be given and maintenance infusion rate increased. Increase in the maintenance infusion rate only, without an additional bolus, results in a very slow increase in plasma lidocaine concentrations, taking more than 6 hrs to reach a new plateau and is therefore not recommended. Another recommended IV dosing is 1.5 mg/kg initially and 0.8 mg/kg at 8-min intervals for three doses. Doses are reduced by about 50% in patients with heart failure.

If the initial bolus of lidocaine is ineffective, up to two more boluses of 1 mg/kg may be administered at 5-min intervals. Patients who require more than one bolus to achieve the therapeutic effect have arrhythmias that respond only to a higher lidocaine plasma concentrations. A greater maintenance dose may be necessary to sustain these higher concentrations. Patients requiring only a single initial bolus of lidocaine should probably receive a maintenance infusion of 30 μg/kg/min, while those requiring two or three boluses may need infusions at 40 to 50 μg/kg/min. Maintenance infusion rates in the range of 1 to 4 mg/kg produce steady state plasma levels of 1 to 5 μg/mL in patients with uncomplicated myocardial infarction, but these rates must be reduced during heart failure or shock and in elderly patients.

Lidocaine is useful because it demonstrates great efficacy against ventricular arrhythmias of diverse etiology, the ability to achieve effective plasma concentrations rapidly, and a fairly wide toxic therapeutic ratio with a low incidence of hemodynamic complications and other side effects. Lidocaine is used primarily for patients with acute myocardial infarction or recurrent ventricular tachyarrhythmias.[9] It is generally ineffective against supraventricular arrhythmias such as AV nodal reentry or AV reentry associated with an accessory pathway. Further, it may accelerate the ventricular response during atrial fibrillation in patients with Wolff-Parkinson-White syndrome who have accessory pathways with a short refractory period.

Most commonly reported adverse effects of lidocaine are dose-related manifestations of central nervous system toxicity, including dizziness, parasthesias, confusion, delirium, stupor, coma and seizures. Occasionally, sinus node depression and His-Purkinje block occur, but they are uncommon.

Mexiletine • Mexiletine is similar to lidocaine in many of its electrophysiologic actions and does not appear to affect the refractory period of human atrial and ventricular muscle significantly. It exerts no major hemodynamic effects and does not depress myocardial performance when given orally. Mexiletine is rapidly and almost completely absorbed orally with an elimination half-life in healthy subjects of approximately 10 and 17 hrs in patients with myocardial infarction. Therapeutic plasma levels of 1 to 2 μg/mL are maintained by oral doses of 200 to 300 mg every 8 hrs. Normally, mexiletine is eliminated metabolically by the liver with less than 10% excreted unchanged in the kidney. Doses should be reduced in patients with cirrhosis and those with left ventricular failure. Total dose should not exceed 1,200 mg daily, and the drug is better tolerated when given with food. In some patients, administration every 12 hrs may be effective.

Mexiletine is effective for treating patients with both acute and chronic ventricular arrhythmias but not in those with supraventricular arrhythmias.[10] Mexiletine combined with other drugs, such as procainamide, ß-blockers, quinidine, disopyramide or amiodarone, can be more effective than mexiletine alone. Adverse effects include tremor, dysarthria, dizziness, paresthesia, diplopia, nystagmus, mental confusion, anxiety, nausea, vomiting and dyspepsia. Adverse effects appear to be dose-related and toxic effects occur at plasma concentrations only slightly higher than therapeutic levels.

Tocainide • Tocainide is a primary amine analog of lidocaine that lacks two ethyl groups which protect it from first pass hepatic elimination and make it effective orally. Its electrophysiologic effects are virtually identical to those of lidocaine and mexiletine. It has a small negative inotropic effect.

Oral regimens of 400 to 600 mg every 8 hrs produce therapeutic plasma concentrations of 4 to 10 µg/mL. Dosing increases should not be made more often than every 3 or 4 days. Doses should be reduced in patients with heart failure, liver or renal disease.

Tocainide has not been very effective in preventing chronic recurrent ventricular tachycardia-ventricular fibrillation and appears less effective than quinidine. Adverse effects are dose-related and similar to those produced by lidocaine. Importantly, hematologic disorders including agranulocytosis, bone marrow depression, leukopenia, hypoplastic anemia, and thrombocytopenia have been reported with an estimated incidence of 0.18%. This agent should probably not be administered if another lidocaine-like agent is required and exerts a beneficial effect.

Phenytoin (Diphenylhydantoin) • Phenytoin's actions resemble those of lidocaine and mexiletine but its value as an antiarrhythmic agent is limited. Orally, phenytoin is given as a loading dose of approximately 1,000 mg the first day, 500 mg on the second and third days, and 400 mg daily thereafter. Maintenance doses can be given once or twice daily. Phenytoin has been used successfully to treat atrial and ventricular arrhythmias caused by digitalis toxicity, but it is much less effective in treating ventricular arrhythmias in patients with ischemic heart disease or atrial arrhythmias not due to digitalis toxicity.

The most common adverse effects are central nervous system problems, such as nystagmus, ataxia, drowsiness, stupor and coma. Nausea, epigastric pain and anorexia are relatively common. Long-term administration may result in hyperglycemia, hypocalcemia, skin rashes, megaloblastic anemia, gingival hypertrophy, lymph node hyperplasia, peripheral neuropathy and drug-induced systemic lupus erythematosus.

Moricizine HCl (Ethmozine) • Moricizine HCl is a phenothiazine developed in the Soviet Union that has recently been approved by the Federal Drug Administration (FDA) for treatment of patients with ventricular tachyarrhythmias. It decreases I_{Na} and therefore the rate of the upstroke of phase 0, action potential amplitude, and action potential duration without changing diastolic potential. It has features of Class 1A, 1B, as well as Class 1C drugs. Moricizine prolongs AV nodal and His-Purkinje conduction time and QRS duration without a significant increase in the corrected QT interval. Ventricular refractoriness prolongs slightly with no consistent atrial change. It exerts few effects on cardiac performance in patients with impaired left ventricular function, therefore exercise tolerance and ejection fraction do not change. Moricizine undergoes extensive first pass metabolism with 95% of the drug protein bound. At least two metabolites are pharmacologically active, but they are in small concentrations and the electrophysiologic actions are due to the parent compound.

The usual adult dose is 600 to 900 mg/d given every 8 hrs in three equally divided doses. Increments of 150 mg/d at 3-day intervals can be tried and some patients can be treated every 12 hrs. Moricizine exerts antiarrhythmic efficacy that appears comparable to quinidine and disopyramide[11] and, in contrast to the effects of flecainide and encainide, does not lead to an increase in mortality in the Cardiac Arrhythmia Suppression Trial. Adverse effects primarily involve the nervous system, followed by gastrointestinal side effects. Proarrhythmic effects occur in about 3%.

Class 1C

Flecainide • Flecainide is approved by the FDA for treatment of patients with life-threatening ventricular arrhythmias. It exerts marked use-dependent depressant effects on the rapid sodium channel, decreasing V_{max} with slow onset and offset kinetics. Significant drug effects occur at physiological heart rates as well. Flecainide shortens the duration of Purkinje fiber action potential, but prolongs it in ventricular muscle. It profoundly slows conduction in all cardiac fibers and prolongs conduction time in the atria, ventricles, AV node, His-Purkinje system and accessory pathways. Minimal increases in atrial and ventricular refractoriness and in the QT interval result.

Flecainide depresses cardiac performance, particularly in patients with compromised myocardial function. Caution is warranted in patients with a history of heart failure. At least 90% of a flecainide dose is absorbed. It has an elimination half-life of approximately 20 hrs, longer in patients with renal disease and heart failure. The starting dose is 100 mg every 12 hrs, increased in increments of 50 mg twice daily, no sooner than every 4 days.

Flecainide is indicated for the treatment of life-threatening ventricular tachyarrhythmias.[12] Therapy should begin in hospital while the ECG is being monitored because of the high incidence of proarrhythmic events. Flecainide prevents electrical induction of ventricular tachyarrhythmias in 20% to 30% of patients and eliminates recurrence of life-threatening ventricular tachyarrhythmias in about 40%. Although recommended for treatment of patients with life-threatening ventricular tachyarrhythmias, as with encainide and all other Class 1 antiarrhythmic drugs, there are no data from control studies to indicate that the drug favorably affects survival or mortality from sudden cardiac death.[13] Flecainide may be very useful in patients with AV nodal and AV reentry tachycardias and other supraventricular tachycardias, although it is not yet approved for these indications.[14]

The dominant adverse effect is a proarrhythmic action, probably due to the marked slowing of conduction. Aggravation of existing ventricular arrhythmias or onset of new ventricular arrhythmias may occur in 5% to 25% of patients, the increased percentage in patients with preexisting sustained ventricular tachycardia, cardiac decompensation and higher doses of the drug. Negative inotropic effects may worsen or cause heart failure. Patients with sinus node dysfunction may experience sinus arrest and those with pacemakers may develop an increase in pacing threshold. Exercise can amplify the conduction slowing of the ventricle produced by flecainide and at times precipitate a proarrhythmic response. In the Cardiac Arrhythmias Suppression Trial, patients treated with flecainide had a 5.1% mortality rate or nonfatal cardiac arrest compared with 2.3% in the placebo group over 10 months.[15]

Encainide* • The electrophysiologic effects of encainide are similar to those of flecainide. It differs in that it has several active metabolites, one of which is more potent than the parent compound and may contribute to its antiarrhythmic efficacy or proarrhythmic action. Approximately 7% of patients lack the enzyme necessary to metabolize encainide and, therefore, develop higher plasma concentrations of the parent compound, with lower concentrations of the metabolites. This difference may not be clinically important. Encainide has minimal negative inotropic action, but it can worsen heart failure in patients with Class 3 and Class 4 heart failure. Its range of efficacy is similar to flecainide.[16,17]

Encainide is generally administered orally three times daily in doses of 100 to 300 mg/d. Changes in dosage should not be made more frequently than every 3 to 4 hrs. Adverse effects include dizziness, diplopia, vertigo, paresthesia, leg cramps and metallic taste in the mouth. Most significant is its potential to cause or exacerbate serious ventricular arrhythmias in approximately 10% of patients. In the Cardiac Arrhythmias Suppression Trial, patients treated with encainide had a 9.6% mortality rate or nonfatal cardiac arrest compared with 3.6% in the placebo group[15] (Figure 3.7).

Propafenone • Propafenone has recently been approved by the FDA for treatment of patients with life-threatening ventricular arrhythmias. It exerts electrophysiologic actions similar to flecainide and encainide.[18] Its active metabolites exert important actions. Negative inotropic effects occur at high concentrations, thus the drug should be given cautiously to patients with significant left ventricular dysfunction and congestive heart failure. More than 95% of the drug is absorbed. Bioavailability increases with the dose and plasma concentration and is therefore nonlinear. A three-fold increase in dose results in a ten-fold increase in plasma concentration, presumably due to saturation of hepatic metabolic mechanisms. The drug is metabolized by an enzyme system similar to that which metabolizes encainide and is absent in 7% of the population. Propafenone exhibits approximately 2.5% to 5% the potency of propranolol in blocking the ß-adrenoreceptor. Since plasma propafenone concentrations may be 50 times or more propranolol levels, these ß-blocking properties can be relevant. Propafenone also blocks the slow calcium channel to a degree about 100 times less than verapamil. Most patients respond to oral doses of 150 to 300 mg every 8 hrs, not exceeding 1200 mg/d. Doses should not be increased more often than every 3 to 4 days. Propafenone increases plasma concentrations of warfarin, digoxin and metoprolol.

The indications for propafenone are similar to those for flecainide. Minor, noncardiac adverse effects occur in about 15% of patients, with dizziness, disturbances in taste and blurred vision being the most common, and gastrointestinal side effects next. Exacerbation of bronchospastic lung disease may occur. Proarrhythmic responses appear in 5% of cases.

Class 2

ß-Adrenoceptor Blocking Drugs • Although 11 ß-adrenoceptor blocking drugs have been approved for use in the United States, only acebutolol (premature ventricular complexes), esmolol (supraventricular tachycardia), metoprolol (postmy-

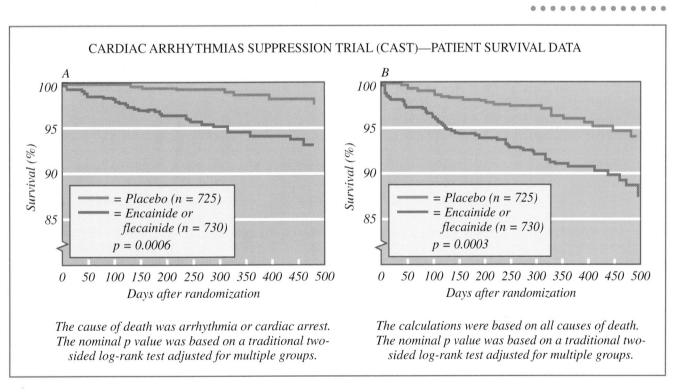

CARDIAC ARRHYTHMIAS SUPPRESSION TRIAL (CAST)—PATIENT SURVIVAL DATA

A

= Placebo (n = 725)
= Encainide or flecainide (n = 730)
p = 0.0006

Days after randomization

The cause of death was arrhythmia or cardiac arrest. The nominal p value was based on a traditional two-sided log-rank test adjusted for multiple groups.

B

= Placebo (n = 725)
= Encainide or flecainide (n = 730)
p = 0.0003

Days after randomization

The calculations were based on all causes of death. The nominal p value was based on a traditional two-sided log-rank test adjusted for multiple groups.

FIGURE 3.7 • Survival plots comparing the primary endpoint of death from arrhythmia or sudden cardiac arrest (A) and from all causes of death (B) among 1455 patients randomly assigned to receive encainide or flecainide, or placebo. (Reproduced with permission. The Cardiac Arrhythmias Suppression Trial (CAST) Investigators: *N Engl J Med* 1989;321:409.)

*Encainide has recently been withdrawn from the market.

ocardial infarction), propranolol (postmyocardial infarction, supraventricular tachycardia, ventricular tachycardia) and timolol (post myocardial infarction) have been approved to treat arrhythmias or to prevent sudden cardiac death after myocardial infarction. It is generally considered that no ß-blocker offers distinctive advantages over the others and that, when titrated to the proper dose, all can be used effectively to treat cardiac arrhythmias, hypertension, or other disorders. However, differences in pharmacokinetic or pharmacodynamic properties that confer safety, reduce adverse effects, or affect dosing intervals or drug interactions, influence the choice of agent.

Beta-receptors can be separated into those that affect predominately the heart ($ß_1$) or the bronchi and blood vessels ($ß_2$). In low doses, selective ß-blockers can block $ß_1$-receptors more than they block $ß_2$- receptors and might be preferable for treating patients with pulmonary or peripheral vascular diseases. In high doses, the selective $ß_1$-blockers also block $ß_2$-receptors. Some ß-blockers exert intrinsic sympathomimetic activity, that is, they slightly activate the ß-receptor. These ß-blockers have not been shown to reduce mortality in patients after myocardial infarction.

Beta blockers can exert an electrophysiologic action by competitively inhibiting catecholamine binding at ß-adrenoceptor sites or by their quinidine-like or direct membrane stabilizing action. The latter is a local anesthetic effect that depresses I_{Na} and occurs at concentrations generally tenfold greater than are necessary to produce ß-adrenoceptor blockade, most likely playing an insignificant antiarrhythmic role. At ß-blocking concentrations, propranolol slows spontaneous automaticity in the sinus node. Concentrations that cause ß-adrenoceptor blockade without local anesthetic effects do not alter normal action potential characteristics significantly. Propranolol slows the sinus discharge rate in humans by 10% to 20%, lengthening the PR interval due to an increase in AV nodal conduction time. His-Purkinje conduction time does not change. The negative inotropic effects produced by propranolol can precipitate or worsen heart failure.

Pharmacokinetics of the various ß-blockers differ substantially. Propranolol undergoes extensive first pass hepatic metabolism. Reduction in hepatic blood flow, as in patients with heart failure, decreases the hepatic extraction of propranolol and decreases its elimination rate. The appropriate dose of propranolol is best determined by a measure of the patient's physiologic response, such as changes in resting heart rate or in prevention of exercise-induced tachycardia, since wide individual differences exist between the observed physiological effect and plasma concentration. Orally, propranolol is given in four divided doses, usually ranging from 40 to 160 mg/d to more than 1 g/d. Generally, if one agent in adequate doses proves to be ineffective, other ß-blockers will be ineffective also. Arrhythmias associated with thyrotoxicosis, pheochromocytoma, exercise or emotion often respond to propranolol therapy. Beta-blocking drugs usually do not convert chronic atrial flutter or atrial fibrillation to normal sinus rhythm, but decrease the ventricular response because of prolongation of AV nodal conduction time and refractoriness. For reentrant supraventricular tachycardias using the AV node

as one of the reentrant pathways, such as AV nodal reentrant tachycardia and reciprocating tachycardias in the Wolff-Parkinson-White syndrome, or for sinus reentrant tachycardia, propranolol can terminate the tachycardia and be used prophylactically to prevent a recurrence. Combining propranolol with digitalis, quinidine or a variety of other agents can be effective when propranolol as a single agent fails. Intravenously the drug is given initially in doses of 0.25 to 0.5 mg and increased to 1 mg if necessary. It is administered every five minutes until either a desired effect or toxicity is produced or a total of 0.15 to 0.2 mg/kg has been given.

Propranolol may be effective for digitalis-induced arrhythmias, ventricular arrhythmias associated with the prolonged QT interval syndrome and with mitral valve prolapse. For patients with coronary heart disease, propranolol generally does not prevent episodes of chronic recurrent ventricular tachycardia that occur in the absence of acute ischemia, but it is effective in some patients, usually at a ß-blocking concentration.[19] It is well accepted that propranolol, timolol and metoprolol reduce the incidence of overall death and sudden cardiac death after myocardial infarction.[20]

Adverse cardiovascular effects from propranolol include hypotension, congestive heart failure and bradycardia, the latter from sinus bradycardia or AV block. Sudden withdrawal of propranolol in patients with coronary heart disease can precipitate angina, arrhythmias or myocardial infarction. Other adverse effects resulting from the administration of ß-blockers include worsening of asthma or chronic obstructive pulmonary disease, intermittent claudication, depression, increased risk of hypoglycemia, easy fatigability and impaired sexual function.

Class 3

Bretylium • Bretylium is a quaternary ammonium compound approved by the FDA for parenteral use only for intensive care patients who have life-threatening recurrent ventricular tachyarrhythmias that have not responded to conventional antiarrhythmic drugs. It is selectively concentrated in sympathetic ganglia and their postganglionic adrenergic nerve terminals. After initially causing norepineprhine release, bretylium prevents norepinephrine release by depressing excitability in the sympathetic nerve terminals without depressing pre- or postganglionic sympathetic nerve conduction, impairing conduction across sympathetic ganglia, depleting the adrenergic neurons of norepinephrine or decreasing the responsiveness of adrenergic receptors. It produces a chemical sympathectomy-like state. The initial release of catecholamines results in several transient electrophysiologic responses, such as an increase in the discharge rates of automatic pacemakers, increases in conduction velocity and excitability and decreases in refractoriness. Initial catecholamine release can aggravate some arrhythmias. Blood pressure can also increase initially. Prolonged drug administration lengthens the duration of action potential and refractoriness of atrial and ventricular muscle and Purkinje fibers, possibly by blocking one or more repolarizing potassium currents. After an initial increase in blood pressure, bretylium may cause significant hypotension, most often when patients are sitting or standing but also supine. Orthostatic hypotension can persist for several days after the drug has been discontinued.

Bretylium is effective orally as well as parenterally, but is absorbed poorly and erratically from the gastrointestinal tract. Elimination half-life is 5 to 10 hrs with fairly wide variability. Bretylium can be given intravenously in doses of 5 to 10 mg/kg body weight, diluted in 50 to 100 mL of 5% dextrose and water and administered over 10 to 20 mins, more quickly in a life-threatening state. The dose can be repeated in 1 to 2 hrs if arrhythmia persists, with a total daily dose probably not exceeding 30 mg/kg. The maintenance IV dose is 0.5 to 2.0 mg/kg. Transient increase in an adrenergic state, followed by hypotension are potentially important side effects.

Amiodarone • Amiodarone is a benzofuran derivative approved by the FDA for the treatment of patients with life-threatening ventricular tachyarrhythmias not responsive to other drugs or when other drugs are not tolerated. When given orally, amiodarone prolongs action potential duration and refractoriness of all cardiac fibers without affecting resting membrane potential. It decreases the slope of diastolic depolarization of the sinus node. Amiodarone also depresses the rate of rise of phase 0 in a rate- or use-dependent manner, that is, it exerts a greater effect at faster rates compared with slower rates. Its metabolite, desethylamiodarone, has relatively greater effects on fast channel tissue and probably contributes importantly to antiarrhythmic efficacy. Amiodarone also noncompetitively antagonizes α- and ß-receptors and blocks conversion of thryoxine (T_4) to triiodothyronine (T_3). Amiodarone exhibits slow channel blocking effects. Chronic oral therapy slows spontaneous sinus nodal discharge rate, prolongs the QT interval, lengthens the effective refractory period, and prolongs conduction in all cardiac tissue. Thus, amiodarone has Class 1 (sodium channel blocking), Class 2 (antiadrenergic) and Class 4 (calcium channel blocking) actions, in addition to Class 3 effects (prolonging action potential).

Amiodarone is a peripheral and coronary vasodilator that exerts some negative inotropic effects. It is slowly, variably and incompletely absorbed and, along with its metabolite, accumulates in multiple tissues, including the myocardium. Plasma clearance is low and renal excretion negligible. While the onset of action after intravenous administration generally occurs within several hours of oral administration, the onset of action may require two to three days, often one to three weeks. Loading doses reduce this time interval. Plasma concentrations relate well to oral doses during chronic treatment, averaging about 0.5 µg/mL for each 100 mg/d at doses between 100 and 600 mg/d. Elimination half-life is multiphasic with an initial 50% reduction in plasma concentration 3 to 10 days after cessation of drug ingestion, followed by a terminal half-life averaging about 50 days. Therapeutic serum concentrations range from 1 to 2.5 µg/mL.

An optimal dosing schedule for all patients has not been achieved. One recommended dose is to treat with 800 to 1,600 mg daily for 1 to 3 weeks, reduce to 800 mg daily for the next 2 to 4 weeks, and then 600 mg daily for 4 to 8 weeks. Finally, after 2 to 3 months of treatment, maintain a dose of 400 mg or less/d. Maintenance drug can be given once or twice daily and should be titrated to the lowest effective dose to minimize the occurrence of side effects.

Amiodarone has been used to suppress a wide spectrum of supraventricular and ventricular tachyarrhythmias in adults and children with an efficacy that equals or exceeds most other antiarrhythmic agents—in the range of 60% to 80% for most supraventricular tachyarrhythmias and 40% to 60% for ventricular tachyarrhythmias. Combining amiodarone with other antiarrhythmic agents may improve efficacy in some patients[21,22] (Figure 3.8).

Adverse effects are reported by about 75% of patients treated with amiodarone for five years, and necessitate drug

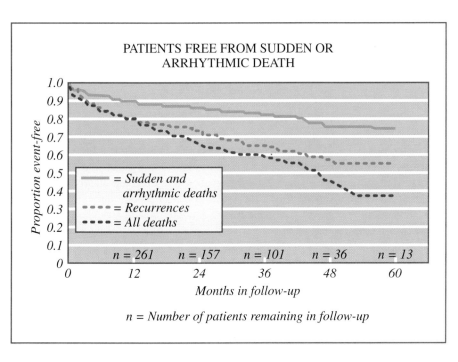

FIGURE 3.8 • Cumulative proportion of patients free from sudden or arrhythmic death, recurrence of sustained ventricular tachycardia or fibrillation, and all types of death—cardiac and noncardiac, sudden and nonsudden. (Reproduced with permission. Herre JM, Sauve MJ, Malone P, et al: *J Am Coll Cardiol* 1989;13:442.)

discontinuation in 18% to 37%. The most frequent side effects requiring drug discontinuation involve pulmonary and gastrointestinal complaints. Of the noncardiac adverse reactions, pulmonary toxicity is the most serious, occurring between 6 days and 60 months of treatment in about 7% of patients. A 10% mortality rate results in patients with pulmonary inflammatory changes.[23] At maintenance doses of less than 300 mg daily, pulmonary toxicity is uncommon. Proarrhythmia occurs in about 3% of patients.

Class 4 Antiarrhythmic Agents

Verapamil • Verapamil, a synthetic papaverine derivative, is one of several drugs that, although heterogeneous in structure, block slow calcium channel in cardiac muscle. Nifedipine exerts minimal electrophysiologic effects at clinical doses, while diltiazem has electrophysiologic actions similar to verapamil. These include reduction in the plateau height of the action potential due to blockade of the slow inward current and suppression of calcium-dependent slow responses, early and late afterdepolarizations, and activity in the sinus and atrioventricular nodes, which are calcium-dependent. The blocking effects of verapamil are more apparent at faster stimulation rates (use-dependency) and in depolarized fibers (voltage-dependency). Clinically, verapamil can slow spontaneous sinus rates slightly and prolong AV nodal conduction time and refractoriness. Because it interferes with excitation-contraction coupling, verapamil inhibits vascular smooth muscle contraction and causes vasodilation in coronary and other peripheral vascular beds. This afterload reduction tends to reduce verapamil's direct negative inotropic actions with resultant reflex sympathetic effects. After single oral doses of verapamil, measurable prolongation of AV nodal conduction time occurs in 30 mins and lasts 4 to 6 hrs. After IV administration, AV nodal conduction delay occurs within 1 to 2 mins. Elimination half-life is 3 to 7 hrs with up to 70% drug excretion by the kidneys. The most commonly used intravenous dose is 10 mg infused over 1 to 2 mins while cardiac rhythm and blood pressure are monitored. A second injection of equal dose may be given 30 mins later.

Intravenous verapamil[24] or diltiazem[25] are the drugs of choice after adenosine for terminating sustained sinus nodal reentry, AV nodal reentry, or reciprocating tachycardias associated with Wolff-Parkinson-White syndrome when one of the reentrant pathways is the AV node. Verapamil should be definitely tried before attempting cardioversion by digitalis administration, pacing, electrical direct current cardioversion or acute blood pressure elevation with vasopressors. Verapamil and diltiazem terminate 60% to more than 90% of episodes of paroxysmal supraventricular tachycardias within several minutes. Both drugs decrease the ventricular response over the AV node during atrial flutter and fibrillation, converting a small number of episodes to sinus rhythm, particularly those of recent onset. In patients with atrial fibrillation associated with Wolff-Parkinson-White syndrome, IV verapamil can accelerate the ventricular response and is therefore contraindicated. In fact, it is preferable to avoid administering IV verapamil to any patient with a wide QRS complex tachycardia. Orally, verapamil can prevent recurrences of AV nodal reentrant and AV reciprocating tachycardias associated with Wolff-Parkinson-White syndrome, as well as help maintain a decreased ventricular response during atrial flutter or atrial fibrillation in patients without an accessory pathway. Its effectiveness appears to be enhanced when given concomitantly with digitalis or propranolol. Verapamil generally is not effective in treating patients with recurrent ventricular tachyarrhythmias, although it may suppress some forms of ventricular tachycardia. Adverse effects include hypotension, bradycardia, AV block and asystole, along with worsening of congestive heart failure, particularly in patients with hemodynamic dysfunction.

Others

Adenosine • Adenosine is an endogenous nucleoside present throughout the body that has recently been approved by the FDA to treat patients with supraventricular tachycardias. It interacts with α_1-receptors present on the extracellular surface of cardiac cells, activating potassium channels in a fashion similar to that produced by acetylcholine. The increase in potassium conductance shortens atrial action potential duration, hyperpolarizes the membrane potential, and decreases atrial contractility. Similar changes occur in the sinus and AV nodes, so that sinus bradycardia and AV block result.[26] Reflex-mediated sinus tachycardia or improved AV nodal conduction can follow adenosine administration. After rapid intravenous administration, elimination half-life is 1 to 6 secs, with most effects produced during the first pass through the circulation.[27] Methyl-xanthines are competitive antagonists and a therapeutic concentration of theophylline totally blocks the exogenous adenosine effect. To terminate a tachycardia, a bolus of adenosine is injected rapidly into a central vein (if possible) at doses of 6 to 12 mg. Adenosine is probably the drug of first choice to acutely terminate a supraventricular tachycardia, such as AV nodal or AV reentry. It produces transient AV nodal block in patients with atrial flutter, atrial fibrillation and some types of atrial tachycardia, facilitating the diagnosis. Adenosine can help differentiate the mechanisms of wide QRS tachycardia since it terminates many supraventricular tachycardias with aberrancy or reveals the underlying atrial mechanism. Furthermore, the agent does not block conduction over the accessory pathway or terminate most ventricular tachycardias. Transient side effects occur in almost 40% of patients and most commonly include transient flushing sensations, dyspnea and chest pressure.

NONPHARMACOLOGIC THERAPY

ABLATION THERAPY

The purpose of catheter ablation therapy is to destroy myocardial tissue by delivering electrical energy in the form of a high energy direct current shock,[28] or radiofrequency energy[29] via electrodes on a catheter placed next to an area of the endocardium that is integrally related to the arrhythmia. Direct current shock delivers energy from an external cardioverter defibrillator and produces barotrauma, electrolysis, heat and flow of current to destroy tissue. Radiofrequency ablation destroys tissue by controlled heat production. These approaches can be used to create heart block for patients with atrial flutter or fibrillation in whom the arrhythmia cannot be suppressed and the ventricular rate cannot be adequately controlled pharmacologically. The therapy makes the patient pacemaker-dependent and does not eliminate other consequences of the arrhythmias, such as the possibility of emboli. It does establish a more physiologic rate with successful responses not requiring drugs in about 75% of patients and another 10% achieving arrhythmia control with drugs. About 15% of patients show no improvement.[30] Immediate complications related to the shock include ventricular tachycardia and fibrillation, pericardial tamponade and transient hypotension. In-hospital mortality rate related to DC shock ablation is 5.6% with a late sudden death rate of 1.8%.[31]

Conduction in the AV node can be modified by careful titration of the radiofrequency energy dose and careful positioning of the ablation catheter. This can result in selective ablation of conduction over the slow or fast pathway involved in AV nodal reentry with preservation of intact AV nodal conduction. Successful elimination of AV nodal reentrant tachycardia occurs in 90% or more of patients with radiofrequency ablation, but the chance of creating complete heart block is 2% to 5%. Similarly, after positioning the catheter near the accessory pathway in patients with the Wolff-Parkinson-White syndrome, one can ablate accessory pathways using DC energy as well as radiofrequency ablation. Success rates and risks are comparable to radiofrequency ablation in AV nodal reentry.

Successful ventricular tachycardia therapy by catheter ablation occurs in about 25% of patients with coronary disease, with total elimination of ventricular tachycardia without the need for antiarrhythmic drugs, and in about 25% with tachycardia suppressed by previously ineffective drugs.[32,33] Procedure-related mortality is 7%. Higher success rates with virtually no mortality occur in patients who have ventricular tachycardia and no structural heart disease.

Chemical ablation with alcohol or phenol of an area of myocardium involved in a tachycardia was first demonstrated in animals[34] and subsequently in patients with ventricular[35] and atrial tachycardias.[36] Angioplasty catheters are used to cannulate the smallest artery perfusing the site to be ablated in order to minimize the amount of myocardium exposed to the alcohol. After test injections with iced saline or lidocaine, alcohol is injected into the tachycardia-related coronary artery. In addition, alcohol has been injected into the AV nodal artery to create AV block in patients not responding to catheter ablation.[37] Excessive myocardial necrosis is the major complication and alcohol ablation should only be considered when other ablative approaches fail.[38]

SURGICAL THERAPY

The objectives of a surgical approach to treating a tachycardia are to excise, isolate or interrupt heart tissue that is critical for the initiation, maintenace or propagation of the tachycardia, while preserving or even improving myocardial function. In addition to a direct surgical approach to correcting an arrhythmia, indirect benefits can be achieved with aneurysmectomy, coronary artery bypass grafting and relief of valvular abnormalities that improve hemodynamics and myocardial blood flow. Cardiac sympathectomy alters adrenergic influences to the heart and has been effective in some patients, particularly those who have recurrent ventricular tachycardia with a long QT syndrome.

Supraventricular Tachycardias

Patients with supraventricular tachycardias are considered surgical candidates if they have symptomatic drug-resistant recurrent tachycardias for which a surgical procedure exists that offers a high probability of success, minimal morbidity and virtually no mortality, and for whom alternative therapies are less desirable or have been unsuccessful. Such patients include those with atrial tachycardias confined to relatively localized areas in the atrium, those with preexcitation syndrome or one of its variants, and those with AV nodal reentry. Electrical or alcohol ablation of AV conduction has virtually replaced open heart surgery as a means of producing AV block in patients without bypass tracts who have uncontrollably rapid ventricular rates during a supraventricular tachycardia, such as atrial flutter or atrial fibrillation. The extremely high success rates of radiofrequency catheter ablation[39,40] has obviated the need for arrhythmia surgery in all but the minority of patients with supraventricular tachycardias. Selected patients with symptomatic drug resistant atrial flutter and atrial fibrillation can be surgical candidates on occasion.

Before surgery, a thorough electrophysiologic evaluation is mandatory to determine the nature of the tachycardia and ascertain areas of the myocardium involved in the arrhythmia. While a more accurate intraoperative evaluation, including mapping, refines the preoperative study, the latter is essential prior to undertaking surgery. For patients with

Wolff-Parkinson-White syndrome, an open heart procedure using hypothermic cardioplegic arrest involves an atriotomy with an endocardial incision above the anulus extended to the AV groove fat pad to interrupt accessory pathways[41] (Figure 3.9). The closed heart technique involves an epicardial dissection extended to the AV groove which is then frozen with the cryoprobe.[42] An atriotomy is required for right anteroseptal pathways, but not for those in the posteroseptal or lateral positions. Normothermic cardiopulmonary bypass is used for anteroseptal pathways and when hypotension occurs during the other dissections. Epicardial and endocardial approaches both achieve close to 100% success with almost no mortality.

The surgical approaches for patients with AV nodal reentry involve either a surgical dissection that isolates the AV node[43] and/or eliminates conduction over the fast or slow pathway,[44] or a cryothermic method that freezes the myocardium entering the AV node.[45] Surgical success exceeds 90% with virtually no mortality. Recurrence rates and heart block are each in the range of 5% to 10%.

Less experience has been acquired with surgical treatment of other supraventricular tachycardias, such as atrial flutter and atrial fibrillation.[46] Atrial isolation procedures, discrete incisions and a complex dissection of the atrium have been used and are under investigation.[47]

Ventricular Tachycardias

In contrast to patients with supraventricular arrhythmias, candidates for surgical therapy of ventricular tachyarrhythmias often have severe left ventricular dysfunction, generally caused by coronary artery disease or cardiomyopathy. Candidates are patients with drug-resistant symptomatic recurrent ventricular tachyarrhythmias who ideally have a localized abnormality, such as scar (usually from a prior myocardial infarction) or an aneurysm with good left ventricular function (Figure 3.10). In patients with ischemic heart disease and ventricular tachycardia, the arrhythmia almost always arises in the left ventricle or on the left ventricular side of the interventricular septum.[48] Careful preoperative and intraoperative mapping techniques

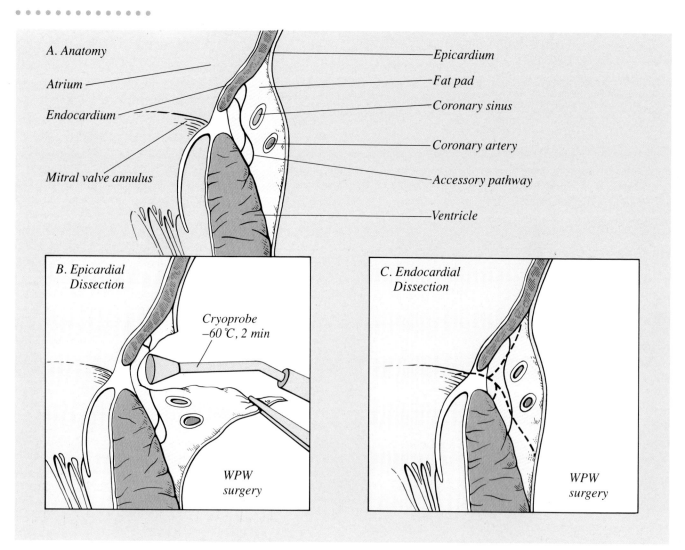

FIGURE 3.9 • Surgical approaches to interrupt an accessory pathway. The anatomy (A). The epicardial approach (B) is a closed heart technique employing cryosurgical ablation following the dissection. The endocardial approach (C) is an endocardial technique requiring open heart surgery and cold cardioplegia.

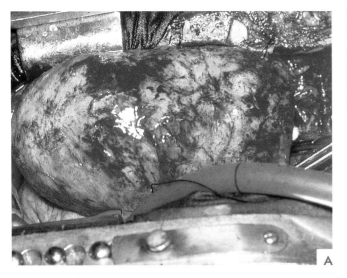

FIGURE 3.10 • Operative view in the surgical treatment of ventricular tachycardia shows a large apical anterior ventricular aneurysm (A). The aneurysm is opened to reveal the thin-walled, scarred myocardium with whitish, thickened endocardium (B). The area of arrthymogenesis is identified and excised along with the aneurysmal sac (C). (Reproduced with permission. Hurst JW, Anderson RH, Becker AE, Wilson BR: *Atlas of the Heart* New York, NY: Gower Medical Publishing;1988:11.4.)

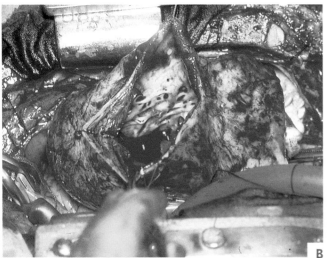

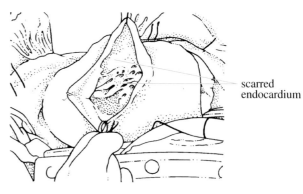

scarred
endocardium

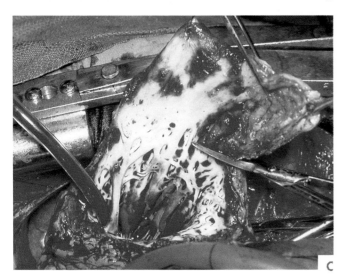

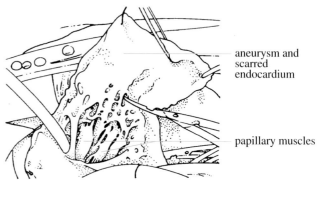

aneurysm and
scarred
endocardium

papillary muscles

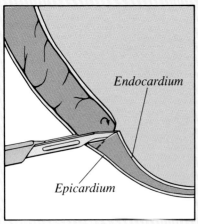

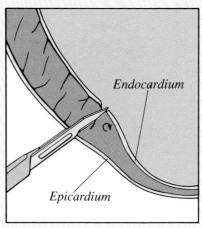

Endocardium

Epicardium

A. Aneurysm Resection

Endocardium

Epicardium

B. Endocardial Ventriculotomy

FIGURE 3.11 • Surgical approaches to treat patients with ventricular tachycardia due to coronary artery disease. Aneurysm resection (A) alone is unsuccessful because the ventricular tachycardia focus is not removed. Encircling endocardial ventriculotomy (B) creates a nontransmural incision to isolate the VT location. This approach is no longer used because it produces myocardial ischemia. The most commonly used techniques involved aneurysm resection, endocardial peeling of the arrhythmogenic site, followed by cryoablation (C,D).

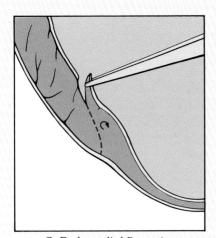

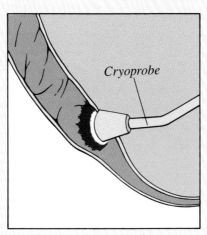

Cryoprobe

C. Endocardial Resection

D. Cryoablation/Isolation

identify an area of the myocardium related to the origin or emergence of the ventricular tachycardia. This area is then resected and/or ablated (Figure 3.11).

In patients without ischemic heart disease, tachycardias can originate in either the right or left ventricle. The type and site or origin of the ventricular tachycardia vary depending on the underlying heart disease.[49] For example, incessant ventricular tachycardia in children may be due to a cardiac tumor that can be resected. In patients who have tetralogy of Fallot, ventricular tachycardia can arise in the region of the right ventricular infundibulectomy scar. Patients with arrhythmogenic right ventricular dysplasia have a right ventricular tachycardia that sometimes can be cryoablated or isolated surgically (Figure 3.12). Patients with prolonged QT or QTU syndrome are considered for left stellate ganglionectomy.

PACEMAKERS AND ANTIARRHYTHMIC DEVICES

A pacemaker is a device that delivers electrical stimuli to the heart, from energy supplied by a battery, over leads with electrodes in contact with the myocardium. Electronic circuitry regulates the timing and characteristics of the stimuli. The power source is a battery, most commonly lithium iodine, while pacing leads are generally made of polyurethane and can be fixated in the atrium or ventricle or sewn to the epicardium or pericardium to deliver shocks. Pacemakers are used to treat patients with bradycardias in order to restore normal heart rates and normal or near normal hemodynamics and, more recently to treat patients with ventricular tachyarrhythmias. The latter devices are capable of delivering pacing stimuli, cardioversion and defibrillation pulses.[50]

Temporary pacing is indicated for patients with symptomatic bradyarrhythmias and prophylactically in patients with a high risk of developing high degree AV block, significant sinus node dysfunction or asystole, when the causal event is likely to be transient and reversible (Table 3.4). Temporary pacing can also be used to terminate tachycardias such as atrial flutter, AV nodal and AV reentry, and sustained ventricular tachycardia. Atrial and ventricular fibrillation and very rapid ventricular tachycardias cannot be treated by pacing techniques. Pacing on occasion can prevent some ventricular tachycardias such as those that are dependent on the

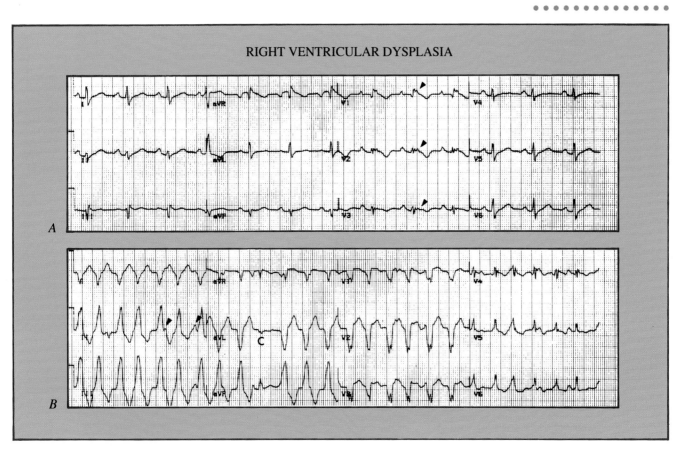

FIGURE 3.12 • 12 lead ECG from a patient with right ventricular dysplasia. Sinus rhythm (A). The arrows point to the epsilon wave that is indicative of right ventricular conduction delay seen in V_1-V_3. Ventricular tachycardia is noted arising in the right ventricle (B). Atrioventricular dissociation is present (P waves indicated by arrows) with a ventricular capture (C).

TABLE 3.4 • INDICATIONS FOR CARDIAC PACING

	Definitely indicated	Probably indicated	Probably not indicated	Defintely not indicated
Complete atrioventricular block				
Congenital (atrioventricular nodal)				
Asymptomatic			X	
Symptomatic	T,P			
Acquired (His-Purkinje)				
Asymptomatic		T,P		
Symptomatic	T,P			
Surgical (persistent)				
Asymptomatic	T	P		
Symptomatic	T,P			
Second degree atrioventricular block				
Type I (atrioventricular nodal)				
Asymptomatic			X	
Symptomatic	T,P			
Type II (His-Purkinje)				
Asymptomatic		T,P		
Symptomatic	T,P			
First degree atrioventricular block				
Atrioventricular nodal				
Asymptomatic				X
Symptomatic			X	
His-Purkinje				
Asymptomatic				X
Symptomatic			X	
Bundle branch block				
Asymptomatic				X
Symptomatic				
Normal measurement of His-Purkinje conduction time		P[5]		
Prolonged measurement of His-Purkinje conduction time	P			
Distal His block at paced atrial rates <130/min	P			
Left bundle branch block during right heart catheterization	T			

T = Temporary pacing

P = Permanent pacing

X = Pacing not indicated

[1]Site and rate of stimulation may influence success

[2]Atrial fibrillation with a rapid ventricular response may be a complication

[3]Prove efficacy with temporary pacing

[4]May accelerate ventricular tachycardia

[5]No other cause found for symptoms

[6]Replaced by radiofrequency catheter ablation

(Reproduced with permission. Zipes DP, Duffin EG: Cardiac pacemakers. In: Braunwald E, ed. *Heart Disease. A Textbook of Cardiovascular Medicine* Philadelphia, Pa: WB Saunders; 1988:718.)

TABLE 3.4 • INDICATIONS FOR CARDIAC PACING (CONT'D)

	Definitely indicated	Probably indicated	Probably not indicated	Defintely not indicated
Acute myocardial infarction				
Newly acquired bifascicular bundle branch block	T			
Preexisting bundle branch block				X
Newly acquired bundle branch block plus transient complete atrioventricular block	T	P		
Second degree atrioventricular block				
Type I (asymptomatic)				X
Type II	T	P		
Complete atrioventricular block	T	P		
Atrial fibrillation with slow ventricular response				
Asymptomatic				X
Symptomatic	T,P			
Sick sinus syndrome				
Asymptomatic			X	
Symptomatic	T,P			
Hypersensitive carotid sinus syndrome				
Asymptomatic			X	
Symptomatic	T,P			
Bradycardia-tachycardia syndrome				
Asymptomatic			X	
Symptomatic	T,P			
Bradycardia-miscellaneous				
Asymptomatic			X	
Symptomatic	T,P			
Tachycardia prevention[1]				
Associated with bradycardia	T,P			
Associated with long Q-T, torsades de pointes	T	P		
Not associated with bradycardia, long Q-T, torsades de pointes (after drug failure)		T	P[3]	
Tachycardia termination (after drug failure)[1,3]				
Atrial flutter	T,P			
Atrial fibrillation				X
Atrioventricular nodal reentry	T,P[6]			
Reciprocating tachycardia in Wolff-Parkinson-White syndrome	T,P[2,6]			
Ventricular tachycardia	T[4]	P[4]		

presence of a bradycardia or those with QT prolongation and torsades de pointes (Figure 3.13). Temporary pacing is most often achieved with a pacing lead introduced through a groin, arm, neck or chest vein but it can also be achieved transcutaneously, by pacing the chest wall.

Permanent pacing is indicated in patients with acquired AV block, AV block associated with myocardial infarction, bundle branch disturbances, sinus node dysfunction, and hypersensitive carotid sinus syndrome as indicated in the accompanying table (refer to Table 3.4).

The most common modes of pacing involve demand pacing in the atrium (AAI), demand pacing in the ventricle (VVI), or dual chamber pacing (DDD). Table 3.5 indicates the explanation for the three letter code. Most recently, rate adaptive pacemakers — designated by an R in the fourth position—have been used in patients who are unable to increase their heart rate to levels that sat-

isfy body needs. End points such as the state of physical activity, blood temperature, respiratory rate and other biologic variables are used to regulate pacemaker discharge rate.[51]

Implantable cardioverter/defibrillators (ICD) are used to treat patients with ventricular tachyarrhythmias.[52] These devices monitor the cardiac rhythm and are capable of delivering competitive pacing stimuli (Figure 3.14) as low and high energy direct current shocks over electrodes in or on the heart (Figure 3.15) to terminate ventricular tachycardia and fibrillation. Indications include the presence of recurrent symptom-producing ventricular tachycardia and ventricular fibrillation that cannot be controlled pharmacologically or with surgery, or the patient is not a candidate for those approaches. The ICDs weigh about 250 to 280 g, but are getting smaller, and usually have 3 to 4 years of effective therapeutic life, with an ability to deliver 100 to 200 shocks depending upon how the device is used by

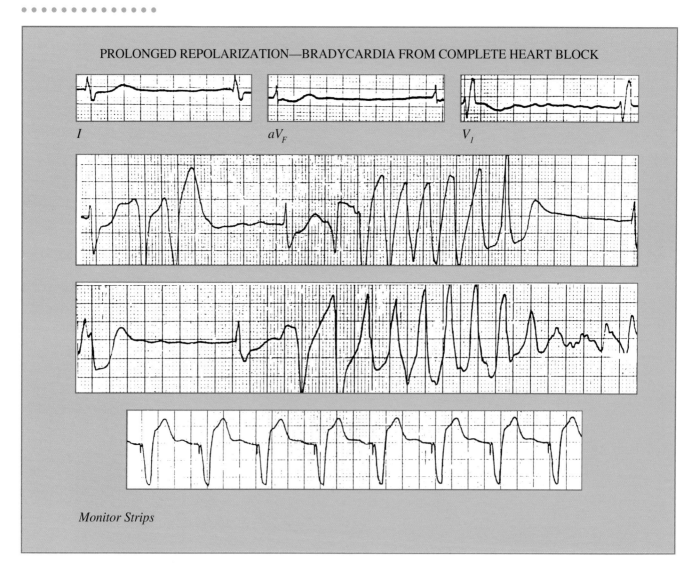

FIGURE 3.13 • Prolonged repolarization due to bradycardia from complete heart block. The patient has atrial fibrillation with complete AV block. The ventricular escape rate is about 35 beats/min. The QT interval is at least 600 msec in V₁. Runs of a polymorphic ventricular tachycardia can be seen and are completely eliminated by pacing at a rate of only 83 beats/min (bottom strip).

TABLE 3.5 • FIVE-POSITION PACEMAKER CODE

I. Chamber paced	II. Chamber sensed	III. Mode of response	IV. Program-mability	V. Tachyarrhythmia functions[1]
V = Ventricle	V = Ventricle	I = Inhibited	P = Programmable rate and/or output	B = Burst
A = Atrium	A = Atrium	T = Triggered	M = Multi-programmable	N = Normal rate competition
D = Atrium and ventricle	D = Atrium and ventricle	D = Atrial triggered and ventricular inhibited	O = None	S = Scanning
			R = Rate adaptive	C = Cardioversion/defibrillation
	0 = None	R = Reverse		E = Externally activated
S = Single chamber	S = single chamber	O = None		O = None

This table provides a shorthand description of pacemaker operation. Symbols placed in the first two positions indicate chambers in which the pacemaker functions. A symbol in the third position represents the mode of operation of the pacemaker. In the fourth position, its programmable characteristics are shown. And finally, its antitachycardia features are demonstrated in the fifth position. For example:

• If the pacing lead were inserted into the ventricle and the pulse generator were a ventricular demand inhibited unit, the chamber paced would be ventricle and the first letter in the five-position code would be V. The chamber sensed would be ventricle and therefore, the second letter in the five position code would also be V. The pacemaker's mode of response would inhibit a pacing spike when spontaneous electrical activity was sensed. Therefore, an I would be in the third position.

• If only the rate and/or output of the pulse generator could be programmed externally, P would be in the fourth position. If the pacemaker were used to treat tachycardias, the tachyarrhythmia function would be indicated in the fifth position. Pulse generators that pace or sense in both atrium and ventricle are indicated by the designation D—dual.

• If the pacemaker does not have a function in one of the classifications, an O is used.

Recently, the letter C has been suggested for the fourth position to indicate a "communicating" function—telemetry, with programmable features assumed.

An S may be used as a manufacturer's designation to label multiprogrammable single-chamber pacemakers adaptable for either atrial or ventricular use.

[1]The fourth or fifth positions are optional, as is a comma separating the third and fourth postions.

(Reproduced with permission. Zipes DP, Duffin EG: Cardiac pacemakers. In: Braunwald E, ed.: *Heart Disease. A Textbook of Cardiovascular Medicine* Philadelphia, Pa: WB Saunders; 1988:721.)

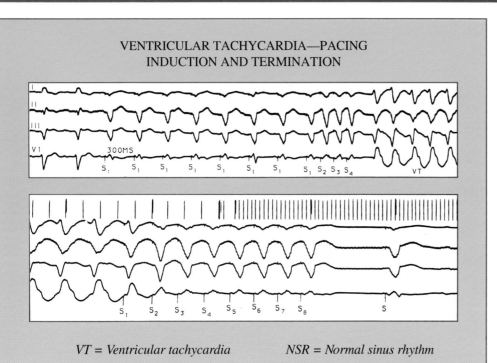

VENTRICULAR TACHYCARDIA—PACING INDUCTION AND TERMINATION

VT = Ventricular tachycardia   NSR = Normal sinus rhythm

FIGURE 3.14 • Pacing induction and termination of ventricular tachycardia (Medtronic PCD). After two sinus beats, a train of eight ventricular stimuli at a cycle length of 300 msec followed by 3 premature stimuli are delivered from the PCD triggered by the external programmer. Ventricular tachycardia (VT) results. The PCD recognizes the VT and delivers eight stimuli at coupling intervals that progressively shorten by 10 msec each. Ventricular tachycardia terminates, ventricular pacing occurs for 1 beat and sinus rhythm follows. (Reproduced with permission. Barold SS, Zipes DP: In: Braunwald E, ed. *Cardiac Pacemakers in Heart Disease: A Textbook of Cardiovascular Medicine* Philadelphia, Pa: WB Saunders;1992. In press.)

an individual patient. Devices are implanted using a thoracotomy or median sternotomy (especially if other cardiac procedures are performed) and a subxiphoid or subcostal incision. Two or three defibrillating patches are applied inside or outside the pericardium, in addition to pacemaker electrodes for rate sensing, pacing and synchronization of the shock. Nonthoracotomy approaches involving right ventricular/superior vena cava/coronary sinus electrodes plus a subcutaneous extrathoracic electrode over the cardiac apex are being investigated.

The type of electrical therapy delivered by most devices is determined by the spontaneous heart rate. For example, the ICD is capable of escalating therapy from competitive pacing to terminate a ventricular tachycardia, deliver a low energy synchronized direct current shock if pacing does not work, and to deliver a high energy asynchronous defibrillating shock should ventricular fibrillation supervene. Combined therapy with drugs and other surgical approaches are often used.

Although no randomized trials on the efficacy of the ICD have yet been published, it is generally considered that the device effectively prevents sudden death, reducing the incidence of arrhythmic death to less than 2% each year. Complications include device malfunction, inappropriate sensing, premature battery depletion and the expected complications following major chest surgery.

EVALUATION OF THE PATIENT WITH A CARDIAC ARRHYTHMIA

The initial evaluation of the patient suspected of having a cardiac arrhythmia begins by obtaining a careful history, specifically questioning the patient regarding the presence of palpitations, syncope, spells of light-headedness, chest pain or symptoms of congestive heart failure. Some patients can reproduce their feelings of palpitations, which is an awareness of the heartbeat, by tapping on their chests, knees or table tops to replicate a perceived heart beat, or may recognize a cadence tapped out by a physician. Such a maneuver may help establish the rate and rhythm of the arrhythmia, narrowing it to a par-

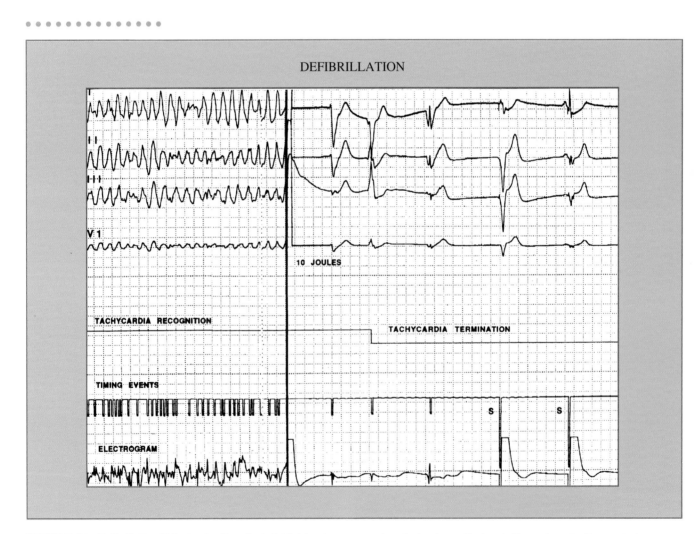

FIGURE 3.15 • Defibrillation (Telectronics Guardian). A 10 J shock delivered over patches placed on the heart terminates ventricular fibrillation. Horizontal line indicates tachycardia recognition and termination sensed by the device. Timing events indicate sensed electrical activity and pacing(s). Electrogram is telemetered from the sensing electrodes on the heart. (Reproduced with permission. Barold SS, Zipes DP: In: Braunwald E, ed. *Cardiac Pacemakers in Heart Disease. A Textbook of Cardiovascular Medicine* Philadephia, Pa: WB Saunders:1992. In press.)

ticular rate range, a regular or irregular arrhythmia, or one in which a regular rhythm is interrupted by premature beats. A rapid irregular tapping may suggest the ventricular response to atrial fibrillation, while a regular tapping may suggest tachycardia—AV nodal or AV reentrant tachycardia in a young person, or a ventricular tachycardia in an older person with coronary artery disease. Information regarding the nature of onset and termination of the rhythm disturbance is particularly important. A sinus tachycardia may begin gradually, while a pathologic tachycardia may have sudden onset. The rate of tachycardia provides important information, and the physician should demonstrate how to determine the pulse rate. Premature atrial or ventricular beats, perceived as dropped or skipped beats by the patient, are probably the most common cause of palpitations. Triggers of the tachycardia should be sought, such as emotionally upsetting events, menses, ingestion of caffeine-containing beverages, cigarette smoking, exercise, excessive alcohol intake or fatigue. A careful diet and drug history may be useful, for example, in revealing that the patient develops palpitations only after using a nasal decongestant that contains a sympathomimetic vasoconstrictor. States conducive to the genesis of arrhythmias should be considered, such as thyrotoxicosis, pericarditis, mitral valve prolapse, diuretics with hypokalemia, administration of antiarrhythmic drugs. Physical findings that can be helpful include signs indicative of AV dissociation and the characteristics of the second heart sound, which points to the presence of a right or left bundle branch block. The response to carotid sinus massage provides important diagnostic information by increasing vagal tone. Sinus tachycardia may gradually slow during carotid sinus massage, returning to the previous rate when massage is discontinued. AV nodal reentry and AV reciprocating tachycardia that involve the AV node may slow slightly, terminate abrupt-ly or not change. The ventricular response to atrial flutter, atrial fibrillation and some atrial tachycardias usually decreases. Carotid sinus massage rarely terminates a ventricular tachycardia.

The ECG remains the most important and definitive single noninvasive diagnostic test. Finding P waves is essential. If they are not clearly visible, special maneuvers may be needed. Occasionally, esophageal (Figure 3.16) or intracavitary right atrial recordings are necessary.

In addressing each arrhythmia, one should ask the following questions:

- Are P waves present?
- What are the atrial and ventricular rates?
- Are they identical?
- Are the P-P and R-R intervals regular or irregular? If irregular, is it a consistent repeating irregularity?
- Is there a P wave related to each ventricular complex?
- Does the P wave precede or follow the QRS complex?
- Is the resultant PR or RP interval constant?
- Are all P waves and QRS complexes identical and normal in contour?
- Are P, PR, QRS and QT durations normal?
- Considering the clinical setting, what is the significance of the arrhythmia? Should it be treated and if so, how?

GENERAL APPROACHES TO THERAPY

The therapeutic approach to a patient with a cardiac arrhythmia begins with an accurate electrocardiographic interpretation of the arrhythmia and continues with determination of the cause

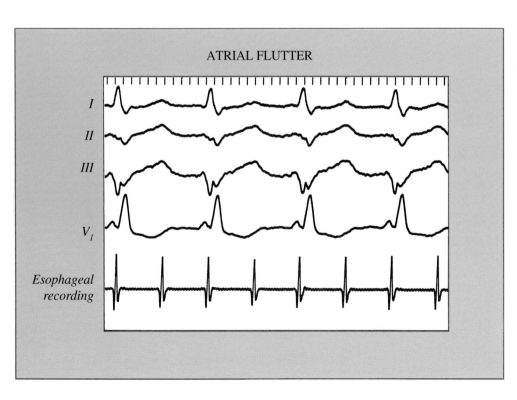

ATRIAL FLUTTER

I

II

III

V₁

Esophageal recording

FIGURE 3.16 • Atrial flutter. During a wide QRS tachycardia with a right bundle branch block contour, no atrial activity was apparent on the scalar ECG. The tachycardia can be diagnosed as atrial flutter with 2:1 conduction from the esophageal recording of atrial activity. The finding of two P waves for each QRS complex excludes the possibility of ventricular tachycardia. (Reproduced with permission. Miles WM, Zipes DP: Electrophysiology of wide QRS tachycardia. *Prog Cardiol* 1988;1/2:77.)

of the arrhythmia, if possible, the nature of the underlying heart disease, if any, and the consequences of the arrhythmia in the individual patient. Most arrhythmias are treated in the context of the entire clinical situation.

When a patient develops a tachyarrhythmia, slowing the ventricular rate is the initial and often the most important therapeutic maneuver. Therapy may differ radically for the same arrhythmia in two different patients because the consequences of the tachycardia in individual patients differs. In a patient without structural heart disease, a ventricular tachycardia may only produce palpitations or fatigue, while in another patient it may precipitate cardiogenic shock.

The etiology of the arrhythmia may influence therapy markedly. Electrolyte imbalance, acidosis or alkylosis, hypoxemia and many drugs can produce rhythm disturbances. Their identification and treatment can abolish or prevent these arrhythmias. Because heart failure can cause arrhythmias, treatment of this condition with digitalis, diuretics or vasodilators can suppress some arrhythmias that accompany cardiac decompensation. Arrhythmias secondary to hypotension may respond to leg elevation or vasopressor therapy. Precipitating or contributing disease states, such as infection, hypokalemia and thyroid disorders should be sought and treated. It is important to remember that antiarrhythmia drugs can cause cardiac arrhythmias and, therefore, one must be certain that the risks of not treating the arrhythmia outweigh the risks of therapy.

INDIVIDUAL CARDIAC ARRHYTHMIAS[53]

SINUS NODAL DISTURBANCES

Normal sinus rhythm is arbitrarily limited to impulse formation originating in the sinus node at rates between 60 and 100 beats/min. Infants and children generally have faster rates than adults do, both at rest and during exercise. The PR interval exceeds 120 msec and may vary slightly with respiration.

Sinus tachycardia in the adult is present when the sinus rate is between 100 and 180 beats/min, but may be higher with extreme exertion (Figure 3.17). Sinus tachycardia generally has a gradual onset and termination. PP intervals are usually regular, but they may vary slightly. Carotid sinus massage and Valsalva or other vagal maneuvers may gradually slow a sinus tachycardia which then accelerates to its previous rate upon cessation of enhanced vagal tone. More rapid sinus rates may fail to slow in response to a vagal maneuver. Sinus tachycardia is the normal reaction to a variety of physiologic or pathophysiologic stresses, such as fever, hypotension, thyrotoxicosis, anemia, anxiety, exertion, pulmonary emboli, myocardial ischemia, congestive heart failure or shock. Drugs, such as catecholamines, atropine, alcohol, nicotine, caffeine or a variety of inflammatory states, can produce sinus tachycardia. Treatment is generally directed toward the cause. Elimination of stimulants, treatment of congestive heart failure, thyrotoxicosis or anemia when indicated is the usual approach.

Sinus bradycardia exists in the adult when the sinus node discharges at a rate of less than 60 beats/min (Figure 3.18). Sinus bradycardia can result from excessive vagal or decreased sympathetic tone as well as from anatomical changes in the sinus node. It is frequently present in healthy young adults, particularly in well trained athletes. During sleep, the normal heart rate may fall to 35 to 40 beats/min. Drugs such as lithium, amiodarone, ß-adrenoceptor antagonists, calcium channel blockers or clonidine can produce sinus bradycardia. Sinus bradycardia can occur in 10% to 15% of patients with acute myocardial infarction—particularly postinferior wall infarction—and is generally associated with a more favorable outcome than is the presence of sinus tachycardia. Bradycardia after resuscitation from cardiac arrest is associated with a poor prognosis.

Treatment of sinus bradycardia is usually not necessary unless the patient is symptomatic. If therapy is required, IV atropine, 0.5 mg, as an initial dose (repeated if necessary) or, in the absence of myocardial ischemia, IV isoproterenol, 1 to 2

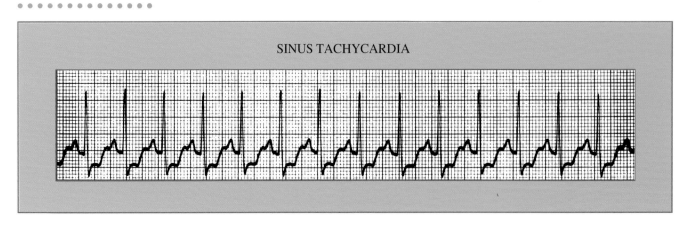

FIGURE 3.17 • Sinus tachycardia. Note the significant ST segment depression indicative of myocardial ischemia. Sinus tachycardia is present at a rate of 125 beats/min.

μ/min, is usually effective. Ephedrine, hydralazine, or theophylline may be used for managing some patients with symptomatic sinus bradycardia. Occasionally, pacemaker implantation is necessary, preferably using atrial pacing to preserve sequential atrial ventricular contraction. As a rule, no available drugs increase the heart rate reliably and safely over long periods without intolerable side effects.

Sinus pause or sinus arrest is recognized by a pause in the sinus rhythm during which the PP interval delimiting the pause does not equal a multiple of the basic PP interval (Figure 3.19). In contrast, sinoatrial exit block is a pause in the sinus rhythm, the duration of which is a multiple of the PP interval (Figure 3.20). Sinus pause or arrest is thought to be due to slowing or cessation of spontaneous sinus nodal automaticity, while sinoatrial exit block is thought to be due to a conduction disturbance during which an impulse within the sinus node fails to depolarize the atria. Therapy is reserved for symptomatic patients as outlined for sinus bradycardia.

HYPERSENSITIVE CAROTID SINUS SYNDROME

This condition is most frequently characterized by ventricular asystole due to the cessation of atrial activity from sinus arrest or sinoatrial exit block in response to carotid sinus massage

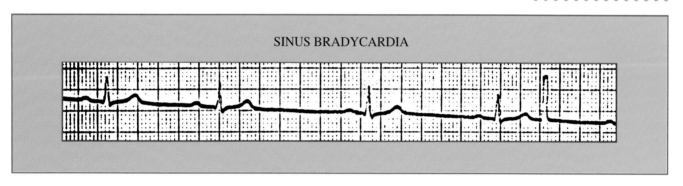

FIGURE 3.18 • Sinus bradycardia (40 to 55 minutes) is shown in this monitor lead recorded during sleep.

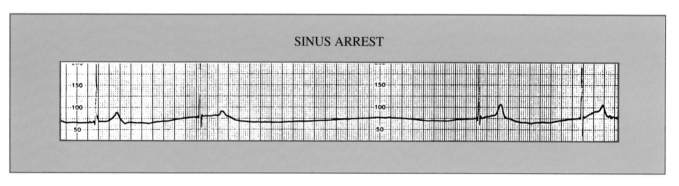

FIGURE 3.19 • Sinus arrest. A diminutive P wave can be seen in front of the first QRS complex and possibly the last QRS complex. No other clear atrial activity exists, although it is possible that P waves are buried within the changing contour of the T waves.

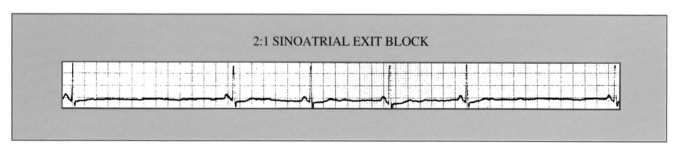

FIGURE 3.20 • 2:1 sinoatrial exit block. The interval between the first and second and last two P waves is twice the interval of the PP cycles in the midportion of the tracing, consistent with 2:1 sinoatrial exit block.

(Figure 3.21). Atrioventricular (AV) block is observed less frequently, probably in part because the absence of atrial activity due to sinus arrest precludes the manifestations of AV block. In symptomatic patients, AV junctional or ventricular escape beats generally do not occur or do so at very slow rates. Two components comprise the hypersensitive carotid sinus syndrome. The cardioinhibitory component refers to the rate change while the vasodepressor component accounts for the decrease in systolic blood pressure without a significant rate change. Hypersensitive carotid sinus reflex is most commonly associated with coronary artery disease. The mechanism is not known, but certainly relates to some sort of autonomic dysfunction causing heightened vagal tone and perhaps decreased sympathetic tone.

Atropine abolishes cardioinhibitory carotid sinus hypersensitivity. However, the majority of patients require pacemaker implantation. Because AV block may occur during periods of hypersensitivity carotid sinus reflex, some form of ventricular pacing, with or without atrial pacing, is generally required. Atropine does not prevent the decrease in systemic blood pressure in the vasodepressor form of carotid sinus hypersensitivity. Similarly, pacing may not prevent this response. Therapy with volume expanders, sympathomimetic amines and the use of support hose may be necessary. Combinations of vasodepressor and cardioinhibitory responses may occur. Vasodepressor responses may cause continued syncope after pacemaker implantation in some patients.

SICK SINUS SYNDROME

Sick sinus syndrome is the term applied to a syndrome encompassing a number of sinus nodal abnormalities that include:
- Persistent sinus bradycardia not caused by drugs and inappropriate for the physiologic circumstance.
- Sinus arrest or exit block.
- Combinations of sinus and AV conduction disturbances.
- Alternations between supraventricular tachycardia and bradycardia—for example, atrial fibrillation and sinus arrest or exit block (Figure 3.22).

Treatment depends on the basic rhythm disturbances, but almost always involves permanent pacemaker implantation to treat the bradycardia in symptomatic patients, combined with drug therapy to treat the tachycardia.

SINUS NODAL REENTRY

The sinus node can participate in a reentrant tachycardia, resulting in P waves that resemble the normal sinus P wave at rates from 80 to 200 beats/min with an average rate of 130 to 140 beats/min (Figure 3.23). The PR interval is related to the tachycardia rate, but generally the RP interval is long and the PR interval is shorter than the RP interval. AV block may occur without affecting the tachycardia. Vagal maneuvers may slow or terminate the tachycardia. Sinus nodal reentry may account for 5% to 10% of supraventricular tachycardia cases requiring therapy. Many patients do not seek medical attention because the rel-

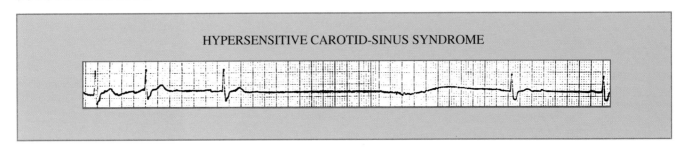

FIGURE 3.21 • Hypersensitive carotid sinus syndrome. Carotid sinus massage instituted at the beginning of the recording produces complete asystole, terminated by a junctional escape and then resumption of sinus rhythm in the last complex of the recording.

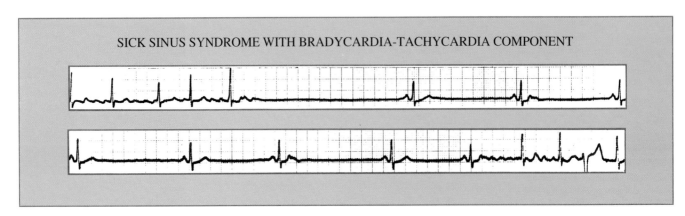

FIGURE 3.22 • Sick sinus syndrome with bradycardia-tachycardia component. Atrial fibrillation spontaneously terminates, followed by a slow sinus rhythm and nonconducted premature atrial complexes. Note the distortion of the T wave in the second complex from the end in the top strip and the third and fifth complexes in the bottom strip. The premature atrial complex in the fifth complex initiates atrial flutter/fibrillation again.

atively slow rate of the tachycardia does not produce serious symptoms. Sinus nodal reentry may be responsible for apparent "anxiety related sinus tachycardia" in some patients. Drugs such as propranolol, verapamil and digitalis may be effective.

PREMATURE COMPLEXES

Premature complexes are one of the most common causes of an irregular pulse. They may originate from any area in the heart, most frequently from the ventricles, less often from the atria and from the atrioventricular (AV) junctional area, and rarely from the sinus node. Although premature complexes arise in normal hearts, they are more often associated with structural heart disease and increase in frequency with age.

Premature Atrial Complexes

Premature atrial complexes can be recognized by a premature P wave with a PR interval exceeding 120 msec and a contour that differs from the normal sinus P wave (Figures 3.24, 3.25). When premature atrial complexes occur early in the cardiac cycle, the premature P waves can be difficult to discern because

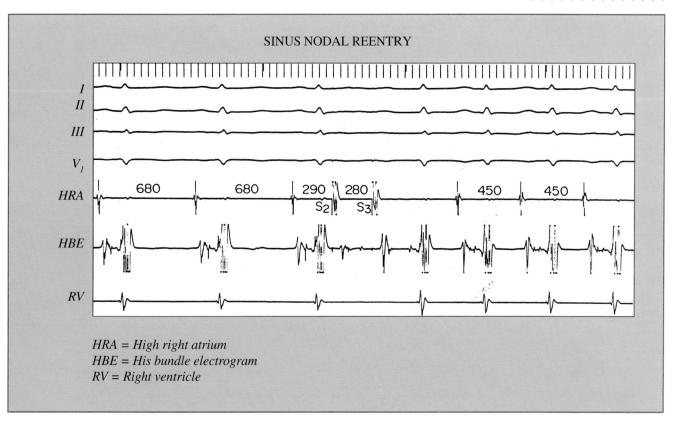

FIGURE 3.23 • Sinus nodal reentry. Following three spontaneous sinus beats at cycle lengths of 680 msec, two premature stimuli are delivered to the atria (S_2-S_3) at coupling intervals of 290 and 280 msec, respectively. They initiate a supraventricular tachycardia—cycle length 450 msec—that produces a high-low atrial activation sequence similar to that in sinus rhythm. Atrial activity begins in the high right atrium (HRA), proceeding to the low right atrium recorded in the His bundle electrogram (HBE). P wave contour in the surface leads is indistinct, but is similar during sinus nodal reentry and sinus rhythm.

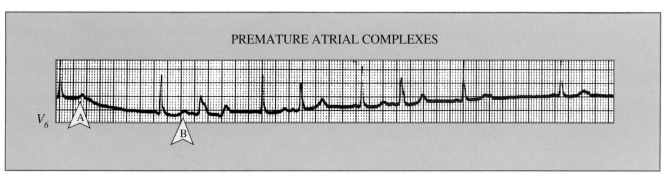

FIGURE 3.24 • Premature atrial complexes. In this V_6 recording, premature atrial complexes that are nonconducted (A) and conducted with a functional left bundle branch block (B) are apparent. Note that functional right bundle branch block aberrancy is far more common than is functional left bundle branch block aberrancy.

they are superimposed on the preceding T wave. Often such a premature atrial complex conducts with a prolonged PR interval or blocks in the AV junction before reaching the ventricle and the rhythm can be misinterpreted as a sinus pause or a sinus exit block. As a general rule, the RP interval is inversely related to the PR interval. Thus, a short RP interval produced by an early premature atrial complex occurring close to the preceding QRS complex is followed by a long PR interval. Some premature atrial complexes can conduct aberrantly in the ventricle, producing either functional right or functional left bundle branch block.

Premature atrial complexes can occur in a variety of situations, such as during infection, myocardial ischemia or heart failure or they can be provoked by a variety of medications or by tobacco, alcohol, or caffeine. Premature atrial complexes can precipitate supraventricular tachycardia and rarely, ventricular tachycardia. Treatment generally is not necessary. In symptomatic patients or when the premature atrial complexes precipitate tachycardias, treatment with digitalis, propranolol or verapamil can be tried. If these drugs are unsuccessful, trials with Class 1A antiarrhythmic drugs can sometimes be worthwhile. Rarely, amiodarone can be used.

ATRIAL FLUTTER

During atrial flutter, the ECG reveals identically occurring regular sawtooth flutter waves, generally at a rate of 250 to 350 beats/min, often best visualized as negative deflections in leads II, III, aV_F or V_1 (Figure 3.26). Ordinarily, the atrial rate is about 300 beats/min and, in untreated patients, the ventricular rate is 150 beats/min. In children, in patients with the Wolff-Parkinson-White syndrome, and occasionally in patients with hyperthyroidism or in those who have atrioventricular (AV) nodes that conduct rapidly, atrial flutter can conduct to the ventricle in a 1:1 fashion, producing a ventricular rate of 300 beats/min. If the AV conduction ratio remains constant, the ventricular rhythm will be regular. If the ratio of conducted beats varies, usually with resultant Wenckebach AV block, the ventricular rhythm will be irregular. Intermittent atrial flutter can occur in patients without structural heart disease while chronic atrial flutter is usually associated with underlying heart disease such as rheumatic or ischemic changes or cardiomyopathy. Atrial dilation from septal defects, pulmonary, mitral or tricuspid valve stenosis or regurgitation, or chronic ventricular failure can produce atrial flutter. Atrial flutter tends to be unstable, reverting to sinus rhythm or atrial fibrillation. Less commonly, the atria may continue to flutter for months or years. Carotid sinus massage generally decreases the ventricular response in multiples, returning in reverse to the former ventricular rate at the termination of carotid massage. Exercise, by enhancing AV nodal conduction, can increase the ventricular response. In flutter, the atria contract can account in part for a lower incidence of systemic emboli than during atrial fibrillation.

Treatment depends upon the clinical situation. In the symptomatic patient, synchronous direct current (DC) cardiover-

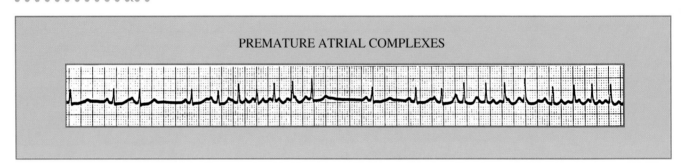

FIGURE 3.25 • Premature atrial complexes precipitate short runs of atrial flutter/fibrillation.

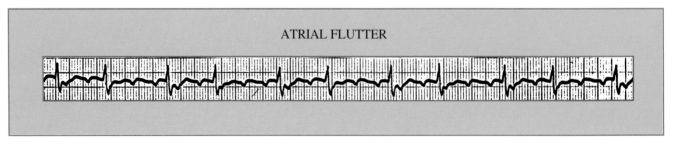

FIGURE 3.26 • Atrial flutter. Flutter waves, normally at a rate of 300 beats/min, occur at a rate of 190 beats/min, having been slowed by quinidine administration. AV conduction varies from 2:1 to 3:1.

sion is commonly the initial treatment of choice with restoration of sinus rhythm usually following low energy—less than 50 J-shocks. If the patient cannot be electrically cardioverted or if electrical cardioversion is contraindicated, for example after administering large amounts of digitalis, rapid atrial pacing can effectively terminate atrial flutter, producing sinus rhythm or atrial fibrillation with a slowing of the ventricular rate and clinical improvement.

If the atrial flutter cannot be terminated, then measures to slow the ventricular response are instituted. A short acting digitalis preparation, such as digoxin can be given intravenously. Frequently, atrial fibrillation develops after digitalis administration and may revert to normal sinus rhythm on withdrawal of digitalis. Verapamil given as an initial 5 to 10 mg IV bolus, followed by a constant infusion rate of 5 µg/kg to slow the ventricular response may be tried. Diltiazem can also be effective. Esmolol, a short acting ß-adrenoceptor block, can be tried acutely. Propranolol effectively diminishes the ventricular response to atrial flutter and can be combined with digitalis in patients whose rate is not decreased after digitalis alone.

If the atrial flutter persists, quinidine sulfate 200 to 400 mg orally every 6 hrs can restore sinus rhythm. Similarly, disopyramide, procainamide, or amiodarone can be tried empirically. If conversion to sinus rhythm results, maintenance doses of the successful drug are continued. It is important to remember that drugs such as quinidine can slow the atrial flutter to rates of 200/min, which can result in 1:1 conduction if prior digitalis, propranolol or verapamil has not been administered. Class 1 drug therapy should be discontinued if the atrial flutter remains. The patient should be treated solely with drugs to slow the ventricular response. Preventing occurrences of atrial flutter may be difficult, but should be approached as outlined for averting recurrences of AV nodal reentry. If occurrences cannot be prevented, therapy is directed toward controlling the ventricular rate when the flutter does occur, as noted earlier. Electrical ablation of the His bundle to produce complete block, and implantation of a rate adaptive pacemaker can be successful. Chronic anticoagulation is not necessary for most patients with atrial flutter in the absence of history of embolic events, mitral or severe congestive heart failure.

ATRIAL FIBRILLATION

Atrial fibrillation is characterized by totally disorganized atrial depolarizations without effective atrial contraction. Electrocardiographically, atrial fibrillation presents as small irregular baseline undulations of variable amplitude and morphology called F waves at a rate of 350 to 650 beats/min (Figure 3.27). The ventricular response is grossly irregular ("irregularly irregular") and, in the untreated patient with normal AV conduction, is usually between 100 and 160 beats/min. In patients with Wolff-Parkinson-White syndrome, the ventricular rate during atrial fibrillation at times may exceed 300 beats/min and lead to ventricular fibrillation. Atrial fibrillation should be suspected when the ECG shows supraventricular complexes at an irregular rhythm and no obvious P waves. When the ventricular rate is very rapid or slow, it may appear to be more regular. It is easier to slow the ventricular rate with drugs, such as digitalis, propranolol and verapamil during atrial fibrillation than during atrial flutter.

Atrial fibrillation may be chronic or intermittent, the former almost always associated with underlying heart disease such as rheumatic valvular heart disease, atrial septal defect, cardiomyopathy, pulmonary emboli, coronary heart disease or as a complication of cardiovascular surgery. Hypertensive cardiovascular disease is the most common antecedent disease, largely because of its frequency in the general population. Occult or manifest thyrotoxicosis should always be considered in a patient with atrial fibrillation of recent onset. Mortality is unchanged in patients who have paroxysmal atrial fibrillation with no other identified cardiovascular impairment. However, paroxysmal atrial fibrillation associated with mitral stenosis incurs a significantly increased mortality.[54] The development of chronic atrial fibrillation is associated with a doubling of overall mortality and of mortality from cardiovascular disease.[55]

Patients with chronic atrial fibrillation are at increased risk of embolic stroke. In the absence of rheumatic heart disease, atrial fibrillation is associated with a more than fivefold increase in the incidence of stroke and an even greater increase in patients with mitral valvular heart disease.[56] Subjects with atrial fibrillation in the absence of recognized structural heart disease ("lone" atrial fibrillation) have an increased

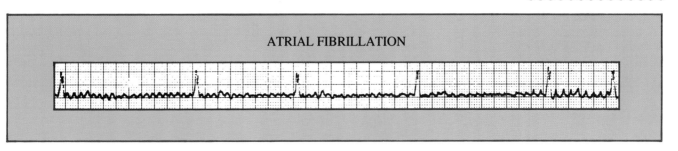

FIGURE 3.27 • Atrial fibrillation. Undulations in the baseline, called F waves, characterize atrial fibrillation in this monitor lead.

risk of stroke, according to the Framingham Heart Study, but not according to a Mayo Clinic study[57] (Figure 3.28).

When one begins treating a patient with atrial fibrillation, it is important to search for the underlying cause, such as thyrotoxicosis, mitral stenosis, pulmonary emboli or pericarditis and to treat it accordingly. The patient's clinical status determines initial therapy, the objective being to slow the ventricular rate and restore atrial systole. If the sudden onset of atrial fibrillation with a rapid ventricular rate results in acute cardiovascular decompensation, electrical cardioversion is the treatment of choice. In the absence of decompensation, the patient can be treated with digitalis and/or a ß-blocker or calcium channel blocker to maintain a resting apical rate of 60 to 80 beats/min that does not exceed 100 beats/min after slight exertion. The speed, route, dosage and type of drug preparation administered is determined by the clinical status of the patient. The ventricular rate must be slowed by digitalis and/or a calcium channel or ß-blocking drug prior to giving quinidine or other Class IA or IC drugs, to prevent an increase in the ventricular rate when the latter drugs are administered. Quinidine, given with digitalis, is often necessary to convert to sinus rhythm. Prior to electrical cardioversion, maintenance doses of quinidine sulfate in the range of 800 to 1,600 mg/d should be administered for a few days. During this time, normal sinus rhythm will resume in 10% to 15% of patients. Electrical cardioversion establishes normal sinus rhythm in over 90% of patients, but sinus rhythm remains for 12 months in only 30% to 50%. Patients treated with quinidine may have an increased risk of sudden death due to possible proarrhythmic actions of quinidine[58] (Figures 3.29, 3.30). Patients with atrial fibrillation

of less than one year's duration and those with left atrial dimensions less than 5.0 cm have a greater chance of maintaining sinus rhythm after cardioversion. Procainamide or disopyramide can be tried in place of quinidine. Amiodarone is effective in preventing recurrences of atrial fibrillation, as is flecainide. Rapid atrial pacing will not terminate atrial fibrillation.

The role of anticoagulation prior to cardioversion is controversial because of imperfect studies. Anticoagulation before drug or electrical cardioversion is ordinarily indicated in patients with a high risk of emboli such as those with mitral stenosis, atrial fibrillation of recent onset, recent or recurrent emboli, the presence of a prosthetic mitral valve, mitral stenosis, low output states and/or cardiomegaly. Some recommend two weeks of anticoagulation before cardioversion of atrial fibrillation present for about one week if no contraindications exist, and to continue anticoagulation for two additional weeks after cardioversion. The incidence of systemic embolization during conversion into normal sinus rhythm is 1% to 2%.[59]

Many elderly patients tolerate atrial fibrillation well without therapy because the ventricular rate is slow as a result of concomitant AV nodal disease. These patients often have associated sick sinus syndrome so development of atrial fibrillation represents a cure of sorts. Such patients may demonstrate supraventricular and ventricular arrhythmias or asystole after cardioversion, hence the likelihood of establishing or maintaining sinus rhythm should be weighed against the risks of cardioversion or other forms of therapy. For patients with nonvalvular chronic atrial fibrillation, aspirin 325 mg once or twice daily or anticoagulation with warfarin, maintaining the pro-

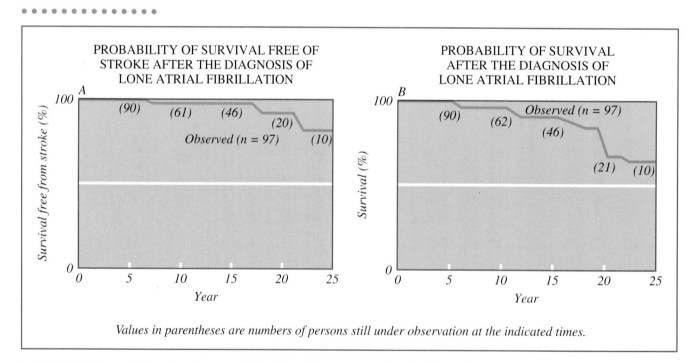

FIGURE 3.28 • The probability of survival free of stroke (A) and the probability of survival (B) after the diagnosis of lone atrial fibrillation.

(Reproduced with permission. Kopecky SL, Gersh BJ, McGoon MD, et al: *N Engl J Med* 1987;317:669.)

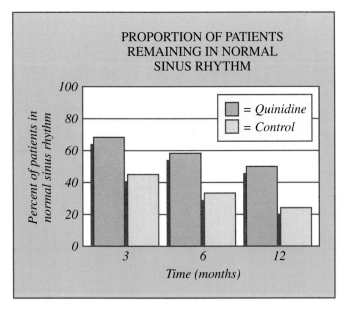

FIGURE 3.29 • Proportion of patients remaining in normal sinus rhythm at 3, 6, and 12 months after cardioversion was greater at all time intervals in the quinidine-treated group compared with the control group. (Reproduced with permission. Coplan SE, Antman EM, Beslin JA, et al: *Circulation* 1990;82:1106.)

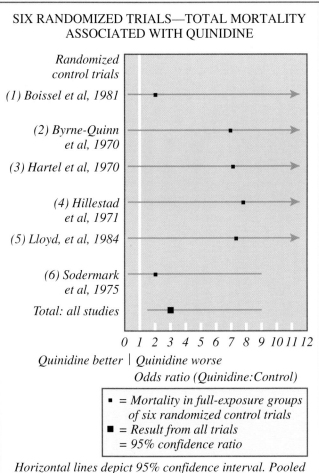

FIGURE 3.30 • Odds ratios (quinidine:control) for total mortality in full exposure groups of six randomized controlled trials. Pooled odds ratio and its 95% confidence interval fall to the right of the vertical line, which indicates a significant increase in total mortality in the quinidine-treated group compared to controls. (Reproduced with permission. Coplan SE, Antman EM, Beslin JA, et al: *Circulation* 1990;82:1106.)

References (1) Boissel JP, Wolf E, Gillet J, et al: Controlled trial of a long-acting quinidine for maintenance of sinus rhythm after conversion of sustained atrial fibrillation. *Eur Heart J* 1981;2:49. (2) Byrne-Quinn E, Wing AJ: Maintenance of sinus rhythm after DC reversion of atrial fibrillation: A Double-blind controlled trial of quinidine bisulphate. *Br Heart J* 1970;32:370. (3) Hartel G, Vouhija A, Konttinen A, et al: Value of quinidine in maintenance of sinus rhythm after electric conversion of atrial fibrillation. *Br Heart J* 1970;32:57. (4) Hillestad L, Bjerkelund C, Dale J, et al: Quinidine in maintenance of sinus rhythm after electroconversion of chronic atrial fibrillation: A controlled clinical study. *Br Heart J* 1971;33:518. (5) Lloyd EA, Gersh BJ, Forman R: The efficacy of quinidine and disopyramide in the maintenance of sinus rhythm after electroconversion from atrial fibrillation. *S Afr Med J* 1984;65:367. (6) Sodermark T, Jonsson B, Olsson A, et al: Effect of quinidine on maintaining sinus rhythm after conversion of atrial fibrillation or flutter: A multicentre study from Stockholm. *Br Heart J* 1975;37:486.

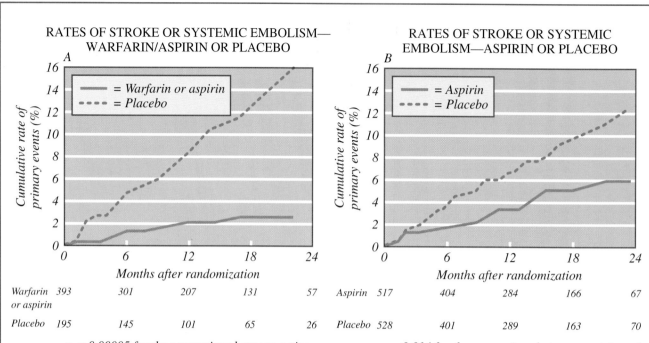

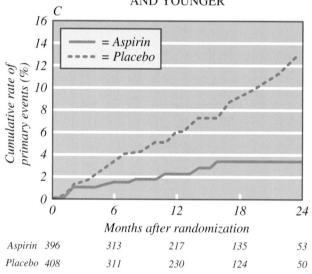

RATES OF STROKE OR SYSTEMIC EMBOLISM—
WARFARIN/ASPIRIN OR PLACEBO

A

= Warfarin or aspirin
= Placebo

Cumulative rate of primary events (%)

Months after randomization

| Warfarin or aspirin | 393 | 301 | 207 | 131 | 57 |
| Placebo | 195 | 145 | 101 | 65 | 26 |

p < 0.00005 for the comparison between active therapy and placebo (risk reduction=81%; 95% confidence interval=56 to 91). The value below the months indicate the number of patients free of events in each group.

RATES OF STROKE OR SYSTEMIC EMBOLISM—ASPIRIN OR PLACEBO

B

= Aspirin
= Placebo

Cumulative rate of primary events (%)

Months after randomization

| Aspirin | 517 | 404 | 284 | 166 | 67 |
| Placebo | 528 | 401 | 289 | 163 | 70 |

p = 0.014 for the comparison between aspirin and placebo (risk reduction=49%; 95% confidence interval=15 to 69). The values below the months indicate the number of patients free of events in each group.

RATES OF STROKE OR SYSTEMIC EMBOLISM—PATIENTS 75 YEARS AND YOUNGER

C

= Aspirin
= Placebo

Cumulative rate of primary events (%)

Months after randomization

| Aspirin | 396 | 313 | 217 | 135 | 53 |
| Placebo | 408 | 311 | 230 | 124 | 50 |

p = 0.0042 for the comparison between aspirin and placebo (risk reduction=65%; 95% confidence interval=34 to 81). The values below the months indicate the number of patients free of events in each group.

FIGURE 3.31 • Rates of stroke or systemic embolism (primary events) in patients given active therapy (warfarin or aspirin) or placebo in Group 1 (A). Rates of stroke or systemic embolism in patients given aspirin or placebo in Groups 1 and 2 combined (B). Rates of stroke or systemic embolism in patients 75 years of age and younger given as-pirin or placebo in Groups 1 and 2 combined (C). The values below the months indicate the number of patients free of events in each group. (Reproduced with permission. Preliminary report of the stroke prevention in atrial fibrillation study. *N Engl J Med* 1990;322:863.)

thrombin time 1.3 to 1.5 more than normal, is probably indicated, if no contraindications exist[60] (Figure 3.31).

ATRIAL TACHYCARDIA

Atrial tachycardia is characterized electrocardiographically by atrial rates of about 150 to 200 beats/min and with a P wave contour different from the sinus P wave. Conduction to the ventricle can be 1:1 or AV nodal block may be present, generally of the Wenckebach type (Figure 3.32). The atrial rate may be irregular and characteristic isoelectric intervals exist between P waves. Common causes include coronary artery disease, cor pulmonale, or digitalis intoxication. AV nodal block can exist without affecting the tachycardia. Vagal maneuvers generally do not terminate the tachycardia even though they may produce AV nodal block or enhance preexisting block. Usually the PR interval is shorter than the RP interval.

Treatment of atrial tachycardia in a patient not receiving dig-

italis is similar to treating other atrial tachyarrhythmias. Depending on the clinical situation, digitalis or a ß-blocker or calcium channel blocker can be administered to slow the ventricular rate. If the atrial tachycardia persists, quinidine, disopyramide, procainamide or other antiarrhythmic drugs can be added. If atrial tachycardia occurs in a patient receiving digitalis, the latter should be assumed initially to be responsible for the arrhythmia. Therapy includes cessation of digitalis, administration of potassium chloride orally or intravenously if serum potassium concentration is low or not abnormally elevated, or use of a drug such as lidocaine, propranolol or phenytoin. Often, the ventricular response is not excessively fast and simply withholding digitalis suffices.

Chaotic (sometimes called multifocal) atrial tachycardia is characterized by atrial rates of 100 to 130 beats/min with marked variation in P wave morphology and totally irregular PP intervals[61] (Figure 3.33). Generally, at least three P wave con-

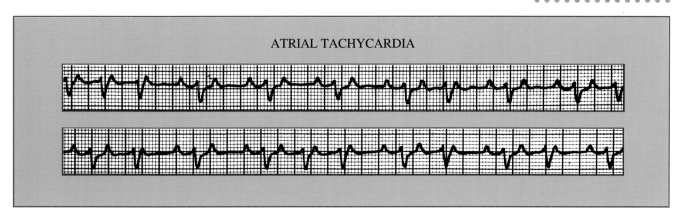

FIGURE 3.32 • Atrial tachcyardia. In this continuous recording, atrial tachycardia is seen at a rate of 150 beats/min and conducts with an AV ratio of 2:1, 3:2 and 4:3. The block is an AV nodal Wenckebach AV block.

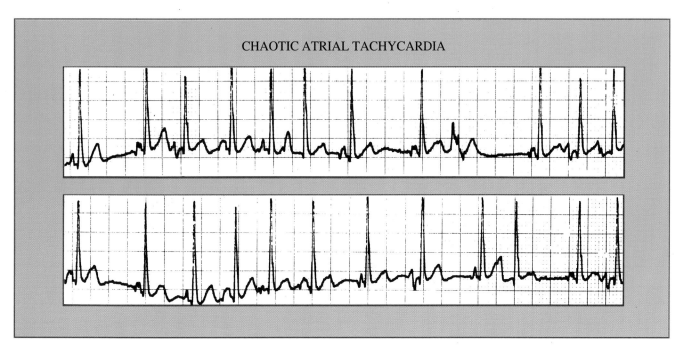

FIGURE 3.33 • Chaotic atrial tachycardia. P waves of at least 3 different contours occurring at irregular intervals characterize this tachycardia.

tours are noted with most P waves conducted to the ventricles. This tachycardia occurs commonly in patients with pulmonary disease who are hypoxic and can eventually degenerate into atrial fibrillation. Digitalis appears to be an unusual cause while theophylline administration has been implicated. Therapy is directed primarily toward the underlying disease. Antiarrhythmic drugs are often ineffective in slowing either the rate of the atrial tachycardia or the ventricular response. Verapamil or a ß-blocker can be useful, but the ß-blocker is often contraindicated in the patient with pulmonary disease.

ATRIOVENTRICULAR JUNCTION ESCAPE BEATS

Automatic fibers that are prevented from initiating depolarization by a pacemaker (such as the sinus node, which possesses a more rapid rate of firing) are called latent pacemakers and are found in various areas of the atrium, atrioventricular (AV) node-His bundle area, right and left bundle branches and Purkinje system. A latent pacemaker can become the dominant pacemaker if there is a decrease in the number of impulses reaching the latent pacemaker site as a result of sinus slowing (Figure 3.34) or

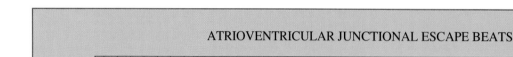

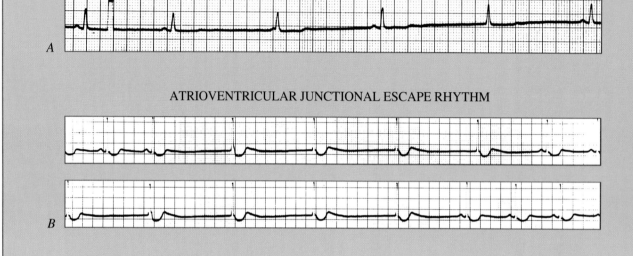

ATRIOVENTRICULAR JUNCTIONAL ESCAPE BEATS

ATRIOVENTRICULAR JUNCTIONAL ESCAPE RHYTHM

FIGURE 3.34 • AV junctional escape beats (A). Because of sinus slowing, the AV junction escapes and is responsible for the third and fifth QRS complexes. The escape rate is constant at approximately 40 beats/min. AV junctional escape rhythm (B). Sinus slowing allows the AV junction to escape at a rate of 35 to 40 beats/min.

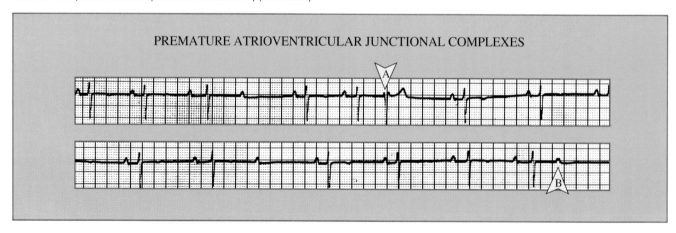

PREMATURE ATRIOVENTRICULAR JUNCTIONAL COMPLEXES

FIGURE 3.35 • Premature AV junctional complexes. In the mid-portion of the top tracing, a premature AV junctional complex arising from the His bundle results (A). Slight aberrancy exists. A compensatory pause follows. On other occasions, the premature junctional (His) discharge occurs but blocks en route to the ventricle. However, it also invades the AV node retrogradely (not seen) so that the latter is refractory to the next sinus P wave, which blocks (B). These are called concealed His extrasystoles. Thus, this ECG demonstrates both manifest and concealed His bundle extrasystoles. (Reproduced with permission. Bonner AJ, Zipes DP: *Arch Intern Med* 1976;136:700.)

AV block. This allows the latent pacemaker to escape and initiate depolarization. Thus, an AV junctional escape beat generally occurs at a rate of 35 to 60 beats/min. The QRS complex is normal in contour and not preceded by a conducted P wave. Treatment, if any, lies in increasing the discharge rate of the higher pacemakers or improving AV conduction and can require pacing. Frequently, no treatment is necessary.

Premature AV junctional complexes are characterized by a premature QRS complex of normal contour that is not preceded by a conducted P wave (Figure 3.35). Premature AV junctional complexes that conduct aberrantly are difficult to distinguish from premature ventricular complexes by scalar electrocardiography. Treatment is generally not necessary.

ATRIOVENTRICULAR JUNCTIONAL RHYTHM

If the atrioventricular (AV) junctional escape beats continue for a period of time, the rhythm is called an AV junctional rhythm (refer to Figure 3.34). It generally occurs at a rate of 35 to 60 beats/min. The AV junctional tissue can assume the role of dominant pacemaker at this rate only by passive default of the sinus pacemaker or because of AV block. The QRS complexes can conduct retrogradely to the atrium or can occur independently of atrial discharge, producing AV dissociation.

The AV junctional escape rhythm can be a normal phenomenon in response to the effects of vagal tone, or it can occur during abnormal sinus bradycardia or heart block. The escape beat or rhythm serves as a safety mechanism to prevent the occurrence of ventricular asystole.

NONPAROXYSMAL ATRIOVENTRICULAR JUNCTIONAL TACHYCARDIA

Enhanced discharge rate of the junctional focus, between 70 and 130 beats/min, with gradual onset and termination and QRS complexes of normal contour characterize nonparoxysmal atrioventricular (AV) junctional tachycardia (Figure 3.36). Although accepted terminology confers the label of tachycardia to rates exceeding 100 beats/min, the term nonparoxysmal AV junctional tachycardia, although not entirely correct, has generally been accepted because rates exceeding 60 beats/min represent, in effect, a tachycardia for the AV junctional tissue. The rhythm is regular and can be slowed by vagal discharge. Although retrograde activation of the atrium can occur, an independent sinus, atrial or, on occasion, a second AV junctional focus commonly control the atria, resulting in AV dissociation. Accelerated automatic discharge in or near the His bundle is probably responsible for this tachycardia. It occurs most commonly in patients with underlying heart disease such as inferior myocardial infarction, myocarditis, after open-heart surgery or from excess digitalis. Exit block from the junctional focus can occur, and when it is of the Wenckebach type, it can produce a regular irregularity of the rhythm.

Therapy is directed toward the underlying cause and support of the cardiovascular system. If the rhythm is regular, the cardiovascular status is not compromised, and if the patient is not taking digitalis, digitalis administration should be considered. Electrical cardioversion can be tried, if necessary, as long as digitalis toxicity is excluded. Theoretically, however, if the nonparoxysmal AV junctional tachycardia is due to enhanced automaticity, electrical cardioversion can be ineffective. If the patient tolerates the arrhythmia well, careful monitoring and attention to the underlying heart disease is usually all that is required. The arrhythmia usually abates spontaneously. If digitalis toxicity is a cause, the drug must be stopped and potassium, lidocaine, phenytoin or propranolol administered.

ATRIOVENTRICULAR NODAL REENTRANT TACHYCARDIA

Atrioventricular (AV) nodal reentrant tachycardia is characterized electrocardiographically by QRS complexes of supraventricular origin—functional aberrancy may be present—with a sudden onset and termination, generally at rates of 150 to 250 beats/min—commonly 180 to 200 beats/min in adults—and a

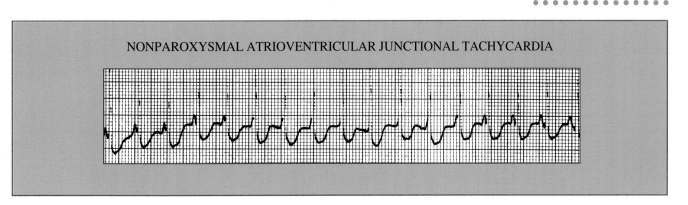

NONPAROXYSMAL ATRIOVENTRICULAR JUNCTIONAL TACHYCARDIA

FIGURE 3.36 • Nonparoxysmal AV junctional tachycardia. A normal QRS tachycardia at a rate of 165 beats/min is present, along with AV dissociation. Atrial activity is indicated by the arrows at the beginning of the recording and can be seen toward the end as well. The AV dissociation is isorhythmic because of the similar rates between atrial and ventricular activity.

regular rhythm (Figure 3.37). Uncommonly, the rate may be as slow as 110 beats/min and occasionally, especially in children, may exceed 250 beats/min. The mechanism is reentry within the AV node, with the anterograde impulse traveling down a slowly conducting AV nodal pathway, and the retrograde impulse returning over a more rapidly conducting fast pathway (Figure 3.38). AV nodal reentry recorded at its onset begins abruptly, often following a premature atrial complex that conducts with a prolonged PR interval. Abrupt termination is sometimes followed by a period of transient asystole or bradycardia. The RR interval may shorten over the course of the first few beats at the onset or lengthen during the last few beats preceding termination of the tachycardia. Carotid sinus massage can slow the tachycardia slightly prior to its termination or, if termination does not occur, can produce only transient, slight slowing of the tachycardia. P waves in most patients occur simultaneously with the QRS complex and therefore are not recognized in the scalar ECG. In approximately 30% of instances, atrial activation begins at the end of, or just after the QRS complex, giving rise to a discrete P wave on the surface ECG. In the most common variety of AV nodal reentrant tachycardia, the VA interval (time interval between onset of QRS complex and onset of atrial activity) is less than 50% of the RR interval and the ratio of AV to VA intervals exceeds 1. Uncommonly, patients can have a long RP and short PR interval because the reentry is traveling in a reverse direction to the ventricles over the fast pathway and to the atria over the slow pathway.

AV nodal reentry commonly occurs in patients who have no structural heart disease. Symptoms frequently accompany the tachycardia and range from feelings of palpitations, nervousness and anxiety, to angina, heart failure, syncope or shock, depending on the duration and rate of the tachycardia and the presence of structural heart disease. Tachycardia can cause syncope because of the rapid ventricular rate, reduced cardiac output and cerebral circulation or because of asystole when the tachycardia terminates, owing to tachycardia-induced depression of sinus node automaticity. Hemodynamic consequences in patients with normal left ventricular function are due primarily to a marked decrease in left ventricular end diastolic and stroke volumes with an increase in ejection rate and cardiac output, without a significant change in ejection fraction as heart rate is increased and the atrial contribution to ventricular filling is lost.

The nature of acute therapy depends on the underlying heart disease, how well the tachycardia is tolerated, and the behavior of previous attacks in the individual patient. For some patients, rest, reassurance and sedation may be all that are required to abort an attack. Vagal maneuvers, including carotid sinus massage, Valsalva and Mueller maneuvers, gagging, and exposing the face to ice water serve as the first line of therapy. These maneuvers may slightly slow the tachycardia rate, which may then speed up the original rate after cessation of an unsuccessful attempt, or they may terminate the tachycardia. Vagal maneuvers should be tried again after each pharmacologic approach. Knowing where drugs exert their actions can be helpful in selection (refer to Figure

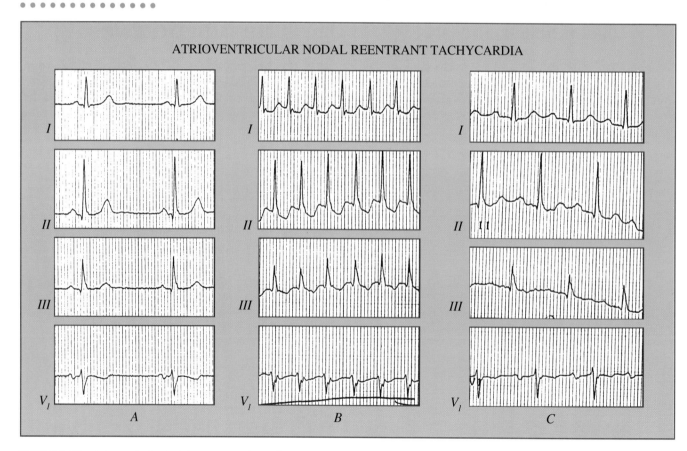

FIGURE 3.37 • Atrioventricular nodal reentrant tachycardia (AVNRT). Normal sinus rhythm (A). AVNRT at a rate of 200 beats/min (B). Normal sinus rhythm after radio frequency ablation (C). Note the increase in the PR interval due to ablation of the fast AV nodal pathway.

3.38). The first drug of choice is IV adenosine given rapidly in doses of 6 to 12 mg. Onset of action is immediate, and successful termination exceeds 90%. Adverse effects are minimal and transient. IV verapamil, 5 to 10 mg, terminates AV nodal reentry successfully in about two minutes in over 90% of instances and should be tried next. Diltiazem produces similar results. Cholinergic drugs, particularly edrophonium chloride (Tensilon), a short-acting cholinesterase inhibitor, can terminate AV nodal reentry when administered initially at a trial of 3 to 5 mg IV and, if unsuccessful, repeated at a dose of 10 mg IV. This onset of action is rapid, of short duration and has minimal side effects. Edrophonium chloride should be used cautiously or not at all in patients who are hypotensive or who have lung disease, especially a history of asthma. Treating arrhythmias is not an FDA approved indication for use of edrophonium chloride.

If these initial approaches are unsuccessful, IV digitalis administration may be attempted using one of the following short-acting digitalis preparations:

- IV ouabain 0.25 to 0.5 mg followed by 0.1 mg every 30 to 60 mins if needed, keeping the total dose less than 1 mg within a 24-hr period or 0.01 mg/kg as a single dose over 10 to 15 mins.
- IV digoxin 0.5 to 1.0 mg given over 10 to 15 mins, followed by 0.25 mg every 2 to 4 hrs, with a total dose less than 1.5 mg within any 24-hr period.
- IV deslanoside 0.8 mg, followed by 0.4 mg every 2 to 4 hrs, restricting the total dose to less than 2.0 mg within a 24-hr period.

Oral digitalis administration to terminate a tachycardia is not indicated. Vagal maneuvers, previously ineffective, may terminate the tachycardia after digitalis administration and therefore should be repeated.

Propranolol given intravenously at a rate of 0.5 to 1.0 mg/min for a total dose of 0.5 to 3.0 mg may be tried if previous therapy is unsuccessful. Higher doses may be used in some patients. A short acting ß-blocker, such as esmolol, is preferable. Beta-blockers must be used cautiously, if at all, in patients with heart

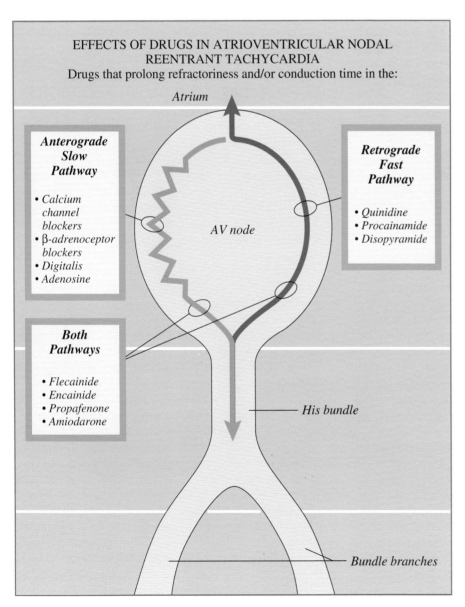

FIGURE 3.38 • Effect of drugs in atrioventricular nodal reentrant tachycardias.

EFFECTS OF DRUGS IN ATRIOVENTRICULAR NODAL REENTRANT TACHYCARDIA
Drugs that prolong refractoriness and/or conduction time in the:

Atrium

Anterograde Slow Pathway
- Calcium channel blockers
- β-adrenoceptor blockers
- Digitalis
- Adenosine

Retrograde Fast Pathway
- Quinidine
- Procainamide
- Disopyramide

AV node

Both Pathways
- Flecainide
- Encainide
- Propafenone
- Amiodarone

His bundle

Bundle branches

failure, chronic lung disease, or history of asthma. Before administering digitalis or ß-blockers, it is advisable to reassess the clinical status of the patient and consider whether DC cardioversion is advisable. DC shock administered to patients who have received excessive amounts of digitalis, can be dangerous and result in serious postshock ventricular arrhythmias. Particularly if there are signs or symptoms of cardiac decompensastion, DC electrical shock should be considered early. DC shock, synchronized to the QRS complex to avoid precipitating ventricular fibrillation, successfully terminates AV nodal reentry with energies in the range of 10 to 50 J. Higher energies may be required in some patients. In the event that digitalis has been given in large doses and DC shock is contraindicated, atrial or ventricular pacing can restore sinus rhythm. In some patients, esophageal or transcutaneous pacing can be used.

Uncommonly, procainamide, quinidine, or disopyramide can terminate AV nodal reentry. Unless contraindicated, DC cardioversion generally should be used before using these agents, which are more often administered to prevent recurrences.

Pressor drugs can terminate AV nodal reentry by inducing reflex vagal stimulation mediated by baroreceptors in the carotid sinus and aorta when the systolic pressures are acutely elevated to levels exceeding 180 mm Hg, but are infrequently used unless hypotension coexists. One of the following drugs, diluted in 5 to 10 mL of 5% dextrose in water, can be given over 1 to 3 minutes:
- Phenylephrine (Neosynephrine), 0.5 to 1.0 mg.
- Methoxamine (Vasoxyl), 3 to 5 mg.
- Metaraminol (Aramine), 0.5 to 2.0 mg.

Pressor drugs should be used cautiously or not at all in the elderly and in patients who have structural heart disease, significant hypertension, hypothryroidism or acute myocardial infarction. This potentially dangerous and almost always uncomfortable procedure is rarely required unless the patient is also hypotensive.

Prevention of recurrences is often more difficult than terminating the acute episode. Initially, one must decide whether the frequency and severity of the attacks warrant long-term drug prophylaxis. If the attacks are infrequent, well-tolerated, and either terminate spontaneously or are easily terminated by the patient, no prophylactic therapy may be necessary. If the attacks are sufficiently frequent to necessitate therapy, the patient may be treated with drugs empirically or on the basis of serial electrophysiologic testing of multiple drugs. The latter approach appears reasonable in some patients with poorly tolerated tachycardias that recur only sporadically. If empirical testing is desirable, the following choices are recommended:
- Digitalis is generally the initial drug of choice. It has the advantages of being well tolerated and requiring administration once daily. The clinical situation determines the speed of digitalization. Using digoxin, rapid oral digitalizaiton can be accomplished in 24 to 36 hrs, with an initial dose of 1.0 to 1.5 mg followed by 0.25 to 0.5 mg every 6 hrs for a total dose of 2.0 to 3.0 mg. The less rapid regimen digitalizes the patient in 2 to 3 days within an initial dose of 0.75 to 1.0 mg, followed by 0.25 to 0.5 mg every 12 hrs for a total dose of 2.0 to 3.0 mg.
- Alternatively, digoxin administered as a maintenance dose of 0.125 to 0.5 mg achieves digitalization in about 1 week. Dig-

itoxin, which has a longer duration of action, may be used instead of digoxin. Oral digitalization with digitoxin may be accomplished in 24 to 36 hrs with an initial dose of 0.5 to 0.8 mg followed by 0.2 mg every 6 to 8 hrs until a total dose of 1.2 mg is reached. A slower approach involves administering 0.2 mg 3 times daily for 2 to 3 days. Complete digitalization can be also accomplished in about one month simply by giving a daily maintenance dose of 0.05 to 0.2 mg.
- If digitalis alone is unsuccessful, one can then add verapamil, 80 to 120 mg every 6 or 8 hrs; diltiazem 30 mg every 6 or 8 hrs to a daily total dose of 180 to 360 mg; quinidine sulfate 200 to 400 mg every 6 hrs; propranolol 10 to 40 mg every 6 hrs. Procainamide, disopyramide, flecainide, encainide, or amiodarone can be used in place of quinidine. In some patients, concomitant administration of several drugs, such as digitalis, propranolol and quinidine may be necessary.
- Infrequently, antitachycardia pacemaker implantation provides acceptable treatment. Surgical isolation of the AV node or cryoablation of atrial inputs to the AV node has eliminated tachycardia while preserving AV nodal conduction. Radiofrequency (RF) modification of the AV node with a strategically placed catheter has been very successful with a risk of heart block of 2% to 5% (refer to Figure 3.37).

REENTRY OVER A RETROGRADELY CONDUCTING (CONCEALED) ACCESSORY PATHWAY

If an accessory pathway conducts from the ventricle to the atrium but not in a reverse direction, its presence is not apparent by analysis of the scalar ECG during sinus rhythm because the ventricle is not preexcited (Figs. 3.39C, 3.40). Therefore, the ECG manifestations of Wolff-Parkinson-White syndrome are absent and the accessory pathway is said to be "concealed." The mechanism responsible for most tachycardias in Wolff-Parkinson-White patients is macro-reentry caused by anterograde conduction over the atrioventricular (AV) node-His bundle pathway and retrograde conduction over an accessory pathway. Even if latter only conducts retrogradely, it can still participate in the reentrant circuit to cause an AV reciprocating tachycardia (Figure 3.39C).

Electrocardiographically, a tachycardia due to this mechanism presents as a regular, normal QRS tachycardia, with a rate of 180 to 220 beats/min with the retrograde P wave occurring after completion of the QRS complex, in the ST segment or early T wave. Therefore, the PR interval exceeds the RP interval. The P wave must follow the QRS complex because, before the propagating impulse can enter the accessory pathway and excite the atrium retrogradely, the ventricle must be activated. Because the atrium may be activated eccentrically, that is, in a manner other than the normal retrograde activation sequence starting at the low right atrial septum from the AV node, the P wave contour may be unusual. For example, many concealed accessory pathways are located in the left lateral position, making the left atrium the first site of retrograde atrial activation and causing the retrograde P wave to be negative in lead 1 and sometimes aVL. Finally, because the tachycardia circuit involves the ventricles, if functional bundle branch block occurs in the same ventricle in which the accessory pathway is located, the cycle

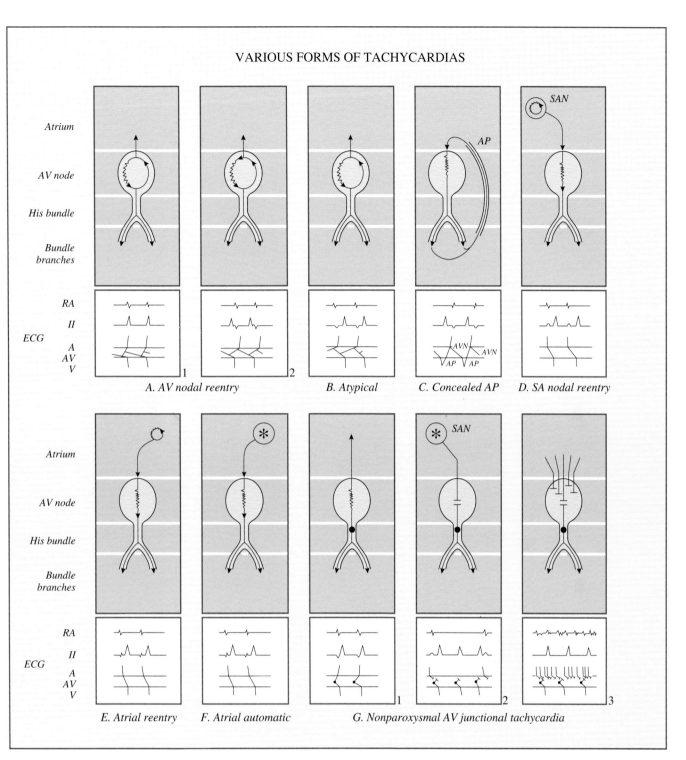

VARIOUS FORMS OF TACHYCARDIAS

A. AV nodal reentry

B. Atypical

C. Concealed AP

D. SA nodal reentry

E. Atrial reentry

F. Atrial automatic

G. Nonparoxysmal AV junctional tachycardia

FIGURE 3.39 • Various forms of tachycardia. In the top portion of each example, the presumed anatomical pathways are shown. The bottom half demonstrates their respective ECG presentations and explanatory ladder diagrams. Atrioventricular (AV) nodal reentry (A). Reentrant excitation is confined to the AV node, with retrograde atrial activity occurring simultaneously with ventricular activity due to anterograde conduction over the slow AV nodal pathway and retrograde conduction over the fast atrioventricular nodal pathway (A1). Atrial activity occurs slightly later than ventriclar activity, owing to retrograde conduction delay (A2). Atypical AV nodal reentry due to anterograde conduction over a fast AV and retrograde conduction over a slow AV pathway (B). Concealed accessory pathway (AP) (C). Reciprocating tachycardia is due to anterograde conduction over the AV node and retrograde conduction over the accessory pathway.

Retrograde P waves occur after the QRS complex. Sinus nodal reentry (D). The tachycardia is due to reentry within the sinus node, which then conducts to the rest of the heart. Atrial reentry (E). Tachycardia is stimulated by reentry within the atrium, which conducts to the rest of the heart. Automatic atrial tachycardia (F). Tachycardia is due to automatic discharge in the atrium, which then conducts to the rest of the heart. This is difficult to distinguish from atrial reentry. Nonparoxysmal AV junctional tachycardia (G). Various presentations of this tachycardia are depicted with retrograde atrial capture (G1), AV dissociation with the sinus node in control of the atria (G2), and AV dissociation with atrial fibrillation (G3). (Reproduced with permission. Zipes DP: Specific arrhythmias: Diagnosis and treatment. In: Braunwald E, ed. *Heart Disease. A Textbook of Cardiovascular Medicine* Philadelphia, Pa: WB Saunders; 1988:668.)

length of the tachycardia could become longer. This important change ensues because the bundle branch block lengthens the reentrant circuit by lengthening the VA interval, which in turn can lengthen the cycle length of the tachycardia. This does not occur in patients with a septal accessory pathway or in patients with AV nodal reentry.

Vagal maneuvers produce a response similar to AV nodal reentry by acting predominately on the AV node and the tachycardia may transiently slow with or without termination. Termination tends to occur in the anterograde direction so that the last retrograde P wave fails to conduct to the ventricles.

Concealed accessory pathways account for about 30% of patients with supraventricular tachycardia referred for electrophysiologic evaluation. The majority of these accessory pathways are located between the left atrium and left ventricle. It is important to be aware of the possibility of a concealed accessory pathway being responsible for apparently "routine" supraventricular tachycardia, since the therapeutic response at times may not follow the usual guidelines. Antiarrhythmic targeting may need to be directed toward drugs that affect the accessory pathway such as Class 1A and 1C agents or amiodarone. Also, interruption of the accessory pathway can be accomplished surgically or with radiofrequency ablation.

The therapeutic approach to terminate this form of tachycardia acutely is as outlined for AV nodal reentry. It is necessary to achieve block of a single impulse from atrium to ventricle or ventricle to atrium. The most successful method is to produce transient AV nodal block. Therefore, vagal maneuvers, adenosine, verapamil or diltiazem, digitalis and propranolol or esmolol are acceptable choices. Antiarrhythmic agents that prolong activation time and refractoriness in the accessory pathway must be considered for chronic therapy to prevent recurrences (refer to preexcitation syndrome). Atrial fibrillation in patients with a concealed accessory pathway should not present a greater therapeutic challenge than it does in patients who lack such a pathway because anterograde AV conduction occurs over the AV node. Verapamil and digitalis are not contraindicated. However, it must be remembered that under some circumstances, such as catecholamine stimulation, anterograde conduction in the apparently concealed accessory pathway can be restored. Radiofrequency catheter ablation should be considered early in the patient with symptomatic recurrent tachycardia.

PREEXCITATION SYNDROME

Preexcitation syndrome occurs when the atrial impulse activates the whole or some part of the ventricle, or the ventricular impulse activates the whole or some part of the atrium, earlier than would be expected if the impulse traveled by way of the normal specific conduction system only. In Wolff-Parkinson-White syndrome, two muscular connections composed of working myocardial fibers exist outside the specialized conducting tissue, and connect the atrium and the ventricle (refer to Figure 3.41). They are named accessory AV pathways or connections—commonly called Kent bundles—and are responsible for the most prevalent variety of preexcitation. Three basic features typify the ECG abnormalities of patients with the usual form of Wolff-Parkinson-White syndrome caused by an atrioventricular (AV) connection:

- PR interval less than 120 msec during sinus rhythm.
- QRS complex duration exceeding 120 msec with a slurred, slowly rising onset of the QRS in some leads (∂ wave) and usually a normal terminal QRS portion.
- Secondary ST-T wave changes that are generally directed opposite to the major Δ and QRS vectors.

The term Wolff-Parkinson-White syndrome is applied when the patient has symptoms, generally due to tach-

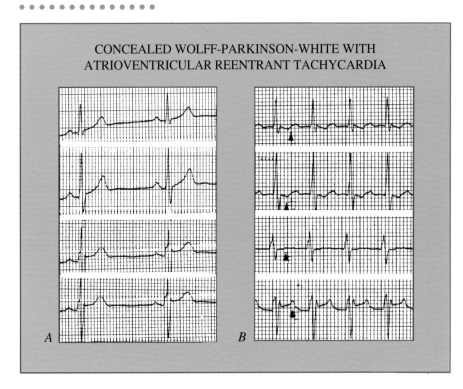

CONCEALED WOLFF-PARKINSON-WHITE WITH ATRIOVENTRICULAR REENTRANT TACHYCARDIA

A   B

FIGURE 3.40 • Concealed Wolff-Parkinson-White syndrome. Normal sinus rhythm with no apparent ∂ wave (A). Concealed Wolff-Parkinson-White with AV reentrant tachycardia (B).

yarrhythmias. The most common tachycardia is characterized by a normal QRS, ventricular rates of 180 to 220 beats/min (generally faster than AV nodal reentry), and sudden onset and termination, behaving in many respects like the tachycardia described for conduction utilizing a concealed accessory pathway. The major difference between the two is the capacity for anterograde conduction over the accessory pathway during atrial flutter or atrial fibrillation. Several anatomical substrates exist that provide the basis for different ECG manifestations of preexcitation syndrome variations. For example, fibers from the atrium to the His bundle that bypass the physiological delay of the AV node are called atriohisian tracts and are associated with a short PR interval and a normal QRS complex. Although demonstrated anatomically, the electrophysiologic significance of these tracts in the genesis of tachycardias with a short PR interval and a normal QRS complex—so-called Lown-Ganong-Levine (LGL) syndrome[2] remains to be established. Indeed, evidence does not support the presence of a specific LGL syndrome comprising a short PR interval, a normal QRS complex and tachycardias related to an atriohisian bypass tract. The short PR interval reported in many patients probably represents one end of the normal AV conduction spectrum. True atriohisian bypass tracts have been reported in several patients with tachycardias, however. Two varieties of Mahaim fibers include those passing from the AV node to the ventricle (nodoventricular or nodofascicular fibers), and those arising in the His bundle or bundle branches and inserting in the ventricular myocardium (fasciculoventricular fibers). For nodoventricular connections, the PR interval can be normal or short and the QRS complex is a fusion beat. Fasciculoventricular connections create a normal PR interval and a fixed, anomalous QRS complex. The existence of these tracts has been reevaluated recently. Several varieties are probably present, including accessory AV connections that conduct more slowly than the usual connections, for instance AV nodal-like properties that simulate nodoventricular connections but still travel from atrium to ventricle (Figure 3.41).

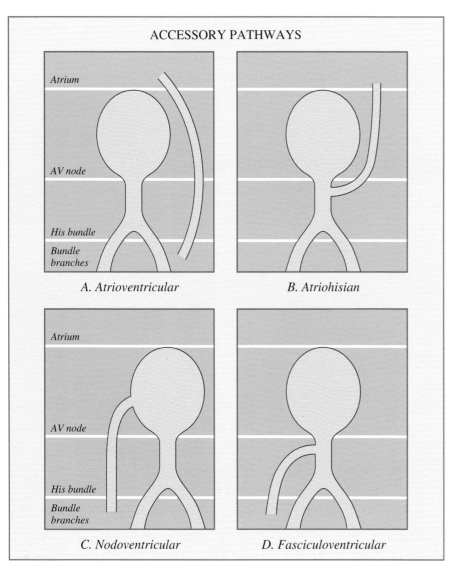

ACCESSORY PATHWAYS

Atrium

AV node

His bundle

Bundle branches

A. Atrioventricular

B. Atriohisian

Atrium

AV node

His bundle

Bundle branches

C. Nodoventricular

D. Fasciculoventricular

FIGURE 3.41 • Accessory pathways. The most common form of atrioventricular (AV) connection (A). An uncommon form of atrio-Hisian connection (B). Nodoventricular connection, which may be explained by atrioventricular pathways with AV nodal-like properties rather than a pathway coming off the AV node (C). Uncommon fasciculoventricular connections (D). (Reproduced with permission. Zipes DP: Specific arrhythmias: Diagnosis and treatment. In: Braunwald E, ed. *Heart Disease. A Textbook of Cardiovascular Medicine* Philadelphia, Pa: Saunders;1988:687.)

If the accessory pathway is capable of anterograde conduction, two routes of AV conduction are possible to the ventricle, one subject to physiological delay over the AV node and the other passing directly without delay from atrium to ventricle. This produces the typical QRS complex that is a fusion beat due to depolarization of the ventricle, in part by the wavefront traveling over the accessory pathway and in part by the wavefront traveling over the normal AV node-His bundle route. The delta wave represents ventricular activation from input over the accessory pathway. The extent of contribution to ventricular depolarization by the wavefront over each route depends upon their relative activation times. If AV nodal conduction delay occurs, for example, because of a rapid atrial pacing rate or a premature atrial complex, more of the ventricle becomes activated over the accessory pathway, and the QRS complex becomes more anomalous in contour. Total activation of the ventricle over the accessory pathway happens when the AV nodal delay is sufficiently long. In contrast, if the accessory pathway is relatively far from the sinus node, for example, in the left lateral ventricle, or if AV nodal conduction time is relatively short, more of the ventricle is activated over the normal pathway. The normal fusion beat during sinus rhythm has a short HV interval or His-bundle activation. This occurs after the onset of ventricular depolarization because part of the atrial impulse bypasses the AV node and activates the ventricle early, at a time when the impulse traveling over the normal route just reaches the His bundle. This finding of a short or negative HV interval occurs only during conduction over an accessory pathway or from retrograde His activation during a ventricular tachycardia.

The position of the accessory pathway can be determined by a careful analysis of the spatial direction of the delta wave in the 12 lead ECG in maximally preexcited beats. A simple ECG algorithm with 90% accuracy localizes left free wall pathways by a Q wave in the lateral precordial leads and right bundle branch block contour, posteroseptal pathways by a Q wave in the inferior leads and either right or left bundle branch block contour, anteroseptal pathways by left bundle branch block and inferior axis and right freewall pathways by left bundle branch block contour and left axis deviation (Figure 3.42).

The usual activation sequence for a reciprocating tachycardia circuit (orthodromic) with a left-sided accessory pathway without functional bundle branch block progresses from:

atrium → AV node-His bundle → right and left ventricles → accessory pathway → atrium and → AV node-His bundle…etc

This tachycardia produces a short RP-long PR relationship (Figs. 3.43, 3.44). If the impulse travels in a reverse direction to the ventricle over the accessory pathway and back to the atrium over the normal AV node-His bundle, so-called antidromic tachycardia, the QRS complex, becomes anomalous due to activation of the ventricle over the accessory pathway. Ten

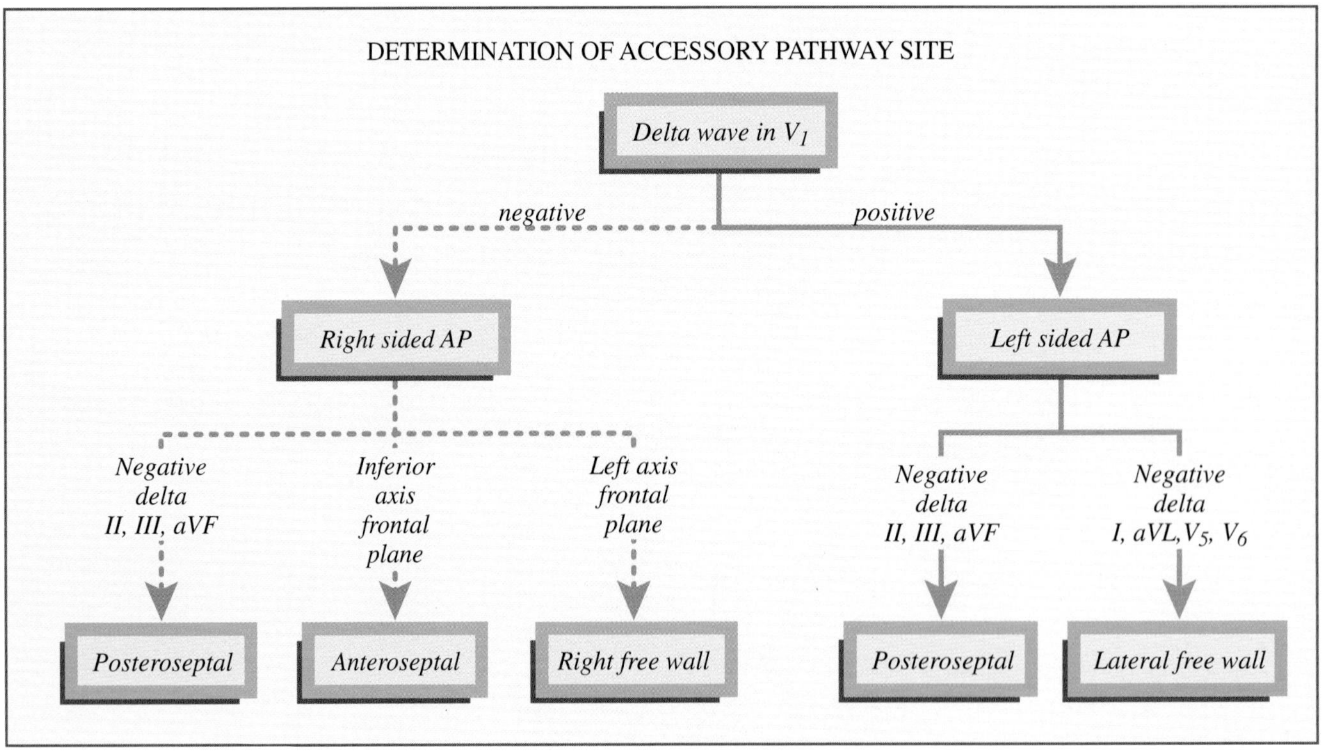

DETERMINATION OF ACCESSORY PATHWAY SITE

FIGURE 3.42 • Electrocardiographic determination of accessory pathway site. This branching diagram indicates how the use of the ECG during full preexcitation can help localize the ventricular quadrant at which the accessory pathway is located with a 90% or greater accuracy.

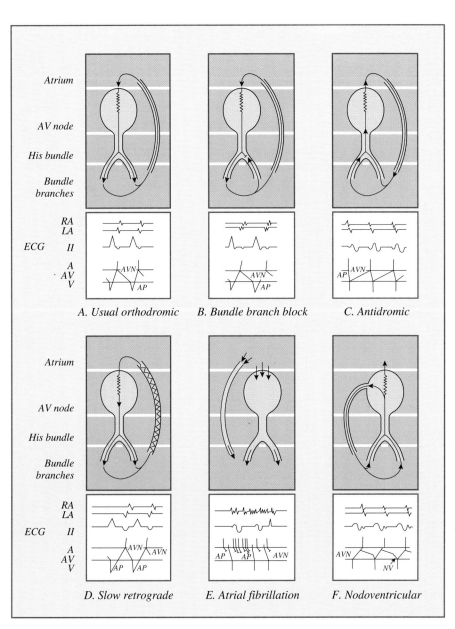

A. Usual orthodromic
B. Bundle branch block
C. Antidromic
D. Slow retrograde
E. Atrial fibrillation
F. Nodoventricular

FIGURE 3.43 • Tachycardias associated with accessory pathways. Orthodromic tachycardia with anterograde conduction over the atrioventricular (AV) node-His bundle route and retrograde conduction over the accessory pathway—left-sided for this example as depicted by left atrium (LA) activation preceding right atrium (RA) activation (A). Orthodromic tachycardia and ipsilateral functional bundle branch block (B). Antidromic tachycardia with anterograde conduction over the accessory pathway and retrograde conduction over the AV node-His bundle (C). Orthodromic tachycardia with a slowly conducting accessory pathway (D). Atrial fibrillation with the accessory pathway as a bystander (E). Anterograde conduction over a portion of the AV node and a nodoventricular pathway and retrograde conduction over the AV node (F). (Reproduced with permission. Zipes DP: Specific arrhythmias: Diagnosis and treatment. In: Braunwald E, ed. *Heart Disease. A Textbook of Cardiovascular Medicine* Philadephia, Pa: WB Saunders;1988:690.)

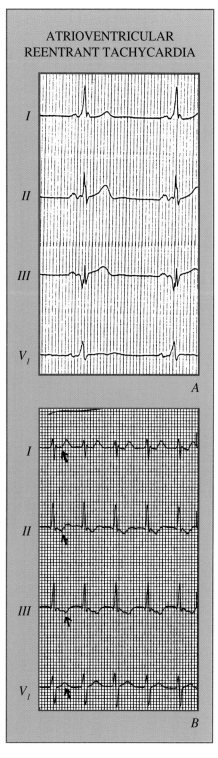

ATRIOVENTRICULAR
REENTRANT TACHYCARDIA

FIGURE 3.44 • Atrioventricular reentrant tachycardia. Preexcitation due to conduction over a left posterolateral accessory pathway (A). Note the retrograde P waves (arrows) (B).

percent to 15% of patients have multiple accessory pathways. On occasion, tachycardia may be due to a reentrant loop anterogradely over one accessory pathway and retrogradely over the other. During atrial fibrillation or atrial flutter, impulses arising in the atrium can travel the normal AV node-His bundle route or over the accessory pathway to the ventricle. Because conduction over the accessory pathway bypasses the normal AV nodal delay, ventricular rates during atrial fibrillation in a patient with Wolff-Parkinson-White syndrome can become quite rapid (Figure 3.45).

An incessant form of supraventricular tachycardia has been recognized—permanent form of AV junctional tachycardia, PJRT—occurs with a long RP interval and shorter PR interval. A posteroseptal accessory pathway that conducts very slowly, possibly due to a long and tortuous route, appears responsible. PJRT is maintained by anterograde AV nodal conduction and retrograde conduction over the accessory pathway. The long anterograde conduction time over the accessory pathway can prevent ECG manifestations of accessory pathway conduction during sinus rhythm (Figure 3.46).

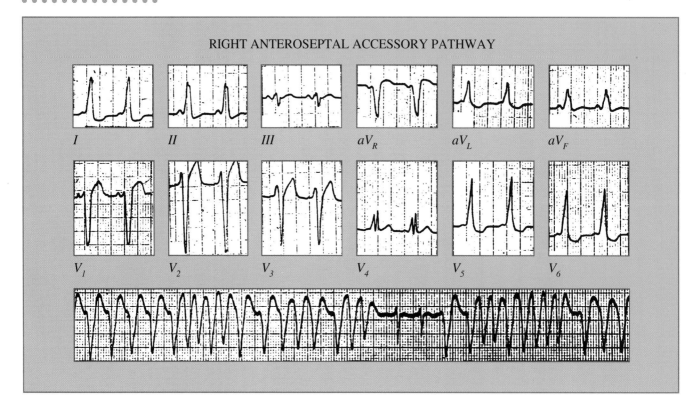

FIGURE 3.45 • The patient has a right anteroseptal accessory pathway that conducts during atrial fibrillation with rates exceeding 300 beats/min at times.

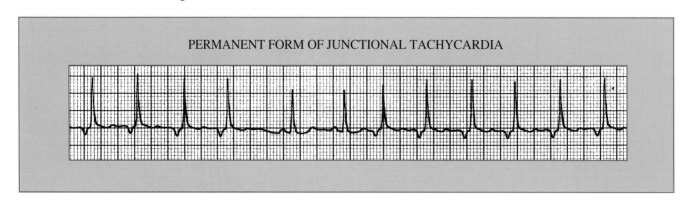

FIGURE 3.46 • Lead 2 recording demonstrates the incessant nature of the permanent form of junctional tachycardia (PJRT), due to an accessory pathway conducting slowly retrogradely (refer to figure 3.43D).

It is important to remember that patients with preexcitation syndrome can have other causes of tachycardia, such as AV nodal reentry, sinus nodal reentry and even ventricular tachycardia unrelated to the accessory pathway. Accessory pathways can conduct only anterogradely or retrogradely. If the pathway conducts only anterogradely, it cannot participate in the usual form of orthodromic reciprocating tachycardia. However, it can participate in antidromic tachycardia as well as conduct to the ventricle during atrial flutter or atrial fibrillation (refer to Figure 3.43).

Wolff-Parkinson-White syndrome is found in all age groups, from the newborn to the elderly, in identical twins and in some animal species. The prevalence is higher in males and decreases with age, apparently due to loss of preexcitation. The majority of adults with preexcitation syndrome have normal hearts, although a variety of acquired and congenital cardiac defects have been reported. Ebstein's anomaly is a congenital malformation caused by a downward displacement of the tricuspid valve into the right ventricle due to anomolous attachment of the tricuspid leaflets. Patients with this anomaly often have multiple accessory pathways, right-sided either in the posterior septum or posterolateral wall, with preexcitation localized to the atrialized ventricle. The reported incidence of preexcitation syndrome averages about 1.5 per 1000 population. Left-sided accessory pathways are more common than right. The frequency of paroxysmal tachycardia apparently increases with age, from 10/100 cases of Wolff-Parkinson-White in a 20 to 39 year age group to 36/100 cases in patients over 60 years of age. Approximately 80% of patients with tachycardia have AV reciprocating tachycardia, 15% to 30% have atrial fibrillation and 5% have atrial flutter. Ventricular tachycardia occurs uncommonly. The anomalous complexes may mask or mimic myocardial infarction, bundle branch block or ventricular hypertrophy. The prognosis is excellent in patients without ' hycardia or an associated cardiac anomaly. It is likely t: .t the accessory pathway occurs congenitally even if its manifestations are detected in later years. Relatives of patients with preexcitation, particularly those with multiple pathways, have an increased prevalence of preexcitation, suggesting a hereditary mode of acquisition. Intermittent preexcitation during sinus rhythm or loss of conduction over the accessory pathway with exercise or with certain drugs suggests that the refractory period of the accessory pathway is long and that the patient is not at a risk of developing a rapid ventricular rate should atrial fibrillation or atrial flutter develop.

Patients with ventricular preexcitation can have no or only occasional tachyarrhythmias unassociated with significant symptoms. These patients do not require electrophysiologic evaluation or therapy. However, if a patient has frequent episodes of tachyarrhythmias and/or infrequent arrhythmias that cause significant symptoms, evaluation and therapy should be considered. Those who suffer significant hemodynamic consequences from the tachyarrhythmia should definitely be considered for electrophysiologic study.

Three therapeutic options exist:
- Electrical ablation of the accessory pathway.
- Surgical ablation of the accessory pathway.
- Pharmacologic treatment.

Drugs are chosen to prolong conduction time and/or refractoriness in the AV node, the accessory pathway or both structures, to prevent rapid rates (Figure 3.47). If successful, drug therapy prevents initiation and/or maintenance of AV reciprocating tachycardia or a rapid ventricular response to atrial flutter or atrial fibrillation. Some drugs can suppress the premature complexes that precipitate the arrhythmias.

Calcium channel blockers, ß-adrenoceptor blockers, and digitalis all prolong conduction time and refractoriness in the AV node. Verapamil and propranolol do not directly affect conduction in the accessory pathway while digitalis has variable effects. Because digitalis has been reported to shorten refractoriness in the accessory pathway and speed the ventricular response in some patients with atrial fibrillation, it is advisable not to use digitalis as a single drug in patients with Wolff-Parkinson-White syndrome who have or may develop atrial flutter or atrial fibrillation. Since many patients can develop atrial fibrillation during the reciprocating tachycardia, this caveat probably applies to all patients who have tachycardia and Wolff-Parkinson-White syndrome. Rather, drugs that prolong the refractory period in the accessory pathway such as Class 1A and 1C drugs should be used. Class 1C drugs and amiodarone can affect both the AV node and the accessory pathway. Lidocaine does not prolong refractoriness of the accessory pathway in patients whose effective refractory period is less than 300 msec. Intravenous verapamil and lidocaine can increase the ventricular rate during atrial fibrillation in patients with Wolff-Parkinson-White syndrome and intravenous verapamil has been known to precipitate ventricular fibrillation in this setting. This does not appear to happen with oral verapamil. Isoproterenol can expose Wolff-Parkinson-White syndrome in patients with concealed accessory pathway conduction and shorten the refractory period of the accessory pathway.

Termination of the acute episode of reciprocating tachycardia, suspected electrocardiographically by a normal QRS complex, regular RR intervals at a rate of 200 beats/min and a retrograde P wave in the ST segment, should be approached as for AV nodal reentry. After adenosine and vagal maneuvers, IV verapamil or diltiazem should be considered as the initial treatment of choice. If atrial flutter or fibrillation follows intravenous administration of IV verapamil, one should be prepared to perform immediate direct current cardioversion. For atrial flutter or fibrillation, the latter suspected by an anomalous QRS complex and grossly irregular RR intervals, drugs that prolong refractoriness in the accessory pathway, often coupled with drugs that prolong AV nodal refractoriness, for example, procainamide and propranolol, must be used. In some patients, particularly those with a very rapid ventricular response and evidence of cardiac decompensation, electrical cardioversion should be the *initial* treatment of choice.

For long-term pharmacologic therapy to prevent a recurrence, it is not always possible to predict which drugs will be most effective for an individual patient. Some drugs actually can increase the frequency of episodes of AV reciprocating tachycardia episodes by prolonging the duration of the antero-grade and not retrograde refractory period of the accessory pathway, thereby making it easier for a premature atrial complex to block anterogradely in the accessory pathway and initiate tachycardia. Oral administration of two drugs, such as quinidine and propranolol or procainamide and verapamil, to decrease conduction capabilities in both limbs of the reentrant circuit can be beneficial. Depending on the clinical situation, empirical drug trials with serial electrophysiology drug testing can be used to determine optimal drug therapy for patients with AV reciprocating tachycardia. For patients who have atrial fibrillation with a rapid ventricular response, induction of atrial fibrillation while the patient is receiving drug therapy is essential to be certain that the ventricular rate is controlled. At times, stressing the patient with exercise or isoproterenol administration is necessary to demonstrate that the effects of catecholamine do not "override" the blocking action of the antiarrhythmic drug. The safest approach is to perform such drug testing during a controlled electrophysiologic study.

Electrical (Figure 3.48) or surgical (refer to Figure 3.9) ablation of the accessory pathway is advisable for patients with frequent symptomatic arrhythmias that are not fully controlled by drugs or with rapid AV conduction over the accessory pathway during atrial flutter or atrial fibrillation, and in whom significant slowing of the ventricular response during tachycardia cannot be obtained by drug therapy. Patients who have accessory pathways with very short refractory periods may be poor candidates for drug therapy since the refractory period may be prolonged insignificantly in response to standard agents. In some patients, ablative therapy should be considered early in the course of treatment to avoid the necessity of lifelong therapy with antiarrhythmic drugs. Because of the ease, safety and high success rate of radiofrequency catheter ablation, it is often recommended at the time of the *initial* electrophysiologic study to effect an immediate cure. Antitachycardia pacing therapy is not recommended for most patients. Interruption of the accessory pathway should be considered before an antitachycardia device is implanted.

PREMATURE VENTRICULAR COMPLEXES

A premature ventricular complex is characterized by the premature occurrence of a QRS complex that is bizarre in shape and has a duration usually exceeding the dominant QRS complex—generally greater than 120 msec. The T wave is commonly large and opposite in direction to the major deflection of the QRS. The QRS complex is not preceded by a premature P wave but may be preceded by a sinus P wave occurring at its expected time but not conducting to the ventricle (Figure 3.49). Retrograde transmission to the atria from the premature ventricular complex occurs frequently, but is often obscured by the

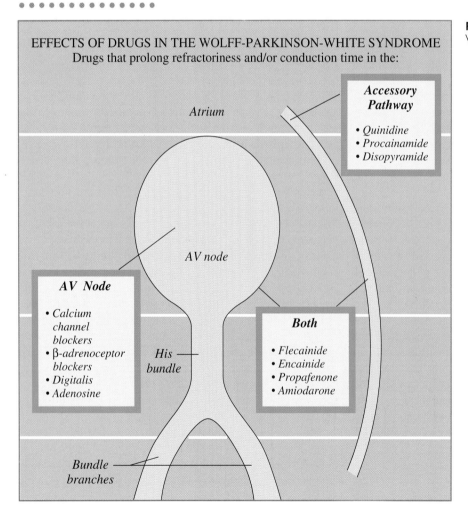

FIGURE 3.47 • Effect of drugs in the Wolff-Parkinson-White (WPW) syndrome.

distorted QRS complex and T wave. If the retrograde impulse discharges and resets the sinus node prematurely, it produces a pause that is not fully compensatory. More commonly, the sinus node and atria are not discharged prematurely by the retrograde impulse because the anterograde impulse conducting from the sinus node collides with the retrograde impulse conducted from the premature ventricular complex. Therefore, a fully compensatory pause usually follows a premature ventricular complex: the RR interval produced by the two sinus-ini- tiated QRS complexes on either side of the premature ventricular complex equals twice the normally conducted RR interval. The premature ventricular complex may not produce any pause and may therefore be interpolated (Figure 3.50). A supraventricular beat or rhythm conducted aberrantly can mimic a ventricular arrhythmia.

Ventricular fusion beats occur when the sinus-initiated beat depolarizes part of the ventricle simultaneously with the premature ventricular complex arising in the ventricle. The resul-

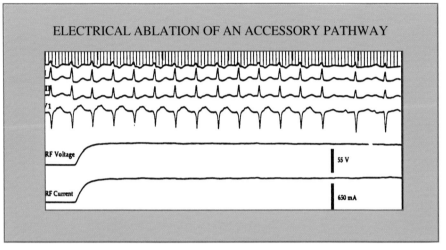

ELECTRICAL ABLATION OF AN ACCESSORY PATHWAY

RF Voltage   55 V

RF Current   650 mA

FIGURE 3.48 • Electrical ablation of an accessory pathway. During atrioventricular reentrant tachycardia, the ablation catheter is positioned next to the accessory pathway, resulting in termination at the tachycardia and elimination of accessory pathway conduction—loss of ∂ wave.

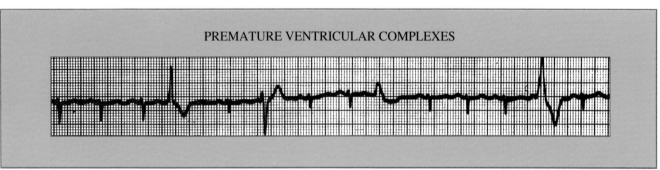

PREMATURE VENTRICULAR COMPLEXES

FIGURE 3.49 • Premature ventricular complexes of four different morphologies, each producing a compensatory pause.

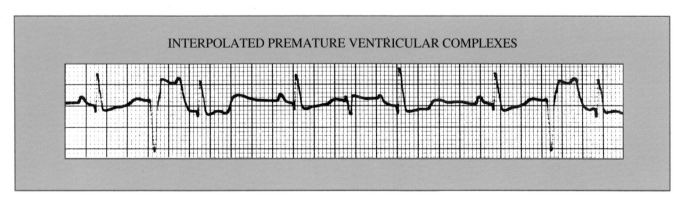

INTERPOLATED PREMATURE VENTRICULAR COMPLEXES

FIGURE 3.50 • Interpolated premature ventricular complexes. In part due to the slow sinus rate, premature ventricular complexes do not block the next sinus P wave. Rather, the latter conducts with a prolonged PR interval. Such premature ventricular complexes are called interpolated. They have no more significance than premature ventricular complexes that produce a compensatory pause except that interpolated premature ventricular complexes do not replace the next sinus initiated QRS complex, but occur in addition to it.

tant QRS complex represents a blend of the features of both beats. Premature ventricular complexes can have different contours and often are called multifocal. More properly they should be called multiform, polymorphic, or pleomorphic because it is not known whether multiple foci are discharging or whether conduction of the impulse originating from one site is merely changing (refer to Figure 3.49). The term bigeminy refers to pairs of complexes and indicates a normal and a premature complex. Trigeminy indicates a premature complex following two normal beats. Quadrigeminy indicates a premature complex following three normal beats. Two successive premature ventricular complexes are termed a pair or a couplet while three successive premature complexes are called a triplet. Arbitrarily, three or more successive premature ventricular complexes are termed ventricular tachycardia.

The importance of premature ventricular complexes varies depending on the clinical setting. In the absence of underlying heart disease, the presence of premature ventricular complexes usually adds no significance regarding longevity or limitation of activity and antiarrhythmic drugs are not indicated. The patient should be reassured if symptomatic. Premature ventricular complexes in middle-aged men and complex ventricular arrhythmias occurring in apparently healthy middle-aged men are associated with the presence of, and greater risk of subsequent death from, coronary heart disease. Similarly, more than three premature ventricular complexes per hour after myocardial infarction is associated with an increased occurence of death. However, it has not been demonstrated that these premature ventricular complexes or complex ventricular arrhythmias play a precipitating role in the genesis of sudden death in these patients and the arrhythmias may simply be a marker of heart disease. No data support the treatment of these ventricular arrhythmias with Class 1 antiarrhythmic drugs. In the Cardiac Arrhythmia Suppression Trial (CAST),[15] it was demonstrated that treatment of asymptomatic ventricular arrhythmias in patients after myocardial infarction with flecainide and encainide increased the incidence of sudden death more than threefold compared with a placebo group. Therefore, as a rule, treatment of premature ventricular complexes is not indicated, particularly in the asymptomatic patient. If the premature ventricular complexes provoke symptoms because of intolerable palpitations or consistently initiate a tachycardia, suppression therapy may be indicated. Chronic treatment should probably begin with a trial of a ß-adrenoceptor blocker, which appears to be safer than Class 1 antiarrhythmic drugs, even though it does not achieve the same degree of efficacy. Occasionally, a calcium channel blocker may be efficacious. Class 1 antiarrhythmic drugs are probably safer in patients without structural heart disease than in those who have structural heart disease, particularly coronary artery disease.

VENTRICULAR TACHYCARDIA

Ventricular tachycardia is a tachycardia that arises distal to the bifurcation of the His bundle, in specialized conduction tissue, in ventricular muscle, or in a combination of both. Ventricular tachycardia is electrocardiographically diagnosed by the presence of three or more consecutive premature ventricular complexes. The RR interval can be regular or can vary. The contour of the QRS complexes can be the same (monomorphic) or changing (polymorphic, pleomorphic, multiform), due to shifting sites of ventricular tachycardia origin or different exit paths from the same origin. Atrial activity can be independent of ventricular complexes (AV dissociation) (Figure 3.51) or the atria can be depolarized by the ventricles retrogradely (VA association) (Figure 3.52). Depending on the particular type of ventricular tachycardia, the rate ranges from 70 to 250 beats/min and the onset can be paroxysmal (sudden) or nonparoxysmal (gradual). Morphology can vary in a more or less:

- Repetitive manner—torsades de pointes.
- Alternate complexes—bidirectional ventricular tachycardia.
- Stable but changing contour—right bundle branch contour changing to left bundle branch block contour.

Ventricular tachycardia can be sustained (defined arbitrarily as lasting more than 30 sec or requiring termination be-

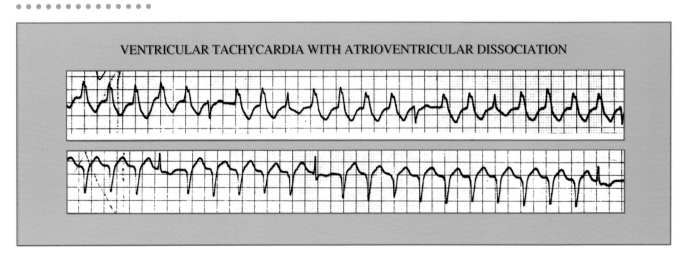

VENTRICULAR TACHYCARDIA WITH ATRIOVENTRICULAR DISSOCIATION

FIGURE 3.51 • Ventricular tachycardia with AV dissociation producing fusion and capture beats. Although atrial activity is not clearly seen, the fact that it results in fusion and capture complexes provides good likelihood that AV dissociation is present.

cause of the hemodynamic collapse) or nonsustained (unsustained, when it stops spontaneously in less than 30 sec).

Distinguishing supraventricular tachycardia with aberration from ventricular tachycardia can be difficult at times, since features of both arrhythmias overlap. Under certain circumstances an aberrantly conducted supraventricular tachycardia can mimic all the criteria established for ventricular tachycardia. Wide QRS complexes indicate only that conduction through the ventricle is abnormal and such complexes can occur in supraventricular rhythms due to preexisting bundle branch block, aberrant conduction during incomplete recovery of repolarization, conduction over accessory pathways and several other conditions. These wide QRS complexes do not necessarily indicate the origin of impulse formation or the reason for the abnormal conduction. Conversely, ectopic beats originating in the ventricle uncommonly can have a fairly normal shape and a duration of less than 120 msec.

The presence of fusion and capture beats provides maximum support for the diagnosis of ventricular tachycardia. Fusion beats indicate activation of the ventricle from two different foci, implying that one focus had a ventricular origin. Capture of the ventricles by the atria with a normal QRS for the captured complex at an RR interval shorter than the tachycardia indicates that the wide QRS complex is of ventricular origin (refer to Figure 3.51). Atrioventricular dissociation has long been considered a hallmark of ventricular tachycardia and, as a general rule, AV dissociation during a wide QRS tachycardia is strong presumptive evidence that the tachycardia is of ventricular origin. However, atrioventricular dissociation can occur uncommonly during supraventricular tachycardias. Also, retrograde VA conduction to the atria from ventricular beats occurs in a fairly large percentage of patients, and therefore ventricular tachycardia may not exhibit AV dissociation. There may be some degree of retrograde VA block, Wenckebach, 2:1, etc. Even if a P wave appears to be related to each QRS complex, it is at times difficult to determine whether the P wave is conducted anterogradely to the next QRS complex, such as supraventricular tachycardia with aberrancy and a long PR interval or retrogradely from the preceding QRS complex— a ventricular tachycardia.

Electrocardiographic features characterizing supraventricular arrhythmias with aberrancy include:
- Consistent onset of the tachycardia with a premature P wave.
- An RP interval less than 100 msec.

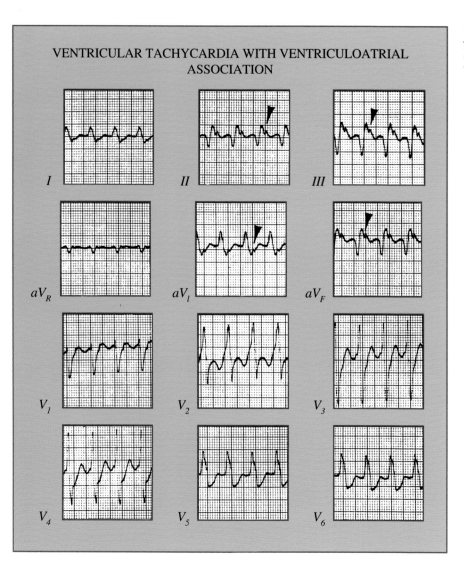

VENTRICULAR TACHYCARDIA WITH VENTRICULOATRIAL ASSOCIATION

FIGURE 3.52 • Ventricular tachycardia with ventriculoatrial association. Arrows point to retrograde atrial capture during ventricular tachycardia.

- QRS configuration the same as that which occurs from known supraventricular conduction at similar rates.
- P and QRS rate and rhythm linked to suggest that ventricular activation depends on atrial discharge—AV Wenckebach.
- Slowing or termination of the tachycardia by vagal maneuvers. It is important to remember that vagal maneuvers can terminate a rare ventricular tachycardia.

Analysis of specific QRS contours may help distinguish aberrant supraventricular conduction from a ventricular tachycardia. QRS contours suggesting a ventricular tachycardia include left axis deviation in the frontal plane and a QRS duration exceeding 140 msec with a QRS of normal duration during sinus rhythm. During ventricular tachycardia with a right bundle branch block appearance:
- The QRS complex is monophasic or biphasic in V_1 with an initial deflection different from sinus initiated QRS complex.
- The amplitude of the R wave in V_1 exceeds the R.
- Small R and large S wave or QS pattern in V_6.

With a ventricular tachycardia having a left bundle branch block contour:
- The axis may be rightward with negative deflections deeper in V_1 than in V_6.
- A broad, prolonged, greater than 40 msec R wave in V_1.
- A small Q, large R wave or QS pattern in V_6.

A QRS complex that is similar in V_1 through V_6, either all negative or all positive, favors a ventricular origin, as does the presence of 2:1 VA block. An upright QRS complex in V_1 through V_6 also can occur due to conduction over a left-sided accessory pathway. Supraventricular beats with aberration often have a triphasic pattern in V_1 with the initial vector of the abnormal complex similar to that of the normally conducted beats, and the aberrant QRS complex terminating a short cycle

that follows a long cycle (long-short cycle sequence). A grossly irregular wide QRS tachycardia with ventricular rates exceeding 200 beats/min should raise the question of atrial fibrillation with conduction over an accessory pathway (refer to Figure 3.45). In the presence of a preexisting bundle branch block, a wide QRS tachycardia with a contour different from that which occurred during sinus rhythm is most likely ventricular tachycardia. Because exceptions exist to all of these criteria, often one must rely on sound clinical judgment, considering the ECG as only one of several helpful ancillary tests.

Symptoms occurring during ventricular tachycardia depend on the ventricular rate, duration of the tachycardia, the presence and extent of the underlying heart disease and peripheral vascular disease. The location of impulse formation and therefore the way the depolarization waves spread across the myocardium also may be important.

More than half of the patients treated for symptomatic recurrent ventricular tachycardia have coronary heart disease. The next largest group has cardiomyopathy—both congestive and hypertrophic—with lesser percentages divided among those with primary electrical disease, mitral valve prolapse, valvular heart disease and miscellaneous causes. In patients resuscitated from sudden cardiac death, 75% have severe coronary artery disease. Ventricular tachyarrhythmias can be induced by premature ventricular stimulation in approximately 75%. When ventricular tachycardia occurs in the ambulatory patient, it is commonly induced by a late premature ventricular complex rather than R on T premature ventricular complexes.

Generally, the most important therapeutic decision is deciding which patient should receive treatment. The relative risks of symptoms or sudden death for each type of ventricular tachycardia determine the course of therapy. Usually patients who have sustained ventricular tachycardia with or without structural heart disease and those who have symptomatic non-sustained ventricular tachycardia, particularly if it is associated

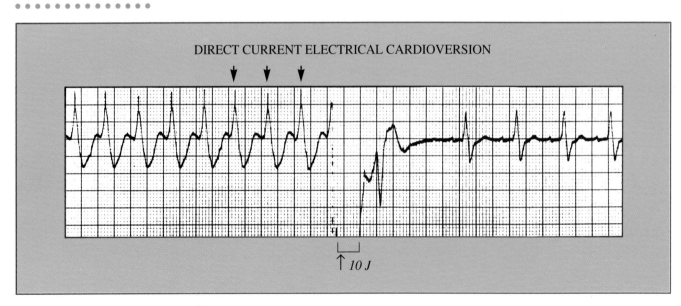

DIRECT CURRENT ELECTRICAL CARDIOVERSION

↑ 10 J

FIGURE 3.53 • Direct current electrical cardioversion with 10 J terminates sustained ventricular tachycardia with restoration of sinus rhythm. The upward arrow indicates delivery of the shock while the downward arrows indicate synchronization of the cardioverter to each QRS complex.

with structural heart disease, are treated. There are no data to support treating asymptomatic patients who have nonsustained ventricular tachycardia, particularly in the absence of structural heart disease. While patients who have structural heart disease and nonsustained ventricular tachycardia are at increased risk for morbidity, there are no data to support treating those patients with antiarrhythmic therapy. Patients who have asymptomatic nonsustained ventricular tachycardia and are otherwise healthy may not need therapy and should be followed closely.

Acute termination of ventricular tachycardia that does not cause hemodynamic decompensation can be attempted by administering IV lidocaine or procainamide according to the doses mentioned earlier. If one of these drugs abolishes the ventricular tachycardia, a continuous IV infusion can be given. Procainamide is more successful than lidocaine. Although quinidine can be used intravenously, great caution is needed because of hypotension. If maximum doses of lidocaine or procainamide are unsuccessful, bretylium can be tried. Amiodarone is effective intravenously, although this method of administration has not been approved by the FDA.

If the ventricular tachycardia does not respond to medical therapy or if it precipitates hypotension, angina, congestive heart failure or symptoms of cerebral hypoperfusion, electrical direct current (DC) cardioversion should be used promptly. Very low en-

ergies can terminate monomorphic ventricular tachycardia, beginning with a synchronized shock of 10 to 25 J (Figure 3.53). Digitalis-induced ventricular tachycardia is best treated pharmacologically. After reversion of the arrhythmia to a normal rhythm, it is essential to institute measures to prevent a recurrence.

Striking the patient's chest, sometimes called "thump version," can terminate ventricular tachycardia mechanically by inducing a premature ventricular complex that presumably interrupts the reentrant pathway necessary to support the ventricular tachycardia. Stimulation at the time of the vulnerable period during ventricular tachycardia can accelerate the ventricular tachycardia or possibly provoke ventricular fibrillation.

In patients with recurrent ventricular tachycardia, a pacing catheter can be inserted into the right ventricle and single, double or multiple stimuli can be introduced competitively to terminate the ventricular tachycardia (Figure 3.54). This procedure incurs the risk of accelerating the ventricular tachycardia to ventricular flutter or ventricular fibrillation. A new catheter electrode has been developed through which synchronized cardioversion can be performed (Figure 3.55). Intermittent ventricular tachycardia, interrupted by several supraventricular beats, is generally best treated pharmacologically.

A search for reversible conditions contributing to the initiation and maintenance of ventricular tachycardia should be

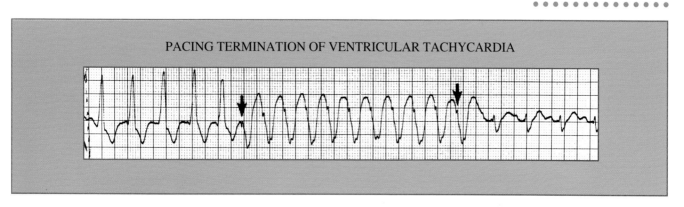

FIGURE 3.54 • Pacing termination of ventricular tachycardia. A ventricular tachycardia at a rate of 125 beats/min is interrupted by 11 paced complexes (between arrows) at a rate of 175 beats/min. Sinus rhythm follows termination of pacing.

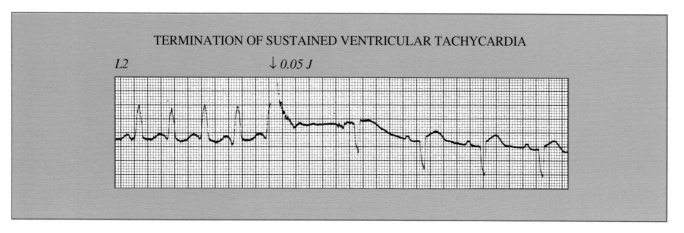

FIGURE 3.55 • A very small amount of energy (0.05 J) delivered over a special catheter placed in the apex of the right ventricle terminates sustained ventricular tachycardia.

made and the conditions corrected if possible. For example, ventricular tachycardia related to ischemia, hypotension or hypokalemia at times may be terminated by antianginal treatment, vasopressors or potassium, respectively. Correction of heart failure can reduce the frequency of ventricular arrhythmias. Slow rates that are caused by sinus bradycardia or AV block can permit the occurrence of premature ventricular complexes and ventricular tachyarrhythmias that can be corrected by administering atropine, or isoproternol temporarily (cautiously), or by transvenous pacing.

Prevention of recurrent ventricular tachycardia is generally more difficult than terminating the acute episode. Initial preventive drug therapy should involve one of the Class 1A drugs such as quinidine, procainamide or disopyramide. Class 1B drugs can be tried next. The Class 1C drugs flecainide and encainide* should be used cautiously. Amiodarone, despite its list of side effects, can be tested.

Specific qualities of a drug can influence choices, and selection is often prejudiced by the drug's side effects. For example, disopyramide should probably not be given to a patient with congestive heart failure, while Class 1B drugs might be chosen early for a patient whose QT interval is prolonged. One group of patients may have a unique form of ventricular tachycardia provoked by activity or catecholamine release, which is suppressed by adenosine, vagal maneuvers, ß-adrenoceptor blockade and verapamil. Verapamil can be effective in some other types of ventricular tachycardia. While propranolol reduces sudden death after myocardial infarction, it does not do so to a greater degree in patients with complex ventricular arrhythmias. This may be because it is effective via an antiischemic mechanism.

When single drugs fail, combinations of drugs with different mechanisms of action can be successful and allow one to use low doses of both agents rather than higher toxic doses of a single drug. Most of the combinations represent empiric trials, but one generally attempts to combine drugs to which the patient has exhibited a partial therapeutic response.

Implantation of a cardioverter/defibrillator that delivers competitive pacing therapy, low energy synchronous cardioversion and high energy defibrillation shocks should be considered for patients with drug-resistant recurrent ventricular tachycardia. Surgical (refer to Figure 3.11) and catheter ablation techniques (Figure 3.56) are effective in some patients. Candidates generally are patients who do not tolerate or whose arrhythmias are not controlled by drugs.

Ventricular Tachycardia Associated with Specific Clinical Syndromes

Coronary artery disease is the most common cause of ventricular tachycardia, with dilated cardiomyopathy as the next most frequent. Ventricular tachycardia can occur in patients with arrhythmogenic right ventricular dysplasia and generally has a left bundle branch block contour, often with right axis deviation. Tetralogy of Fallot with ventricular tachycardia at the site of previous surgery, hypertrophic cardiomyopathies, mitral valve prolapse, catecholamine sensitive ventricular tachycardia and ventricular tachycardia occurring in the absence of recognizable structural heart disease are all well-established clinical entitites.

Several fairly specific types of ventricular tachycardia have been identified, related either to a constellation of distinctive electrocardiographic and electrophysiologic features or to a specific set of clinical events.

Accelerated Idioventricular Rhythm • The ventricular rhythm rate, often 70-110 beats/min, usually is within 10 beats of the sinus rate so that ventricular tachycardia and sinus tachycardia commonly interchange. Fusion and capture beats are common (Figure 3.57). Onset of this arrhythmia is often gradual and occurs when the sinus rate slows or AV block develops,

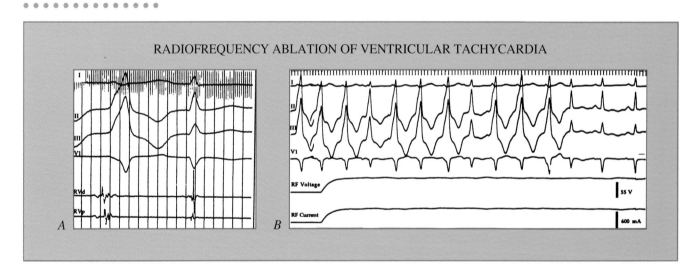

FIGURE 3.56 • Radiofrequency ablation of ventricular tachycardia. Positioning the catheter electrode at the site of ventricular tachycardia origin (A) is followed by delivery of radiofrequency energy with elimination of the ventricular tachycardia (B). (Reproduced with permission. Zipes DP: Management of cardiac arrhythmias. In: Braunwald E, ed. *Heart Disease. The Textbook of Cardiovascular Medicine* Philadelphia, Pa: WB Saunders; 1992. In press.)

*Withdrawn from the market

allowing escape of the ventricular tachycardia. Suppressive therapy rarely is necessary because the ventricular rate is ordinarily less than 100 beats/min and well tolerated. Often simply increasing the sinus rate with atropine or atrial pacing suppresses the accelerated idioventricular rhythm, if therapy is necessary.

Torsades de Pointes • The term torsades de pointes refers to a ventricular tachycardia characterized by QRS complexes of changing amplitude that appear to twist around the isoelectric line and occur at rates of 200 to 250 beats/min (Figure 3.58). Torsades de pointes connotes a syndrome—not simply an ECG description of a polymorphic ventricular tachycardia—that includes prolonged ventricular repolarization with QT intervals exceeding 440 to 470 msec. The U wave may also become prominent but its role in the syndrome and in the long QT syndrome in general is not clear. Striking T wave alternans can be present

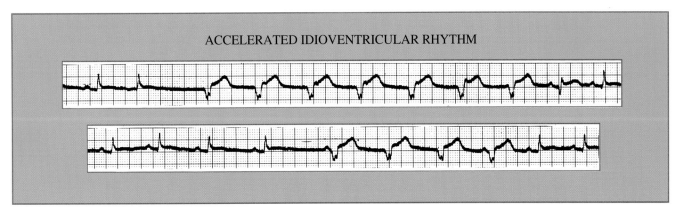

FIGURE 3.57 • Accelerated idioventricular rhythm. In this continuous recording of lead 2, a premature atrial complex in the top strip provides a sufficient pause for the escape of an accelerated idioventricular rhythm which terminates as the sinus rate speeds to regain control. In the bottom recording, sinus slowing allows the accelerated idioventricular rhythm to become manifest for a short while. Fusion complexes (second from the end in the top strip) and capture complexes (second from the end in the bottom strip) are common.

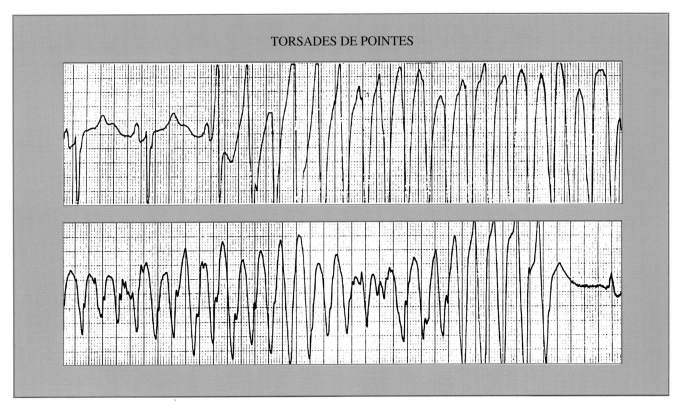

FIGURE 3.58 • Torsades de pointes. Patient developed syncope after being treated with amiodarone. 24-hour electrocardiographic recording revealed the presence of a long QT interval and episodes of polymorphic ventricular tachycardia characteristic of torsades de pointes. (Reproduced with permission. Zipes DP: Assessment of electrical abnormalities. In: Hurst JW, Schlant RC, Rackley CE, et al, eds. The Heart New York, NY: McGraw Hill; 1990:347.)

(Figure 3.59). Premature ventricular complexes may discharge during the termination of the T wave, precipitating successive bursts of ventricular tachycardia during which the peaks of the QRS complexes appear successively on one side and then on the other side of the isoelectric baseline, giving the typical twisting appearance with continuous and progressive changes in QRS contour and amplitude. Ventricular tachycardia often starts with a short interval following a long RR interval and terminates with progressive prolongation of cycle lengths and larger, more distinctly formed QRS complexes. Two primary causes have been recognized: congenital (idiopathic) and acquired, most commonly due to severe bradycardia, potassium depletion and drugs such as quinidine and disopyramide.

Management consists of an increase in the heart rate by atrial or ventricular pacing, or isoproterenol administered cautiously if pacing is not available. IV magnesium has been shown to suppress the acquired torsades de pointes. In the congenital form, long-term ß-adrenoceptor blockade, left stellate surgical interruption, long-term pacing at increased rates and an implantable cardioverter/defibrillator may be indicated.

The Long QT Syndrome • The long QT syndrome is characterized by a corrected QT interval exceeding 440 msec, according to the worldwide QT registry, but longer than 460 msec for men and 470 msec for women, according to other information. Two major causes are responsible. Primary or idio-

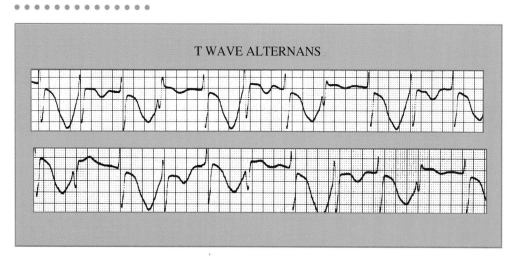

FIGURE 3.59 • T wave alternans. Striking T wave alternation can be seen during this junctional rhythm. The QT interval exceeds 600 msec.

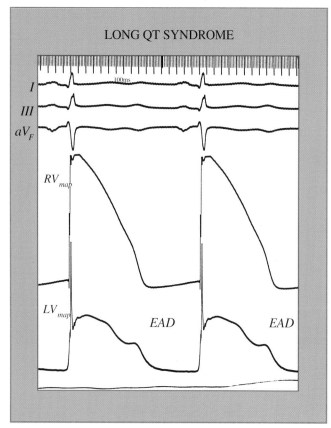

FIGURE 3.60 • Long QT syndrome and early afterdepolarizations. Right and left ventricular endocardial recordings in a patient with the idiopathic (congenital) long QT syndrome reveals a prominent "hump" during repolarization in the left ventricular recording characteristic of an early afterdepolarization.

pathic long QT syndrome is a congenital abnormality, often familial, sometimes but not always associated with deafness. Patients have the long QT syndrome from birth. The second cause is acquired due to:

- Various drugs such as quinidine, disopyramide, phenothiazine or tricyclic antidepressants.
- Metabolic abnormalities such as hypokalemia or hypocalcemia, the consequences of liquid protein diets and starvation.
- Central nervous system lesions, autonomic nervous system dysfunction, coronary artery disease with myocardial infarction.
- Cardiac ganglionitis and mitral valve prolapse.
- Severe bradycardia.

Symptomatic patients with long QT syndrome develop ventricular tachycardias that in many instances are due to torsades de pointes (refer to Figure 3.58). Should the ventricular tachycardia become sustained, sudden death may result. Patients with congenital long QT syndrome who are at increased risk for sudden death include those who have family members who died suddenly at an early age and those who have experienced syncope. Electrocardiograms should be obtained for all family members when the propositus presents with symptoms. The patient should undergo prolonged ECG recording with various stresses designed to evoke ventricular arrhythmias, such as auditory stimuli, psychological stress, cold pressor stimulation and exercise. Valsalva may lengthen the QT interval and cause T wave alternans. Catecholamines may produce ventricular arrhythmias as may stellate ganglion stimulation. Cardiac recordings can reveal the presence of early afterdepolarizations (Figure 3.60).

Treatment in asymptomatic patients with complex ventricular arrhythmias or a family history of premature sudden cardiac death consists of ß-blockers at maximally tolerated doses. Patients with syncope receive ß-blockers at maximally tolerated doses at times combined with phenytoin and phenobarbital. Syncope despite drug treatment requires further therapy, often left-sided cervicothoracic sympathetic ganglionectomy that interrupts the stellate ganglion and the first three or four thoracic ganglia, implantation of cardioverter/defibrillator, or chronic pacing.

Bidirectional Ventricular Tachycardia • This is an uncommon ventricular tachycardia characterized by QRS complexes with a right bundle branch block pattern, alternating polarity in the frontal plane from -60° to -90°, to +120° to +130° and a regular rhythm (Figure 3.61). Digitalis excess is a common cause and requires prompt treatment with cessation of digitalis, and administration of lidocaine, potassium, phenytoin or propranolol.

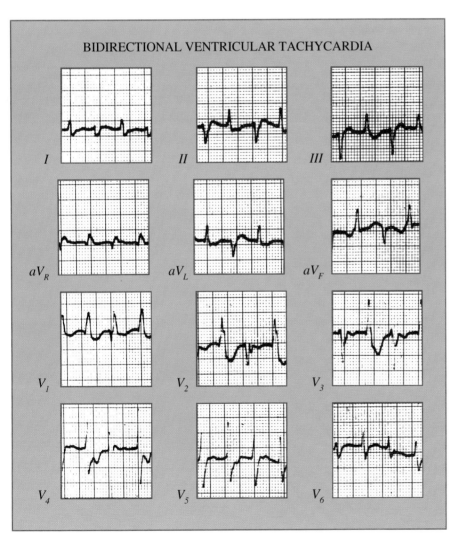

BIDIRECTIONAL VENTRICULAR TACHYCARDIA

I   *II*   *III*

aV_R aV_L aV_F

V_1 V_2 V_3

V_4 V_5 V_6

FIGURE 3.61 • Bidirectional ventricular tachycardia. Characteristic electrocardiographic presentation (refer to text) of this ventricular tachycardia due, in this instance, to digitalis toxicity. (Reproduced with permission. Morris SN, Zipes DP: *Circulation* 1973;48:323.)

Repetitive Monomorphic Ventricular Tachycardia • Repetitive monomorphic ventricular tachycardia is defined as three or more consecutive premature ventricular complexes with only brief periods of intervening sinus complexes. Ventricular complexes generally occur in groups of 3 to 15, but occasionally the ventricular tachycardia may be almost continuous. Ventricular tachycardia is often regular, with rates of 100 to 150 beats/min, sometimes becoming as rapid as 250 beats/min. Episodes of ventricular tachycardia tend to cluster around certain time periods for an individual patient. Often no or minimal structural heart disease is present and the patient is young. The right ventricular outflow tract may be the site of the ventricular tachycardia. Often, it is benign and the outlook is favorable, with infrequent arrhythmia related deaths. The arrhythmia may disappear with time, perhaps accounting for its reduced prevalence in older populations. Therapy is reserved for patients who are symptomatic with palpitations, syncope or near syncope and is the same as for ventricular tachycardia. Catheter radiofrequency ablation can be particularly effective in selected patients.

Bundle Branch Reentrant Ventricular Tachycardia • Ventricular tachycardia due to bundle branch reentry is characterized by a QRS morphology determined by the circuit established over the bundle branches. Retrograde conduction over the left bundle branch system and anterograde conduction over the right bundle branch is most common and creates a QRS complex with a left bundle branch block contour and a frontal plane axis of about +30°. Bundle branch reentrant ventricular tachycardia has been demonstrated to occur more frequently in patients who have dilated cardiomyopathy and can be interrupted by ablation of the right bundle branch.

VENTRICULAR FLUTTER/FIBRILLATION

Ventricular flutter (Figure 3.62) and fibrillation (Figure 3.63) represent severe derangements of the heart beat, usually resulting in syncope, seizures and apnea, eventually followed by death within 3 to 5 min unless stopped. Blood pressure is unobtainable and heart sounds are absent. Ventricular flutter presents as a sine wave with regular large oscillations at 150 to 300 beats/min, while ventricular fibrillation has irregular undulations of varying contour and amplitude without distinct QRS complexes, ST segments and T waves. Ventricular flutter and fibrillation occur in a variety of clinical situations, most commonly associated with coronary artery disease and as a terminal event.

Treatment consists of immediate nonsynchronized DC electrical shock using 200 to 400 J. Cardiopulmonary resuscitation is employed only until defibrillation equipment is ready. Time should not be wasted with cardiopulmonary resuscitation maneuvers if electrical defibrillation can be done promptly. If the circulation is markedly inadequate despite return to sinus rhythm, closed chest massage with artificial ventilation as needed should be instituted. Anesthesia during the electrical shock is generally not indicated because the patient is uncon-

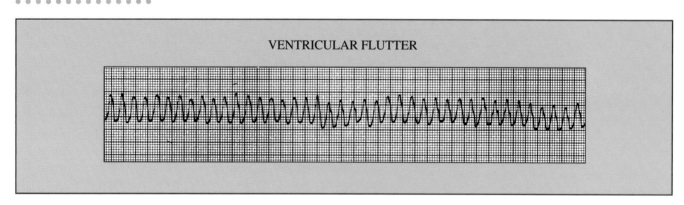

FIGURE 3.62 • Ventricular flutter. Sine wave in appearance, ventricular flutter presents at a rate of more than 300 beats/min.

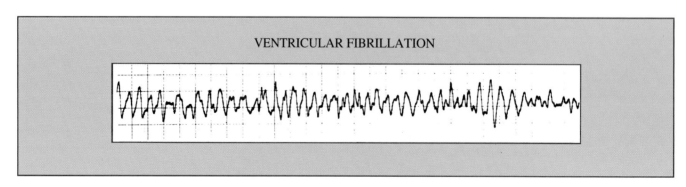

FIGURE 3.63 • Ventricular fibrillation. Large irregular chaotic undulations without any clear QRS complex or T wave characterize ventricular fibrillation.

For asymptomatic patients with congenital complete AV block who maintain an escape rate exceeding 50 beats/min over a 24-hr period, generally no therapy is indicated. If they have syncope, near syncope or ventricular rates less than 50 beats/min, permanent pacing generally is indicated. For patients with symptomatic, chronic type 1 second degree AV block or asymptomatic, type 2 second degree or third degree (Figure 3.69) AV block, pacing is indicated.

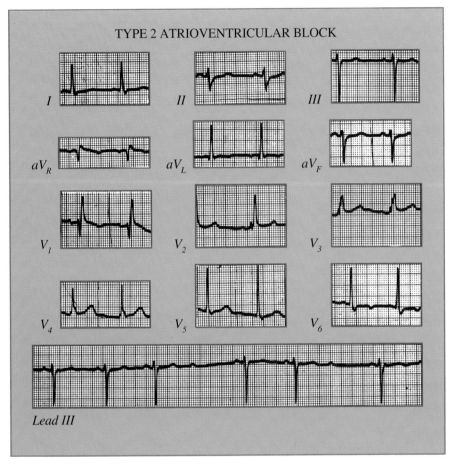

TYPE 2 ATRIOVENTRICULAR BLOCK

I
II
III
aV$_R$
aV$_L$
aV$_F$
V$_1$
V$_2$
V$_3$
V$_4$
V$_5$
V$_6$

Lead III

FIGURE 3.67 • Type 2, second degree atrioventricular block, right bundle branch block and left anterior hemiblock is present in this 12 lead ECG. In the rhythm strip below, nonconducted P waves occur without antecedent PR prolongation.

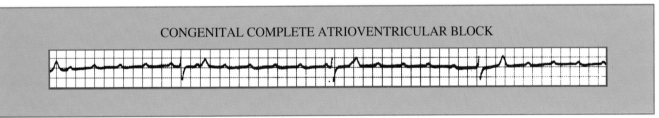

CONGENITAL COMPLETE ATRIOVENTRICULAR BLOCK

FIGURE 3.68 • Congenital complete atrioventricular (AV) block. A normal QRS complex occurs at a rate of about 20/min in this youngster with symptomatic AV nodal congenital complete AV block.

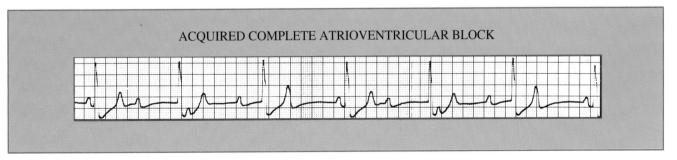

ACQUIRED COMPLETE ATRIOVENTRICULAR BLOCK

FIGURE 3.69 • Acquired complete atrioventricular (AV) block. Ventricular escapes at a rate of 38 beats/min characterize this example of acquired complete AV block due to disease in the His-Purkinje system.

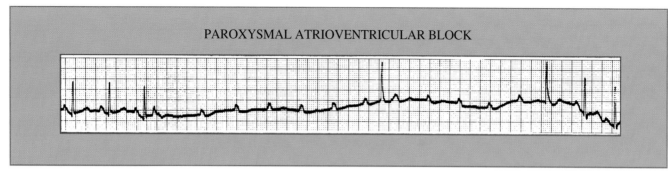

PAROXYSMAL ATRIOVENTRICULAR BLOCK

FIGURE 3.70 • Paroxysmal atrioventricular (AV) block during sinus rhythm. A nonconducted premature atrial complex initiates a period of paroxysmal AV block punctuated by two escape beats and then resumption of sinus rhythm.

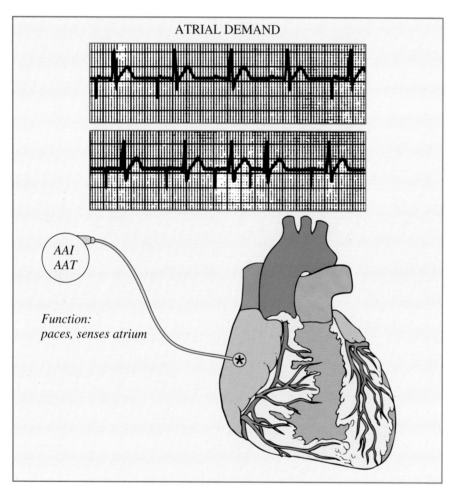

ATRIAL DEMAND

AAI
AAT

Function:
paces, senses atrium

FIGURE 3.71 • Atrial demand pacemakers (AAI, AAT). The atrial demand pacemaker is connected to the right atrium (A). The lead termination is marked with (o) to indicate that the pacemaker senses atrial cardiac activity and an (*) indicates that it stimulates in the atrium. Representative ECGs produced by atrial inhibited (AAI, upper tracing) and atrial triggered (AAT, lower tracing) pacing. In the upper tracing, the first, second, and fifth atrial complexes are pacemaker-induced. The third and fourth atrial complexes are spontaneous and reset pacemaker timing while inhibiting delivery of the stimulus. In the lower tracing, the first, second, and fifth atrial complexes are pacemaker-induced. The third and fourth atrial complexes are spontaneous and reset pacemaker timing while triggering delivery of the stimulus into refractory atrial tissue. Note that the stimulus is delivered after the onset of the third and fourth P waves but initiates the other P waves. (Reproduced with permission. Zipes DP, Duffin EG: Cardiac pacemakers. In: Braunwald E, ed *Heart Disease. A Textbook of Cardiovascular Medicine* Philadephia, Pa: WB Saunders; 1988:722.)

Less common forms of AV block, such as paroxysmal AV block (Figure 3.70) do not have clear electrophysiologic explanation but result in near syncope and syncope and require permanent pacing (Figures 3.71-3.73).

PARASYSTOLE

Parasystole is due to (probable) automatic discharge of a focus in the atrium, ventricle or specialized tissue which produces a regular discharge that is independent of, and partially or fully protected from, discharge by the dominant cardiac rhythm. Parasystole is most likely due to phase 4 diastolic depolarization and the discharge rate and rhythm can be modified by the dominant rhythm (Figure 3.74). Electrocardiographically, parasystole produces:

- Varying coupling intervals between the parasystolic complex and the dominant, generally sinus initiated, complex.
- A common minimal time interval between manifest interectopic intervals so that the longer interectopic intervals are multiples of the minimum interval.
- Fusion complexes.
- The presence of the parasystolic initiated depolarization whenever the cardiac chamber in which it originates is excitable.

Parasystole with exit block may result when the parasystolic discharge focus fails to appear even though the chamber in which it originates is fully excitable (refer to Figure 3.74). Usually, therapy is not required.

ANTIARRHYTHMIC OPTIONS IN THE FUTURE

In this chapter on treatment of arrhythmias and conduction abnormalities, I have reviewed the various therapeutic antiarrhythmic options—beginning with general discussions on drug selections, followed by current nonpharmacologic choices, and ending with specific treatments for the individual cardiac arrhythmias. The wide array of therapeutic options—never before available—is a culmination of knowledge that has evolved over several decades. As our understanding of cardiac electrophysiology continues to evolve, further advances will be possible.

In the future, newer antiarrhythmic agents, particularly potassium channel blockers, may further improve drug efficacy. However, because antiarrhythmic drugs often exhibit an

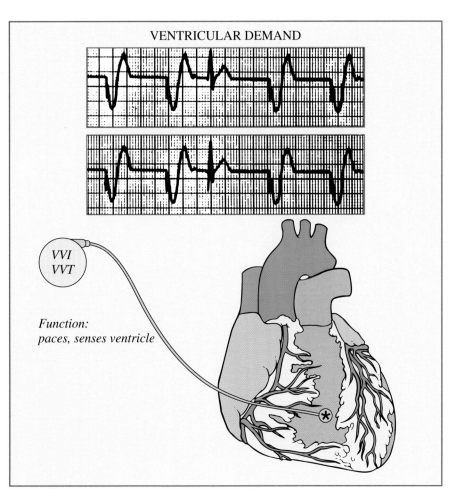

VENTRICULAR DEMAND

VVI
VVT

Function:
paces, senses ventricle

FIGURE 3.72 • Ventricular demand pacemakers (VVI, VVT). The ventricular demand pacemaker is connected to the right ventricle, with a (o) and an (*) at the lead termination to indicate that the pacemaker senses ventricular cardiac activity and stimulates in the ventricle (A). Representative ECGs produced by ventricular inhibited (VVI, upper tracing) and ventricular triggered (VVT, lower tracing) pacing. In the upper tracing, the first, second, fourth, and fifth ventricular complexes are pacemaker-induced. The third ventricular complex results from normally conducted sinus activity. This ventricular complex resets the pacemaker timing and inhibits delivery of the ventricular stimulus. In the lower tracing, the first, second, fourth, and fifth ventricular complexes are pacemaker-induced. The third ventricular complex results form normally conducted sinus activity. This ventricular complex resets pacemaker timing and triggers delivery of the stimulus into the refractory ventricular tissue. Note that the stimulus is delivered after the onset of the third QRS complex but initiates the other QRS complexes. (Reproduced with permission. Zipes DP, Duffin EG: Cardiac pacemakers. In: Braunwald E, ed. *Heart Disease. A Textbook of Cardiovascular Medicine* Philadephia, Pa: WB Saunders; 1988:722.)

unacceptably high degree of inefficacy in patients with serious tachyarrhythmias, and because patients often develop drug intolerance, nonpharmacologic therapies have achieved increased interest and application.

During the next decade, the implantable cardioverter-defibrillator for patients with life-threatening ventricular tachyarrhythmias, will become more sophisticated, providing in their memories and recording systems a wealth of information on tachycardia onset and response to treatment, improved accuracy in tachycardia recognition and identification, as well as flexibility in therapeutic choices—pacing, cardioversion, and defibrillation. Furthermore, device size will diminish and nonthoracotomy placement will become the preferred implantation route. Ultimately, prophylactic insertion in patients at high risk of developing ventricular fibrillation may occur.

The latest advance—one that is revolutionizing clinical electrophysiology—is the use of radiofrequency ablation with a catheter in the heart to eradicate cardiac tissue that is a necessary substrate for the tachycardia. In patients with artrioventricular (AV) nodal and AV reentrant tachycardias, and selected patients with ventricular tachycardias, successful elimination of tachycardias by RF ablation is high, with minimal risks and side effects. In the future, this form of therapy will be offered increasingly as an initial therapeutic option for patients with many kinds of symptomatic recurrent tachycardias.

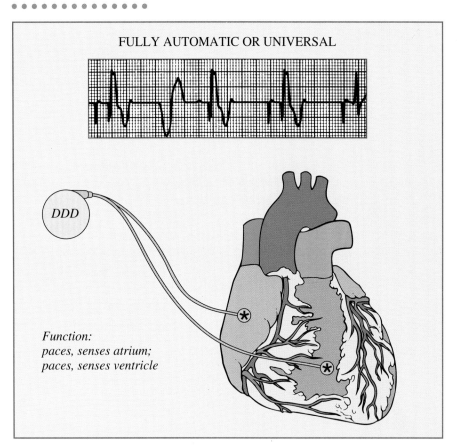

FULLY AUTOMATIC OR UNIVERSAL

DDD

Function:
paces, senses atrium;
paces, senses ventricle

FIGURE 3.73 • Fully automatic or universal pacemaker (DDD). DDD pacemaker with leads connected to the right atrium and ventricle. (*) and (o) at the atrial and ventricular lead terminations indicate that the pacemaker paces and senses in both atrium and ventricle (A). Representative ECG produced by DDD pacing. The first and fourth cardiac cycles, each preceded by two stimulus artifacts, are produced by atrial and ventricular sequential stimulation. The second QRS complex is a PVC, which resets all pacemaker timing and inhibits pacing. The third QRS complex is the result of ventricular pacing triggered by the pacemaker's sensing of the preceding sinus atrial event. The fifth QRS complex is the normally conducted result of atrial pacing. (Reproduced with permission. Zipes DP, Duffin EG: Cardiac pacemakers. In: Braunwald E, ed. *Heart Disease. A Textbook of Cardiovascular Medicine* Philadephia, Pa: WB Saunders;1988:725)

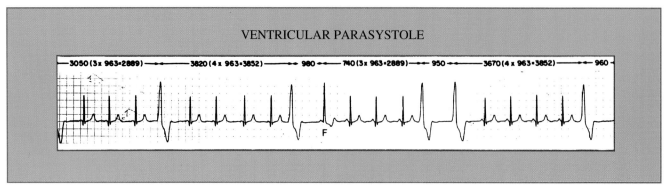

VENTRICULAR PARASYSTOLE

FIGURE 3.74 • Ventricular parasystole. Measured intervals between premature ventricular complexes are indicated in msec. Numbers in parentheses indicate multiples of a basic cycle length determined as the main interval between parasystolic discharge. (Reproduced with permission. Zipes DP: Cardiac electrophysiology: Promises and contributions. *J Am Coll Cardiol* 1989;13:1329.)

REFERENCES

1. Hurst JW, Anderson RH, Becker AE, Wilcox BR: *Atlas of the Heart.* New York, NY: Gower Medical Publishing; 1988.

2. Zipes DP, Jalife J, eds.: *Cardiac Electrophysiology. From Cell to Bedside.* Philadelphia, Pa: WB Saunders; 1990.

3. Woosley RL, Funck-Brentano C: Overview of the clinical pharmacology of antiarrhythmic drugs. *Am J Cardiol* 1988;61:61A.

4. Singh B, Courtney KP: The classification of antiarrhythmic mechanisms of drug action: Experimental and clinical considerations. In: Zipes DP, Jalife J, eds. *Cardiac Electrophysiology. From Cell to Bedside* Philadelphia, Pa: WB Saunders;1990:882.

5. Hondeghem LM: Molecular interactions of antiarrhythmic agents with their receptor sites. In: Zipes DP, Jalife J, eds. *Cardiac Electrophysiology. From Cell to Bedside.* Philadelphia, Pa: WB Saunders; 1990:865.

6. Davidenko JM, Cohn L, Goodrow R, et al.: Quinidine-induced action potential prolongation, early afterdepolarizations, and triggered activity in canine Purkinje fibers. Effects of stimulation rate, potassium and magnesium. *Circulation* 1989;79:674.

7. Roden DM, Hoffman BF: Action potential prolongation and induction of abnormal automaticity by low quinidine concentrations in canine Purkinje fibers. *Circ Res* 1985;56:857.

8. Gorgels APM, van den Doll A, Hofs A, et al.: Procainamide is superior to lidocaine in terminating sustained ventricular tachycardia. *Circulation* 1989;80:652.

9. MacMahon S, Collins R, Peto R, et al.: Effects of prophylactic lidocaine in suspected acute myocardial infarction. *JAMA* 1988;260:1910.

10. Kim SG, Mercando AD, Tam S, et al.: Combination of disopyramide and mexiletine for better tolerance and additive effects for treatment of ventricular arrhythmias. *J Am Coll Cardiol* 1989;13:659.

11. Dorian P, Echt DS, Mead RH, et al.: Ethmozine: Electrophysiology, hemodynamics and antiarrhythmic efficacy in patients with life-threatening ventricular arrhythmias. *Am Heart J* 1986;1112:327.

12. Capparelli EV, Kluger J, Regnier JC, Chow MS: Clinical and electrophysiologic effects of flecainide in patients with refractory ventricular tachycardia. *J Clin Pharm* 1988;28:268.

13. Yusuf S, Wittes J, Friedman L: Overview of results of randomized clinical trials in heart disease. 1. Treatments following myocardial infarction. *JAMA* 1988;260:2088.

14. Anderson JL, Pritchett ELC: International symposium on supraventricular arrhythmias: focus on flecainide. *Am J Cardiol* 1988;62:1D.

15. The Cardiac Arrhythmias Suppression Trial (CAST) investigators: Preliminary report: effective encainide and flecainide on mortality in a randomized trial of arrhythmia suppression after myocardial infarction. *N Engl J Med* 1989;321:406.

16. The Encainide-Ventricular Tachycardia Study Group: Treatment of life-threatening ventricular tachycardia with encainide hydrochloride in patients with left ventricular function. *Am J Cardiol* 1988;62:571.

17. Miles WM, Zipes DP, Rinkenberger RL, et al.: Encainide for treatment of atrioventricular reciprocating tachycardia in the Wolff-Parkinson-White syndrome. *Am J Cardiol* 1988;62:20L.

18. Funck-Brentano C, Kroemer HK, Lee JT, et al.: Propafenone. *N Engl J Med* 1990;322:518.

19. Duff HJ, Mitchell LB, Wyse DG: Antiarrhythmic efficacy of propranolol: Comparison of low and high serum concentrations. *J Am Coll Cardiol* 1986;8:959.

20. Furberg GCD, Byington RP: Beta adrenergic blockers in patients with acute myocardial infarction. *Cardiovasc Clin* 1989;20:235.

21. Herre JM, Sauve MJ, Malone P, et al.: Long-term results of amiodarone therapy in patients with recurrent sustained ventricular tachycardia or ventricular fibrillation. *J Am Coll Cardiol* 1989;13:442

22. Weinberg B, Dusman R, Stanton M, et al.: Five year follow-up of 590 patients treated with amiodarone. *PACE* 1989;12:642.

23. Dusman RE, Stanton MS, Miles WM, et al.: Clinical features of amiodarone-induced pulmonary toxicity. *Circulation* 1990;82:51.

24. Belhassen B, Glick A, Laniado S: Comparative clinical and electrophysiologic effects of adenosine triphosphate and verapamil on paroxysmal reciprocating junctional tachycardia. *Circulation* 1988;77:795.

25. Huycke EC, Sung RJ, Dias VC, et al.: Intravenous diltiazem for termination of reentrant supraventricular tachycardia: A placebo-controlled, randomized, double-blind multicenters study. *J Am Coll Cardiol* 1989;13:538.

26. Belardinelli L: Cardiac electrophysiology and pharmacology of adenosine. *J Cardiovasc Electrophys* 1990.

27. DiMarco JP: Electrophysiology of adenosine. *J Cardiovasc Electrophys* 1990.

28. Scheinman MM, Morady F: Catheter ablation for treatment of supraventricular arrhythmias. In: Zipes DP, Jalife J, eds. *Cardiac Electrophysiology. From Cell to Bedside* Philadelphia, Pa: WB Saunders; 1990:970.

29. Borggrefe M, Hindricks G, Haverkamp W, et al.: Radiofrequency ablation. In: Zipes DP, Jalife J, eds. *Cardiac Electrophysiology. From Cell to Bedside.* Philadelphia, Pa: WB Saunders; 1990:997.

30. Evans GT, Scheinman MM, Zipes DP, et al.: The percutaneous cardiac mapping and ablation registry: Final summary of results. *PACE* 1988;11:1621.

31. Evans GT, Scheinman MM, Akhtar M, et al.: In-hospital mortality after direct current catheter ablation of the atrioventricular junction: A prospective international multi-center study. Submitted.

32. Borggrefe M, Breithardt G, Podozeck A, et al.: Catheter ablation of ventricular tachycardia using defibrillator pulses: electrophysiological findings and long-term results. *Eur Heart J* 1989;10:591.

33. Fontaine G, Frank R, Tonet J, et al.: Full duration of chronic ventricular tachycardia: Results of 47 consecutive cases with a follow-up ranging from 11 to 65 months. In: Zipes DP, Jalife J, eds. *Cardiac Electrophysiology. From Cell to Bedside.* Philadelphia, Pa: WB Saunders; 1990: 978.

34. Inoue H, Waller BE, Zipes DP: Intracoronary ethyl alcohol or phenol injection ablates a conitine-induced ventricular tachycardia in the dog. *J Am Coll Cardiol* 1987;10:1342.

35. Brugada P, Deswart H, Smeets J, et al.: Transcoronary termination and ablation of ventricular tachycardia. *Circulation* 1989;79:475.

36. Sosa EM, Arie S, Scanavacca MI, et al.: Transcoronary chemical ablation of incessant atrial tachycardia. *J Cardiovasc Electrophys* 1990;1:116.

37. Brugada P, DeSwart H, Smeets J, et al.: Transcoronary chemical ablation of atrioventricular conduction. *Circulation* 1990;81:757.

38. Zipes DP: Targeted drug therapy. *Circulation* 1990;81:1139.

39. Calkins H, Sousa J, El-Attassi R, et al: Diagnosis and cure of the Wolff-Parkinson-White syndrome, paroxysmal supraventricular tachycardias during a single electrophysiologic test. *N Engl J Med* 1991;324:1612

40. Jackman WM, Wang X, Friday KJ, et al: Catheter ablation of accessory atrioventricular pathways (Wolff-Parkinson-White syndrome) biradiofrequency current. *N Engl J Med* 1991;324:1605

41. Ferguson TB, Cox JL: Surgical treatment for Wolff-Parkinson-White syndrome. The endocardial approach. In: Zipes DP, Jalife J, eds. *Cardiac Electrophysiology. From Cell to Bedside* Philadelphia, Pa: WB Saunders; 1990: 897.

42. Guiraudon GM, Klein GJ, Sharma AD, et al.: Surgery for the Wolff-Parkinson-White syndrome: The epicardial approach. In: Zipes DP, Jalife J, eds. *Cardiac Electrophysiology. From Cell to Bedside* Philadelphia, Pa: WB Saunders; 1990:907.

43. Guiraudon GM, Klein GJ, Sharma AD, et al.: Skeletonization of the atrioventricular node. Surgical alternative for AV nodal reentrant tachycardia. Experience with 32 patients. *Ann Thorac Surg* 1990;49:565.

44. Johnson DC, Ross DL, Uther JB: The surgical cure of atrioventricular junctional reentrant tachycardia. In: Zipes DP, Jalife J, eds. *Cardiac Electrophysiology. From Cell to Bedside* Philadelphia, Pa: WB Saunders; 1990:921.

45. Cox JL, Holman WL, Caine ME: Cryosurgical treatment of atrioventricular node reentrant tachycardia. *Circulation* 1987;76:1329.

46. Guiraudon GM, Klein GJ, Sharma AD, et al.: Surgery for atrial flutter, atrial fibrillation and atrial tachycardia. In: Zipes DP, Jalife J, eds. *Cardiac Electrophysiology. From Cell to Bedside* Philadelphia, Pa: WB Saunders; 1990:915.

47. Cox JL, Scheussler RB, Caine ME, et al.: Surgery for atrial fibrillation. *Seminars in Thoracic and Cardiovascular Surgery* 1989;1:67.

48. Cox JL: Patient selection criteria and results of surgery for refractory ischemic ventricular tachycardia. *Circulation* 1989;79:I163.

49. Lawrie G, Pacifico A, Kaushik R: Results of direct surgical ablation of ventricular tachycardia not due to ischemic heart disease. *Ann Surg* 1989;209:716.

50. Furman S, Hayes DL, Holmes DR. *A Practice of Cardiac Pacing* Mt. Kisco, NY: Futura Publishing; 1989.

51. Barold SS, Zipes DP: Cardiac pacemakers in heart disease. In: Braunwald E, ed. *A Textbook of Cardiovascular Medicine* Philadelphia, Pa: WB Saunders; 1992. In press.

52. Winkle RA: The implantable defibrillator: progression from first- to third- generation devices. In: Zipes DP, Jalife J, eds. *Cardiac Electrophysiology. From Cell to Bedside* Philadelphia, Pa: WB Saunders Co.; 1990:963.

53. Zipes DP: Specific arrhythmias: Diagnosis and treatment. In: Braunwald E, ed. *Heart Disease: A Textbook for Cardiovascular Medicine* Philadelphia, Pa: WB Saunders; 1992. In press.

54. Stein B, Halperin JI, Fuster V: Should patients with atrial fibrillation be anticoagulated prior to and chronically following cardioversion. *Cardiovasc Clin* 1990;21:231.

55. Wolf PA, Abbott RD, Kannel WB: Atrial fibrillation: a Major contributor to strike in the elderly. The Framingham Study. *Arch Intern Med* 1987;147:1561.

56. Petersen P: Thromboemboembolic complications in atrial fibrillation. *Stroke* 1990;21:4.

57. Kopecky SL, Gersh BJ, McGoon MD, et al.: The natural history of lone atrial fibrillation. A population based study over 3 decades. *N Eng J Med* 1987;317:669.

58. Coplen SE, Antman EM, Beslin JA, et al: Efficacy and safety of quinidine therapy for maintenance of sinus rhythm over cardioversion. A metaanalysis of randomized trials. *Circulation* 1990;82:1106.

59. Dunn M, Alexander J, deSilva R, et al: Antithrombotic therapy in atrial fibrillation. *Chest* 1989;95 (Suppl.)1185.

60. Preliminary report of the stroke prevention in atrial fibrillation study. *N Engl J Med* 1990;322:863.

61. Scher DL, Asura EL: Multifocal atrial tachycardia: Mechanisms, clinical correlates, and treatment. *Am Heart J* 1989;118:574.

4
ETIOLOGIES AND TREATMENT OF HYPERLIPIDEMIA

SCOTT M. GRUNDY, MD, PhD

Synopsis of Chapter Four

INTRODUCTION

During the past decade, overwhelming evidence has accumulated to link high serum cholesterol levels to coronary heart disease (CHD). This link can now be said to be bidirectional (Figure 4.1). This is to say that as serum cholesterol concentrations increase, the risk for CHD likewise rises, whereas, as the level falls, so does the risk. The documentation of this bidirectional relationship has led to a broad consensus that a national effort to reduce serum cholesterol is warranted. This consensus is the foundation of the establishment of a National Cholesterol Education Program (NCEP).[1] The NCEP has taken a two-pronged approach to control elevated cholesterol levels. One is the high-risk strategy in which patients with high cholesterol levels or other dyslipidemias are identified and treated. The other is the public health approach which encourages the general public to modify life styles to reduce average cholesterol concentrations.

This chapter will concentrate on high risk strategy—and will look at the following:
- A review of the basic pathways of lipids and lipoproteins.
- A rationale for treatment of high-risk patients.
- The current modes of therapy.
- The various subgroups of patients that are candidates for lipid-modifying therapy.

LIPID METABOLISM

CHOLESTEROL METABOLISM

Cholesterol is a water insoluble molecule that is an essential component of most cell membranes of the body (Figure 4.2). Several other of its important functions include being:
- A critical constituent of plasma lipoproteins.
- A precursor of bile acids, adrenal steroids and sex hormones.

Daily cholesterol intakes average 250 to 500 mg, with about 50% being absorbed.[2] Whole-body synthesis of cholesterol ranges from 500 to 1000 mg/d.[3,4] The major route of cholesterol excretion is into bile, either as cholesterol itself or after conversion into bile acids.[5] About one third of newly synthesized cholesterol or newly absorbed cholesterol is converted into bile acids.[3,4]

Absorption of cholesterol by the intestine is incomplete because cholesterol is highly insoluble in aqueous solutions. Moderate amounts of cholesterol are brought into solution by mixed micelles containing bile acids, monoglycerides, and lysolecithin[6] (Figure 4.3). Intestinal lumen cholesterol exists in the unesterified (free) form, but when it enters the intestinal mucosa, it becomes esterified with a fatty acid. Along with newly synthesized triglycerides, cholesterol ester is incorporated in-

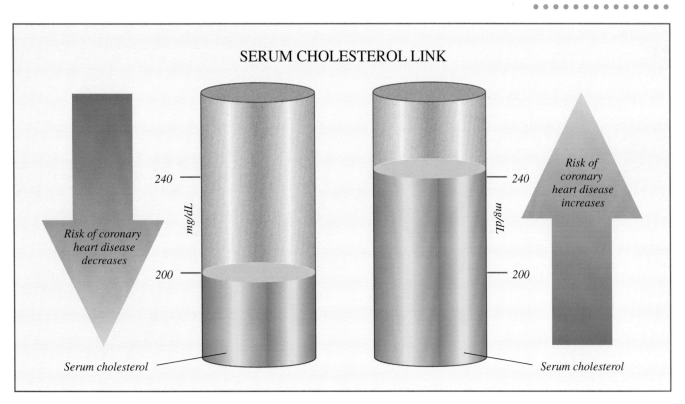

FIGURE 4.1 • The bidirectional link—as serum cholesterol concentrations increase, so does the risk for coronary heart disease. As the level falls, the risk also decreases.

to chylomicrons. These lipoproteins enter intestinal lymphatics, and from there they pass into the peripheral circulation. After partial catabolism of chylomicrons, their residual products (chylomicron remnants) carry newly absorbed cholesterol into the liver.

Hepatic cholesterol has both three sources and three fates.[2] It can arise from new synthesis, from newly absorbed cholesterol, and via uptake of serum lipoproteins. Cholesterol in the liver can be incorporated into lipoproteins which are secreted into plasma. It can also be secreted directly into bile as cholesterol itself, or it can be converted into bile acids. The latter likewise are secreted into the bile. In the intestine, bile acids promote the absorption of fat and cholesterol. They pass into the lower small intestine where they are reabsorbed into the por-

tal circulation and return to the liver. The rate of hepatic cholesterol synthesis is regulated by amounts of cholesterol in the liver, whereas bile acid synthesis is determined by the quantity of bile acids returning to the liver in the enterohepatic circulation.

LIPOPROTEIN METABOLISM

The primary function of lipoproteins is to transport lipids—cholesterol and triglycerides—from one organ (or tissue) to another. The basic structure of a typical lipoprotein is shown in Figure 4.4. All lipoproteins contain a core of neutral lipids—

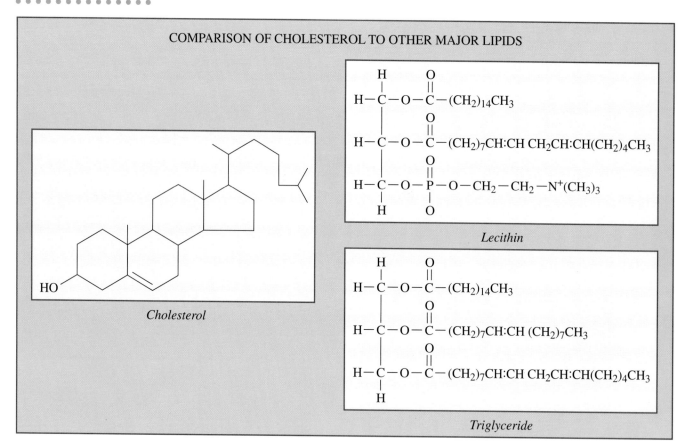

COMPARISON OF CHOLESTEROL TO OTHER MAJOR LIPIDS

Cholesterol

Lecithin

Triglyceride

FIGURE 4.2 • Structure of cholesterol in comparison with structures of other major lipids, lecithin and triglyceride.

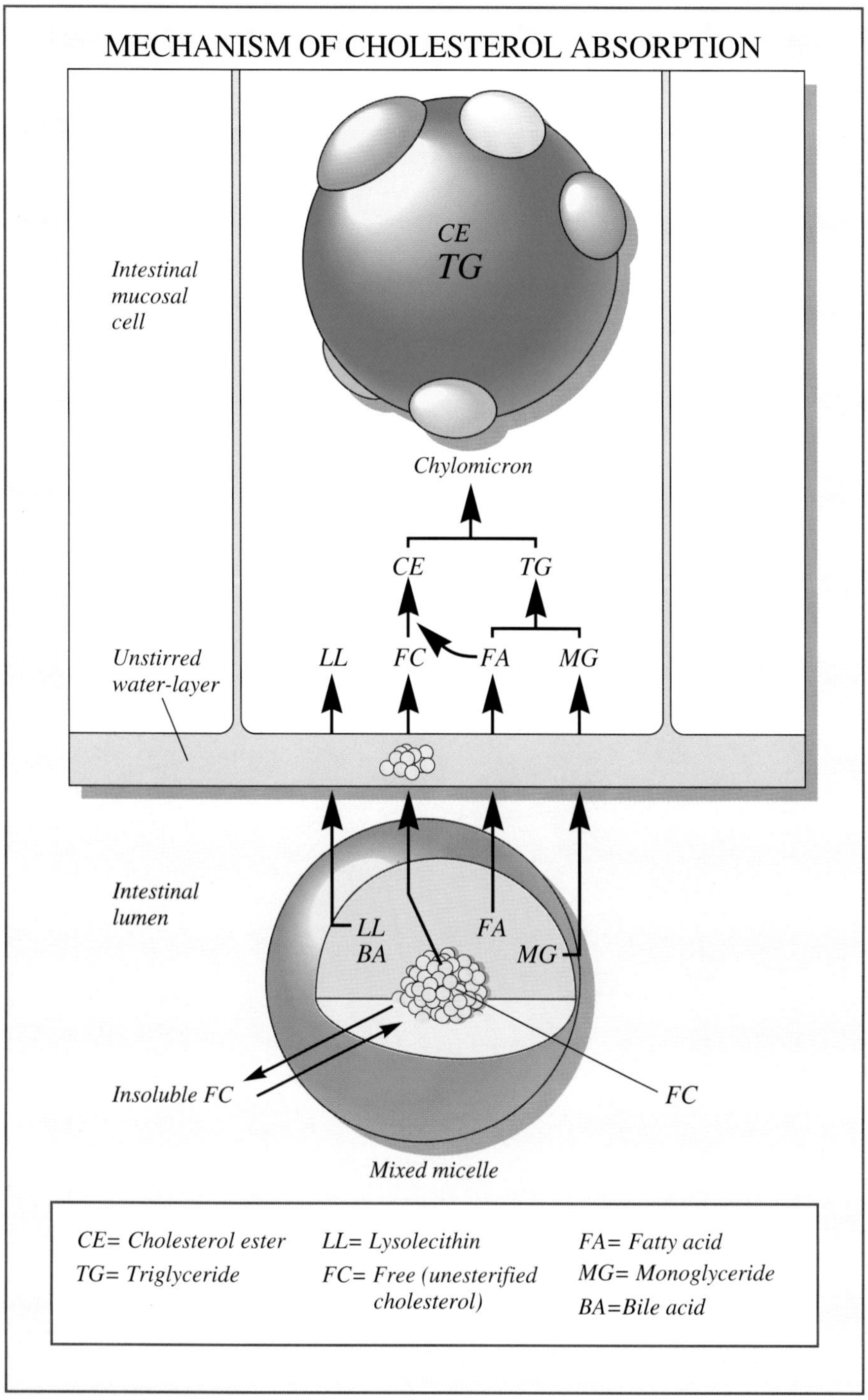

MECHANISM OF CHOLESTEROL ABSORPTION

Intestinal mucosal cell

CE
TG

Chylomicron

CE   TG

LL   FC — FA   MG

Unstirred water-layer

Intestinal lumen

LL
BA   FA
MG

Insoluble FC

FC

Mixed micelle

CE= Cholesterol ester	LL= Lysolecithin	FA= Fatty acid
TG= Triglyceride	FC= Free (unesterified cholesterol)	MG= Monoglyceride
		BA=Bile acid

FIGURE 4.3 • Mechanism of cholesterol absorption.

(cholesterol esters and triglycerides), a surface coat consisting of polar lipids (unesterified cholesterol and phospholipids), and apolipoproteins. The major classes of lipoproteins include (Table 4.1):

• Chylomicrons.
• Very low density lipoproteins (VLDL).
• Intermediate density lipoproteins (IDL).
• Low density lipoproteins (LDL).
• High density lipoproteins (HDL).

The lipoproteins are classified by their density and are variously derived from the intestine, liver, or catabolism of other lipoproteins.

APOLIPOPROTEINS

There are four major classes of apolipoproteins—apo B's, apo A's, apo C's (Figure 4.5) and apo E's (Table 4.2). The apolipoproteins have several functions. Apo B-48 is the major structural apoprotein for chylomicrons,[7] and apo B-100 serves

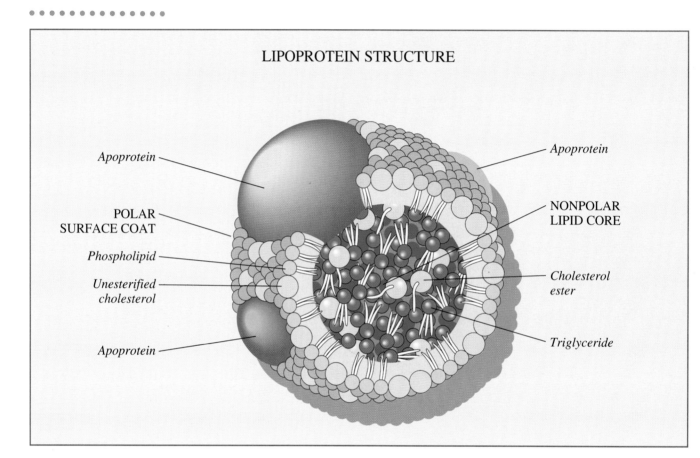

FIGURE 4.4 • Basic structure of lipoproteins.

TABLE 4.1 • CLASSIFICATIONS OF LIPOPROTEINS		
Lipoprotein	**Density (g/mL)**	**Sources**
Chylomicrons	~0.98	Intestine
Very low-density lipoproteins (VLDL)(prebetalipoproteins)	0.98–1.006	Liver
Intermediate-density lipoproteins (IDL)	1.006–1.019	Catabolism of VLDL
Low-density lipoproteins (LDL)(betalipoproteins)	1,019–1.063	Catabolism of IDL
High-density lipoproteins (HDL)(alphalipoproteins)	1.063–1.21	Liver, intestine, other

the same function for VLDL, IDL, and HDL. Apo C-II is required to activate the enzyme that hydrolyzes lipoprotein triglycerides.[8] The apo E's promote receptor-mediated clearance of chylomicrons and VLDL,[9] and the apo A's are the major apoproteins of HDL.

CHYLOMICRONS

Chylomicrons are synthesized in the intestine and contain mainly triglycerides (Figures 4.6, 4.7). Their surface coat is rich in apolipoproteins that include apo B-48, apo A's, Apo C's, and apo E's. When chylomicrons enter the peripheral circulation, they come in contact with lipoprotein lipase, an enzyme located on the surface of capillary endothelial cells. The triglycerides are hydrolyzed to free fatty acids, and during lipolysis, apo A's and apo C's are released into the circulation and are temporarily "stored" in HDL. Removal of most triglycerides transforms chylomicrons into chylomicron remnants, which are rich in cholesterol esters. Chylomicron remnants are taken up by the

FIGURE 4.5 • Gel electrophoresis of the C-apoproteins from the patient (left) and a control (right). The patient shows a missing upper band which is apoprotein CII. (Reproduced with permission. Galton DJ, Krone W: *Hyperlipidaemia in Practice* London: Gower Medical Publishing; 1991.)

TABLE 4.2 • CLASSIFICATION OF APOPROTEINS

Apoprotein	Molecular weight (daltons)	Sources	Lipoproteins
Apoprotein B's			
B-48	264,000	Intestine	Chylomicrons
B-100	550,000	Liver	VLDL, IDL, LDL
Apoproteins A's			
A-I	28,000	Intestine, liver	HDL, chylomicrons
A-II	17,000	Intestine, liver	HDL, chylomicrons
A-IV	46,000	Intestine	HDL, chylomicrons
Apoprotein C's			
C-I	5,800	Liver	Chylomicrons, VLDL, IDL, HDL
C-II	9,100	Liver	Chylomicrons, VLDL, IDL, HDL
C-III	8,750	Liver	Chylomicrons, VLDL, IDL, HDL

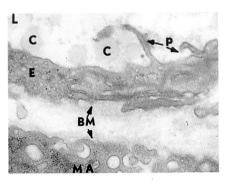
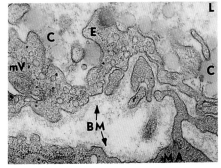
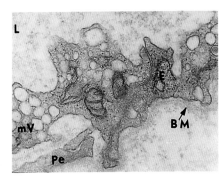

FIGURE 4.6 • An electron micrograph showing chylomicrons (C) binding to the endothelial lining (E) of capillaries which during hydrolysis fill up with fat vacuoles. L = lumen; BM = basement membrane. (Reproduced with permission. Galton DJ, Krone W: *Hyperlipidaemia in Practice* London: Gower Medical Publishing; 1991.)

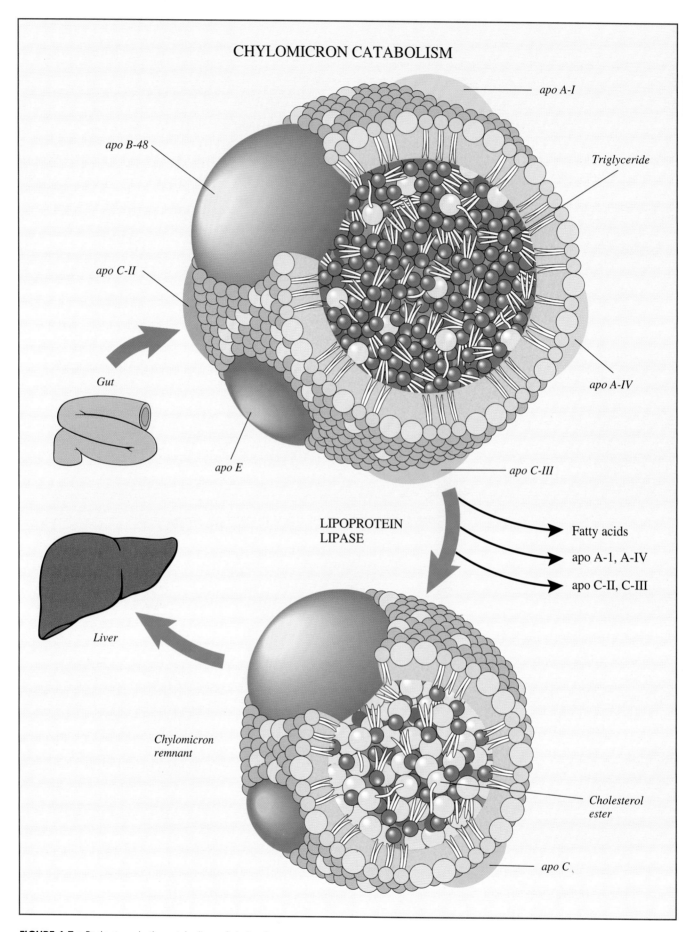

FIGURE 4.7 • Basic steps in the catabolism of chylomicrons.

Treatment of Hyperlipidemias

scious. After reversion to sinus rhythm, cardiac rhythm monitoring is necessary, along with a search for conditions contributing to the initiation of ventricular flutter and fibrillation and an attempt to prevent a recurrence if necessary.

Metabolic acidosis quickly follows cardiovascular collapse and must be remedied by sodium bicarbonate. Artificial ventilation, if necessary, is adequately accomplished by means of a tight fitting rubber face mask and an AMBU bag. Time should not be wasted on endotrachial intubation by inexperienced personnel. Initial medical approaches to prevent a recurrence of ventricular fibrillation include intravenous administration of drugs such as lidocaine, bretylium, procainamide, quinidine, disopyramide or amiodarone. Intravenous epinephrine in doses of 0.5 to 1.0 mg can be tried. IV lidocaine 1 mg/kg, IV bretylium 5 mg/kg may also be useful, and can be repeated if necessary (Figure 3.64).

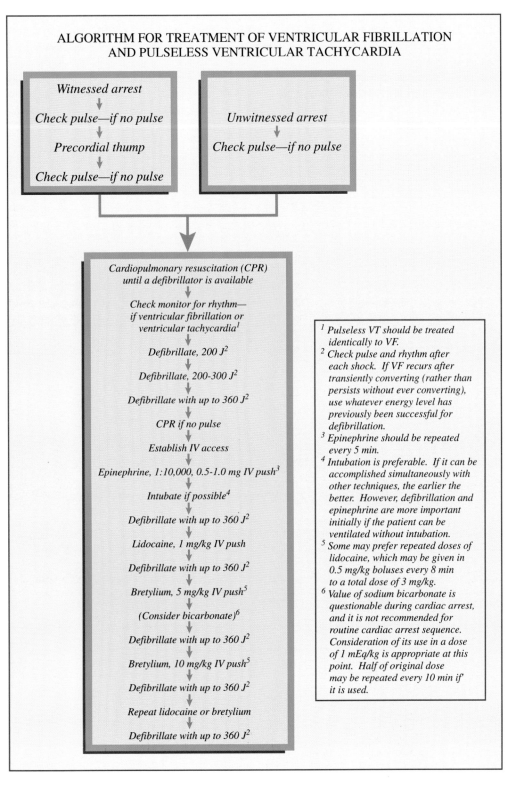

ALGORITHM FOR TREATMENT OF VENTRICULAR FIBRILLATION AND PULSELESS VENTRICULAR TACHYCARDIA

Witnessed arrest
↓
Check pulse—if no pulse
↓
Precordial thump
↓
Check pulse—if no pulse

Unwitnessed arrest
↓
Check pulse—if no pulse

Cardiopulmonary resuscitation (CPR) until a defibrillator is available
↓
Check monitor for rhythm— if ventricular fibrillation or ventricular tachycardia[1]
↓
Defibrillate, 200 J[2]
↓
Defibrillate, 200-300 J[2]
↓
Defibrillate with up to 360 J[2]
↓
CPR if no pulse
↓
Establish IV access
↓
Epinephrine, 1:10,000, 0.5-1.0 mg IV push[3]
↓
Intubate if possible[4]
↓
Defibrillate with up to 360 J[2]
↓
Lidocaine, 1 mg/kg IV push
↓
Defibrillate with up to 360 J[2]
↓
Bretylium, 5 mg/kg IV push[5]
↓
(Consider bicarbonate)[6]
↓
Defibrillate with up to 360 J[2]
↓
Bretylium, 10 mg/kg IV push[5]
↓
Defibrillate with up to 360 J[2]
↓
Repeat lidocaine or bretylium
↓
Defibrillate with up to 360 J[2]

[1] *Pulseless VT should be treated identically to VF.*
[2] *Check pulse and rhythm after each shock. If VF recurs after transiently converting (rather than persists without ever converting), use whatever energy level has previously been successful for defibrillation.*
[3] *Epinephrine should be repeated every 5 min.*
[4] *Intubation is preferable. If it can be accomplished simultaneously with other techniques, the earlier the better. However, defibrillation and epinephrine are more important initially if the patient can be ventilated without intubation.*
[5] *Some may prefer repeated doses of lidocaine, which may be given in 0.5 mg/kg boluses every 8 min to a total dose of 3 mg/kg.*
[6] *Value of sodium bicarbonate is questionable during cardiac arrest, and it is not recommended for routine cardiac arrest sequence. Consideration of its use in a dose of 1 mEq/kg is appropriate at this point. Half of original dose may be repeated every 10 min if it is used.*

FIGURE 3.64 • This sequence was developed to assist in the understanding of treating a broad range of patients with ventricular fibrillation (VF) and pulseless ventricular tachycardia (VT). Some patients may require care not specified in this algorithm—it should not be construed as prohibiting flexibility. The flow of the algorithm presumes that VF is continuing. (Reproduced with permission. *JAMA* 1986;255:2905)

HEART BLOCK

Heart block is a disturbance of impulse conduction that can be permanent or transient and is most commonly recognized as occurring between the sinus node and atrium (SA exit block), between the atria and ventricles (AV block), within the atria (intra-atrial block) or within the ventricles (intraventricular block). AV block can occur in the AV node, His bundle or bundle branches. First degree heart block at any site is characterized by prolonged conduction time but all impulses are conducted. Second degree heart block occurs in two forms: type 1 (Wenckebach) and type 2. Type 1 heart block is denoted by a progressive lengthening of the conduction time, until an impulse is not conducted. Type 2 heart block exhibits occasional or repetitive sudden block of conduction of an impulse without prior measurable lengthening of the conduction time. Complete or third degree heart block indicates that no impulses are conducted. Some investigators use the term advanced AV block when two or more consecutive P waves are blocked.

During first degree AV block, every atrial impulse conducts to the ventricles, but the PR interval exceeds 200 msec in the adult (Figure 3.65). Therapy in the asymptomatic patient is not indicated. Typical type 1 second degree AV block is characterized by a progressive PR prolongation culminating in a nonconducted P wave (Figure 3.66). Type 1 AV block with a normal QRS complex almost always occurs within the AV node and is generally benign without progression to more advanced forms of AV conduction disturbance or the production of symptoms. If a bundle branch block is present, one cannot tell from the ECG whether the AV block is located in the AV node or in the His-Purkinje system. In older people, type 1

AV block with or without a bundle branch block has been associated with a clinical picture similar to type 2 AV block. Type 2 second degree AV block occurs almost always in the setting of a bundle branch block with a fixed PR interval before the blocked P wave. Type 2 AV block usually antedates the development of Adams-Stokes syncope and can progress to complete AV block.

In the patient with acute myocardial infarction, type 1 AV block usually accompanies inferior infarction, is transient and does not require temporary pacing, whereas type 2 AV block is more common in a setting of an acute anterior myocardial infarction, can require temporary or permanent pacing, and is associated with a high rate of mortality generally due to ventricular failure. Type 2 AV block is usually localized in the His-Purkinje system (Figure 3.67). Type 1 AV nodal Wenckebach block unrelated to infarction can be a normal phenomenon in well-trained athletes and healthy normal children, probably related to an increase in resting vagal tone, while true type 2 AV block is never normal.

Complete AV block is present when no atrial activity conducts to the ventricles. The ventricular escape focus usually is located just below the region of block, which may be above or below the His bundle bifurcation. Characteristically, in congenital complete AV block, the escape focus is located in the His bundle because the block occurs within the AV node (Figure 3.68). In contrast, in acquired complete AV block, the escape focus is distal to the His bundle because the site of block is in the bundle branch-Purkinje system. Ventricular escape rates are usually less than 40 beats/min in acquired complete AV block, and the QRS has a bundle branch block contour. In congenital complete AV block, the escape rate is faster.

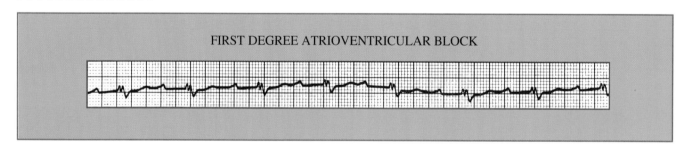

FIGURE 3.65 • First degree AV block. The PR interval is about 360 msec with each P wave conducting to the ventricles. In the setting of a wide QRS complex, the conduction delay can be in AV node and/or in the His Purkinje system. This degree of PR prolongation implies that the AV node is involved but does not exclude some conduction delay in the His Purkinje system.

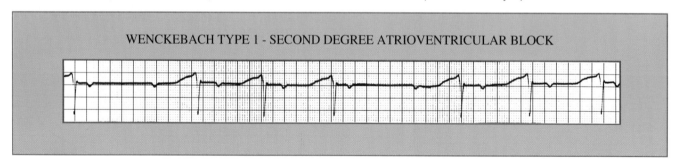

FIGURE 3.66 • Wenckebach type 1, second degree AV block. A 4:3 conduction ratio is present. Note that the PP interval is constant—there is a progressive increase in the PR interval but the absolute increase decreases in the third (conducted) PR interval compared with the second PR interval. Further, there is a decrease in the RR interval preceding the nonconducted P wave, characteristic of classic Wenckebach block.

liver, probably by specific receptors that are yet to be identified. Newly absorbed cholesterol thus passes into the liver with chylomicron remnants, whereas fatty acids of chylomicron triglycerides are released into the peripheral circulation. The fatty acids are bound to albumin and can be used by muscle for energy, resynthesized into triglycerides in adipose tissue, or taken up by the liver for incorporation into lipoprotein triglycerides (Figure 4.8).

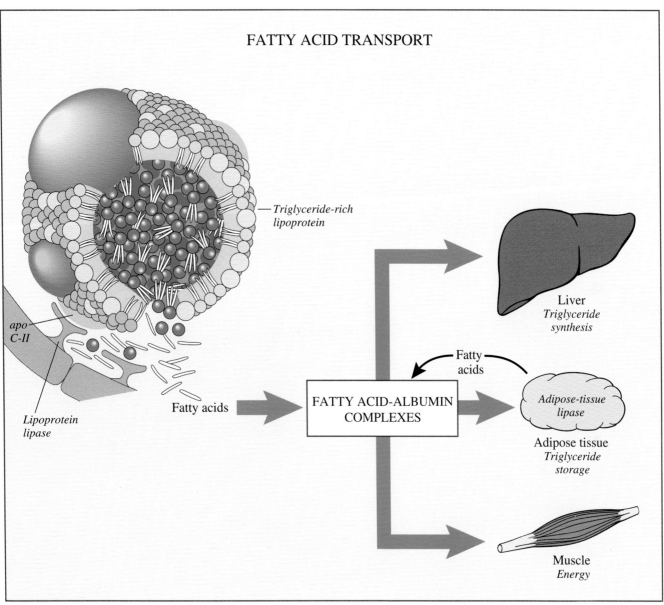

FIGURE 4.8 • Fatty-acid transport and the possible fates of fatty acids.

METABOLISM OF VERY LOW-DENSITY (VLDL)

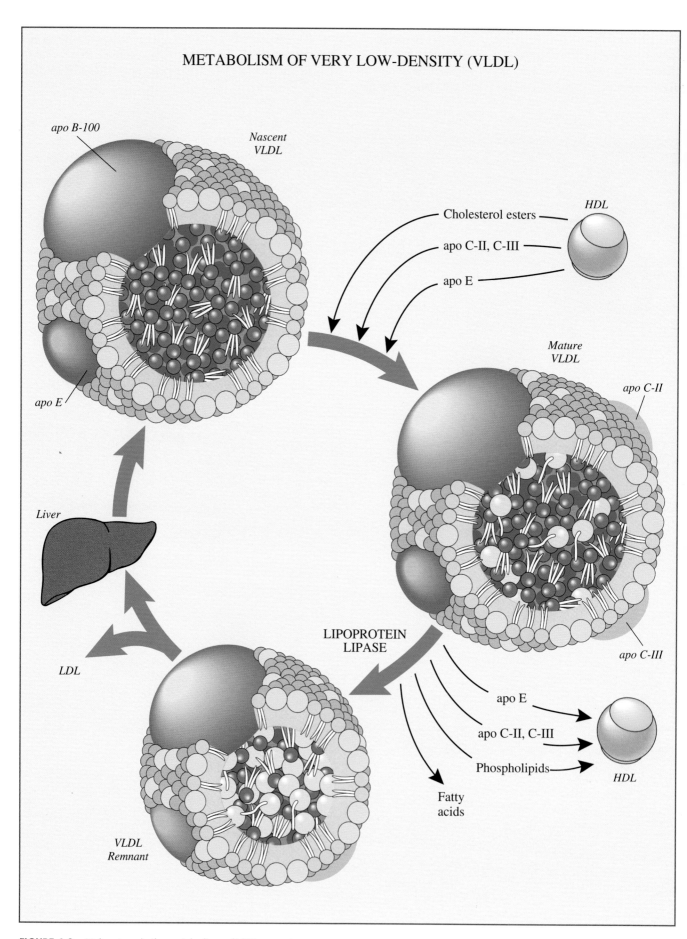

FIGURE 4.9 • Major steps in the metabolism of VLDL.

VERY LOW DENSITY LIPOPROTEINS (VLDL)

The liver, like the gut, produces a triglyceride-rich lipoprotein, VLDL (Figure 4.9). This lipoprotein is secreted as a nascent particle and contains apo B-100 and apo E's on its surface coat.[10] As VLDL particles circulate, they acquire cholesterol esters, apo C's and apo E's from HDL and thereby are transformed into mature VLDL. The latter interact with lipoprotein lipase and are converted into VLDL remnants, which can either be taken up by the liver, or converted to LDL through interaction with hepatic triglyceride lipase (Figure 4.10).

• • • • • • • • • • • • • •

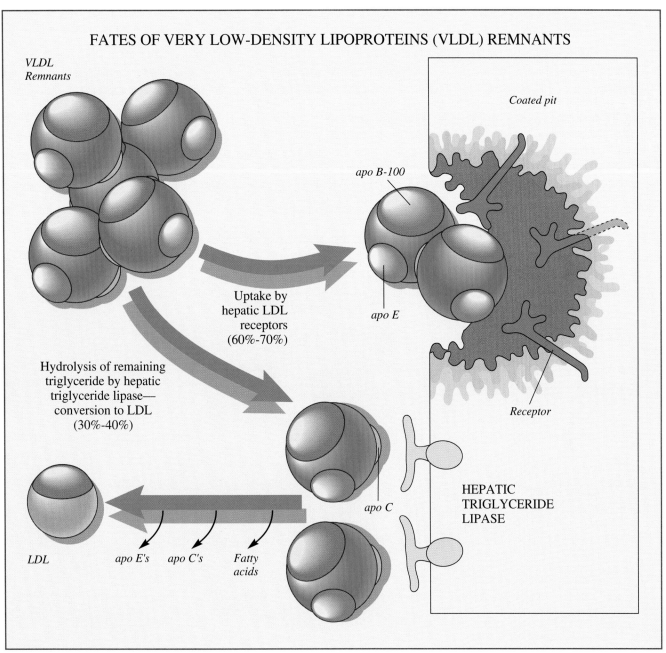

FATES OF VERY LOW-DENSITY LIPOPROTEINS (VLDL) REMNANTS

VLDL Remnants

Coated pit

apo B-100

Uptake by hepatic LDL receptors (60%-70%)

apo E

Hydrolysis of remaining triglyceride by hepatic triglyceride lipase— conversion to LDL (30%-40%)

Receptor

apo C

HEPATIC TRIGLYCERIDE LIPASE

LDL

apo E's   *apo C's*   *Fatty acids*

FIGURE 4.10 • Possible fates of VLDL remnant—uptake by the liver or transformation into low-density lipoproteins.

LOW DENSITY LIPOPROTEINS (LDL)

The LDL are the major cholesterol-carrying lipoprotein in the plasma (Figure 4.11). They contain almost exclusively cholesterol ester in their cores and have only one apolipoprotein—apo B-100—on their surface.[10] LDL can be cleared from the circulation either by the liver or by extra hepatic tissues. Approximately 75% of circulating LDL is cleared by the liver,[11,12] mostly by a receptor-mediated pathway.[13–15] In the liver cell, LDL-receptors are synthesized in the endoplasmic reticulum. They are then transported to the Golgi complex, and from there, to the surface of the cell (Figure 4.12). At the cell surface, LDL-receptors aggregate in coated pits where they bind to circulating LDL and VLDL remnants. These pits become enclosed by the cell membrane and are internalized to form coated vesicles. As these vesicles are transformed into endosomes, receptors dissociate from LDL and recirculate to the surface of cells to be used again. Endosomes change into lysosomes where LDL is degraded. Apo B-100 is hydrolyzed into its amino acids, and cholesterol ester is hydrolized into free cholesterol. When free cholesterol builds up in cells, it down regulates the synthesis of both LDL-receptors and cholesterol, the latter by reducing activity of HMG-CoA reductase, a key enzyme in cholesterol formation.

The concentration of LDL-cholesterol is determined by several factors (Figure 4.13).[16] The formation of LDL is equal to the production rate of VLDL minus hepatic removal of VLDL remnants—shunt pathway. The remaining VLDL remnants are converted to LDL. Levels of LDL also depend on the rate of LDL clearance by the liver or other sites. Clearance of LDL is mediated largely by LDL-receptors.[13–15] The rate of receptor synthesis, therefore, represents a key determinant of LDL-cholesterol concentrations.

HIGH DENSITY LIPOPROTEINS (HDL)

The smallest lipoprotein particles are the HDL. Several steps are involved in the formation of HDL. These steps can be called the maturation of HDL (Figure 4.14). The liver and gut

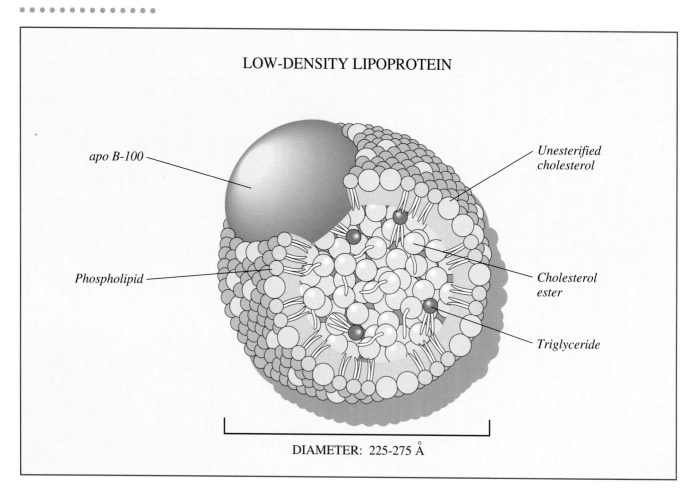

LOW-DENSITY LIPOPROTEIN

apo B-100

Unesterified cholesterol

Phospholipid

Cholesterol ester

Triglyceride

DIAMETER: 225-275 Å

FIGURE 4.11 • Structure of a low-density lipoprotein (LDL).

secrete precursor particles called nascent HDL that consist largely of apo A's and phospholipids.[17] They are disc-shaped particles. As they circulate in plasma, they acquire unesterified cholesterol that becomes esterified by receiving a fatty acid from lecithin. This reaction is catalyzed by an enzyme—lecithin-cholesterol acyl transferase (LCAT).[18] Cholesterol esters enter the core of the lipoprotein to produce a spherical particle called HDL_3. This lipoprotein contains both apo A-I and apo A-II. HDL_3 can acquire more cholesterol ester to become HDL_2. The latter contains more apo A-I than apo A-II, but it also has small quantities of apo C's and apo E's.

HDL_3 and HDL_2 undergo interconversions that can be called the HDL cycle[19] (Figure 4.15). The first product of further enrichment of HDL_3 with cholesterol esters is HDL_{2a}. Some of the cholesterol ester in HDL_{2a} is transferred to VLDL in exchange for triglycerides; this exchange is mediated by cholesterol-ester transfer protein (CETP).[20] Enrichment of HDL_2 with triglycerides leads to HDL_{2b}, the triglycerides of which are then hydrolyzed by HTGL, converting HDL_{2b} back to HDL_3. The HDL cycle plays a key role in reverse cholesterol transport, the process whereby cholesterol in peripheral tissues is returned to the liver for excretion (Figure 4.16). HDL apparently acquires unesterified cholesterol from peripheral tissues and esterifies it. The resulting cholesterol ester can be returned to the liver either directly by hepatic uptake of HDL or indirectly via transfer to VLDL.

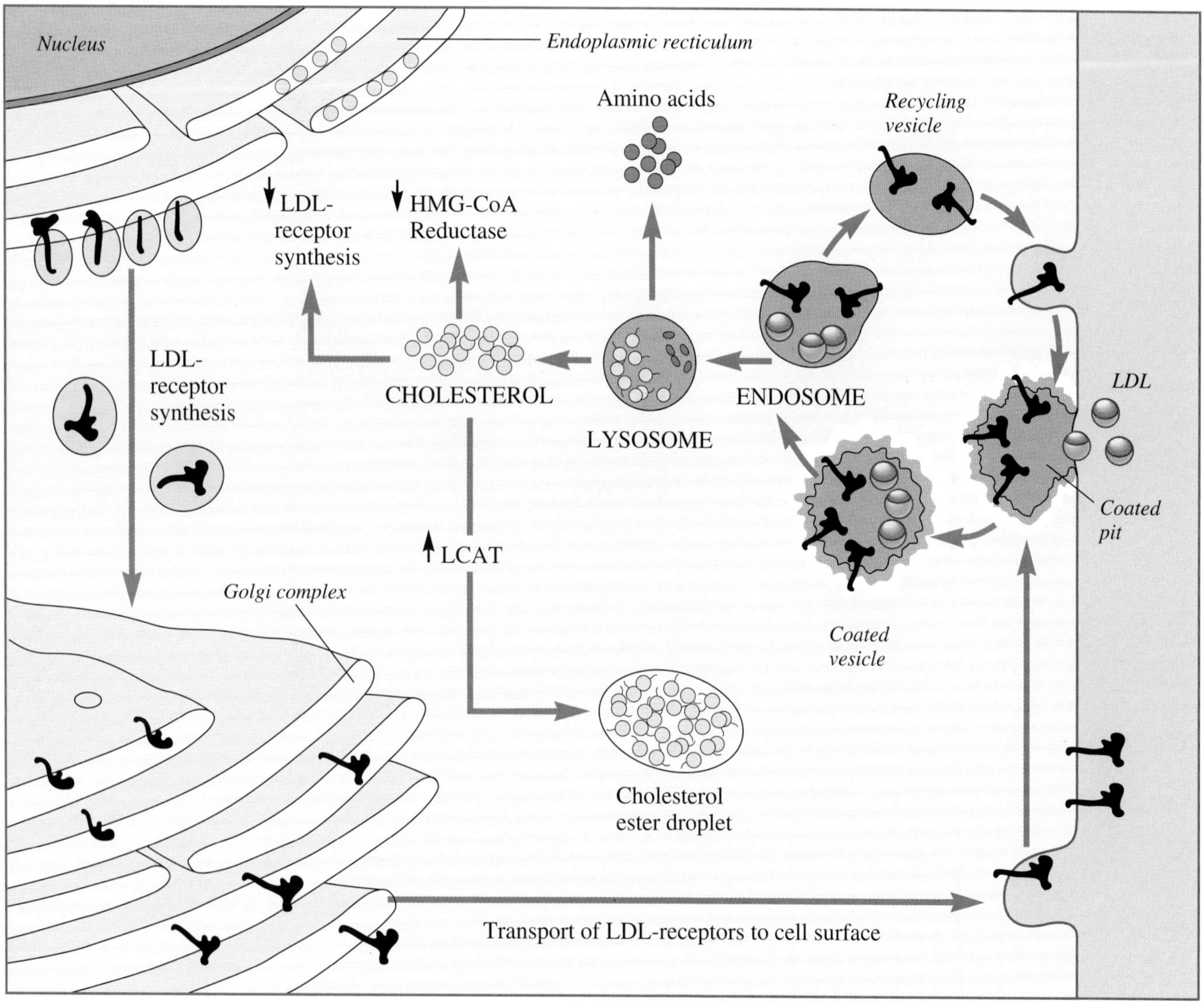

FIGURE 4.12 • Receptor-mediated clearance of LDL. Pathways for uptake and degradation of LDL at the cellular level. Release of LDL-cholesterol in the cell leads to activation of LCAT (storage of cholesterol ester), down regulation of HMG-CoA reduction (inhibition of cholesterol synthesis), and suppression of LDL-receptor synthesis.

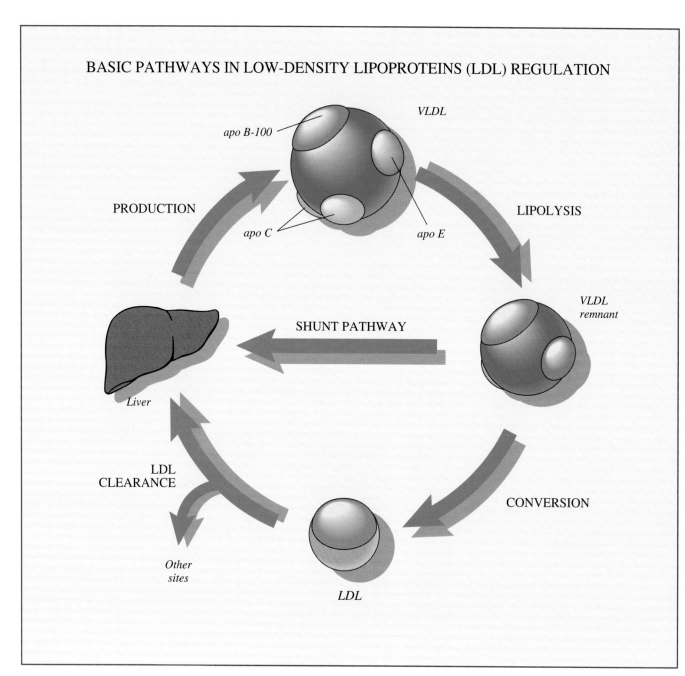

BASIC PATHWAYS IN LOW-DENSITY LIPOPROTEINS (LDL) REGULATION

VLDL

apo B-100

PRODUCTION

LIPOLYSIS

apo C

apo E

VLDL remnant

SHUNT PATHWAY

Liver

CONVERSION

LDL CLEARANCE

Other sites

LDL

FIGURE 4.13 • Basic pathways of the origins and fates of serum LDL.

Treatment of Hyperlipidemias

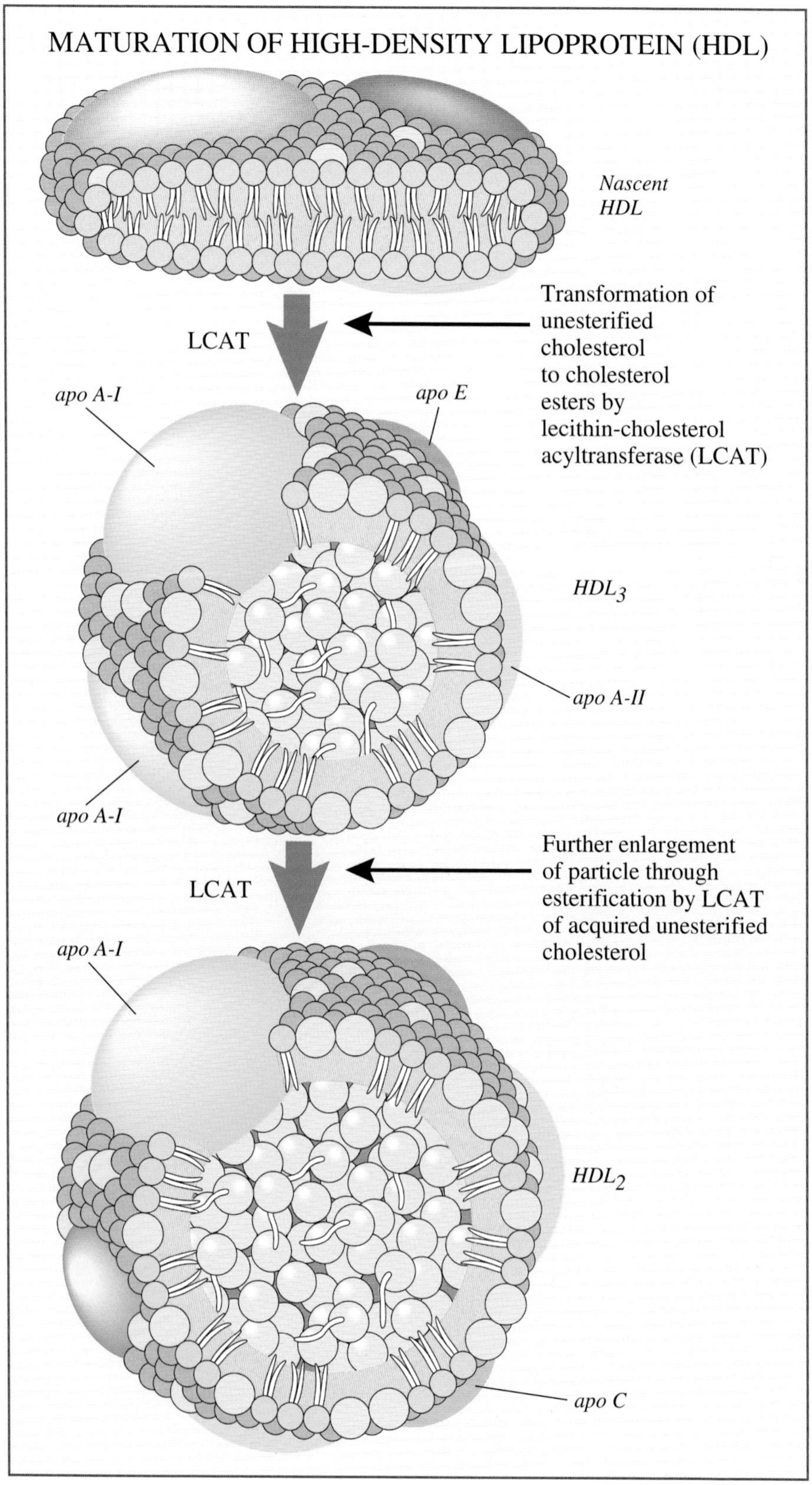

MATURATION OF HIGH-DENSITY LIPOPROTEIN (HDL)

Nascent HDL

LCAT

Transformation of unesterified cholesterol to cholesterol esters by lecithin-cholesterol acyltransferase (LCAT)

apo A-I

apo E

HDL_3

apo A-II

apo A-I

LCAT

Further enlargement of particle through esterification by LCAT of acquired unesterified cholesterol

apo A-I

HDL_2

apo C

FIGURE 4.14 • Basic steps in HDL maturation.

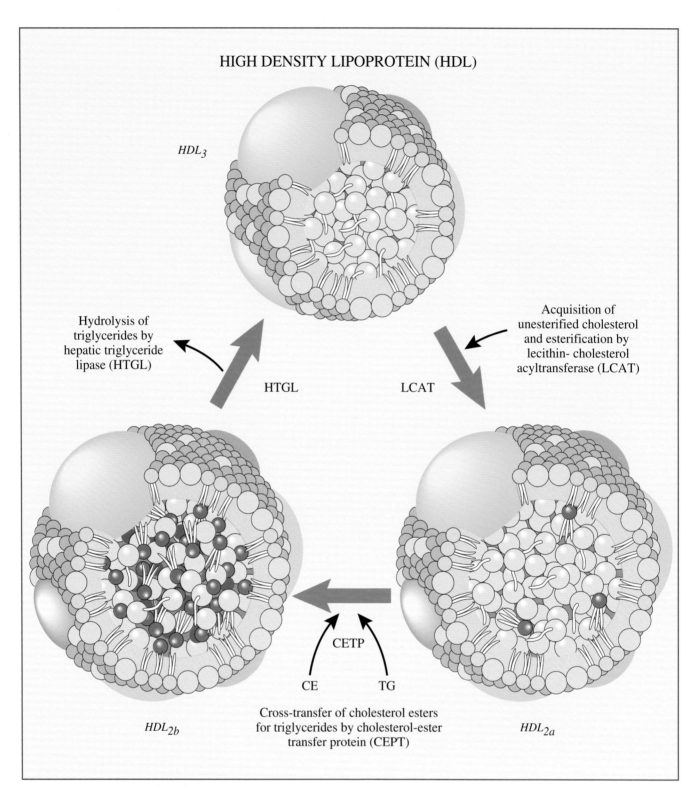

HIGH DENSITY LIPOPROTEIN (HDL)

HDL₃

Hydrolysis of triglycerides by hepatic triglyceride lipase (HTGL)

Acquisition of unesterified cholesterol and esterification by lecithin- cholesterol acyltransferase (LCAT)

HTGL

LCAT

CETP

CE   TG

Cross-transfer of cholesterol esters for triglycerides by cholesterol-ester transfer protein (CEPT)

HDL₂ᵦ

HDL₂ₐ

FIGURE 4.15 • Basic steps in the HDL cycle.

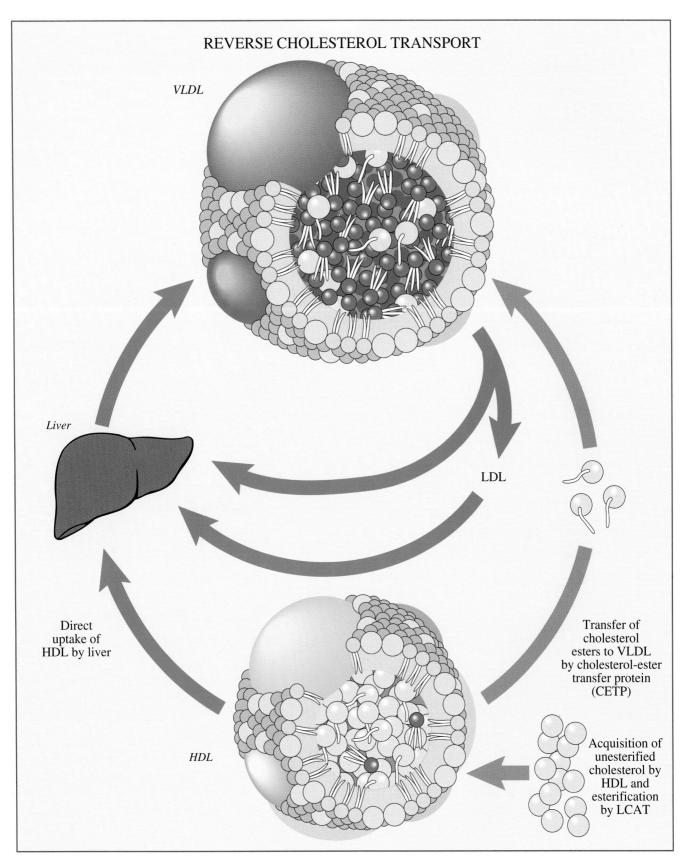

FIGURE 4.16 • Two mechanisms for reverse cholesterol transport. Direct uptake of HDL by the liver and transfer of HDL-cholesterol esters to VLDL—with subsequent hepatioc uptake of VLDL and LDL

ROLE OF LIPOPROTEINS IN ATHEROGENESIS

According to current views,[1] the major atherogenic lipoprotein is LDL. The fundamental premise of the NCEP is that LDL is the primary target for treatment in patients with high serum cholesterol levels. Most of the cholesterol in plasma is carried in LDL, and several lines of evidence indicate that much of the cholesterol in atherosclerotic plaques is derived from circulating LDL. The first step in atherogenesis is the filtration of LDL from the arterial lumen into the arterial wall and its entrapment[21] (Figure 4.17). The second step is the modification of LDL, either by oxidation or chemical derivation[22] (Figure 4.18). This modification of LDL allows it to be recognized by

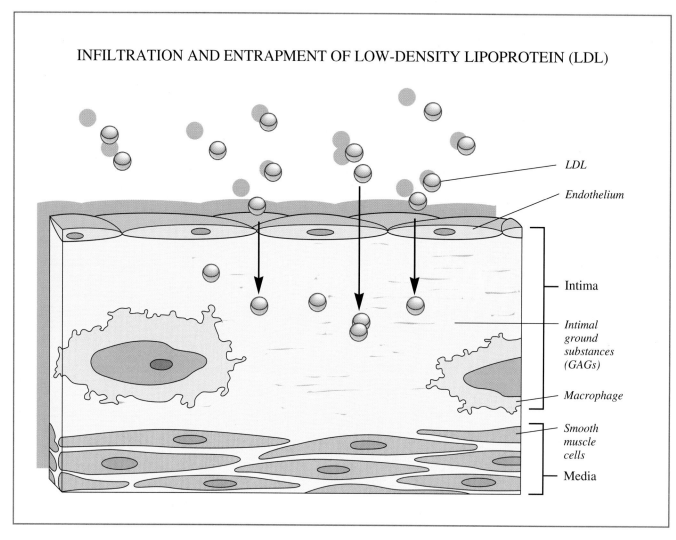

INFILTRATION AND ENTRAPMENT OF LOW-DENSITY LIPOPROTEIN (LDL)

LDL
Endothelium
Intima
Intimal ground substances (GAGs)
Macrophage
Smooth muscle cells
Media

FIGURE 4.17 • First step in atherogenesis. Infiltration of LDL particles through endothelium of arterial wall into intimal layer where some are entrapped.

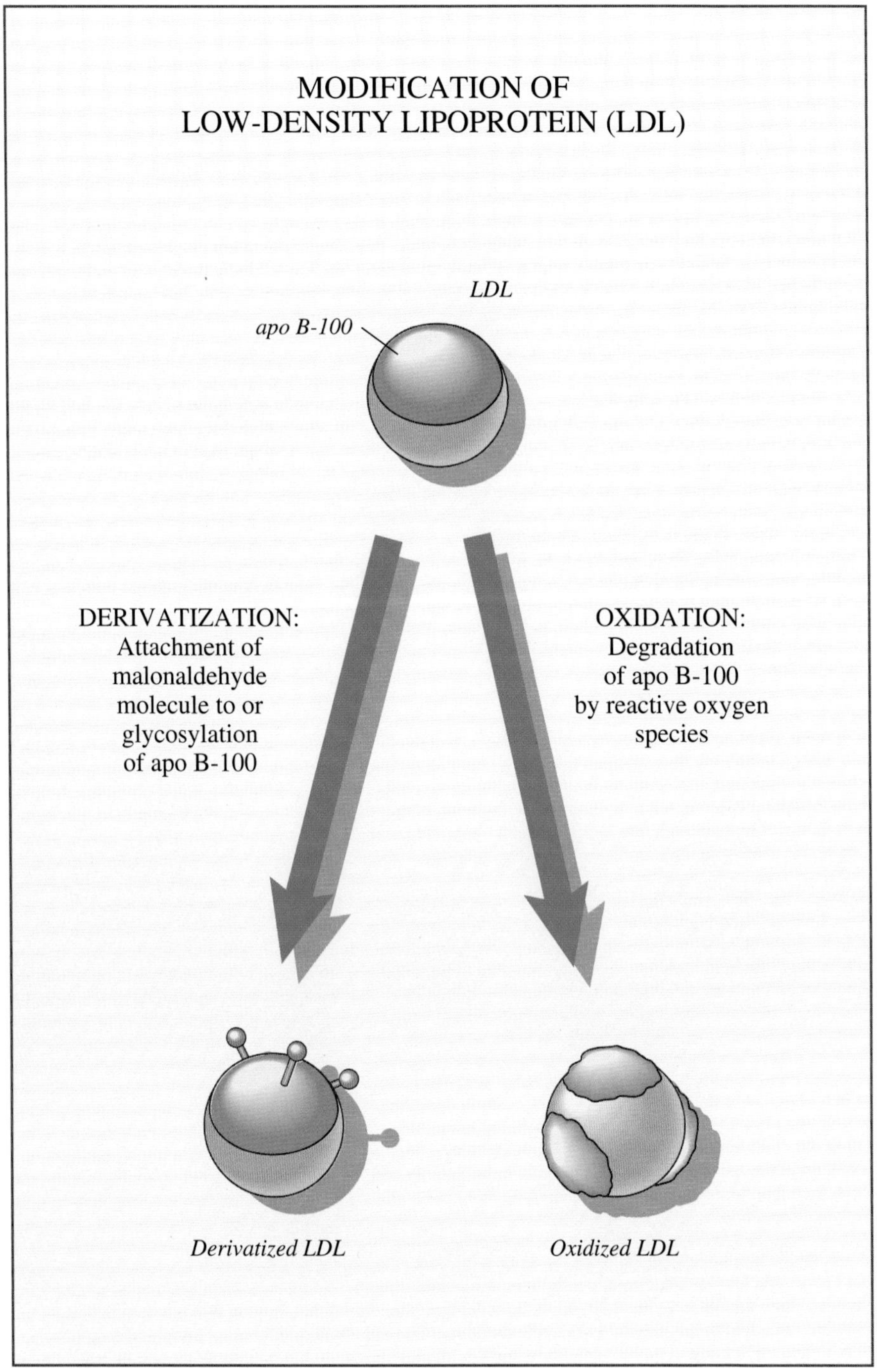

FIGURE 4.18 • Steps in atherogenesis—modification of LDL by oxidation or derivatization.

MODIFICATION OF
LOW-DENSITY LIPOPROTEIN (LDL)

LDL

apo B-100

DERIVATIZATION:
Attachment of
malonaldehyde
molecule to or
glycosylation
of apo B-100

OXIDATION:
Degradation
of apo B-100
by reactive oxygen
species

Derivatized LDL

Oxidized LDL

arterial-wall macrophages so that LDL-cholesterol can be internalized through scavenger pathways (Figure 4.19). Uptake of LDL via this pathway leads to cholesterol accumulation and hence to foam-cell formation, the hallmark of the atherosclerotic lesion (Figure 4.20).

Many investigators believe that VLDL, like LDL, is atherogenic. One form of VLDL that certainly is atherogenic is beta VLDL, or cholesterol-enriched VLDL.[23] Such particles accumulate in the plasma of many cholesterol-fed laboratory animals.[24] They also are found in certain human dyslipidemias.[23] These lipoproteins seemingly promote foam cell formation without the requirement for modification that is necessary for LDL.[24] Even "normal" VLDL remnants may promote foam-cell formation, although it is not clear whether they require modification before incorporation into foam cells. If not, VLDL remnants could be even more atherogenic than LDL.

Finally, high levels of HDL actually may protect against atherosclerosis. One mechanism could be through promotion of reverse cholesterol transport. HDL might enhance removal of cholesterol from the arterial wall, thereby preventing its accumulation.[18] HDL also may prevent the modification of LDL,[25,26] which likewise may retard atherogenesis. In addition, a low HDL level could accompany other mechanisms that independently promote development of atherosclerosis. For example, when HDL concentrations are low, levels of VLDL remnants often are high,[27] and the latter may also be an atherogenic factor.

RATIONALE FOR THERAPY OF DYSLIPIDEMIA

Evidence for a bidirectional link between serum cholesterol and coronary heart disease (CHD) underlies the rationale for therapy of elevated serum cholesterol and other forms of dyslipidemia. This rationale is bolstered by studies in laboratory an-

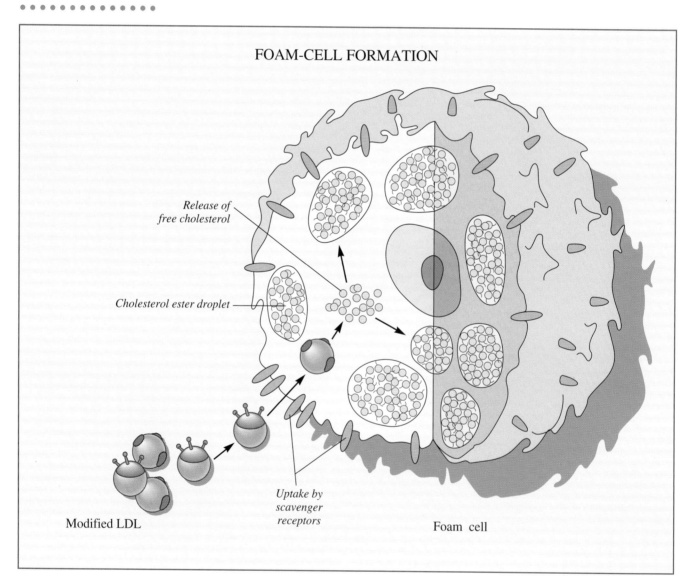

FOAM-CELL FORMATION

Release of free cholesterol

Cholesterol ester droplet

Uptake by scavenger receptors

Modified LDL

Foam cell

FIGURE 4.19 • Steps in atherogenesis. Ingestion of modified LDL by macrophages which initiate the formation of foam cells.

imals that reveal a similar relationship. For human studies, epidemiologic data and clinical trials provide the justification for therapy of various dyslipidemias. Both types of evidence deserve review.

EPIDEMIOLOGIC EVIDENCE

Epidemiologic data of three kinds indicate that high serum cholesterol levels increase risk for CHD:
- Between-country studies.[28]
- Migration studies.[29]
- Within-country studies.[30,31]

Many studies of each type are available, but only a few need be mentioned. The first type is illustrated by the Seven Countries Study.[28] Ancel Keys and associates examined the association between total cholesterol levels and rates of CHD in different populations among seven countries (Figure 4.21). A strong, positive correlation between the two was noted. Because of its magnitude and design, this study has been one of the most influential in establishing a link between high serum cholesterol and CHD.

The best known migration study is the Ni-Hon-San Study.[29] This investigation compared cholesterol levels and CHD rates

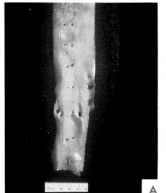 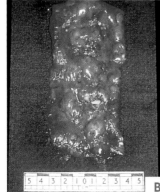

FIGURE 4.20 • An arterial wall affected with minimal atheroma (fatty streaks) (A) and severe atheroma (B).

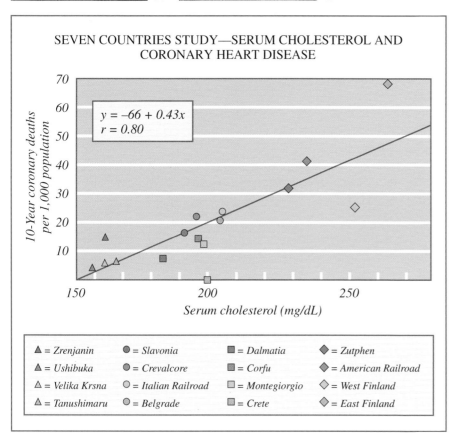

FIGURE 4.21 • Epidemiologic evidence supporting high levels of serum cholesterol as a major risk factor for coronary heart disease (CHD)—The Seven Countries Study. (Reproduced with permission. Hjermann I, Velve Byre K, Holme I, et al. *Lancet* 1981;2:1303.)

TABLE 4.3 • COMPARISON OF CHOLESTEROL LEVELS AND CORONARY HEART DISEASE (CHD) RATES IN JAPANESE LIVING IN JAPAN, HAWAII, AND SAN FRANCISCO			
	Japan	Hawaii	San Francisco
Serum cholesterol (mg/dL)	181	218	228
CHD rate (per 1,000)	25.4	34.7	44.6

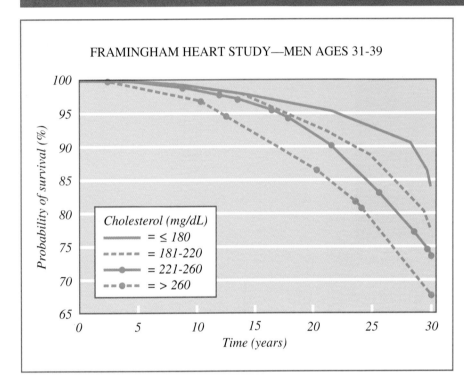

FIGURE 4.22 • Thirty-year mortality by serum cholesterol level for men in the Framingham Heart Study. (Reproduced with permission. Anderson KM, Castelli WP, Levy DL:I. *JAMA* 1987;257:2176.)

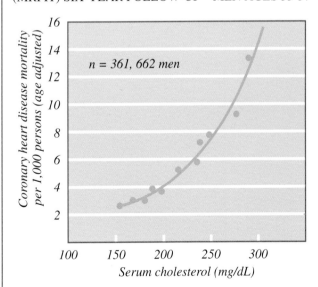

FIGURE 4.23 • Epidemiologic evidence supporting high total cholesterol as a powerful risk factor for coronary heart disease (CHD)—follow-up survey of 360,000 men screened for Multiple Risk Factor Intervention Trial (MRFIT). (Reproduced with permission. Stamler J, Wentworth D, Neaton J: *JAMA* 1986;256:2823

Treatment of Hyperlipidemias

in Japanese living in Japan, Honolulu, and San Francisco. It showed a progressive rise in both cholesterol levels and rates of CHD in these three locations, respectively, suggesting that as Japanese adopted Western lifestyles their serum cholesterol levels rose, which in turn increased their CHD risk (Table 4.3).

The most notable example of an epidemiologic study within a single country is the Framingham Heart Study.[30] In this ongoing study, the population of Framingham Massachusetts has been followed for many years, and cardiovascular risk factors have been related to rates of CHD. This study has documented that serum cholesterol levels are correlated with CHD rates, again implicating elevated cholesterol concentrations in the causation of CHD. One of the advantages of this study has been its long duration. For example, a 30-year follow-up of Framingham participants revealed that long-term survival is inversely related to function of serum total cholesterol at entry[32] (Figure 4.22).

Another investigation in the United States is remarkable for its large number of participants. In the Multiple Risk Factor Intervention Trial (MRFIT), over 360,000 middle-aged men were screened and followed for 6 years for CHD mortality[31] (Figure 4.23). This follow-up showed a strong, positive curvilinear correlation between cholesterol levels at initial screening and subsequent CHD mortality, again indicating that high total cholesterol is a powerful risk factor for CHD.

The Framingham Heart Study[33] has the additional advantage in that it examined the relationship between individual lipoprotein fractions and CHD rates. Support for the concept that LDL is highly atherogenic is the observation that the likelihood ratio for CHD reveals the strength of association between a risk factor and CHD. In the analysis of likelihood ratios, LDL-cholesterol has a greater ratio than does total cholesterol (Figure 4.24). This relationship supports the rationale for using LDL-cholesterol as the primary target of therapy in patients with high serum cholesterol.

Several epidemiologic studies[34] indicate that serum triglycerides, which are a reflection of VLDL concentrations, also are correlated with CHD risk. The same correlation holds for VLDL-cholesterol, as shown by the Framingham Heart Study[35] (Figure 4.25). In this study, VLDL-cholesterol was a stronger predictor for CHD in women than in men, although recent data indicate a stronger link between triglyceride levels and CHD in men than originally observed. The precise nature of the correlation between serum triglyceride levels and CHD remains to be determined. Triglyceride itself does not accumulate in atherosclerotic plaques, which contain mainly cholesterol. Thus, the metabolic consequences of hypertriglyceridemia may represent the key to an understanding of the link. In patients with hypertriglyceridemia, several defects in lipoprotein metabolism are present. These include an increase in chy-

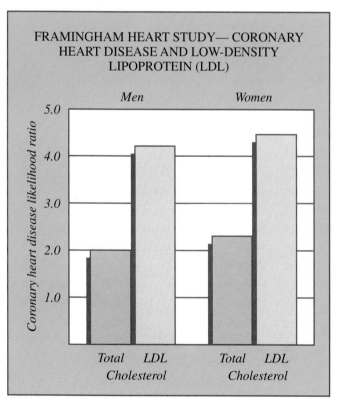

FIGURE 4.24 • Likelihood ratios for coronary heart disease (CHD) of total cholesterol compared with LDL-cholesterol in men and women in the Framingham Heart Study. (Reproduced with permission. Kannel WB, Castelli WP, Gordon T: *Ann Intern Med* 1979;90:85.)

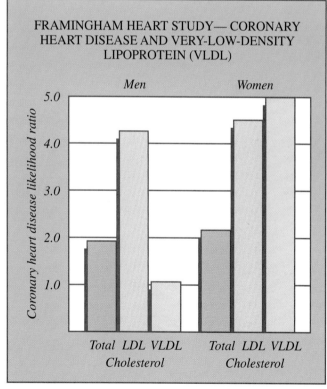

FIGURE 4.25 • Likelihood ratios for coronary heart disease (CHD) of VLDL-cholesterol compared with total cholesterol and LDL-cholesterol in men and women in the Framingham Heart Study. (Reproduced with permission. Castelli WP: *Am Heart J* 1986;112:432.)

lomicron remnants, VLDL remnants, IDL, and small dense lipoproteins[34] (Figure 4.26). All of these lipoproteins have been reported to have a high atherogenecity. In addition, HDL-cholesterol levels usually are reduced in patients with hypertriglyceridemia. Thus, elevated triglycerides per se may not be atherogenic, but they may generate other lipoprotein species that promote the development of atherosclerosis.

The Framingham Heart Study[33,36] has also provided valuable information about the relationship between HDL and CHD. The association is negative, that is, the lower the HDL-cholesterol level, the greater the CHD risk, and vice versa. In fact, among the lipoprotein fractions, HDL levels provided the strongest association. This is revealed by the likelihood ratios for CHD in the Framingham study (Figure 4.27). Another way to examine the relation between HDL and CHD is to compare it with the total cholesterol connection (Figures 4.28, 4.29). For example, increasing the total cholesterol level from 200 to 250 mg/dL approximately doubles the risk for CHD, whereas reducing HDL-cholesterol from 45 to 25 mg/dL also doubles risk. Thus, for every 1.0 mg/dL decrease in HDL-cholesterol, the risk for CHD rises by 2% to 3%.[37]

CLINICAL TRIAL EVIDENCE

Whereas epidemiologic studies provide strong evidence that serum lipoproteins contribute to development of atherosclerosis, clinical trial data generally are held as final proof of efficacy and safety of cholesterol lowering for prevention of CHD. In the past decade, several clinical trials have been completed that strengthen the rationale for therapy of dyslipidemia for preventing CHD. Some of these trials have used dietary therapy, and others have employed drugs. Some studies have been primary prevention trials, such as those designed to prevent the first occurrence of cardiovascular events, whereas the purpose of other trials was to prevent subsequent coronary events in patients with established CHD (secondary trials). Several trials have demonstrated that CHD rates can be reduced by modifying serum lipoproteins, although, generally, a reduction in overall mortality has not been proven. A lack of decrease in

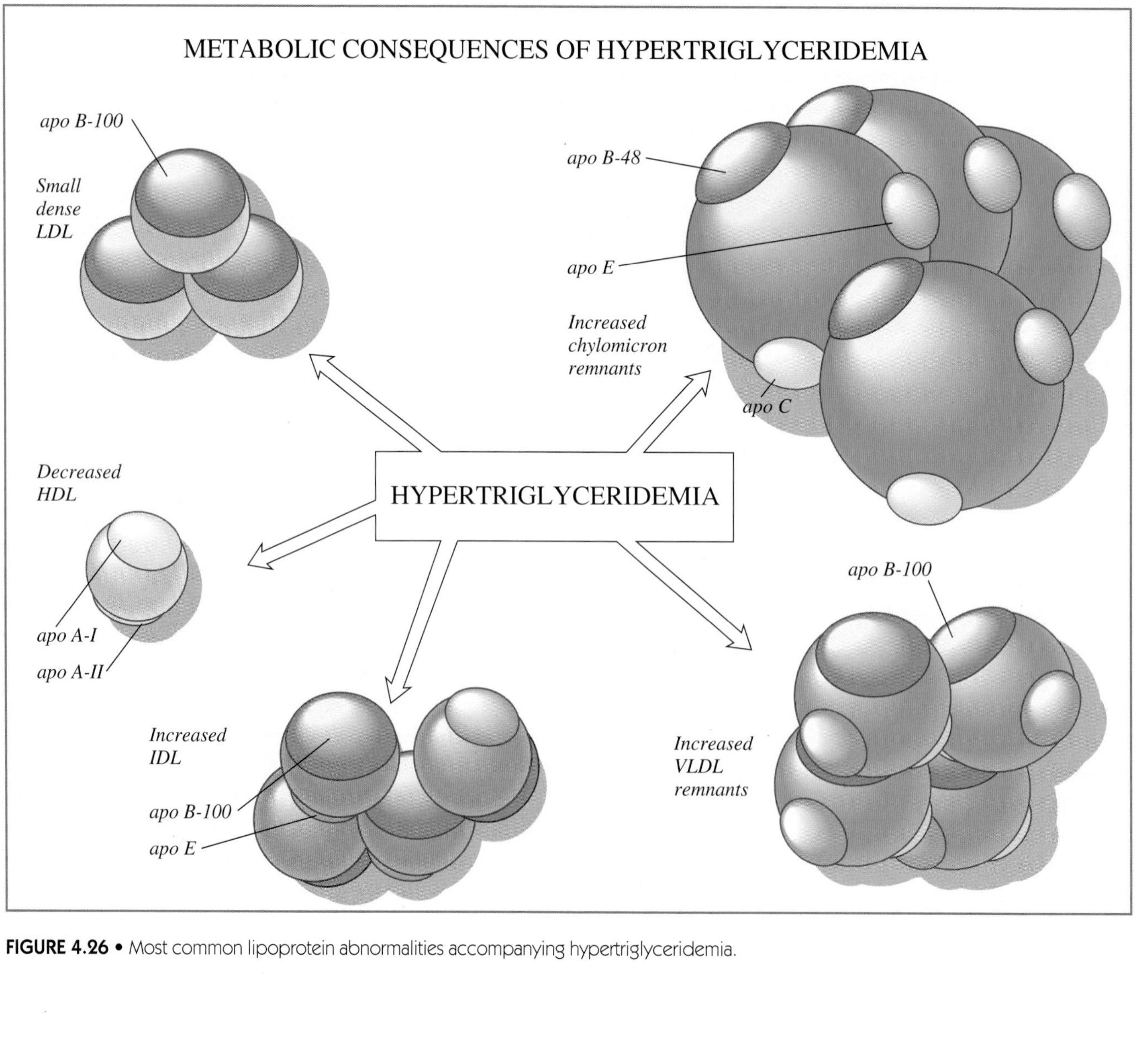

FIGURE 4.26 • Most common lipoprotein abnormalities accompanying hypertriglyceridemia.

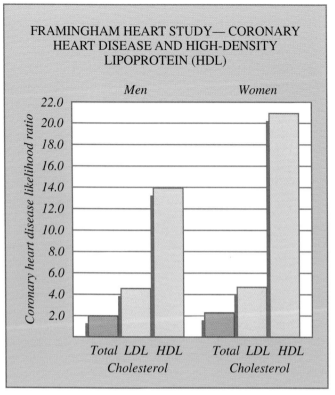

FRAMINGHAM HEART STUDY— CORONARY HEART DISEASE AND HIGH-DENSITY LIPOPROTEIN (HDL)

FIGURE 4.27 • Likelihood ratios for coronary heart disease (CHD) of HDL-cholesterol compared with total cholesterol and LDL-cholesterol in men and women in the Framingham Heart Study.

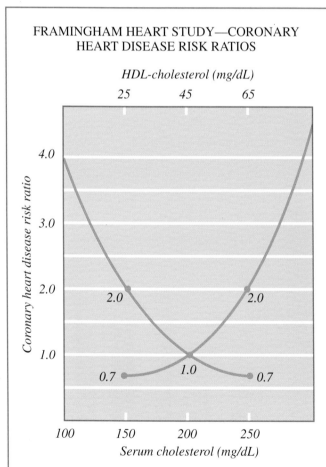

FRAMINGHAM HEART STUDY—CORONARY HEART DISEASE RISK RATIOS

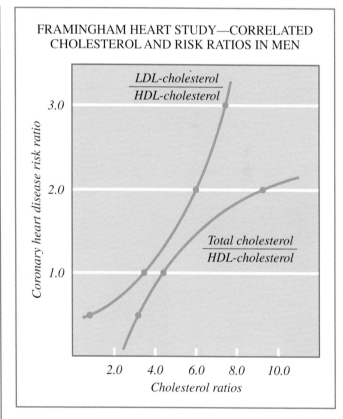

FRAMINGHAM HEART STUDY—CORRELATED CHOLESTEROL AND RISK RATIOS IN MEN

FIGURE 4.29 • Cholesterol ratios—LDL-cholesterol/HDL-cholesterol and total cholesterol/HDL-cholesterol—correlated with risk ratios for coronary heart disease (CHD) in the Framingham Heart Study. (Reproduced with permission. Gordon DJ, Probstfeld JL, Garrison RJ, et al: *Circulation* 1989;79:8.)

FIGURE 4.28 • Risk ratios for coronary heart disease (CHD) of total cholesterol and HDL-cholesterol. Data from the Framingham Heart Study.

overall mortality, however, does not mean that lipid-lowering therapy is ineffective. Clinical trials usually last only a few years, but it is likely that long-term cholesterol lowering will be required to decrease overall mortality (refer to Figure 4.22). Also of importance, prevention of CHD as an end in itself may justify efforts to lower lipid levels regardless of long-term survival; in other words, reduction of morbidity, even without a change in mortality, probably is a sufficient reason to treat dyslipidemia. A review of clinical trial results is in order.

One early secondary prevention trial was the Coronary Drug Project (CDP),[38] a placebo-controlled, double-blind study of men with established CHD. In this trial, patients were treated with a lipid-lowering drug—clofibrate or nicotinic acid for 6 years. Those who had received nicotinic acid had 29% fewer new heart attacks than the placebo group at the end of the trial. A follow up review of overall mortality in this group was determined nine years later.[39] Those who had received nicotinic acid during the trial experienced 11% fewer deaths than found in the placebo group. This difference is statistically significant.

Another secondary prevention trial was the Stockholm Ischemic Heart Disease Study.[39] Participants in this trial also had established CHD. They were randomized into a placebo group and a drug treatment group. The latter received a combined drug regimen—clofibrate and nicotinic acid. The study period was 5 years. Overall, the drug treatment group experienced 26% fewer deaths than the placebo group, and 36% fewer deaths from CHD.

Two other trials have examined the effects of drug therapy on progression of coronary atherosclerosis in patients with definite CHD. In the National Heart, Lung, and Blood Institute (NHLBI) Type II Coronary Intervention Study,[41] patients with

hypercholesterolemia received either a high dose of cholestyramine or placebo. Pre- and posttreatment coronary angiograms were carried out. Posttreatment angiograms showed that coronary artery disease had progressed in 49% of the placebo group, but only in 32% of the cholestyramine-treatment group, a statistically significant difference.

The Cholesterol Lowering Atherosclerosis Study (CLAS)[42] was carried out in 162 men who had recently had coronary artery bypass surgery. The patients were randomized to dietary therapy alone and high-dose, combined drug therapy—nicotinic acid and colestipol. Progression of coronary arterial disease was assessed by angiography. Follow-up coronary angiograms revealed that 61% of the drug-treatment group had either no change in coronary atherosclerosis or regression of lesions, whereas only 39% of the placebo group manifested lack of progression. A recent follow-up of patients in this study showed continued better response in the drug treatment group (Figure 4.30).[43]

Another study similar to CLAS is the Familial Atherosclerosis Treatment Study (FATS) (Figure 4.31).[44] It too examined coronary angiograms in patients with established CHD who were treated with two drugs in combination. The results of this study indicated that cholesterol lowering with drug therapy significantly retarded the progression of coronary atherosclerosis, and in some cases apparently caused reversal of coronary lesions. Efficacy of combined drug therapy for preventing progression of coronary atherosclerosis in patients with high serum cholesterol has been reported by Kane et al[45] (Figure 4.32).

A series of primary prevention trials have further revealed the benefit of lowering cholesterol. One of these was the Oslo Study Diet and Antismoking Trial.[46] The intervention group reduced smoking and modified their diet compared with a control

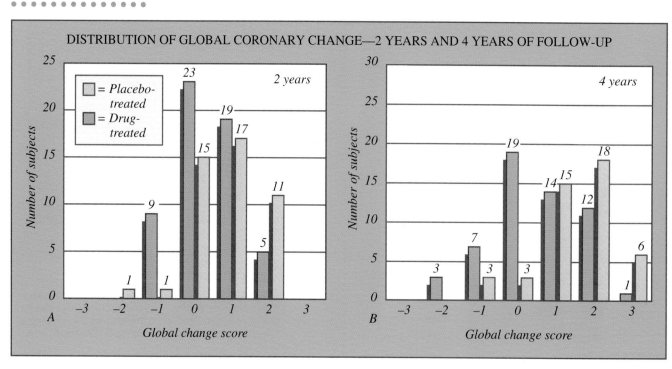

FIGURE 4.30 • Distribution of global coronary change score by treatment group at 2 years of follow-up (A) and at 4 years of follow-up (B). (Reproduced with permission. Blankenhorn DH, Nessim SA, Johnson RL, et al: *JAMA* 1987;257:3233-3240. Cashin-Hemphill et al: *JAMA* 1990;264:3013

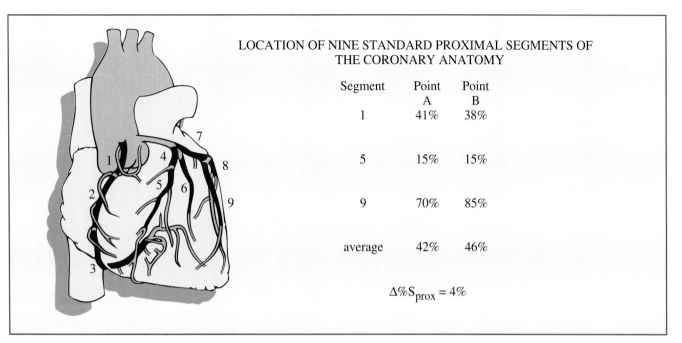

LOCATION OF NINE STANDARD PROXIMAL SEGMENTS OF
THE CORONARY ANATOMY

Segment	Point A	Point B
1	41%	38%
5	15%	15%
9	70%	85%
average	42%	46%

$$\Delta\%S_{prox} = 4\%$$

FIGURE 4.31 • Location of the nine standard proximal segments of the coronary anatomy. The lesion causing the greatest stenosis in each of these segments was measured. The average percent stenosis among these segments was computed, and the mean change in this value between the two studies (time points A and B) was deter- mined ($\Delta\%S_{prox}$). This estimate of the mean change in the severity of proximal stenosis (4%) was made for each patient. (Reproduced with permission. Brown G, Albers JJ, Fisher LD, et al: *N Engl J Med* 1990;323:1291.)

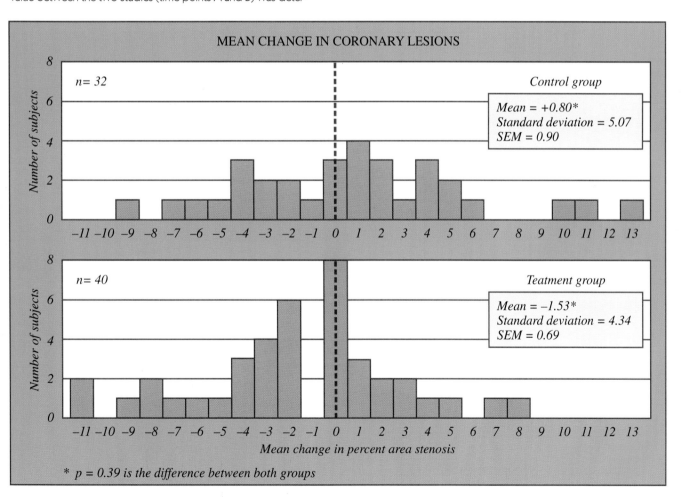

FIGURE 4.32 • Distribution of within-patient mean change in coronary lesions as percent area stenosis in the control (A) and treatment (B) groups. (Reproduced with permission. Kane JP, Malloy MJ, Ports TA, et al: *JAMA* 1990;264:3007.)

group. After five years, the incidence of clinical CHD events in the intervention group was 47% below that of the control group. This significant trend was maintained for another four years in follow-up study. The authors attributed about 75% of the benefit to the cholesterol-lowering diet, and 25% to reduction in smoking.

A major drug trial for primary prevention of CHD was the Lipid Research Clinics (LRC) Coronary Primary Prevention Trial (CPPT).[47,48] This trial randomized more than 3,800 mid-dle-aged, hypercholesterolemic men into placebo and cholestyramine-treatment groups. After seven years of treatment, the cholestyramine group experienced 19% fewer CHD events than the placebo group (Figure 4.33). This difference also extended to other coronary end points. Thus the cholestyramine group had 20% lower new-onset angina pectoris, 25% fewer new positive exercise tests, and a 21% reduction in coronary artery surgery. A life-table cumulative incidence showed a 2-year lag before the benefit of cholestyramine therapy

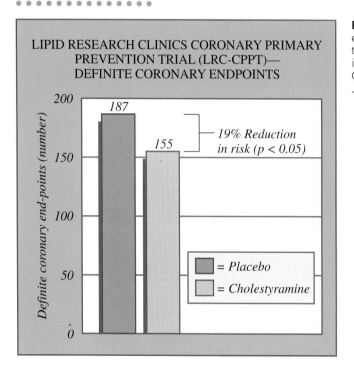

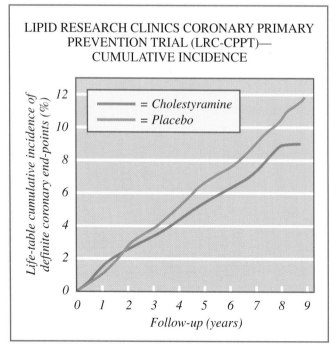

FIGURE 4.33 • Comparison of the incidence of definite coronary end-points—definite coronary heart disease (CHD) death and nonfatal myocardial infarction—in the cholestyramine and placebo groups in the Lipid Research Clinics Coronary Primary Prevention Trial (LRC-CPPT). (Reproduced with permission. Lipid Research Clinics Program: *JAMA* 1984;251:351.)

FIGURE 4.34 • Life-table cumulative incidence of primary end-points in the cholestyramine and placebo groups in the Lipid Research Clinics Coronary Primary Prevention Trial (LRC-CPPT). (Reproduced with permission. Lipid Research Clinics Program: *JAMA* 1984;251:351.)

Treatment of Hyperlipidemias

emerged (Figure 4.34). Further analysis showed a wide range of response depending on drug compliance (Figure 4.35). Those who complied best to drug therapy had the greatest reductions in both LDL-cholesterol levels and CHD events.

Another influential drug trial was the recent Helsinki Heart Study.[49,50] This study compared a fibric acid, gemfibrozil, with placebo in 4,081 middle-aged Finnish men. The patients had elevated total cholesterol concentrations with various lipoprotein patterns. In all patients, nonHDL-cholesterol (VLDL and LDL) exceeded 200 mg/dL at entry. Treatment with gemfibrozil produced a reduction in serum triglycerides and cholesterol and a rise in LDL-cholesterol. Over the 5-year period of the trial, the gemfibrozil group had a 34% reduction in major coronary events—sudden coronary deaths plus fatal and nonfatal myocardial infarctions—compared with placebo. As with the LRC-CPPT, there was a 2-year lag phase before benefit of therapy became apparent. Thereafter, CHD rates declined progressively compared with placebo (Figure 4.36). A reduction in CHD rates were observed in patients with pure hypercholesterolemia and with mixed hyperlipidemia—elevated cholesterol and triglyceride. The authors attributed the reduction of CHD risk to multiple

changes in lipoprotein fractions, such as reduced total cholesterol, triglycerides, LDL-cholesterol, and a rise in HDL-cholesterol.

Another primary prevention trial, the World Health Organization (WHO) Study[51] compared clofibrate with placebo in hypercholesterolemic men. This trial gave a significant reduction in rates of new CHD, compared with placebo, but for unexplained reasons, total mortality was greater in the clofibrate group than in the placebo group. The overall results support the concept that lipid lowering will effectively reduce CHD risk, but it raised the possibility that long-term use of clofibrate is dangerous. A similar disadvantageous response was not recorded to gemfibrozil in the Helsinki Heart Study.

In summary, the aggregate data from these several clinical trials and others indicate that lowering cholesterol levels in hypercholesterolemic patients will reduce risk for CHD, either in primary or secondary prevention (Figure 4.37). When the results of these studies are combined, it can be seen that reduction in CHD risk is proportional to the reduction in serum cholesterol level. This figure thus summarizes the argument that serum cholesterol lowering will decrease CHD risk, a result that strengthens the rationale for treatment of dyslipidemia.

• • • • • • • • • • • • • • •

FIGURE 4.35 • Relationship between the percentage reduction in LDL-cholesterol and the percentage reduction in coronary heart disease (CHD) risk, by the Cox proportional hazards model, for participants in the Lipid Research Clinics Coronary Primary Prevention Trial (LRC-CPPT).

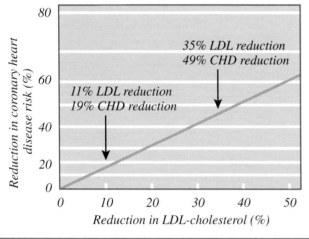

LIPID RESEARCH CLINICS CORONARY PRIMARY PREVENTION TRIAL (LRC-CPPT)—REDUCING LDL AND CORONARY HEART DISEASE RISK

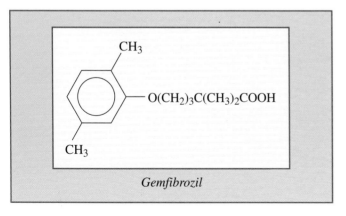

FIGURE 4.36 • Structural formula of gemfibrozil.

WORKUP OF PATIENT WITH DYSLIPIDEMIA

CLASSIFICATION OF SERUM CHOLESTEROL

All adults over age 20 should be tested for total serum cholesterol.[1] This measurement also should be carried out on children over age 5 in whom parents have premature coronary heart disease (CHD) or in families with genetic hyperlipidemias. For adults, three categories of serum total cholesterol were defined by the National Cholesterol Education Program (NCEP) (Figure 4.38). A total cholesterol below 200 mg/dL is called **desirable**. In the range of 200 to 239 mg/dL is designated **borderline-high serum cholesterol**, and 240 mg/dL and above, **high serum cholesterol**.

When the total cholesterol is in the desirable range, CHD risk from serum cholesterol is relatively low, and repeat measurement is not required for five years. However, the patients should be advised to follow a cholesterol-lowering diet to maintain the desirable range. Some authorities recommend a full lipoprotein profile on all adults regardless of the total cholesterol concentration, but the consensus view is that relatively few people with desirable cholesterol levels have serious dyslipidemias.[52]

About 40% of American adults have borderline high serum cholesterol.[1] In this range, CHD risk is increased compared

with desirable levels, although only moderately[31] (refer to Figure 4.23). With a level in this range, repeat measurement for confirmation is indicated. Further workup depends on the overall evaluation of the patients. Patients who are deemed to be at low risk do not require further testing of lipoproteins. However, those considered to be at high risk require additional testing. The NCEP defined the high risk patient as one having definite CHD or two other CHD risk factors. These risk factors include:

- Male
- Cigarette smoking.
- Hypertension.
- Diabetes mellitus.
- Low HDL-cholesterol (less than 35 mg/dL).
- Family history of premature CHD.
- History of any type of atherosclerotic disease.
- Severe obesity

A total cholesterol exceeding 240 mg/dL requires further workup of the lipoprotein pattern regardless of the overall risk status.

SCREENING FOR RISK FACTORS

A relatively high level of total cholesterol appears to be a requirement for the development of clinically significant coronary atherosclerosis. Cholesterol is a major element of

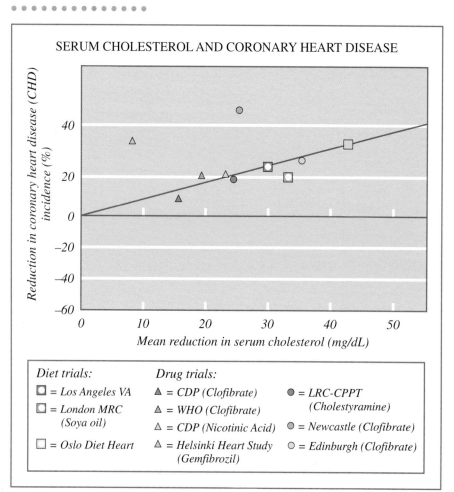

FIGURE 4.37 • Clinical-trial evidence supporting a connection between serum cholesterol and coronary heart disease (CHD). Therapeutic lowering of cholesterol levels in hypercholesterolemic patients reduces risk for CHD. (Reproduced with permission. Basil Rifkind, personal communication.)

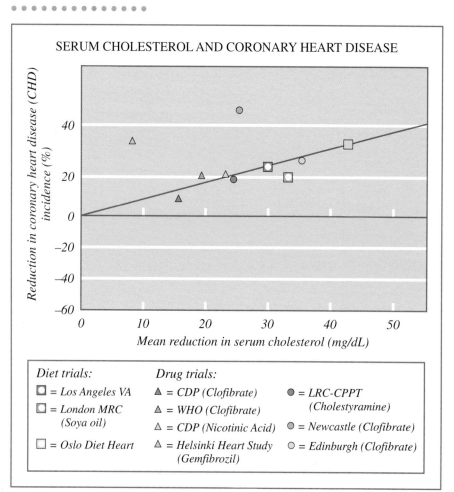

SERUM CHOLESTEROL AND CORONARY HEART DISEASE

Reduction in coronary heart disease (CHD) incidence (%)

Mean reduction in serum cholesterol (mg/dL)

Diet trials:
☐ = Los Angeles VA
☐ = London MRC (Soya oil)
☐ = Oslo Diet Heart

Drug trials:
▲ = CDP (Clofibrate)
▲ = WHO (Clofibrate)
△ = CDP (Nicotinic Acid)
△ = Helsinki Heart Study (Gemfibrozil)

● = LRC-CPPT (Cholestyramine)
◐ = Newcastle (Clofibrate)
○ = Edinburgh (Clofibrate)

the atherosclerotic plaque, and most of it is derived from plasma lipoproteins.[21] In populations having low serum cholesterol levels, rates of CHD are relatively low even when other risk factors are common.[28,29] On the other hand, the presence of other risk factors substantially increases the danger of CHD in populations with higher cholesterol levels.[53] Indeed, there is a strong interaction of the coronary risk factors (Figure 4.39). This figure shows how combining other risk factors with increasing serum cholesterol levels leads to incremental rises in CHD risk. Thus, it is mandatory not to view serum cholesterol in isolation. A thorough search for other risk factors is essential, and an effort should be made to

modify these factors as well as to lower the serum cholesterol level. Consideration will be given subsequently on how to manage an elevated serum cholesterol in patients with other risk factors.

LIPOPROTEIN PROFILE

The essential lipoprotein profile includes serum total cholesterol, total triglycerides, LDL-cholesterol and HDL-cholesterol.[1] The total cholesterol and triglycerides are best measured on fasting serum. The HDL-cholesterol is determined after precipitation of VLDL and LDL. LDL-cholesterol is estimated by the following equation:

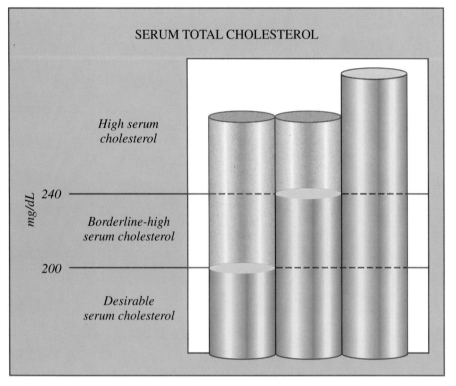

FIGURE 4.38 • Categories of serum cholesterol as defined by the National Cholesterol Education Program (NCEP).

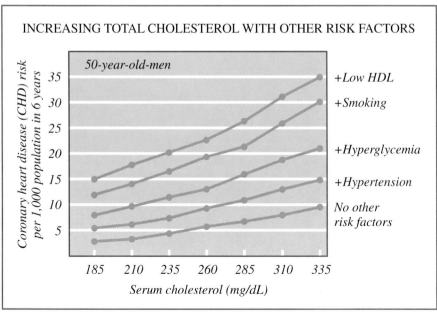

FIGURE 4.39 • Effects of increasing total cholesterol levels on the risk of coronary heart disease (CHD) in the presence of other risk factors in men aged 50 years.

**LDL-cholesterol =
(total cholesterol) - (triglyceride/5) - (HDL-cholesterol)**

This equation is valid when the triglyceride level is below 400 mg/dL. At levels above this, the serum should be subjected to ultracentrifugation to remove excess triglyceride.

Lipoprotein analysis provides a detailed picture of the patient's lipoprotein status which is valuable both in assessment and management. First, the patient's serum triglyceride concentration should be classified (Figure 4.40). A triglyceride level below 250 mg/dL can be called "normal," although some investigators believe that below 150 mg/dL is safer than be-

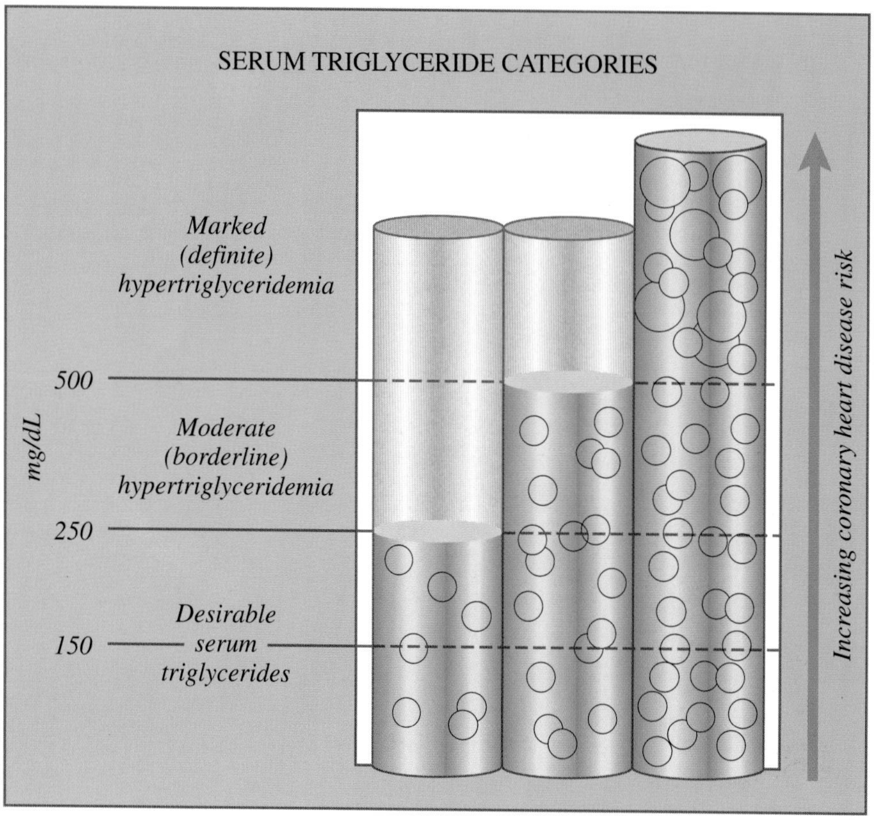

• • • • • • • • • • • • • • • •

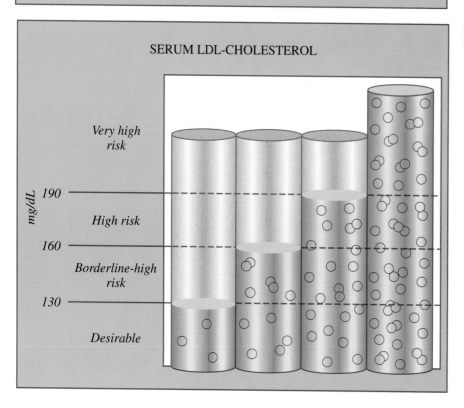

SERUM TRIGLYCERIDE CATEGORIES

Marked (definite) hypertriglyceridemia

Moderate (borderline) hypertriglyceridemia

Desirable serum triglycerides

mg/dL

500

250

150

Increasing coronary heart disease risk

FIGURE 4.40 • Categories of serum triglyceride levels and their relation to increasing risk of coronary heart disease (CHD).

SERUM LDL-CHOLESTEROL

Very high risk

High risk

Borderline-high risk

Desirable

mg/dL

190

160

130

FIGURE 4.41 • Categories of serum LDL-cholesterol.

Treatment of Hyperlipidemias

tween 150 and 250 mg/dL. Concentrations in the range of 250 to 500 mg/dL can be called moderate, or "borderline," hypertriglyceridemia.[54] These levels confer increased risk for CHD, at least in some patients.[34,55] When serum triglycerides exceed 500 mg/dL, both VLDL and chylomicrons usually are present, and the patient has increased risk for acute pancreatitis. The danger increases markedly when triglyceride levels exceed 1500 mg/dL.[56]

The analysis of lipoproteins also allows for a classification of the patient's LDL-cholesterol (Figure 4.41). According to the NCEP[1], serum LDL-cholesterol is called **desirable**. Between 130 and 159 mg/dL is **borderline high risk**, and above 160 mg/dL is **high risk**. When the LDL-cholesterol exceeds 190 mg/dL, it can be called **very high risk**. As implied by the terminology, the risk for CHD increases progressively at higher levels of LDL-cholesterol.

Finally, the lipoprotein profile gives the level of HDL-cholesterol, and provides for classification (Figure 4.42). The NCEP defines a low HDL-cholesterol as a level below 35 mg/dL, but as shown in Figure 4.29, the inverse relationship between HDL and CHD risk is a continuous function. The NCEP makes use of an arbitrary level for low HDL-cholesterol to set targets for treatment of hypercholesterolemia. Causes of reduced HDL-cholesterol are presented in Table 4.4. Perhaps the three most common causes of low HDL-cholesterol are cigarette smoking, obesity, and lack of exercise. Thus, it should be possible to reverse a low HDL level in most people by lifestyle modification. Less common causes are drugs and androgenic steroids. Beta-adrenergic blocking agents will reduce HDL levels in some patients, and when anabolic steroids are taken in high doses, HDL concentrations can be severely depressed.

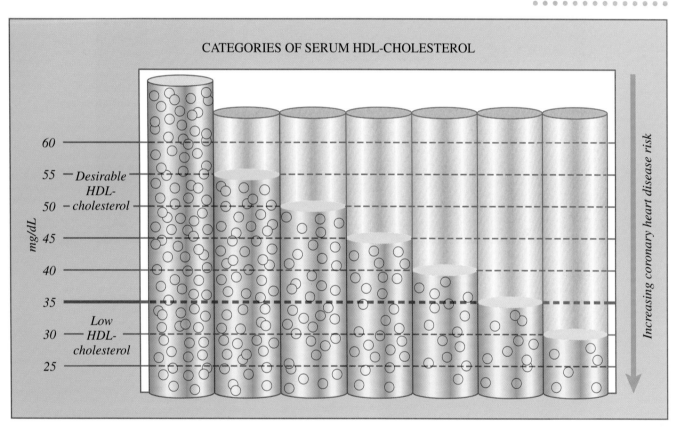

FIGURE 4.42 • Categories of serum HDL-cholesterol and their relation to increasing risk of coronary heart disease (CHD).

TABLE 4.4 • CAUSES OF REDUCED HDL-CHOLESTEROL		
Cigarette smoking	Androgenic and related steroids	ß-adrenergic blocking agents
Obesity	• Androgens	Genetic factors
Lack of exercise	• Progestational steroids	• Primary
	• Anabolic steroids	hypoalphalipoproteinemia

ASSESSMENT OF NUTRITIONAL STATUS AND EATING HABITS

The physician or staff should make an assessment of the patient's previous and current eating habits. The patient's current weight and weights at significant ages should be recorded. The desirable weight should be calculated, and the degree of overweight, if present, can be determined. The following information about dietary habits needs to be determined:

• Patterns of meals during the day.

• Whether meals are routinely skipped.
• Time of largest meal.
• Where meals are prepared, such as home, restaurant, work cafeteria, fast foods, deli, etc..
• Foods that are especially liked or disliked.
• Foods that are difficult to avoid.
• A rough estimate should be made of percentage intake of saturated fatty acid and daily intake of cholesterol in milligrams.

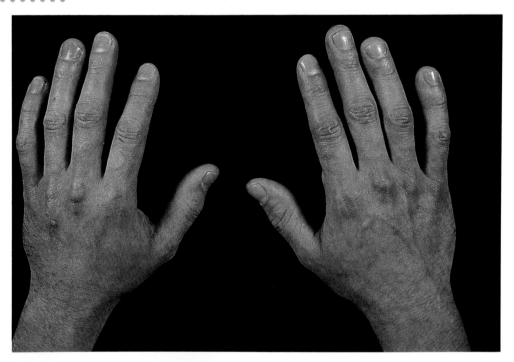

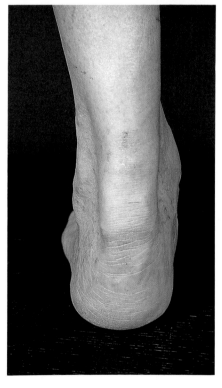

FIGURE 4.43 • Tendon xanthomas secondary to familial hypercholesterolemia. (Courtesy of Jean Davignon, MD, Montreal, Quebec, Canada)

Treatment of Hyperlipidemias

FAMILY SCREENING

If a patient is found to have hyperlipidemia that cannot be explained by secondary causes, the chances are high that genetic factors contribute significantly to elevated lipids. Therefore, lipid testing in first-degree relatives is in order. These include parents, siblings, and children. Such testing may help to define the type of hyperlipidemia, which could facilitate decisions about management. In addition, other family members requiring lipid-lowering therapy may be identified.

IDENTIFICATION OF SECONDARY HYPERLIPIDEMIAS

Before initiating lipid-lowering therapy, secondary causes of hyperlipidemia should be ruled out. These causes include hypothyroidism, diabetes mellitus, chronic renal failure, nephrotic syndrome, obstructive liver disease, corticosteroid excess, dysproteinemias (for example, multiple myeloma, benign monoclonal gammopathy), and certain drugs (for example, ß-adrenergic blocking agents). Appropriate laboratory tests should be carried out in patients suspected of having any of these disorders or conditions.

CLASSIFICATION OF PRIMARY HYPERLIPIDEMIAS
Hypercholesterolemia

In this chapter, the term "hypercholesterolemia" is defined as an increase in either LDL-cholesterol or VLDL and LDL-cholesterol. The term is modified according to severity— mild, moderate, or severe (refer to Figure 4.41). In general, mild hypercholesterolemia is considered to be of dietary origin, whereas the term "primary" is applied to moderate and severe hypercholesterolemias. Genetic factors frequently contribute to primary hypercholesterolemia, and a genetic origin can be divided into two categories—monogenic and polygenic.

Two types of monogenic hypercholesterolemia have been identified. One of these is called familial hypercholesterolemia (FH). The underlying defect in FH is a deficiency of LDL-receptors.[13-15] Normally, two functioning LDL-receptor genes are inherited, one from each parent. Both are required to maintain a normal level of LDL-cholesterol. One in 500 people inherit a defective gene for the LDL receptor, and hence they have only half the normal number of LDL-receptors. Such people are said to have heterozygous FH, and their LDL-cholesterol concentrations are twice normal. In recent years, a large number of defects in the gene encoding for LDL-receptors has been identified, and each of these produces the syndrome of heterozygous FH. As a result of the deficiency of LDL-receptors, hepatic clearance of both LDL and VLDL remnants is impaired. Patients with heterozygous FH often have tendon xanthomas[57] (Figure 4.43). FH men frequently develop premature CHD in their thirties and forties, whereas FH women commonly manifest CHD in their fifties and sixties (Figure 4.44). Rare individuals, one in a million, inherit two abnormal genes for LDL-receptors, and they develop extreme elevations of LDL-cholesterol. These individuals are said to have homozygous FH.

Another monogenic hypercholesterolemia is familial defective apo B-100 (FDB).[58-62] In this disorder, apo B-100, which normally binds to LDL-receptors, fails to interact with receptors. Consequently, serum LDL levels are increased. In contrast to FH, VLDL remnants of FDB patients bind normally to receptors because they contain apo E, which also has the capacity to interact with receptors. Like FH, there are two alleles for apo B-100, one from each parent. Thus, most patients with FDB are heterozygotes, that is, half of their LDL particles bind normally to receptors, but the other half do not. To date, only one mutation in apo B-100 has been identified as causing FDB. This is an arginine-for-glutamine substitution at position 3500 of the apo B-100 molecule.[61] In all likelihood, other defects in apo B-100 structure will be identified in the future. Defects also impair apo B binding to LDL-receptors. Although LDL levels usually are not as high in FDB patients as in FH patients, tendon xanthomas and premature CHD have been reported with this condition.

Most patients with primary hypercholesterolemia do not have monogenic varieties. Instead, for most, seemingly two or more abnormal genes are inherited that raise LDL concentrations into the elevated range. The defect in each of these genes apparently is relatively minor so that the presence of a single abnormal gene is not sufficient to produce detectable hypercholesterolemia. However, the simultaneous occurrence of several of these abnormalities will produce a definitely increased LDL-cholesterol. This condition therefore is called

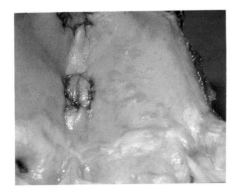

FIGURE 4.44 • A close-up view of fatty streaks in the root of the aorta in a patient with familial hypercholesterolemia. (Reproduced with permission. Galton DJ, Krone W: *Hyperlipidaemia in Practice* London: Gower Medical Publishing; 1991.)

polygenic hypercholesterolemia[63–65] or if only two defective genes are present, oligogenic hypercholesterolemia.[66] The characteristics of these mildly defective genes have not been defined, but they may result in abnormal regulation in synthesis of LDL-receptors (for example, hyperabsorption of cholesterol, defective conversion of cholesterol into bile acids, defective control of the promotor region of the LDL receptor), abnormalities in apo E structure, and overproduction of apo B-100. In the majority of cases, the result is moderate hypercholesterolemia, but in some instances, severe hypercholesterolemia can occur.[66]

Hypertriglyceridemia

Mild hypertriglyceridemia can be defined as a total triglyceride in the range of 150 to 250 mg/dL, with many investigators defining this range as "high-normal." Levels of 250 to 500 mg/dL can be called moderate hypertriglyceridemia. They also have been labeled "borderline" hypertriglyceridemia, although this is a confusing term. Triglyceride levels over 500 mg/dL are designated severe hypertriglyceridemia (Figure 4.45). An increase in plasma triglycerides can occur in either VLDL or chylomicron fractions. An increase in VLDL alone is called type 4 hyperlipoproteinemia (HLP), whereas an increase in VLDL plus chylomicrons is type 5 HLP.[67] Type 4 HLP also has been designated "endogenous" hypertriglyceridemia because VLDL are derived mainly from the liver.

Secondary causes of hypertriglyceridemia include diabetes mellitus, chronic renal failure, and excess cortiscosteroids. Beta-adrenergic blocking agents can accentuate hypertriglyceridemia in some patients. The same is true for obesity and excess alcohol intake.

Primary hypertriglyceridemia usually has a genetic component. Type 4 HLP occurring on a genetic basis is called familial hypertriglyceridemia.[63–65] Rare patients appear to have familial type 5 HLP.[68] Two general mechanisms appear to underlie the development of familial hypertriglyceridemia. Some patients appear to have hepatic overproduction of VLDL triglycerides,[69] whereas others have defective lipolysis of triglyceride-rich lipoproteins.[70] The latter is most dramatic in complete absence of lipoprotein lipase,[68] also called type 1 HLP,[67] but this disorder is rare, occurring only once in a million people. Much more common are milder defects in lipolysis producing type 4 HLP.[70]

Hypertriglyceridemia can be combined with elevated total cholesterol giving mixed hyperlipidemia. As described before, hypercholesterolemia can be mild, moderate, or severe. Multiple factors can contribute to development of mixed hyperlipidemia. Both elevated triglycerides and cholesterol can be the result of genetic factors (primary), secondary to other conditions, or of dietary origin. One form of mixed hyperlipidemia that appears to be of genetic origin is familial combined hyperlipidemia.[63–65,71] This hyperlipidemia is characterized by the presence of multiple lipoprotein phenotypes occurring in a single family. There are two theories of the origin of familial combined hyperlipidemia. Some investigators believe that it is monogenic,[63–65] with the underlying defect being overproduction of VLDL apo B-100 by the liver.[69,72] Alternatively, it could be polygenic in origin—there could be a combination of defects in a single family, overproduction of VLDL triglycerides, defective lipolysis of triglyceride-rich lipoproteins, and a deficiency of LDL-receptors. If this latter mechanism pertains, a single family presumably would have inherited several abnormal genes affecting both serum cholesterol and triglycerides. This mechanism is analogous to polygenic hypercholesterolemia in which several gene abnormalities combine to produce an elevated LDL-cholesterol concentration.

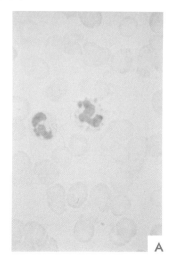

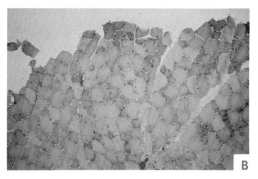

FIGURE 4.45 • White blood cells showing early accumulation of triglyceride vacuoles (A). Muscle biopsy showing abnormal accumulation of tryglycerides (B). (Reproduced with permission. Galton DJ, Krone W: *Hyperlipidaemia in Practice* London: Gower Medical Publishing; 1991.)

DIETARY THERAPY

SERUM CHOLESTEROL-RAISING FACTORS IN THE DIET

Three factors in the diet are known to increase serum cholesterol levels:
- Dietary cholesterol.
- Certain fatty acids.
- Obesity.

The relative contributions of each to higher serum cholesterol levels in high-risk populations depend on several variables, and at present, one dietary factor cannot be called more "hypercholesterolemic" than another. For example, dietary cholesterol and obesity seemingly raise serum cholesterol more in younger adults than in older people. In contrast, dietary fatty acids apparently have similar effects on cholesterol levels at all ages. Nonetheless, all three factors contribute to the "mass hypercholesterolemia" of Americans, and the key to effective dietary control of elevated serum cholesterol is to modify each of these factors. The following reviews each briefly.

Dietary Cholesterol

Feeding cholesterol to many animal species, such as rabbits and monkeys, produces marked hypercholesterolemia.[73-75] This finding led to the hypothesis that dietary cholesterol is atherogenic in humans. Studies in humans, however, showed that people in general are more resistant to dietary cholesterol than several other species, including primates.[76] High intakes of cholesterol usually cause only mild-to-moderate elevations of serum total cholesterol.[77] Some investigators[78-80] have even claimed that for most people dietary cholesterol is without significant effect on serum cholesterol. The better investigations[81-88] however, reveal that increasing cholesterol intake will raise serum cholesterol in most people. The extent of rise is illustrated by studies carried out by three different groups[81-83] (Figure 4.46). The relationship between cholesterol intake and the increase in serum cholesterol was similar, although not identical. When data from the major studies are pooled, the serum total cholesterol increases approximately 8 to 10 mg/dL for every 100 mg of dietary cholesterol/1,000 calories.[77] For example, increasing cholesterol intakes from 300 to 500 mg/dL on the average will raise the serum total cholesterol by 8 to 10 mg/dL. Because risk for coronary heart disease (CHD) rises about 1% for every 1 mg/dL increment in total cholesterol, the effect of a cholesterol intake of 500 mg/dL on overall CHD risk is not trivial.

Most of the increment in serum total cholesterol resulting from an increase in dietary cholesterol occurs in the LDL fraction. This increase is primarily due to a suppression of LDL receptor activity.[89,90] The synthesis of LDL-receptors by liver cells is a function of the hepatic cholesterol content. When the cholesterol content increases, LDL-receptor synthesis is suppressed. This action is believed to be mediated by the formation of an oxysterol that acts in the nucleus of the cell to suppress the activation of the promoter for the LDL-receptor gene.[91] The consequences for serum LDL metabolism are outlined in Figure 4.47. Reduced LDL receptor activity raises LDL levels in two ways:
- By retarding direct clearance of LDL.
- By inhibiting uptake of VLDL remnants, leading to conversion of more VLDL remnants to LDL.

• • • • • • • • • • • • • • •

FIGURE 4.46 • Studies of Keys, Mattson, and Hegsted, and their colleagues, showing the relationship between increases in the cholesterol content of the diet and rises in serum cholesterol levels. (Results from Keys A, Anderson JT, Grande F: *Metabolism* 1965;13:759. Hegsted DM, McGandy RB, Myers ML, et al: *Am J Clin Nutr* 1965;17:281. Mattson FH, Erickson, Klingman AM: *Am J Clin Nutr* 1972;25:589.)

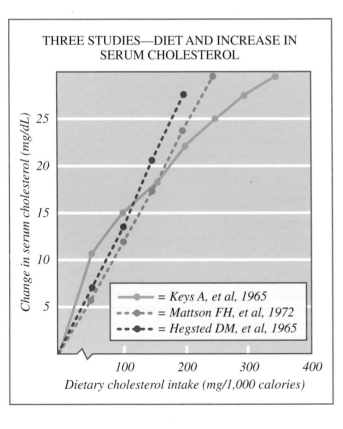

THREE STUDIES—DIET AND INCREASE IN SERUM CHOLESTEROL

= Keys A, et al, 1965
= Mattson FH, et al, 1972
= Hegsted DM, et al, 1965

Change in serum cholesterol (mg/dL)

Dietary cholesterol intake (mg/1,000 calories)

High intakes of cholesterol also can raise levels of VLDL-cholesterol and HDL-cholesterol. The significance of the increase in HDL-cholesterol is unknown, although the rise in LDL-cholesterol and VLDL-cholesterol should enhance CHD risk. Moreover, newly absorbed cholesterol, associated with chylomicrons and chylomicron remnants, likewise could be atherogenic.[92] Finally, previous cholesterol-balance studies have shown that increased intake of cholesterol causes enhanced absorption of cholesterol. Thus, unless compensatory mechanisms are precise, increased cholesterol absorption will expand body stores of cholesterol.[93] This "loading" of the body with cholesterol might have several adverse effects. For example, it might contribute to the rise of cholesterol with age, because increasing body pools of cholesterol should down-regulate LDL receptor activity. It also might retard reverse cholesterol transport, thereby directly promoting development of atherosclerosis. In support of these hypotheses, several epidemiologic studies[94] suggest that high intakes of cholesterol predispose to CHD independently of their effects on fasting lipoprotein concentrations.

The average intake of cholesterol for adult American men is about 450 mg/d, and for women, about 300 mg/d. The difference in cholesterol intake between men and women relates mainly to differences in total caloric intake. Dietary cholesterol

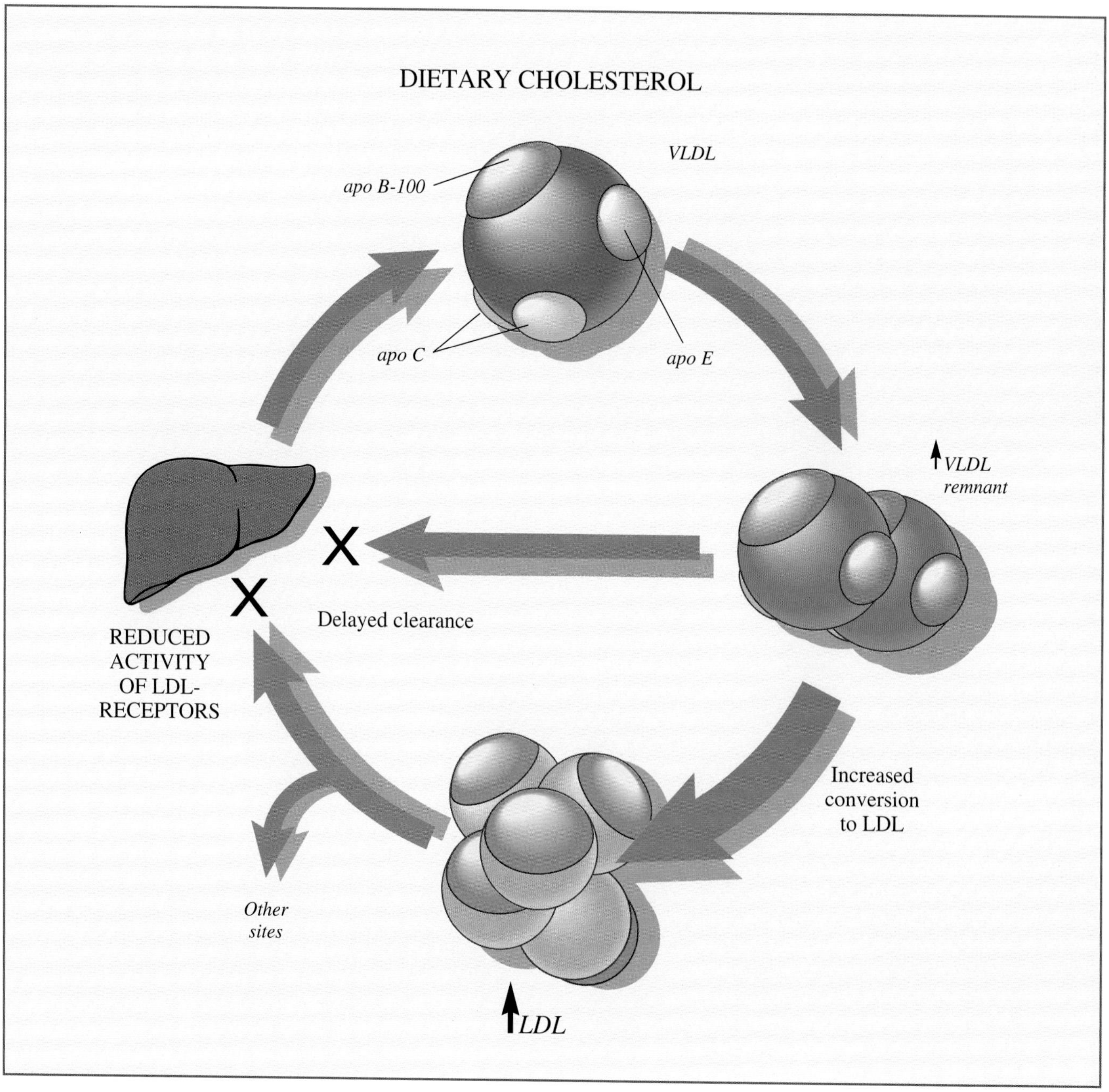

FIGURE 4.47 • Effects of high intakes of dietary cholesterol on the basic pathways of lipoprotein metabolism.

comes about equally from eggs, meat, and animal fats, including milk and milk products.[95] Among fats, butterfat and its products —whole milk, butter, cream, and cheese—are especially rich in cholesterol. Lean meat has only about 70 to 80 mg cholesterol/3 ounces. Organ meats—liver, pancreas, kidneys, brains, and heart—are very high in cholesterol. Most fish and shellfish have approximately the same content per weight as lean meat. The exception is shrimp, which contains about 166 mg cholesterol/3 ounces.

Cholesterol-Raising Fatty Acids

The saturated fatty acids as a group have been shown to increase serum cholesterol levels. Epidemiologic studies, such as the Seven Countries Study,[28] strongly suggest that dietary saturated fatty acids raise the serum cholesterol (Figure 4.48). Supportive evidence comes from studies in laboratory animals,[96,97] and definite proof has been obtained in metabolic ward studies in humans.[98–100] The diet normally contains a variety of saturated fatty acids of different chain lengths (Figure 4.49).

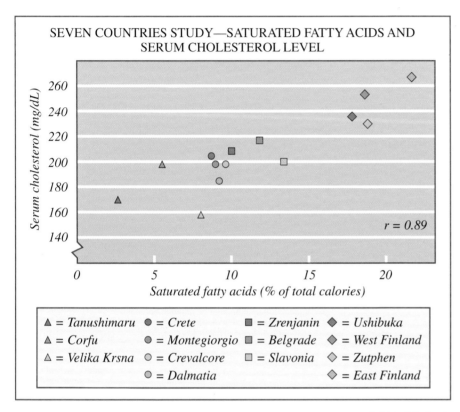

FIGURE 4.48 • Epidemiologic evidence showing the relationship between intakes of saturated fatty acids and serum cholesterol levels—the Seven Countries Study. (Reproduced with permission. Keys A: *Circulation* 1970;41(suppl 1):1.)

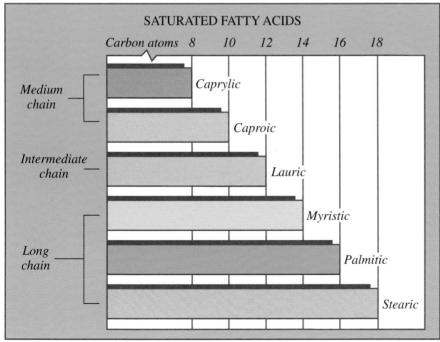

FIGURE 4.49 • Carbon-chain lengths of common saturated fatty acids of the diet.

Most saturated fatty acids come from animal fats, but tropical plant oils also are rich in these acids. Palmitic acid (16:0) is the major saturated acid in the diet, but various sources of dietary fat differ in their patterns of saturated fatty acids. Although all saturated fatty acids have been widely assumed to be "hypercholesterolemic," there is growing evidence that some fatty acids do not raise cholesterol levels. In this latter category are medium-chain fatty acids, caprylic (8:0) and caproic (10:0)[101,102] acids, and long-chain stearic acid (18:0).[99–105] This leaves the major cholesterol-raising saturates as palmitic acid, myristic acid (14:0), and lauric acid (12:0).

The mechanisms whereby the latter three saturated fatty acids increase the serum cholesterol are not fully understood. Recent data, however, suggest that they reduce LDL-receptor clearance of apo B-containing lipoproteins (refer to Figure 4.26).[96,97] Whether they suppress the synthesis of LDL-receptors in liver cells, or reduce the activity of these receptors at the surface of liver cells has not been determined with certainty. Regardless, they raise cholesterol levels in almost everyone tested. Although people may vary in their responsiveness to saturated fatty acids, on the average, for every 1% of total calories of saturated fatty acids substituted for other nutrients, the serum total cholesterol level rises about 2.7 mg/dL.[99,100]

The major sources of saturated fatty acids in the diet are milk products (28%), meats and meat products (33%), baked goods (9%), and miscellaneous foods (30%) (Figure 4.50).[95] The latter includes various cooking fats and oils, snack foods, mixed dishes, and fried foods. Thus, the relatively high intake of saturated fatty acids in the American diet comes from a variety of sources, and elimination of one source is not sufficient to achieve an acceptable reduction. Milk fat in the form of butter, cheese, ice cream, and cheese is the most hypercholesterolemic

of fats because of its high content of palmitic and myristic acids. Although beef fat is the single largest source of saturated fat in the American diet, its high content of stearic acid makes it less hypercholesterolemic than milk fat.

Recently, another category of fatty acid has been identified as a serum cholesterol raiser. This category includes trans-monounsaturated fatty acids.[106,107] The major acid of this class is elaidic acid, which has 18 carbon atoms and one double bond located at the omega-9 position—the double bond is in the trans-configuration. Other trans-fatty acids have double bonds at other locations up and down the carbon chain. Trans-fatty acids are formed from hydrogenation of linoleic acid (18:2), and they are found in various margarines and shortenings. The trans-double bond gives them a rigid structure, similar to that of a saturated fatty acid, and this "saturated" structure may account for their ability to raise the serum cholesterol level.

Obesity

A third dietary factor that increases the serum cholesterol is obesity. Obesity appears to be more hypercholesterolemic in younger adults than in older ones, but at all ages being overweight raises cholesterol levels.[108–113] The greatest increments in cholesterol levels appear to occur with moderate weight gain so that mild-to-moderate obesity is about as hypercholesterolemic as severe obesity. The higher serum cholesterol in obese people occurs both in the VLDL and LDL fractions.

The mechanism for the rise in both VLDL and LDL is an overproduction of apo B-containing lipoproteins by the liver.[114–116] Some obese people have predominant hypertriglyceridemia (Figure 4.51), whereas others have mainly hypercholesterolemia (Figure 4.52). In other individuals, obesity causes mixed hyperlipidemia. Not only does obesity raise

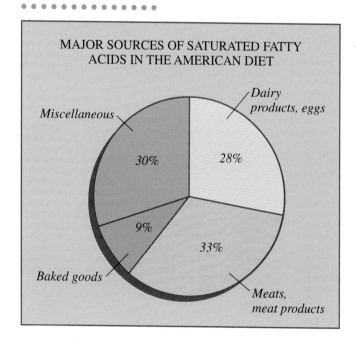

FIGURE 4.50 • Major sources of saturated fatty acids in the American diet.

VLDL-cholesterol and LDL-cholesterol, but it also reduces HDL-cholesterol.[117] Thus, in contrast to dietary cholesterol and saturated fatty acids, the adverse action of obesity on lipoprotein metabolism is not confined to raising LDL. When the unfavorable effects of obesity on lipoprotein metabolism are added to its other undesirable actions (for example, raising blood pressure, increasing blood glucose), obesity seems to be the major nutritional problem promoting the development of cardiovascular disease.

UNSATURATED FATTY ACIDS

This category includes monounsaturated and polyunsaturated fatty acids. The former have one double bond, the latter, two or more. The major monounsaturated fatty acid is oleic acid

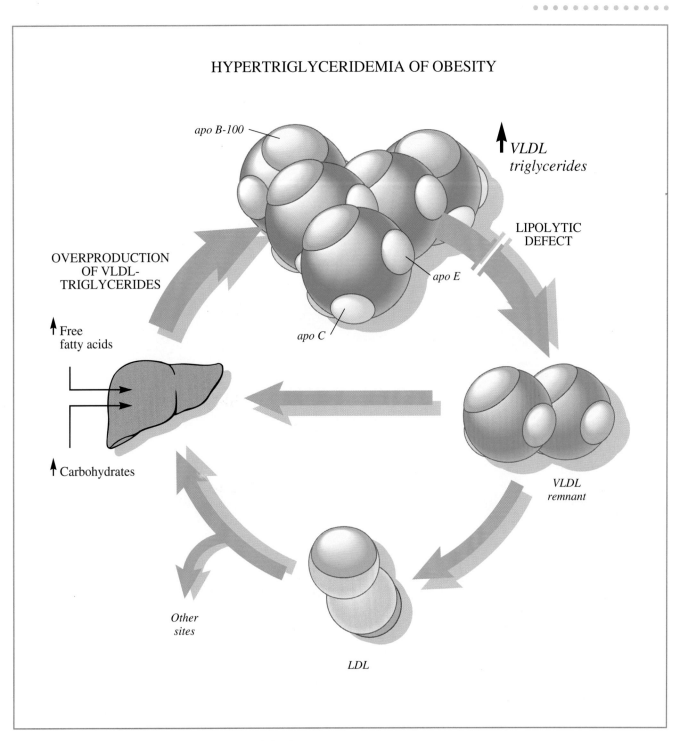

HYPERTRIGLYCERIDEMIA OF OBESITY

FIGURE 4.51 • Mechanisms of hypertriglyceridemia of obesity.

(Table 4.5). It has 18 carbon atoms, one double bond located in the ω9 position, that is, 9 carbon atoms from the terminal end of the molecule. The double bond is in the cis-configuration.

The predominate polyunsaturated fatty acid in the diet is linolenic acid (18:2ω6), but another important group includes the ω3 polyunsaturates—linoleic acid (18:3:ω3), eicosapentaenoic acid (20:5ω3) (EPA), and docosahexaenoic acid (DHA) (22:6ω3). Each different type of polyunsaturate apparently has different effects on lipoprotein metabolism.

POLYUNSATURATED FATTY ACIDS

Linoleic acid is a common constituent of vegetable oils. For many years, dietary linoleic acid was considered to have a unique property to lower LDL-cholesterol levels, and for this reason, it was widely recommended for cholesterol lowering diets. More recent evidence[118,119] has thrown this concept into doubt, and it now appears that linoleic acid is "neutral" with respect to LDL-cholesterol, neither raising nor lowering the level. On the other hand, when linoleic acid is consumed in large quantities, it causes a moderate lowering of HDL-cholesterol levels.[118,120–122]

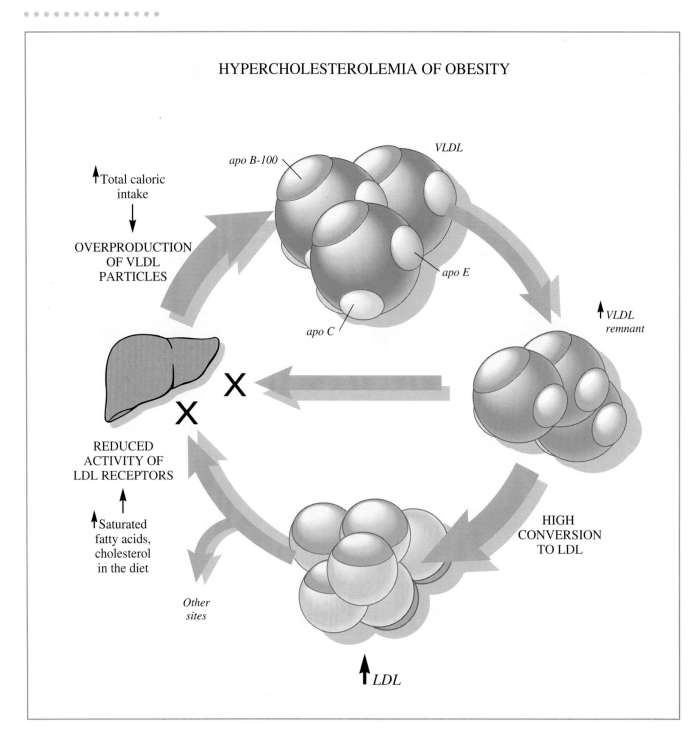

FIGURE 4.52 • Mechanisms of hypercholesterolemia of obesity.

Treatment of Hyperlipidemias

Other findings with linoleic acid have dampened enthusiasm for its use. It suppresses the immune system in laboratory animals and promotes development of tumors. In humans, linoleic acid may increase risk for cholesterol gallstones in some patients, and recent data[123,124] indicate that it promotes oxidation of LDL, possibly a critical step in atherogenesis. For these several reasons, most investigators recommend limiting intake of linoleic acid to less than 10% of total calories, and possibly to less than 7%.[125]

The very-long-chain, ω3 fatty acids—eicosapentaeonic acid (EPA) and dicosahexaenoic acid (DHA)—occur mainly in fish oils. They too appear to be neutral with respect to LDL-cholesterol levels, and may have mild HDL-lowering properties. Their major action, however, is to suppress hepatic secretion of VLDL triglycerides.[126,127] Consequently, they may have some utility for treating hypertriglyceridemia. In contrast, they probably are of little value for lowering serum cholesterol levels. Even so, they may have other beneficial effects for CHD prevention, notably for inhibiting coronary thrombosis because of their action to prevent platelet aggregation.

MONOUNSATURATED FATTY ACIDS

For many years, oleic acid was ignored as a potentially valuable nutrient for cholesterol-lowering diets. This was because it was considered to be neutral with respect to cholesterol levels, whereas polyunsaturated fatty acids were believed to lower the cholesterol levels. Because of recent evidence that linoleic and oleic acids have similar effects on LDL levels,[118,119] oleic acid has received increased attention. One great advantage of oleic acid over linoleic acid is that large quantities of oleic acid have been consumed for centuries in Mediterranean countries where rates of CHD are relatively low.[28] In addition, dietary oleic acid apparently does not suppress the immune system or promote development of tumors in animals, it does not enhance LDL oxidation, nor does it lower HDL-cholesterol with high intakes. When all factors are taken into consideration, high intakes of oleic acid thus may be preferable to high intakes of linoleic acid for diets designed to prevent CHD.

CARBOHYDRATES

The diet contains a variety of carbohydrates, including simple sugars—monosaccharides, disaccharides—and complex carbohydrates—starches, cellulose, and soluble fibers. The sources of dietary carbohydrates are fruits, vegetables, cereals, legumes, and processed foods. In the American diet, which is relatively high in fat, intake of digestible carbohydrates averages about 45% of total calories. In many other countries in which fat intake is relatively low, carbohydrates constitute between 50% and 75% of total calories. In many of the latter countries, rates of CHD are low, leading many researchers to the conclusion that low-fat, high-carbohydrate diets will protect against CHD. Serum cholesterol levels typically are in the desirable range in these populations, and they have a low prevalence of obesity. Both of these effects have been attributed to low-fat, high-carbohydrate diets. Other factors, however, may contribute to less obesity and lower cholesterol levels in these populations, and thus the diet may not deserve all the credit. Nonetheless, the American Heart Association[128] and the National Cholesterol Education Program (NCEP)[1] have recommended that a major part of the reduction in saturated fatty acids recommended for the American diet be replaced by carbohydrate.

Low-fat, high-carbohydrate diets have several actions on the metabolism of serum lipoproteins, as compared with the typical American diet (Figure 4.53). They stimulate the synthesis of VLDL triglycerides,[129–131] and may reduce the activity of lipoprotein lipase[132–133]. These two changes can lead to higher levels of VLDL triglycerides. The mechanisms whereby a low-fat diet lowers LDL-cholesterol concentrations are not fully understood,[134] but replacement of saturated fatty acids by carbohydrates may remove suppression of synthesis of LDL-receptors. High-carbohydrate diets can cause a lowering of HDL-cholesterol,[135–140] apparently by reducing the secretion of apo A-I by the liver.[141]

Nondigestible carbohydrates include the insoluble fibers—cellulose—and soluble fibers—pectins, gums, and psyllium. The insoluble fibers apparently have little or no effect on serum-cholesterol levels, but soluble fibers have been reported

Fatty Acid	Designation
TABLE 4.5 • UNSATURATED FATTY ACIDS OF THE DIET	
Omega-9	
• Oleic acid	18:1ω9
Omega-6	
• Linoleic acid	18:2ω6
Omega-3	
• Linolenic acid	18:3ω3
• Eicosapentaenoic acid (EPA)	20:5ω3
• Dicosahexaenoic acid (DHA)	20:6ω3

to lower LDL-cholesterol concentrations. When relatively high intakes are consumed, serum-total cholesterol concentrations fall in the range of about 3% to 5%. The mechanism for this effect is not known.

ALCOHOL

The intake of alcohol in the American diet averages about 5% of total calories, although for many people it is much higher than this amount. Alcohol has a variety of adverse effects,

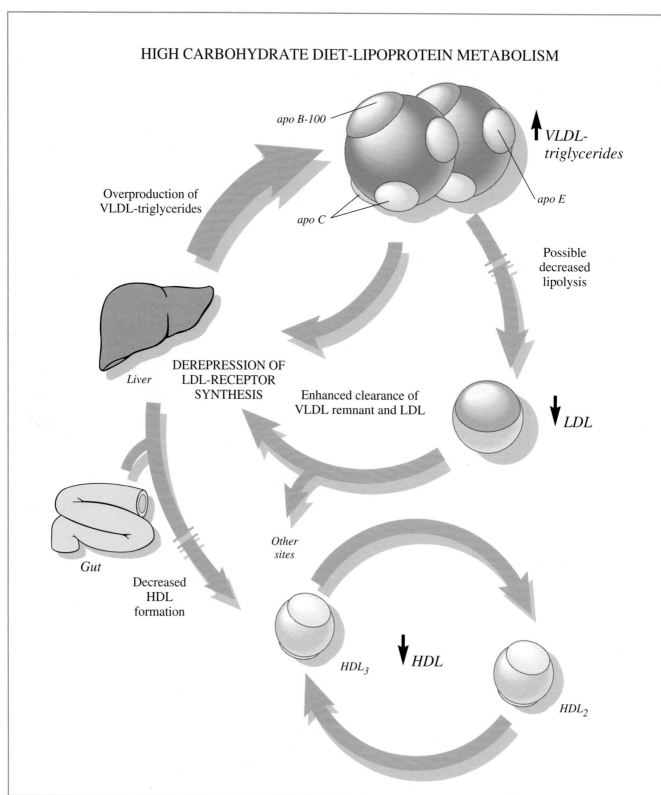

HIGH CARBOHYDRATE DIET-LIPOPROTEIN METABOLISM

FIGURE 4.53 • Major actions of a high-carbohydrate diet on the basic pathways of lipoprotein metabolism.

both social and physiological, but in addition it has several actions on lipoprotein metabolism (Figure 4.54). It stimulates the production of VLDL-triglycerides by the liver, which can raise triglyceride levels.[142-145] In addition, it often raises the HDL-cholesterol concentration, seemingly by stimulating the secretion of apo A-I. Although some investigators[146] speculate that daily ingestion of alcohol may reduce risk for CHD, most workers take the position that the known ad-

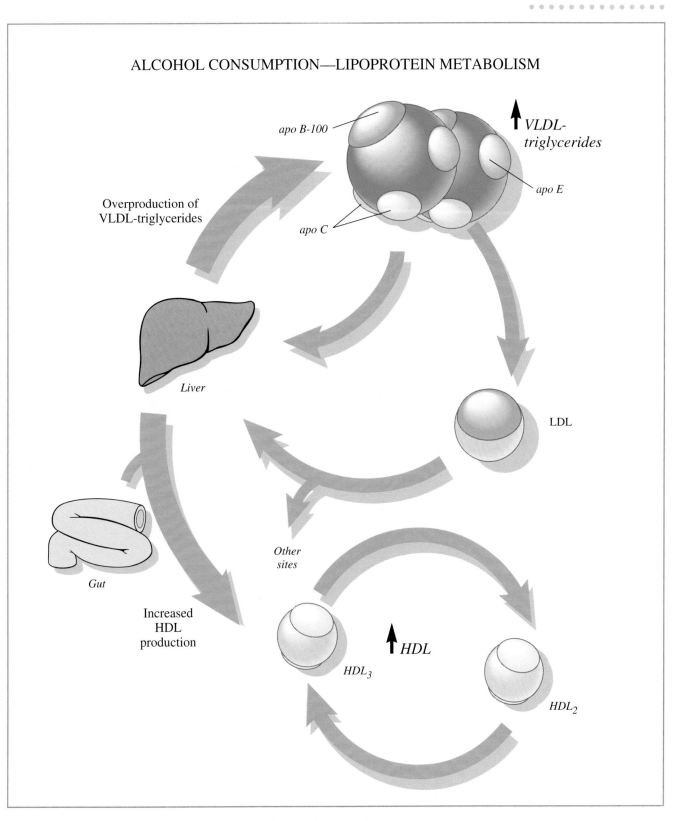

ALCOHOL CONSUMPTION—LIPOPROTEIN METABOLISM

FIGURE 4.54 • Major actions of alcohol consumption on lipoprotein metabolism.

verse effects of high alcohol intake far outweigh any theoretical advantages.

RECOMMENDED DIETS FOR DYSLIPIDEMIA

The NCEP[1] has set forth recommendations for treatment of high serum cholesterol in the clinical setting. To some extent, these diets are applicable for patients with other forms of dyslipidemia. Essentially the same diet is recommended by the American Heart Association. The basic principle of the recommended diet is a threefold change in eating habits, namely, a decreased intake of cholesterol-raising fatty acids, a reduced intake of cholesterol, and weight reduction to achieve a desirable body weight. The cholesterol-raising fatty acids usually are equated with saturated fatty acids, but for reasons outlined before, the identification of specific fatty acids that increase cholesterol levels is more reasonable. A reduction in cholesterol-raising fatty acids and cholesterol occurs in two steps:

- The Step I diet calls for dietary saturated fatty acids of less than 10% of total calories, and cholesterol intake of less than 300 mg/d (Figure 4.55, Table 4.6).
- The Step II diet further reduces saturated fatty acids to less than 7%, and dietary cholesterol to less than 200 mg/d (Table 4.7).

The recommendation indicates that total fat intake should be 30% or less of total energy, although this recommendation is

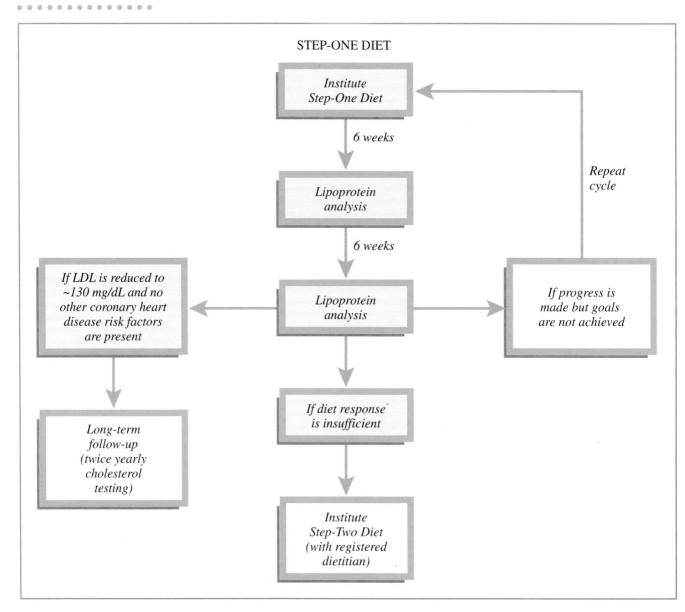

FIGURE 4.55 • The Step-One Diet

less well-founded on scientific evidence. A somewhat higher fat intake, up to 35% of calories, is justified provided that the increment consists of monounsaturated fatty acids.

In practical terms, adherence to a cholesterol-lowering diet requires attention to several food groups. Within each group, some types of food should be chosen and others should be decreased. These groups include fish, meats, and poultry; dairy products; breads and cereals; eggs, fruits and vegetables; and fats and oils (Table 4.8). By making the changes outlined in Table 4.8, a substantial reduction in saturated fatty acid and cholesterol intakes should be achieved. These changes will produce a decrease in serum total cholesterol levels of approximately 20 mg/dL in most patients. If weight reduction is carried out in obese people, a further 10 to 15 mg/dL reduction in total cholesterol level should be obtained.

DRUG THERAPY

In the past two decades, significant advances have been made in the use of drugs used for treatment of hyperlipidemia. Some of these drugs indeed have been shown to reduce the risk of coronary heart disease (CHD). Although all drugs have adverse effects, the side effect profile for lipid-lowering drugs has been determined, and in general most side effects do not appear to be

TABLE 4.6 • COMPOSITION OF THE STEP-ONE DIET

Nutrient	Recommendations (percent of total calories)
Total fat	≤ 30%
• Saturated fatty acids	< 10%
• Polyunsaturated fatty acids	< 10%
• Monosaturated fatty acids	10%-15%
Carbohydrates	50%-60%
Protein	15%

Reduce total calories ⟶	To achieve desirable weight
Cholesterol ⟶	< 300 mg/d

TABLE 4.7 COMPOSITION OF STEP-TWO DIET

Nutrient	Recommendations (percent of total calories)
Total fat	≤ 30%
• Saturated fatty acids	< 7%
• Polyunsaturated fatty acids	< 10%
• Monosaturated fatty acids	10%-15%
Carbohydrates	50%-60%
Protein	15%

Reduce total calories ⟶	To achieve desirable weight
Cholesterol ⟶	< 200 mg/d

Fish, Meats, and Poultry

Choose
- Fish
- Shellfish
- Poultry without skin
- Lean cuts of beef, pork, lamb
- Veal

Decrease
- Fatty cuts of beef, lamb, or pork
- Spareribs
- Organ meats
- Processed meats— cold cuts, bacon, sausages, hot dogs
- Sardines, roe

Dairy products

Choose
- Skim milk or low fat (1%-2% milk), buttermilk
- Low fat varieties of yogurt, cottage cheese, and cheeses
- Sherbet
- Sorbet

Decrease
- Whole milk—4% fat
- Whole-milk yogurt and cottage cheese
- Cream, half-and-half
- Cream cheese
- Sour cream
- Ice cream
- Natural cheeses

Fruits and Vegetables

Choose
- Fruits: fresh, frozen, canned, dried
- Vegetables

Decrease
- Fruits with cream or ice cream
- Vegetables prepared in butter, cream, or other sauces

Fats and Oils

Choose
- Unsaturated vegetable oils
- Margarines and shortenings made from vegetable oils
- Mayonnaise and salad dressings made from vegetable oils
- Seeds and nuts

Decrease
- Butter
- Lard (bacon fat)
- Coconut oil
- Palm oil
- Palm kernel oil
- Chocolate
- Coconut

Breads and Cereals

Choose
- Homemade baked goods (using unsaturated oils)
- Angel food cake
- Low-fat crackers and cookies
- Rice, pasta
- Whole-grain breads and cereals

Decrease
- Commercial baked goods: pies, cakes, doughnuts, croissants, pastries, biscuits
- High fat crackers and cookies
- Egg noodles
- Egg-containing breads

Eggs

Choose
- Egg whites (2 egg whites = 1 whole egg in recipes)
- Cholesterol-free egg substitutes

Decrease
- Egg yolks (restricted to 3 per week)

serious. Because of increased potency of new drugs or use of older drugs in combination, it is now possible to normalize serum lipid levels in most patients with hyperlipidemia. In this section, currently available lipid-lowering drugs will be reviewed.

BILE ACID SEQUESTRANTS

These drugs are resins that bind bile acids in the intestinal tract. Two available sequestrants are cholestyramine and colestipol (Figure 4.56). Their action is limited entirely to the intestinal tract; this action is to inhibit the reabsorption of bile acids and thereby to interrupt their enterohepatic circulation.[146] A reduction in return of bile acids to the liver releases the feedback inhibition of bile acids on the conversion of cholesterol into bile acids. This action lowers the hepatic content of cholesterol, which promotes the synthesis of LDL-receptor. As a result, the plasma concentration of LDL falls. Theoretically, this mechanism should produce a marked reduction in LDL levels, but in fact, the degree of LDL reduction is limited by a compensatory increase in synthesis of cholesterol. Even so, at moderate intakes of bile acid sequestrants, LDL-cholesterol levels fall by 15% to 25%. The degree of reduction of LDL levels increases with higher doses, although at higher doses, the increment in cholesterol reduction declines. Thus, at a dose of cholestyramine of 8 g/d (colestipol 10 g/d), a fall in LDL-cholesterol levels of 15% to 20% is typical, whereas at twice this dose, decreases usually range from 20% to 25%. In general, the lower dose is much better tolerated than the higher dose.

The major side effects of bile acid sequestrants are constipation and gastrointestinal distress—bloating, epigastric fullness, nausea, flatulence, and occasionally diarrhea. These side effects are particularly troublesome in patients who have underlying gastrointestinal disease—chronic constipation, hemorrhoids, peptic ulcer disease, and persistent esophageal reflux. Constipation may be controlled by increasing dietary fiber or by stool softeners. Laxatives should usually be avoided.

Sequestrants can interfere with the absorption of digitalis products, warfarin, thyroxine, thiazide diuretics, and ß-adrenergic blocking agents. These drugs should be administered either one hour before or four hours after administration of bile acid sequestrants. The absorption of fat-soluble vitamins may be reduced, but vitamin deficiency is rare. Transitory increases in hepatic transaminases or alkaline phosphatase have been reported in patients taking sequestrants, but these changes probably are not causally related. Sequestrant therapy can raise triglyceride levels by stimulating the synthesis of VLDL triglycerides. These drugs are contraindicated in patients with severe hypertriglyceridemia, because of the risk of acute pancreatitis.

The effectiveness of bile acid sequestrants for reducing the risk of CHD has been demonstrated in the Lipid Research Clinic Coronary Primary Prevention Trial,[47,48] with supporting evidence from the National Heart, Lung, and Blood Institute (NHLBI) Type II study,[41] the CLAS trial,[42,43] and the Familial Atherosclerosis Treatment Study (FATS) trial.[44] The National

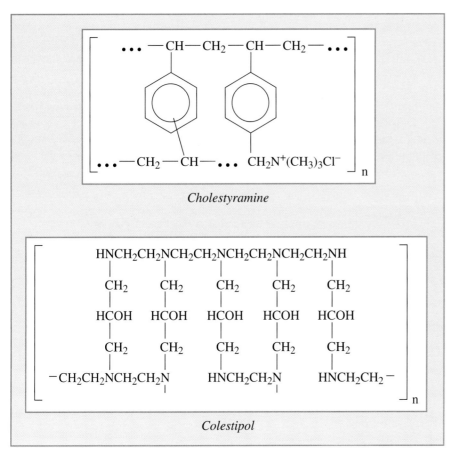

FIGURE 4.56 • Structural formulas of cholestyramine and colestipol.

Cholesterol Education Program (NCEP)[1] thus designated bile acid sequestrants as a first-line drug for treatment of hypercholesterolemia (Figure 4.57).

NICOTINIC ACID

This agent is a B vitamin and is required in small amounts in the diet. At high intakes, nicotinic acid is a cholesterol-lowering drug, and should not be considered a vitamin. Because high doses may have significant and potentially serious side effects, the drug should be administered only by a physician. Nicotinic acid can be purchased in health-food stores as a vitamin, but people should be discouraged from self-medication. Many different preparations of nicotinic acid are available in health food stores, but the quality of these preparations is poorly monitored. Slow-release preparations may reduce flushing and mitigate gastrointestinal side effects, but hepatotoxicity appears to be increased.

The mechanisms of cholesterol-lowering action of nicotinic acid are not well understood. Available evidence suggests that it decreases the production of VLDL particles by the liver (Figure 4.58). This action leads to a reduction of both VLDL and LDL levels, and secondarily to an increase in HDL-cholesterol concentrations. The drug may have other actions, such as inhibition of release of free fatty acids by adipose tissue and stimulation of the activity of lipoprotein lipase. Both of these effects should lower VLDL triglycerides, and secondarily, raise HDL levels.

Reductions in serum lipid levels are proportional to dose. To obtain optimal reductions, a dose of 4.5 g or 1,500 mg three times daily usually is required. Some patients sustain a good response at 3.0 g/d. To enhance drug tolerance, it should be started in low doses, for example, 100 mg three times daily, with a gradual increase in dose over a period of a few weeks. At higher doses, LDL-cholesterol levels typically fall by 15% to 25%, and increases of HDL-cholesterol of 20% to 30% are common.

Although nicotinic acid is inexpensive and highly effective, its utility is limited by several side effects. Only 50% to 60% of patients can tolerate full doses of the drug. Many patients are not able to tolerate its irritation of the upper gastrointestinal tract. The drug should be used with caution in patients with a history of peptic ulcer or chronic bowel disease because these may be reactivated. Nicotinic acid can cause several cutaneous responses—flushing and itching of the skin, rash and, rarely, acanthosis nicricans. Hepatotoxicity, apparently, is more likely to occur with delayed release preparations. The drug usually heightens hyperglycemia in diabetic patients and may precipitate frank diabetes in patients with glucose intolerance. The uric acid level usually rises, which can precipitate an episode of acute gout. Visual changes may indicate toxic amblyopia, and occasional patients may manifest cardiac arrhythmias.

The NCEP[1] designated nicotinic acid as a first-line drug for treatment of dyslipidemia. This was done for several reasons. First, long experience has shown that the drug is highly efficacious for lowering serum cholesterol and triglycerides, and although it has numerous side effects, they rarely are serious or irreversible. Further, the drug appeared to reduce risk for CHD and to prolong life in patients in the Coronary Drug Project.[38,39] On the other hand, the high prevalence of side effects cannot be ignored, and at most, only 50% to 60% of patients who are started on the drug will be able to tolerate it at therapeutically effective doses on a long-term basis.

HMG-CoA REDUCTASE INHIBITORS

These drugs are a new class of agents that hold great promise for treatment of hyperlipidemia. Their primary action is to inhibit the conversion of 3-hydroxy-3-methylglutaryl (HMG) coenzyme A (CoA) to mevalonic acid. This conversion is a rate-limiting step in cholesterol synthesis, and it is catabolized by the enzyme HMG-CoA reductase. The HMG-CoA reductase inhibitors contain a structure that is analogous to HMG and thereby compete with HMG for the enzyme. The structures of the major HMG-CoA reductase inhibitors are shown in Figure 4.59.

The prototype drug of this class is mevastatin (compactin). It was discovered in Japan in 1976,[147,148] and subsequently was shown to be effective for lowering cholesterol levels in both animals[149,150] and humans.[151,152] The derivative, lovastatin, was developed in the United States,[153] and was approved by the Food

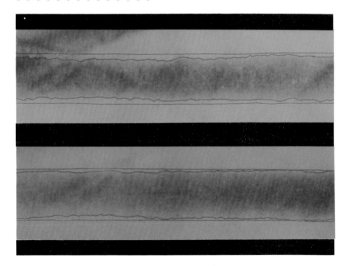

FIGURE 4.57 • Femoral angiograms showing the effect on atherosclerotic lesions of lowering blood cholesterol levels for 22 months. Before treatment (A). After treatment with cholestyramine (B). Note the improvement of the endothelial irregularity after treatment. (Reproduced with permission. Galton DJ, Krone W: *Hyperlipidaemia in Practice* London: Gower Medical Publishing; 1991.)

and Drug Administration in 1987. At present, over two million patients in the United States are taking lovastatin. Other agents that recently became available in the United States are simvastatin and pravastatin. Another agent under investigation is fluvastatin. Future studies will be required to determine whether these agents have relative advantages or disadvantages compared with the others.

Lovastatin can be given in three doses—20, 40, and 80 mg/d. It can be given either once or twice per day. At 20 mg/d, the LDL-cholesterol level falls about 25%; at 40 mg/d, the level declines by approximately 30%, and by 35% at 80 mg/d. Pravastatin has a similar potency as lovastatin. Simvastatin has approximately twice the potency, but toxicity likewise is doubled.

The HMG-CoA reductase inhibitors act primarily in the liver. Inhibition of HMG-CoA reductase reduces the cholesterol content of the liver cell, which in turn, stimulates the synthesis of LDL-receptors[154–156] (Figure 4.60). The consequences of this action for serum lipoproteins are shown in Figure 4.61. The clearance of LDL is enhanced, thus lowering LDL-cholesterol levels. In addition, the direct removal of VLDL remnants is increased because these lipoproteins likewise are recognized by LDL-receptors that result in two changes:

• First, fewer VLDL remnants are converted to LDL, further lowering the LDL level.
• Secondly, VLDL remnant concentrations are reduced, which results in a fall in serum triglyceride levels.

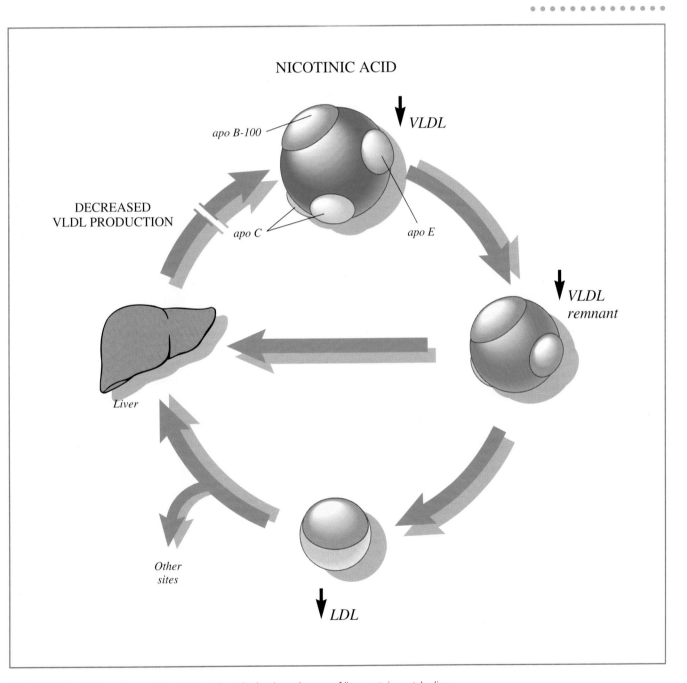

FIGURE 4.58 • Major actions of nicotinic acid on the basic pathways of lipoprotein metabolism.

3-HYDROXY-3-METHYLGLUTARYL COENZYME A (HMG-CoA) REDUCTASE INHIBITORS

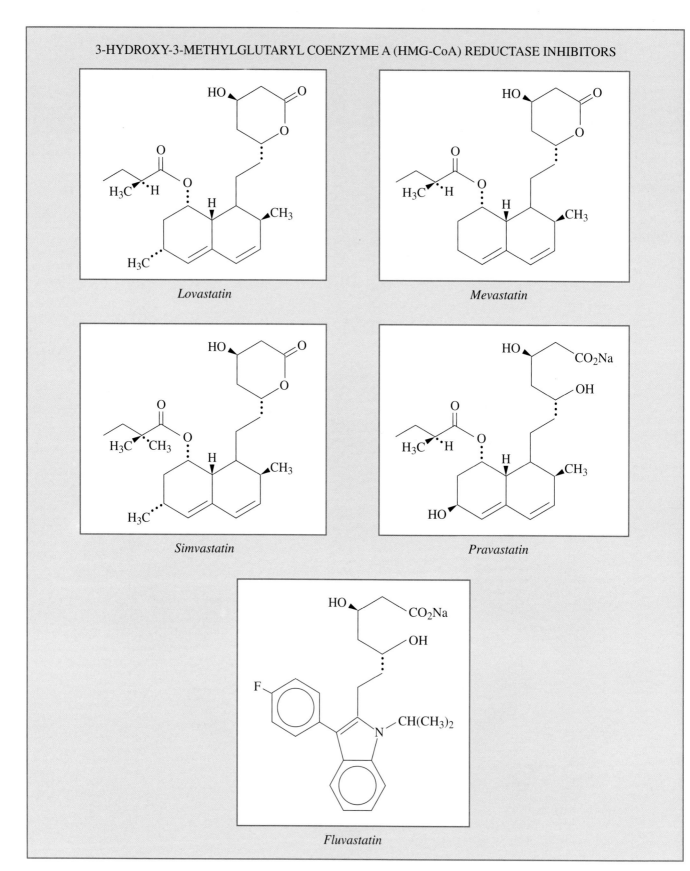

Lovastatin

Mevastatin

Simvastatin

Pravastatin

Fluvastatin

FIGURE 4.59 • Structural formulas of the HMG-CoA reductase inhibitors.

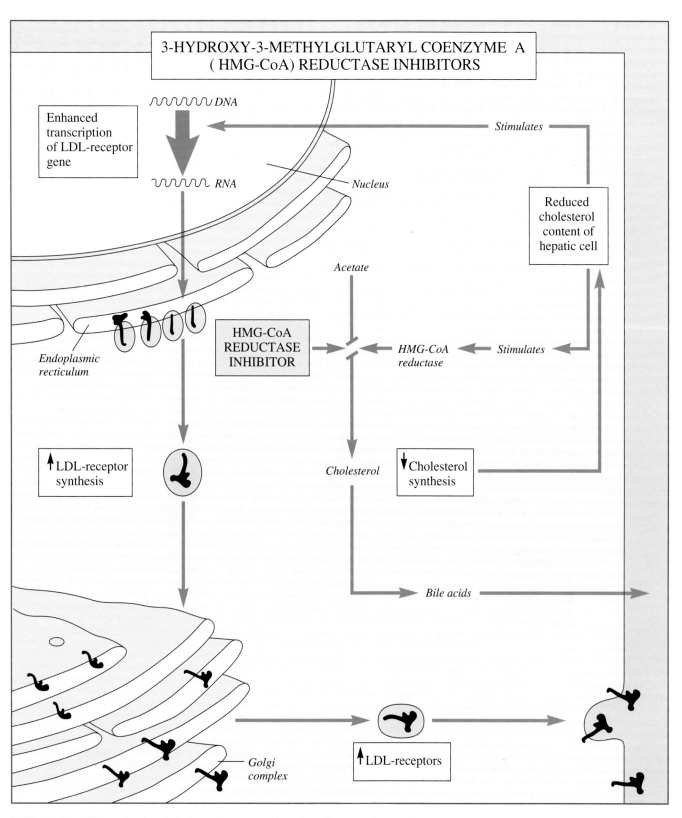

FIGURE 4.60 • Effects of reduced cholesterol content of hepatic cells, secondary to the actions of HMG-CoA reductase inhibitors on the synthesis of cholesterol and LDL-receptors.

Some investigators[157,158] suggest that HMG-CoA reductase inhibitors reduce the formation and secretion of apo B-containing lipoproteins by the liver. Such an effect might be secondary to inhibition of cholesterol synthesis, a key constituent of lipoproteins. This putative mechanism, however, remains to be documented with certainty, and a study from our laboratory throws it into question.[159] Finally, the reduction of LDL and VLDL remnants can lead to a secondary rise in HDL levels.

The HMG-CoA reductase inhibitors have proven to be remarkably free of side effects for most patients. This apparent safety probably is due to the fact that most of the newly absorbed drug is removed in its first pass through the liver, which is the primary target organ. The high first-pass clearance of reductase inhibitors is fortuitous because there is growing evidence that high systemic levels can produce significant side effects. A few patients have gastrointestinal side effects, but the most common adverse effect is hepatotoxicity. The mechanism for hepatotoxicity is unknown, but it presumably is due to inhibition of cholesterol synthesis in the liver. The incidence of hepatotoxicity is proportional to dose. At 80 mg/d, approximately 1.0% of patients have significant clinical hepatotoxicity, whereas at 20 mg/d, only 0.1% have this reaction.[160] In general, hepatotoxicity cannot be detected by clinical signs, but

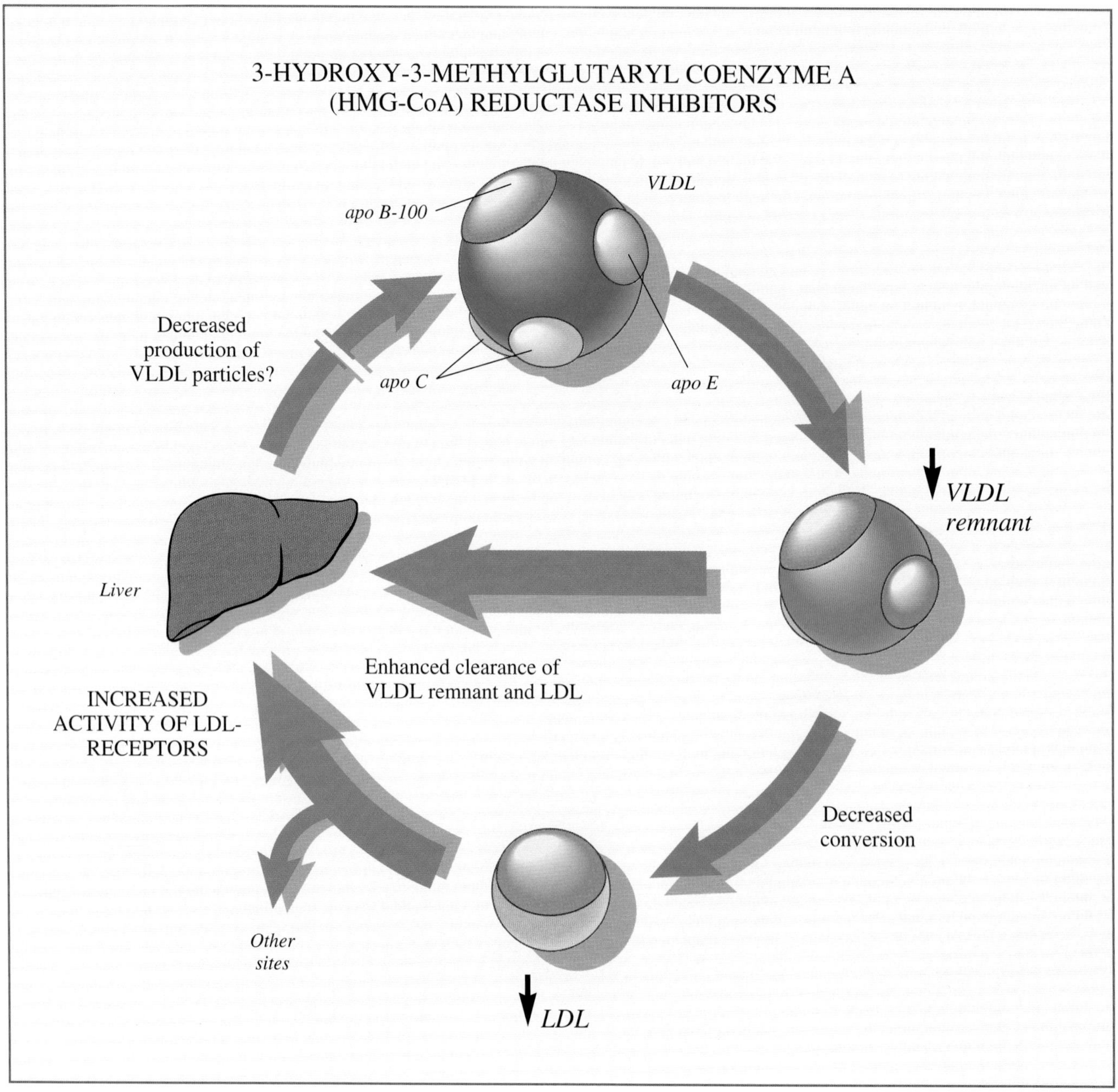

FIGURE 4.61 • Major actions of the HMG-CoA reductase inhibitors on the basic pathways of lipoprotein metabolism.

must be recognized by laboratory measurements. Periodic measurements of liver function tests are necessary because it is theoretically possible that long-term, undetected hepatotoxicity could lead to chronic liver disease.

If significant amounts of HMG-CoA reductase inhibitors pass into the systemic circulation, then other organ-specific side effects can occur. High blood levels of drug can occur in the presence of liver disease or with drugs that prevent hepatic destruction and excretion of drugs (for example, cyclosporine). One adverse effect is myopathy and can occur in three forms:

- Mild muscle symptoms (myalgia).
- Mild-to-moderate increases in creatine kinase.
- Severe myopathy. The latter, fortunately, is rare because it can lead to myoglobinemia and acute tubular necrosis. Passage of drug into the brain may lead to insomnia and sleep disorders. Likewise, perfusion of the skin by drug can lead to various cutaneous reactions. Thus, HMG-CoA reductase inhibitors are potentially toxic, but fortunately, systemic toxicity is relatively rare because of efficient hepatic clearance. Even this toxicity may be further reduced in the future by development of drugs that have a low uptake in extra hepatic tissues.

Since HMG-CoA reduction inhibitors are relatively new agents, they have not been tested adequately for their efficacy in preventing CHD. Recent preliminary results, however, are suggestive that they may be effective for this purpose. For this reason, they should be used with the recognition of this lack of information. On the other hand, their high efficacy and apparent safety justify their use in patients with severe hypercholesterolemia or in those with moderate hypercholesterolemia who are at high risk from other causes. Future research, moreover, may reveal their utility for other conditions, namely, hypertriglyceridemia, hypoalphalipoproteinemia, and various secondary dyslipidemias.

FIBRIC ACIDS

Drugs of this class have been used for treatment of hyperlipidemia for almost three decades.[161] They are remarkably effective for some forms of hyperlipidemia, but are largely ineffective in others. Their use has been marked with controversy, especially because of the apparently unfavorable results with clofibrate in the WHO trial,[162] but their outlook has improved with the positive outcome of the Helsinki Heart Study with gemfibrozil.[49,50] The fibric acids currently in use throughout the world are shown in Figure 4.62. Among these, clofibrate and gemfibrozil are currently approved for use in the United States. There is disagreement whether the therapeutic or side-effect profiles differ among the fibric acids. Very few direct comparisons have been carried out, and it is difficult to compare efficacy and safety between various trials carried out under different conditions.

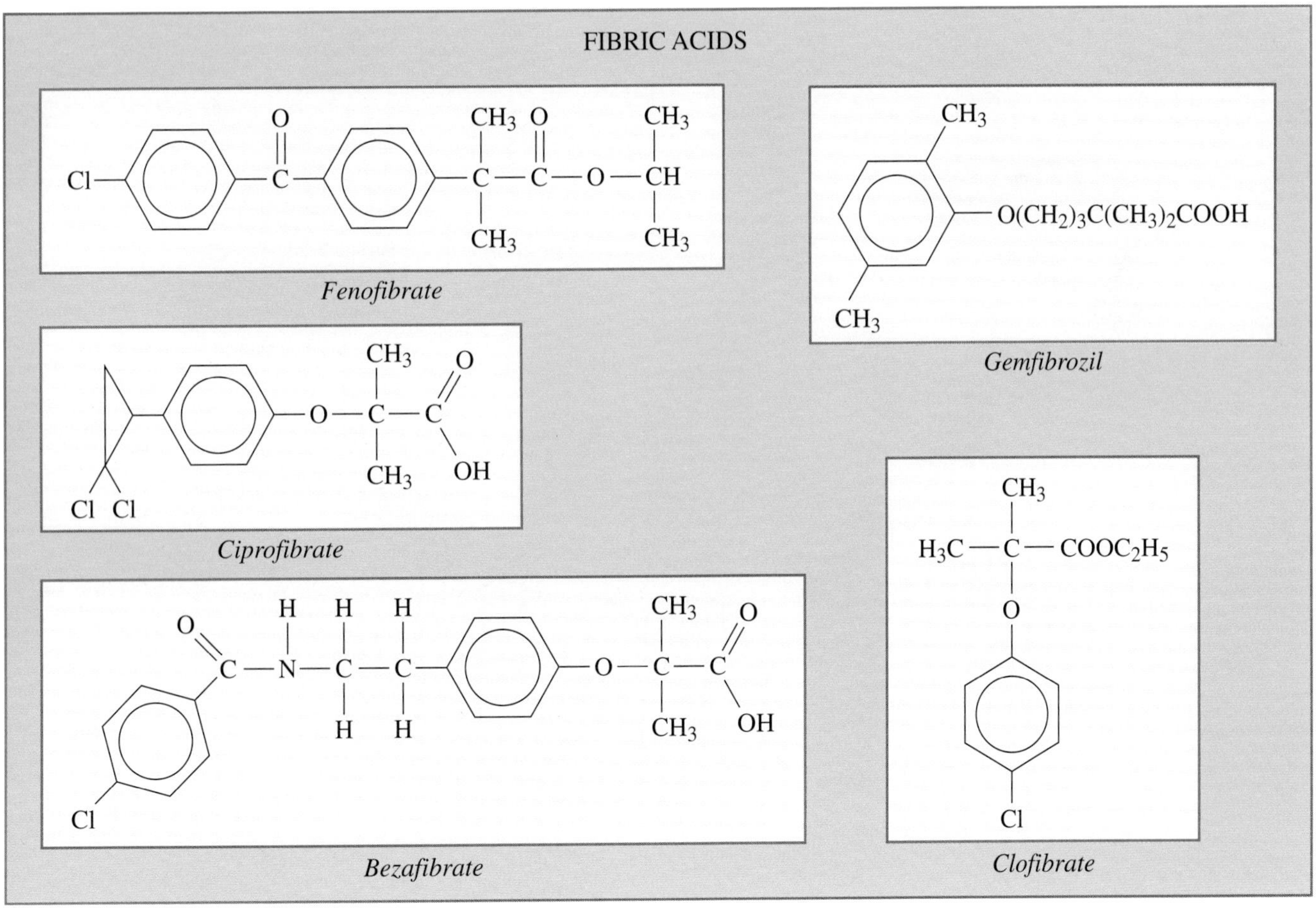

FIBRIC ACIDS

Fenofibrate

Gemfibrozil

Ciprofibrate

Bezafibrate

Clofibrate

FIGURE 4.62 • Structural formulas of currently used fibric acids.

The essential mechanism of action of fibric acids is unknown. A variety of actions have been reported in humans or animals. These agents have been reported to inhibit the synthesis of triglycerides in the liver,[163] to stimulate the activity of lipoprotein lipase,[164-166] to interfere with release of free fatty acids from adipose tissue, reduce synthesis of cholesterol and bile acids,[167,168] to enhance the secretion of cholesterol into bile,[169-171] to increase the activity of LDL-receptors,[172] and to stimulate the synthesis of apo A-I.[173,174] Whether there is a common underlying mechanism to account for all of these effects or instead fibric acids truly have multiple actions remains to be determined. Regardless, they affect concentrations of all lipoprotein fractions—VLDL, LDL and HDL.

Fibric acids are most effective in patients with hypertriglyceridemia. They have been reported to have two effects on triglyceride metabolism, namely, to interfere with production of VLDL triglycerides and to promote lipolysis of triglyceride-rich lipoproteins (Figure 4.63). Fibric acids often cause marked reductions of triglyceride levels in patients with severe hypertriglyceridemia, although there are some chylomicronemic patients who are resistant to their action.

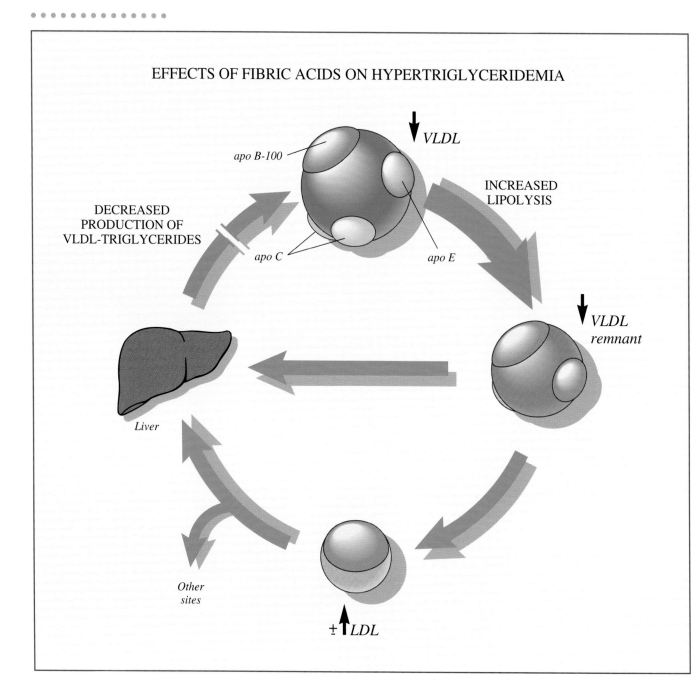

FIGURE 4.63 • Major actions of gemfibrozil in lowering the serum triglyceride levels in hypertriglyceridemia.

The drugs also will effectively lower levels of VLDL in patients with type IV HLP, and ß-VLDL in type III HLP. In patients with type IV HLP, they are less effective for lowering total cholesterol than triglycerides.[175] A decline in VLDL-cholesterol often is accompanied by a rise in LDL-cholesterol. Levels of total apo B, are likewise reduced minimally in type IV HLP.[176] A fall in triglycerides frequently results in an increase in HDL-cholesterol,[174] but this response is by no means invariable, and usually is relatively small.

In patients with pure hypercholesterolemia (type IIA HLP), fibric acids typically reduce LDL-cholesterol levels by 10% to 15%, and by 20% in a few patients. They seemingly enhance clearance of LDL from the circulation[172] (Figure 4.64). Whether enhanced LDL clearance is secondary to changes in metabolism of triglyceride-rich lipoproteins, or to modification of hepatic cholesterol metabolism, remains to be determined. In patients with type IIA HLP, levels of HDL-cholesterol are increased on an average by about 10%. Because fibric acids can raise HDL levels, their use has been suggested for normolipidemic patients with low HDL-cholesterol concentrations. Many patients with CHD have this pattern of dyslipidemia. Limited data, however, are available

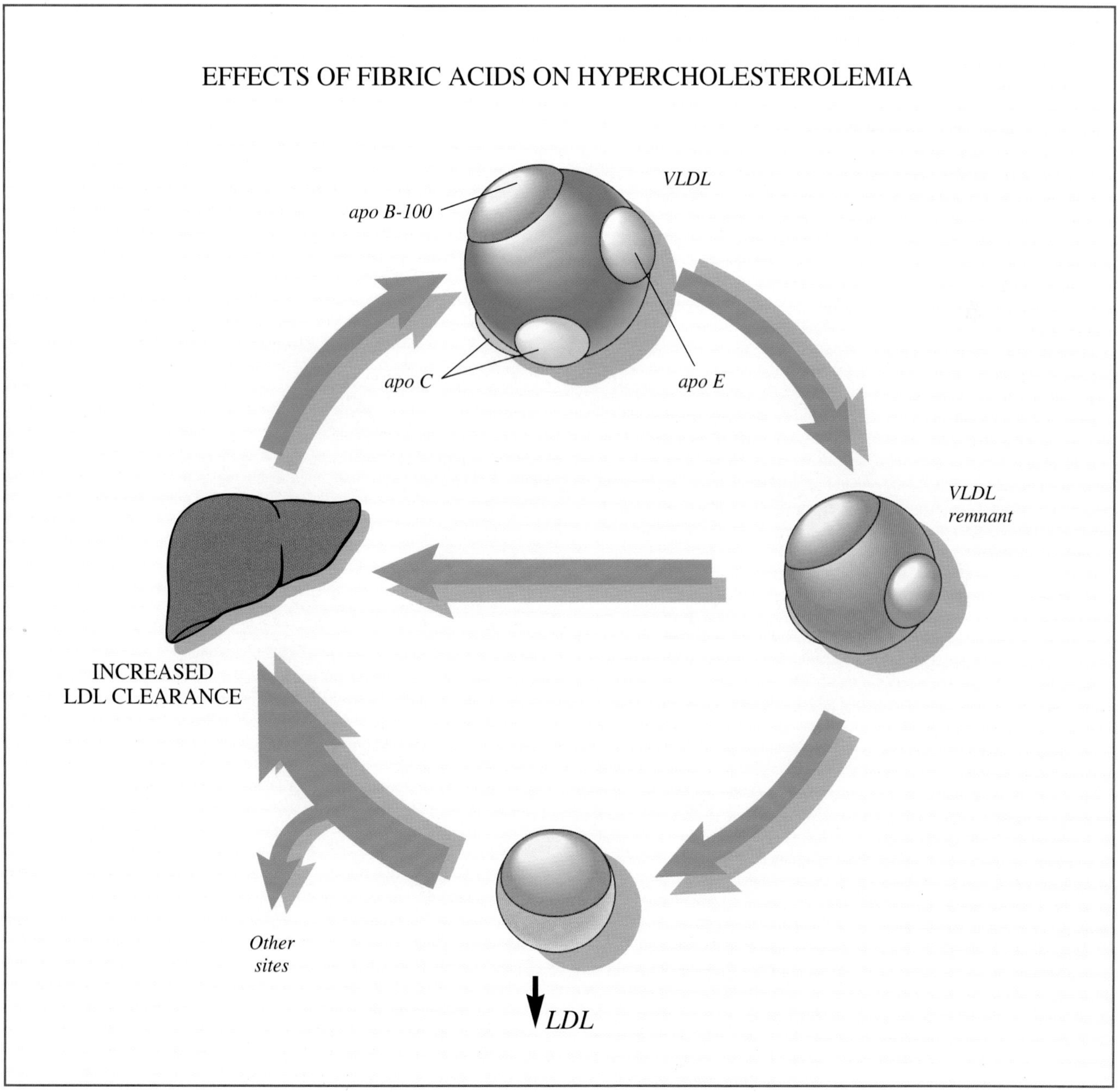

FIGURE 4.64 • Major actions of gemfibrozil in lowering the LDL-cholesterol levels in hypercholesterolemia.

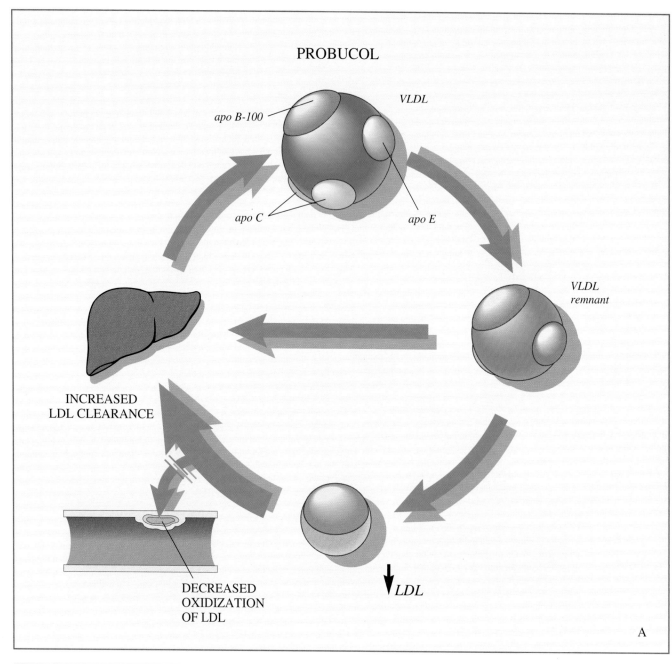

PROBUCOL

VLDL

apo B-100

apo C

apo E

VLDL
remnant

INCREASED
LDL CLEARANCE

DECREASED
OXIDIZATION
OF LDL

↓LDL

A

FIGURE 4.65 • Major actions of probucol on the basic pathways of lipoprotein metabolism (A). The chemical structure of probucol (B).

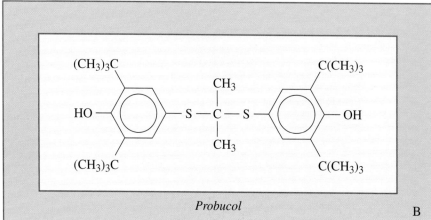

Probucol

B

Treatment of Hyperlipidemias

on their efficacy for raising HDL levels in patients of this type. Studies from our laboratory[177] indicate that the ability of fibric acids to raise HDL-cholesterol in low-HDL patients is limited, increasing levels by only about 3 mg/dL on the average.

Fibric acids have numerous side effects, most of which are not serious. One adverse effect is an increased risk for cholesterol gallstones and may occur as a result of enhanced secretion of cholesterol in bile. Hypertriglyceridemic patients are already prone to gallstone formation, and their risk is increased further during fibric acid therapy. Approximately 5% of patients treated with these drugs will develop gallstones. Fibric acids can cause transient elevations of hepatic enzymes, but it is not necessary to monitor liver function tests on a long-term basis. Neutropenia, but not agranulocytosis, is relatively common. Weight gain due to water retention, secondary to increased antidiuretic hormone, has been reported. Occasionally, patients may develop myopathy. The risk for serious myopathy is greatly increased in patients with chronic renal failure, and fibric acids probably should be avoided in such patients. The WHO trial[162] raised the possibility that fibric acids may increase the risk for cancer, but no specific type of cancer was identified. An increased cancer rate was not confirmed with gemfibrozil in the Helsinki Heart study.[49]

PROBUCOL

This is a cholesterol-lowering drug that has been available for almost two decades. It is given in a dose of 1 g/d. Probucol lowers LDL-cholesterol levels by 10% to 15%, but the mechanism is unknown. Limited data suggest that it promotes clearance of LDL via non-receptor pathways[178] (Figure 4.65). Probucol also lowers HDL-cholesterol and apo A-I concentrations, possibly by reducing the synthesis of apo A-I. Whether the reduction in HDL level increases risk for CHD is unknown. Probucol can reverse xanthomas in some patients with familial hypercholesterolemia, especially the homozygous variety. This finding raises the possibility that the HDL-lowering effect of probucol is not dangerous, and in fact, the drug could retard or reverse atherogenesis.

Support for the latter concept comes from the observation that probucol interferes with the oxidation of LDL by active oxygen species[179–181] (Figure 4.65). The oxidation of LDL within the arterial wall may enhance cellular uptake of LDL-cholesterol, thus promoting development of atherosclerosis.[22] If probucol prevents LDL oxidation, it could retard atherogenesis. In support, studies in rabbits with genetic hypercholesterolemia have shown that probucol administration prevents the atherosclerosis that normally occurs in these animals.[182] This finding suggests the need for a clinical trial to examine the potential of probucol for preventing CHD.

Research with probucol raises the possibility that other antioxidants might retard atherogenesis. Two naturally occurring antioxidants are tocopherol (vitamin E) and ascorbic acid (vitamin C). Studies carried out in our laboratory and others indicate that these vitamins also will prevent the oxidation of LDL.[180,181] If they are effective *in vivo* they might have utility for the nutritional prevention of CHD.

MANAGEMENT OF DYSLIPIDEMIA

Since dyslipidemia can vary in type, depending on abnormalities in lipid and lipoprotein metabolism, appropriate management of dyslipidemia requires a working knowledge of lipoproteins plus good clinical judgement. A general knowledge of the relationship between lipoprotein fractions and risk for coronary heart disease (CHD), as this relationship depends on age and sex, is required.

Special attention must be given to patients with clinically manifest coronary artery disease because these patients have already demonstrated propensity for coronary atherosclerosis. As a general principle, dietary therapy is the first line of therapy for most types of dyslipidemia, and drug therapy should be used only if diet modification fails to provide an adequate response. Still, certain patients are strong candidates for drug therapy, and in these patients appropriate drugs should not be withheld. In this section, the various forms of dyslipidemia will be examined, and a rational strategy for their management will be developed.

PRIMARY HYPERCHOLESTEROLEMIA
Severe Hypercholesterolemia

This condition was defined as an LDL-cholesterol exceeding 210 mg/dL, with triglyceride levels below 250 mg/dL. It can either be monogenic or polygenic in origin, and risk for CHD is increased approximately four fold above that with desirable LDL levels.[31] Dietary therapy is indicated for all patients with this condition, and for most adults, drug therapy will be required as well. Drug therapy especially is required for adult men. In fact, for most patients use of drugs in combination is required to achieve a "normalization" of cholesterol levels. Two therapeutic regimens have been used with success. The first is the combination of a bile acid sequestrant and nicotinic acid[45,183] (Figure 4.66). This combination has the advantage of being relatively inexpensive and of raising HDL levels as well as lowering LDL. On the other hand, the side effects of nicotinic acid cannot be tolerated by many patients.

An alternative is a bile acid sequestrant plus an HMG-CoA reductase inhibitor, which produces a 50% to 60% reduction in LDL-cholesterol when full doses are taken[184,185] (refer to Figure 4.66). This combination, in addition, is better tolerated than that with nicotinic acid. Finally, an HMG-CoA reductase inhibitor alone, in relatively high doses, is sufficient in some patients with severe hypercholesterolemia, but in most, it will not reduce cholesterol levels to the desirable range.

Postmenopausal women with severe elevations of LDL-cholesterol deserve the same therapy as men. Premenopausal women are protected to some extent against CHD because of their sex, and if they have no other risk factors, use of a bile acid sequestrant alone may be sufficient and prudent. However, if they are at high risk because of other factors, such as smoking or poorly controlled hypertension, they should be treated with the same regimen as men. Teenagers with heterozygous FH probably should receive a bile acid sequestrant, but HMG-CoA reductase inhibitors should be withheld until more information about their safety is available. An exception may be teenage boys with total cholesterol levels in the range of 400 to 500 mg/dL who may be considered candidates for HMG-CoA reductase inhibitors.

Moderate Hypercholesterolemia

Multiple factors contribute to development of moderate hypercholesterolemia, both dietary and poorly defined genetic factors.[186,187] LDL-cholesterol levels range from 160 to 210 mg/dL, with triglycerides below 250 mg/dL. All patients with moder-

ate hypercholesterolemia deserve maximal dietary therapy in an attempt to achieve the goals outlined by the National Cholesterol Education Program (NCEP).[1] If these goals are not achieved, drug therapy can be considered, but drugs are by no means mandated in all patients. Factors that favor use of cholesterol-lowering drugs, and the choice of drugs, can be reviewed. As a general rule, patients with highest risk are those most in need of drug treatment.

Consideration can be given first to treating men with moderate hypercholesterolemia. Men at greatest risk are those who

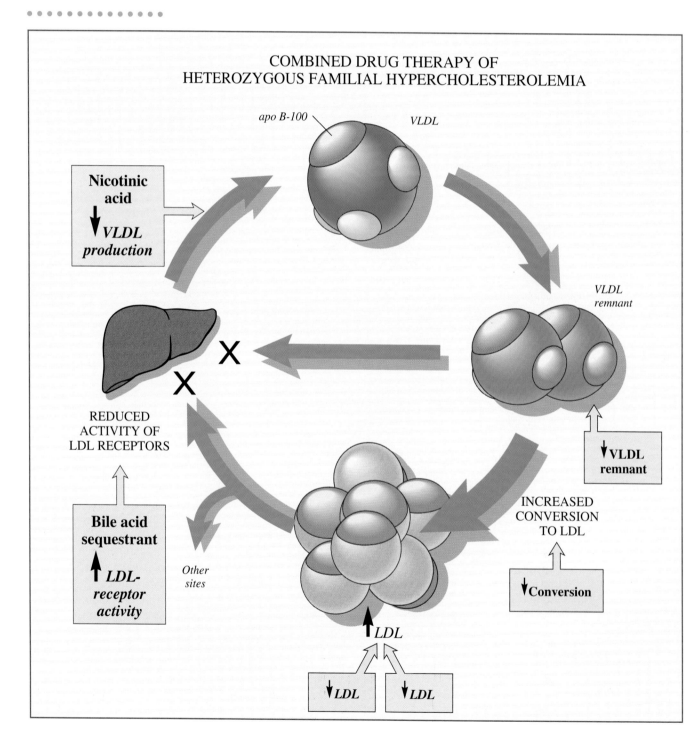

FIGURE 4.66 • Major actions of combined therapy with a bile acid sequestrant and nicotinic acid on the lipoprotein abnormalities found in heterozygous familial hypercholesterolemia.

have clinical coronary artery disease, either angina pectoris or previous myocardial infarction. Such men have already manifest a propensity to develop coronary atherosclerosis, and their prognosis depends, in part, on the rate of progression of their coronary lesions. For this reason, efforts to prevent coronary atherogenesis are justified; these efforts should include maximal reduction of LDL-cholesterol levels. Some authorities suggest that LDL-cholesterol levels should be reduced to below 100 mg/dL in CHD patients, and this view seems reasonable. In some patients, a single cholesterol-lowering drug may achieve this aim, but in others, combined drug therapy may be required. This is not to say that all patients with established CHD require cholesterol-lowering drugs, but the general principle of maximal LDL lowering in such patients is reasonable. Certainly clinical trials are needed to test the utility of this approach.

Other high-risk patients without documented CHD may be candidates for drug therapy if they have moderate hypercholesterolemia. This is true for both men and women, especially if they have two CHD risk factors. Because male sex counts as a risk factor, a man with one additional risk factor must come under consideration for drug treatment. For example, men who smoke cigarettes and have elevated LDL-cholesterol concentrations may require drugs, especially if they are unable to stop smoking. Although the risk for future myocardial infarction may not be as high in such patients as in those with documented coronary artery disease, their risk nonetheless is substantially increased. Again, the goal of therapy should be to produce a maximal lowering of LDL-cholesterol levels. In some patients, a bile acid sequestrant may be sufficient therapy, but others may respond better to an HMG-CoA reductase inhibitor. If the patient concomitantly has a low HDL-cholesterol as an additional risk factor, consideration can be given to using nicotinic acid. Finally, another approach is to use relatively low doses of two drugs in combination, for example, a bile acid sequestrant and an HMG-CoA reductase inhibitor.

Special consideration must be given to young-adult and middle-aged men who have moderate hypercholesterolemia but no other risk factors. Although these patients may be at increased risk for CHD, in many cases, their risk is not raised sufficiently to justify the use of cholesterol-lowering drugs. Maximal dietary therapy should be utilized first. This includes Step II dietary therapy and weight reduction—if the patient is overweight. Drug therapy should not be instituted immediately, but instead, dietary treatment should be continued for a period of at least six months in the attempt to obtain a maximal response. If a patient maintains relatively high LDL-cholesterol levels, especially in the range of 180 to 210 mg/dL, a reasonable approach is to use a bile acid sequestrant in low doses, such as cholestyramine, 8 g/d. The patient should be followed carefully, and if other risk factors should develop, more aggressive drug therapy, as outlined in the preceding paragraph, must be brought into consideration. However, the institution of life-long drug therapy in a patient with only moderate hypercholesterolemia should be instituted with reluctance because of its relatively high cost and the possibility of long-term side effects.

Older men, such as those over age 60, probably should be considered separately. There is growing evidence that hypercholesterolemia remains a significant risk factor in elderly men.[188] In fact, in terms of attributable risk, the total impact of hypercholesterolemia in older men may be greater than it is in young and middle-aged men[188] (Figure 4.67). The first line of therapy in older men, of course, is dietary therapy. However, because the nutrition of many elderly persons is of marginal quality, care must be taken not to recommend a diet that will worsen the patient's overall health. For this reason, a careful dietary history should be taken before starting a cholesterol-lowering diet. Once a nutritious cholesterol-lowering diet has been started and the response monitored, the possibility of drug therapy can be entertained if the response to diet is not sufficient. In general, drug therapy should be utilized only in older men who otherwise are relatively healthy and have an overall good prognosis. Certainly, drug therapy can be recommended more highly for men in their 60's than for those in their 70's or 80's. To obtain a significant reduction in CHD risk by

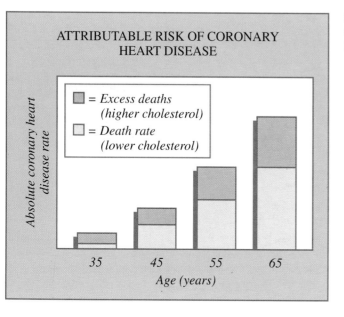

ATTRIBUTABLE RISK OF CORONARY HEART DISEASE

☐ = Excess deaths (higher cholesterol)
☐ = Death rate (lower cholesterol)

Absolute coronary heart disease rate

Age (years)
35   45   55   65

FIGURE 4.67 • Attributable risk of coronary heart disease (CHD) at different ages in the MRFIT follow-up study. (Reproduced with permission. Denke MA, Grundy SM *Ann Intern Med* 1990;112:780.)

cholesterol lowering in the elderly, a substantial decrease in LDL-cholesterol is required. This requirement may justify use of an HMG-CoA reductase inhibitor in older men. However, it must be noted that efficacy of reductase inhibitors for prevention of CHD events in older men remains to be documented.

Postmenopausal women constitute an extremely large group of subjects with moderate hypercholesterolemia. Approximately 40% of all postmenopausal women have LDL-cholesterol levels exceeding 160 mg/dL.[1] This high percentage may be related to loss of estrogen-stimulated synthesis of LDL-receptors after menopause. Unfortunately, limited data are available on the effectiveness of different forms of cholesterol-lowering therapy in women of this age group. Dietary therapy can be expected to lower LDL-cholesterol concentrations by about 20 mg/dL, but such a reduction may not be sufficient in many women. If a woman has other CHD risk factors, she can be treated as outlined above for high-risk patients. If no other risk factors are present, and if dietary therapy does not produce a satisfactory reduction in LDL levels, consideration must be given to drug therapy. Certainly, CHD is the number one killer of older women.[188] On the other hand, onset of CHD is delayed in women by about 10 years, compared with men. Thus, even with a high prevalence of hypercholesterolemia in older women, life expectancy for women in general exceeds that of men, not to mention the inability of our social structure to sustain a high quality of life in very old people. Consequently, a decision to use cholesterol-lowering drugs in elderly women with no other CHD risk factors must be made judiciously.

Even more caution is needed for premenopausal women with moderate hypercholesterolemia. These women are largely protected against premature CHD, provided they are devoid of other risk factors. There is growing evidence that the presence of diabetes mellitus removes the premenopausal protection against CHD in women. Whether the same holds for cigarette smoking or poorly controlled hypertension is not clear, but these factors can be taken into account when deciding about drug therapy. If no other risk factors are present, however, it is probably wise to avoid using drugs for treatment of moderate hypercholesterolemia in premenopausal women.

A similar level of caution extends to children and adolescents with moderate hypercholesterolemia. For any child with cholesterol levels in this range, dietary modification should be encouraged. In teenage boys with cholesterol concentrations approaching the severely elevated range, use of bile acid resins, but not HMG-CoA reductase inhibitors, can be considered. Boys should be urged to begin an exercise program as well as dietary modification to facilitate reduction of LDL levels. Further, boys should be monitored both for response and trends of cholesterol levels. If hypercholesterolemia extends into young adulthood, the approach outlined above for adults can then be followed.

Mild Hypercholesterolemia

This condition is synonymous with borderline-high risk LDL-cholesterol—a level of 130 to 159 mg/dL. If a patient with borderline-high risk LDL-cholesterol does not have other risk factors, he/she can be given general advice to modify the diet to lower the LDL level to the desirable range.[1] If two other risk factors or clinical coronary artery diseases are present, more aggressive lowering of LDL-cholesterol levels is in order. Espe-

cially for patients with coronary artery disease, a reduction of LDL-cholesterol to below 100 mg/dL is reasonable.

PRIMARY HYPERTRIGLYCERIDEMIA
Severe Hypertriglyceridemia

Severe elevations of serum triglycerides, with total triglycerides exceeding 1,000 mg/dL are found with Types I and V HLP. With Type I HLP, chylomicrons are mainly increased, whereas with Type V HLP, both chylomicrons and VLDL are raised.[67] When serum triglycerides are in the range of 500 to 1,000 mg/dL, chylomicrons usually are present, justifying the diagnosis of Type V HLP. The most immediate danger of triglyceride levels exceeding 1,000 mg/dL is acute pancreatitis, and thus, the primary goal of therapy is to decrease this risk. Patients with Type I HLP do not appear to be at increased risk for CHD, but many patients with Type V HLP have premature CHD, perhaps due to an elevation of VLDL-cholesterol. In Type V HLP, therefore, consideration also must be given to reducing risk for CHD.

The primary mode of therapy of Type I HLP is to reduce dietary fat, the source of circulating chylomicrons. Drug therapy is not effective. Intake of total fat should be reduced to less than 10% of total dietary energy. Some of the fat in the diet can be replaced by medium-chain triglycerides, because medium-chain fatty acids do not become incorporated into chylomicrons. If triglyceride levels can be maintained consistently below 1,000 mg/dL, the risk for acute pancreatitis is greatly reduced. Unfortunately, even a single fat-rich meal can precipitate an attack of pancreatitis in a patient with severe hypertriglyceridemia.

Multiple factors, such as genetic, diabetes mellitus, obesity, and excess alcohol intake, often combine to produce Type V HLP. An approach to management of Type V HLP is outlined in Figure 4.68. Dietary therapy should be used first and this includes:
- Weight reduction.
- Restriction of alcohol intake.
- Decreased consumption of dietary fat.

If the patient has diabetes mellitus, reduction of glucose levels by specific therapy may significantly lower triglyceride levels. If the triglyceride level is not reduced to below 1,000 mg/dL with diet alone, drug therapy must be considered. Nicotinic acid is the first line of therapy. If nicotinic acid is not well tolerated, a fibric acid—clofibrate or gemfibrozil—can be utilized. In most patients with type V HLP, triglyceride levels are lowered sufficiently to reduce risk for pancreatitis. Whether triglyceride lowering will reduce risk for CHD is a question that has not been resolved.

Moderate Hypertriglyceridemia

Moderate hypertriglyceridemia includes serum triglycerides in the range of 250 to 500 mg/dL. Elevated triglycerides can be due to genetic factors, secondary diseases—diabetes mellitus, renal disease—or dietary factors—obesity, alcohol, or excess dietary carbohydrates. Any secondary condition should be treated, which may lower triglyceride levels. Alcohol should be avoided, and if the patient is overweight, caloric restriction is indicated. Triglyceride-lowering drugs can be considered in patients in whom other risk factors for CHD are present—established coronary artery disease, strong family history of CHD, persistent smoking, diabetes mellitus, and poorly controlled hypertension (Figure 4.69).

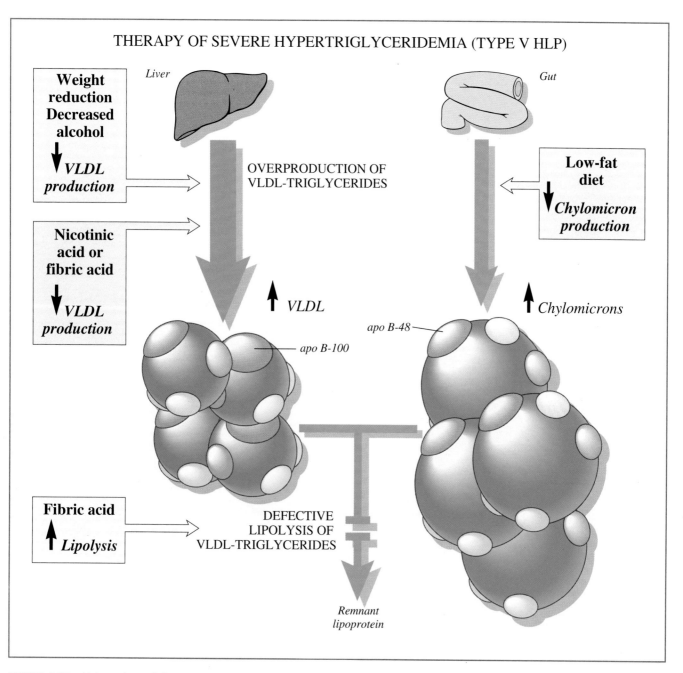

THERAPY OF SEVERE HYPERTRIGLYCERIDEMIA (TYPE V HLP)

Liver

Gut

Weight reduction Decreased alcohol

↓ *VLDL production*

OVERPRODUCTION OF VLDL-TRIGLYCERIDES

Low-fat diet

↓ *Chylomicron production*

Nicotinic acid or fibric acid

↓ *VLDL production*

↑ *VLDL*

↑ *Chylomicrons*

apo B-48

apo B-100

Fibric acid

↑ *Lipolysis*

DEFECTIVE LIPOLYSIS OF VLDL-TRIGLYCERIDES

Remnant lipoprotein

FIGURE 4.68 • Major actions of dietary modification and drug therapy with either nicotinic acid or gemfibrozil on the lipoprotein abnormalities characterizing severe hypertriglyceridemia (Type V HLP).

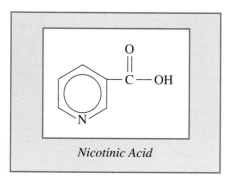

Nicotinic Acid

FIGURE 4.69 • Structural formula of nicotinic acid (niacin).

Several alternate drugs can be used (Figures 4.70, 4.71). Nicotinic acid is the drug of choice, although it frequently is not well tolerated. If glucose intolerance is present, nicotinic acid may precipitate diabetes mellitus. Gemfibrozil is useful for patients in whom cholesterol levels are in the desirable range. If cholesterol levels are raised to the borderline range, 200 to 240 mg/dL, an HMG-CoA reductase inhibitor may be preferable.[176] Gemfibrozil has little effect on total cholesterol levels in patients

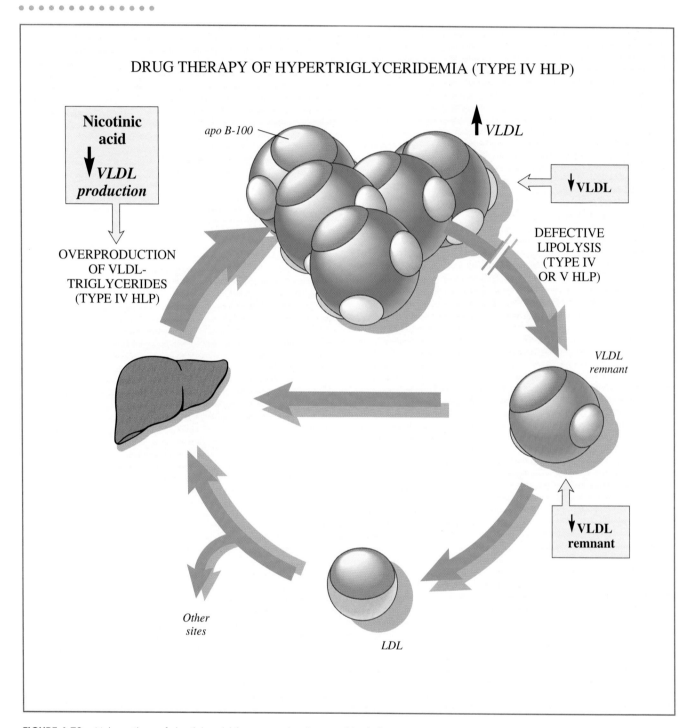

FIGURE 4.70 • Major actions of nicotinic acid therapy on the abnormalities in lipoprotein metabolism found in moderate hypertriglyceridemia (Type IV HLP).

with primary hypertriglyceridemia, and it may shift VLDL-cholesterol to LDL, thus raising LDL-cholesterol. Unfortunately, clinical trials that document the efficacy for reducing CHD risk by triglyceride lowering have not been carried out.

Primary Mixed Hyperlipidemia

An increase in both total cholesterol (greater than 240 mg/dL) and triglycerides (greater than 250 mg/dL) can be called mixed hyperlipidemia. Multiple factors can contribute to both eleva-

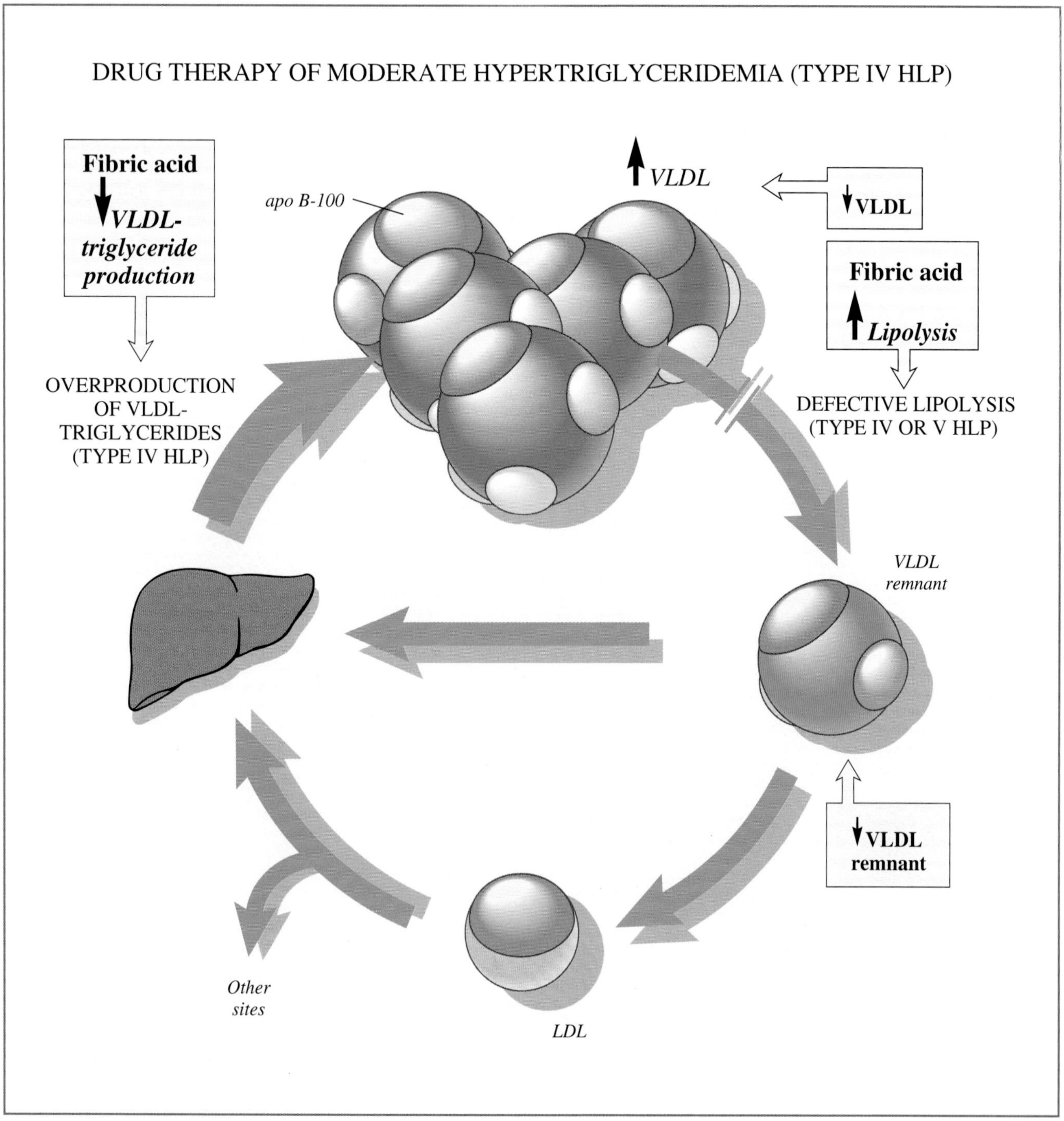

DRUG THERAPY OF MODERATE HYPERTRIGLYCERIDEMIA (TYPE IV HLP)

FIGURE 4.71 • Major actions of therapy with gemfibrozil on the lipoprotein abnormalities found in moderate hypertriglyceridemia (Type IV HLP).

tions (Figure 4.72), and when these include dietary or secondary factors, they should be modified appropriately. If mixed hyperlipidemia persists after these modifications, it can be called "primary." Severe hypertriglyceridemia often is accompanied by elevations of total cholesterol, but this condition was discussed above. Therefore, in the following, the term "mixed hyperlipidemia" will be restricted to conditions in which triglycerides are moderately elevated—250 to 500 mg/dL.

Familial Combined Hyperlipidemia

This disorder is characterized by multiple lipoprotein phenotypes in a single family (Figure 4.73). One clinical manifestation of familial combined hyperlipidemia is mixed hyperlipidemia. Reduction in intakes of saturated fatty acids and cholesterol, and weight reduction, may reduce serum lipids in this disorder, but

to achieve desirable levels, drug therapy often is required. Nicotinic acid is the drug of choice, because it lowers both cholesterol and triglycerides (Figure 4.74). An alternative to nicotinic acid is gemfibrozil. In the Helsinki Heart Study,[49] gemfibrozil appeared to reduce risk for CHD in patients with mixed hyperlipidemia. A recent study from our laboratory[189] indicated that lovastatin is effective for lowering both cholesterol and triglycerides in this condition, and it can be used as an alternative, particularly when total cholesterol levels are markedly elevated (Figure 4.75). Two studies from our laboratory[189,190] have shown that the combination of lovastatin and gemfibrozil are highly effective for lowering both cholesterol and triglyceride levels, and for raising HDL concentrations in familial combined hyperlipidemia. Unfortunately, this combination is accompanied by a relatively high risk for severe myopathy and thus must be used

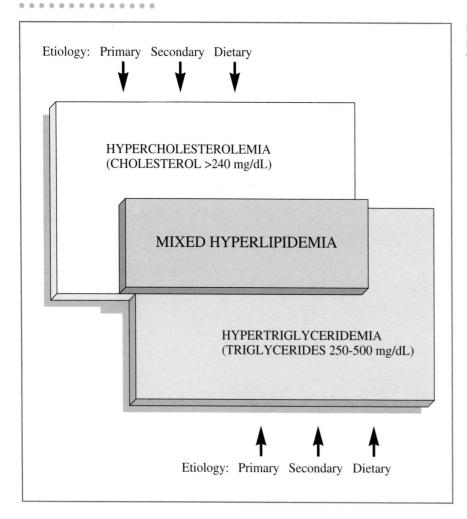

FIGURE 4.72 • Complex interaction of primary, secondary, and dietary factors contributing to mixed hyperlipidemia.

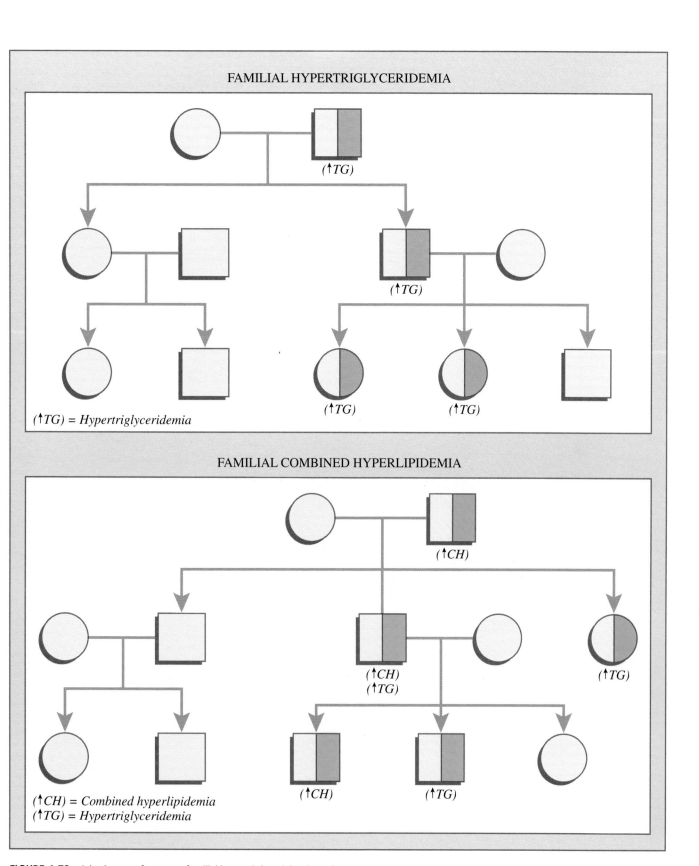

FAMILIAL HYPERTRIGLYCERIDEMIA

(↑TG)

(↑TG)

(↑TG)

(↑TG)

(↑TG)

(↑TG) = Hypertriglyceridemia

FAMILIAL COMBINED HYPERLIPIDEMIA

(↑CH)

(↑CH)
(↑TG)

(↑TG)

(↑CH)

(↑TG)

(↑CH) = Combined hyperlipidemia
(↑TG) = Hypertriglyceridemia

FIGURE 4.73 • Inheritance of patterns familial hypertriglyceridemia and familial combined hyperlipidemia as a monogenic-dominant disorder.

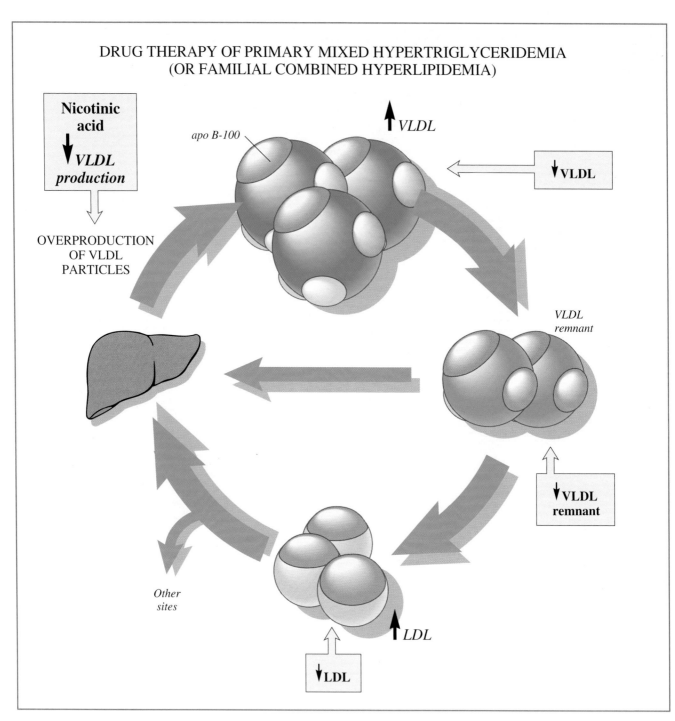

FIGURE 4.74 • Major actions of nicotinic acid therapy on the disordered metabolic pathways found in primary mixed hyperlipidemia or familial combined hyperlipidemia.

DRUG THERAPY OF PRIMARY MIXED HYPERLIPIDEMIA
(MULTIPLE LIPOPROTEIN DEFECTS)

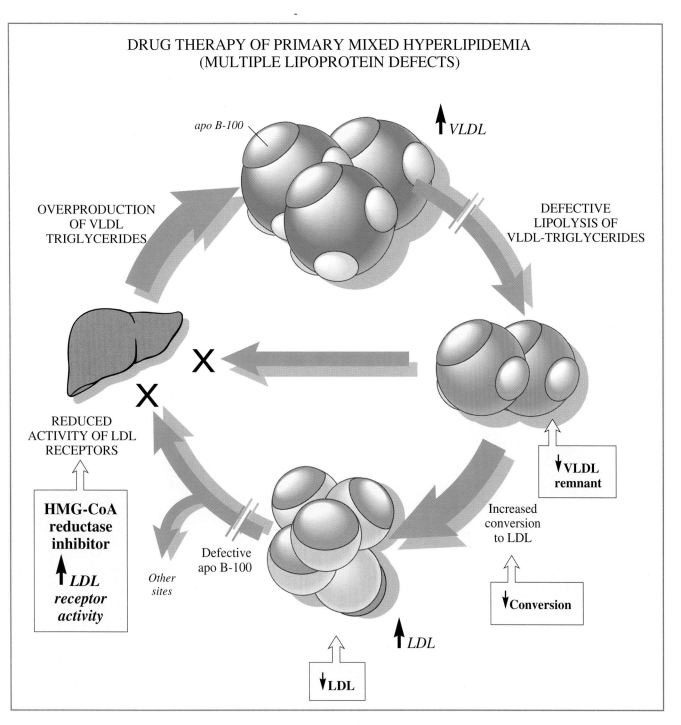

FIGURE 4.75 • Major actions of therapy with an HMG-CoA reductase inhibitor on the multiple lipoprotein defects found in primary mixed hyperlipidemia.

with caution.[191] Other drug combinations, such as a bile acid sequestrant plus nicotinic acid or gemfibrozil, can be tried with less risk of serious side effects (Figure 4.76). In some patients with mixed hyperlipidemia, it is not possible to prove the presence of familial combined hyperlipidemia in first-degree relatives, but the principles of therapy outlined here still pertain.

FAMILIAL DYSBETALIPOPROTEINEMIA (TYPE III HLP)

This variant of mixed hyperlipidemia is characterized by an increase in ß-VLDL. One prerequisite for an elevation of ß-VLDL is a defect in apo E, usually the apo E$_2$ isoform, which prevents binding of VLDL remnants to hepatic receptors. Most

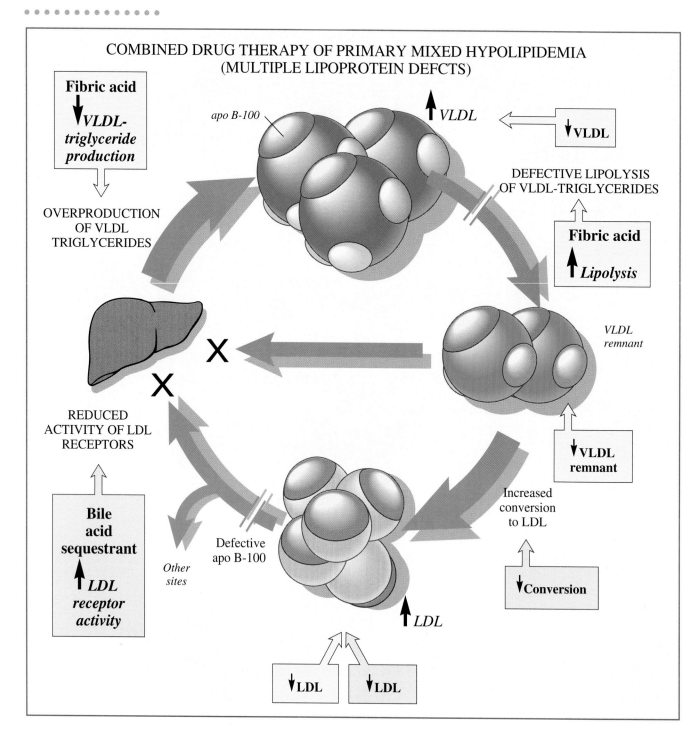

FIGURE 4.76 • Major actions of combined therapy with a bile acid sequestrant and gemfibrozil on the multiple lipoprotein defects found in primary mixed hyperlipidemia.

Treatment of Hyperlipidemias

patients have a second disorder of triglyceride metabolism that accentuates the accumulation of ß-migrating VLDL. The approach to treatment of type III HLP generally is that described for mixed hyperlipidemia—nicotinic acid (Figure 4.77), gemfibrozil (Figure 4.78), or HMG-CoA reductase inhibitor (Figure 4.79). All have proven effective for reducing concentrations of ß-VLDL. Some patients may respond better to one drug, while other patients may respond better to another. Nicotinic acid is the preferred drug, but often is poorly tolerated. Gemfibrozil is more effective when hypertriglyceridemia is predominant, whereas lovastatin is preferable when hypercholesterolemia predominates.

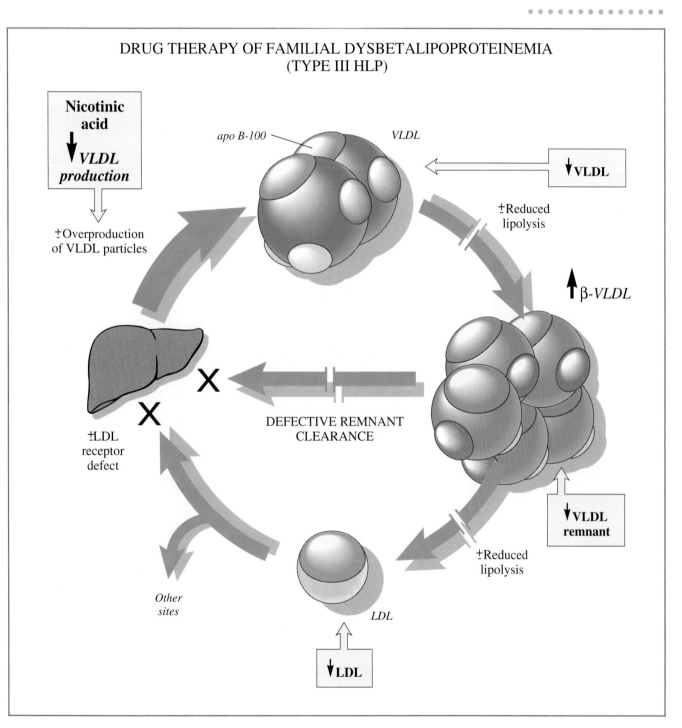

FIGURE 4.77 • Major actions of nicotinic acid therapy on the disordered pathways found in familial dysbetalipoproteinemia (Type III HLP).

HYPOALPHALIPOPROTEINEMIA

Several factors contribute to low HDL-cholesterol:

- Obesity.
- Hyperlipidemia.
- Lack of exercise.
- Smoking.
- Androgenic and related steroids.
- Genetic factors.

In patients with low HDL-cholesterol, modifiable factors should be changed appropriately. Among drugs for treatment of hyperlipidemia, nicotinic acid is the most effective for simultaneously raising triglyceride levels. The utility of treatment of low HDL-cholesterol in the absence of secondary causes is a matter of controversy.[52] Some investigators favor use of drugs, particularly if the patient is at high risk for CHD, or has established coronary artery disease. If drugs are to be used for rais-

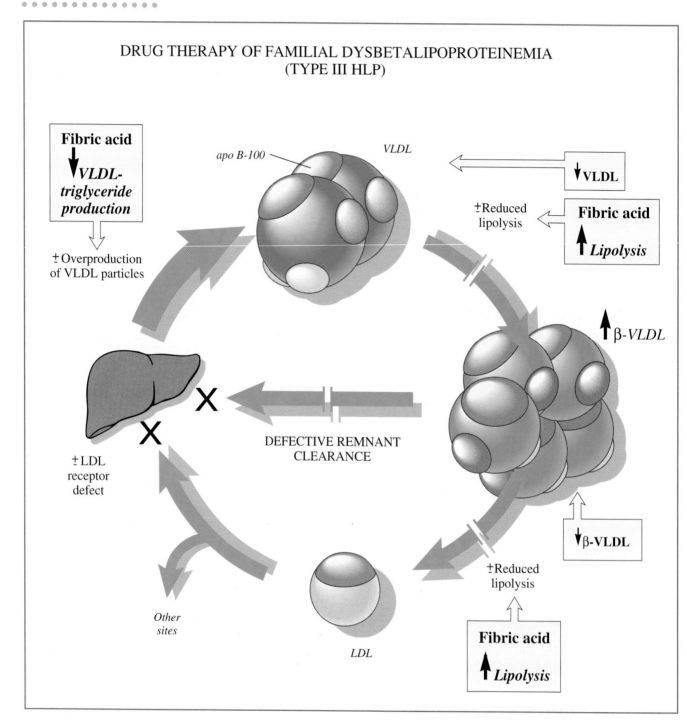

FIGURE 4.78 • Major actions of therapy with gemfibrozil on the abnormalities in lipoprotein metabolism found in familial dysbetalipoproteinemia (Type III HLP).

Treatment of Hyperlipidemias

ing HDL levels, nicotinic acid probably will be the most effective. Gemfibrozil has been recommended because the raising of HDL was considered to be one factor responsible for reduction in CHD risk in the Helsinki Heart Study. However, a recent study from our laboratory[177] revealed that lovastatin was just as effective as gemfibrozil in raising HDL levels in patients with primary hypoalphalipoproteinemia, and lovastatin therapy was more effective for lowering total cholesterol, LDL-cholesterol, and LDL/HDL ratios. Thus, in our view, an HMG-CoA reductase inhibitor is preferable to a fibric acid for treatming primary hypoalphalipoproteinemia if the patient cannot tolerate nicotinic acid.

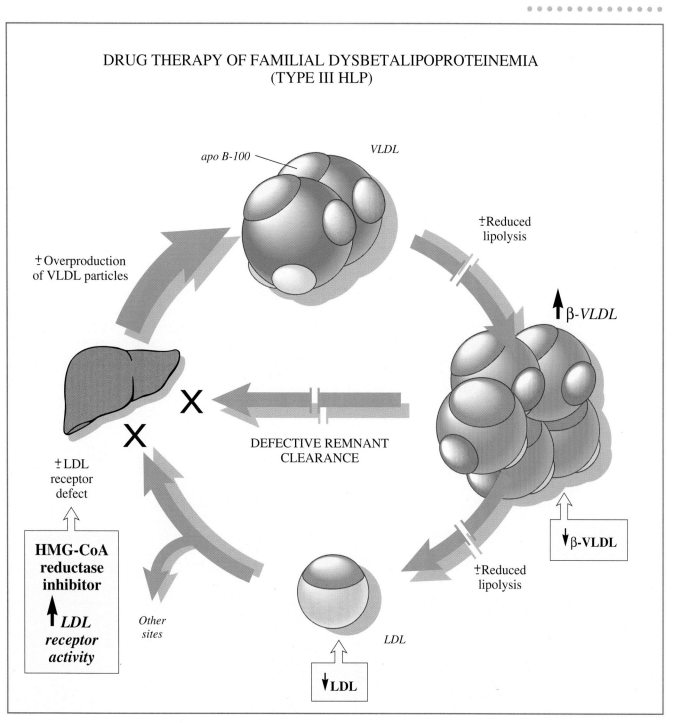

DRUG THERAPY OF FAMILIAL DYSBETALIPOPROTEINEMIA (TYPE III HLP)

apo B-100

VLDL

±Reduced lipolysis

↑β-VLDL

± Overproduction of VLDL particles

DEFECTIVE REMNANT CLEARANCE

↓β-VLDL

±LDL receptor defect

HMG-CoA reductase inhibitor

↑*LDL receptor activity*

Other sites

±Reduced lipolysis

LDL

↓LDL

FIGURE 4.79 • Major actions of therapy with an HMG-CoA reductase inhibitor on the disordered metabolic pathways of familial dysbetalipoproteinemia (Type III HLP).

CONCLUSIONS

High serum cholesterol is a major risk factor for coronary heart disease (CHD). Recently there is growing evidence that lowering elevated serum cholesterol will reduce the risk for CHD. Even though a simple cholesterol-CHD link is firmly established, however, it has become increasingly apparent that the transport of cholesterol in the serum is a complicated process. When the clinical management of hypercholesterolemia is required for individuals, a general knowledge of the cholesterol-transport system is needed.

Low density lipoprotein (LDL) appears to contribute more to development of atherosclerosis than any of the other lipoproteins. High density lipoprotein (HDL) actually may protect against CHD through its action to promote reverse cholesterol transport. There is dispute whether triglyceride-rich lipoproteins—chylomicrons and very low density lipoprotein (VLDL)—are atherogenic. In recent years, however, evidence has been growing that VLDL at least has atherogenic potential. For most patients with hypercholesterolemia, the increase in serum cholesterol occurs mainly in LDL, and LDL lowering is the major target of therapy.

The lipid risk factors interact with other risk factors—smoking, hypertension, diabetes mellitus, and obesity—to promote development of atherosclerosis. For this reason, management of dyslipidemia should depend on the number of other CHD risk factors present. If established CHD or two or more nonlipid risk factors are present in a single patient, efforts to modify abnormal lipoprotein patterns should be more aggressive.

Evidence to support active therapy to modify dyslipidemia to reduce risk for CHD is of several types. These include studies showing that increasing cholesterol levels, particularly LDL-cholesterol, are accompanied by increased development of coronary atherosclerosis and CHD risk. Other studies indicate that lowering cholesterol levels will reduce risk for CHD. Recent clinical trial data has demonstrated that reduction of cholesterol levels in individuals with hypercholesterolemia decreases CHD risk. Thus a strong case can be made for aggressive therapy in patients with significant abnormalities in lipoprotein metabolism, particularly elevations of LDL-cholesterol. Furthermore, treatment of dyslipidemia is especially important when patients already have manifest clinical evidence of CHD, or have two or more other CHD risk factors in the absence of clinical CHD.

All adults over age 20 should be tested for total serum cholesterol. A total cholesterol below 200 mg/dL is called **desireable**.The range of 200 to 239 mg/dL is designated **borderline-high cholesterol**, and over 240 mg/dL is high serum cholesterol. If a patient has borderline high cholesterol, and manifest CHD or two other CHD risk factors—smoking, hypertension, diabetes mellitus, low HDL-cholesterol, obesity, peripheral vascular disease or male sex—a lipoprotein profile —total cholesterol, triglycerides, LDL cholesterol and HDL cholesterol—should be obtained. In addition, a lipoprotein profile should be obtained on all people who have high serum cholesterol over 240 mg/dL. Secondary causes of hyper-cholesterolemia—hypothyroidism, renal disease, liver disease, or drug-induced causes—should be ruled out. Further, in patients with elevated LDL-cholesterol levels, testing of first-degree relatives should be done to rule out familial disorders of lipoprotein metabolism.

The goal for LDL-cholesterol lowering depends upon an overall assessment of the patient's risk status. If no other CHD risk factors are present, the LDL-cholesterol level should be reduced at least to below 160 mg/dL. If two other risk factors coexist, the goal for LDL lowering is an LDL-cholesterol level below 130 mg/dL. Some authorities believe that the LDL-cholesterol concentration in patients with manifest CHD should be below 100 mg/dl, although there is not universal agreement on this question, particularly if this level of LDL lowering requires drug therapy. At the present time, specific therapy to raise HDL-cholesterol levels, especially with drugs, cannot be recommended on the basis of clinical trial evidence. However, in patients with low HDL-cholesterol levels, it may be prudent to attempt further lowering of LDL-cholesterol levels. For patients with serum triglyceride levels in the range of 250 to 500 mg/dL, the total cholesterol can be used as the target of therapy since much of the serum cholesterol is carried in the VLDL fraction. If no other risk factors are present, the total cholesterol should be reduced to below 240 mg/dL, and if CHD or two other factors are present, the goal for total cholesterol should be less than 200 mg/dL.

The first approach to treatment of dyslipidemia is dietary therapy. Three factors in the diet are known to increase serum cholesterol levels:

- Dietary cholesterol
- Certain fatty acids
- Obesity.

All three factors contribute to the "mass hypercholesterolemia" which is seen in this country. For individuals with high LDL-cholesterol levels, modification of all is required. The first stage of management of high cholesterol by diet is called the Step I Diet. If the target for cholesterol lowering is not obtained by the Step I Diet, a further reduction may be obtained by moving to the Step II Diet. Implementation of the Step II diet is best achieved by consultation with a qualified dietitian. Achievement of desirable body weight is advocated for both the Step I and Step II Diets. If the goals for cholesterol lowering are not achieved with either of these two diets, drug therapy can be considered. However, for most patients, it is prudent to continue dietary therapy for at least 6 months before resorting to drug therapy.

Most patients with moderate hypercholesterolemia—LDL-cholesterol between 160 to 210 mg/dL—can be treated effectively with bile acid sequestrants. This is particularly the case when no other risk factors are present, or if the LDL-cholesterol level is in the range of 160 to 190 mg/dL Bile acid sequestrants have been proven to be effective for reducing risk of CHD in the Lipid Research Clinics Coronary Primary Prevention Trial, and they can be given with a minimum of side effects. However, because of their bulk and inconvenience and their tendency to produce constipation, not all patients can tolerate these drugs on a long-term basis. Still, for many patients with moderate hypercholesterolemia, the bile acid sequestrants are well tolerated and may be sufficient to bring cholesterol levels to the target range.

Another drug that is effective for treatment of moderate hypercholesterolemia is nicotinic acid—niacin. This drug inhibits the formation of lipoproteins in the liver, and consequently it lowers VLDL and LDL levels and raises HDL levels. The drug is especially useful for hypercholesterolemic patients with moderate hypertriglyceridemia or low HDL-cholesterol levels. It was shown to be effective in prevention of CHD in the Coronary Drug Project. Unfortunately, nicotinic acid has a variety of side effects that limits its utility. These include flushing and itching of the skin, skin rash, hepatotoxicity, gastrointestinal distress, worsening of glucose tolerance, and hyperuricemia. Only 50% to 60% of patients can be maintained on nicotinic acid for long periods. Nonetheless, for those patients who can tolerate the drug, it can be highly effective.

Another class of drugs for treatment of hypercholesterolemia include the HMG-CoA reductase inhibitors. These drugs inhibit the synthesis of cholesterol in the liver and thereby increase the formation of LDL-receptors. They also may inhibit the secretion of lipoproteins to a moderate degree. The HMG-CoA reductase inhibitors are highly effective for lowering LDL-cholesterol and VLDL-cholesterol levels. However, no clinical trials have been carried out to demonstrate their ability to reduce risk for CHD. In the Familial Atherosclerosis Treatment Study, these drugs in combination with bile acid sequestrants were shown to slow the development of new coronary artery lesions. The HMG CoA reductase inhibitors have a low level of toxicity, although rare patients develop drug-induced hepatitis or myopathy. These drugs appear to hold great promise for the treatment of hypercholesterolemia, especially in its more severe forms. The combination of a bile acid sequestrant and an HMG-CoA reductase inhibitor can be highly effective for treatment of familial hypercholesterolemia.

One class of drugs that is useful for treating patients with hypertriglyceridemia is the fibric acids, such as clofibrate, gemfibrozil, bezafibrate, and fenofibrate. These agents enhance the activity of lipoprotein lipase which promotes lipolysis of VLDL-triglycerides. The lowering of triglycerides often is accompanied by increases in HDL-cholesterol. Gemfibrozil therapy was shown to be effective for reducing risk of CHD in patients with mixed hyperlipidemia—elevated cholesterol and triglycerides—in the Helsinki Heart Study. Unfortunately, triglyceride lowering is not accompanied by a major reduction in cholesterol levels. However, when a fibric acid is combined with an HMG-CoA reductase inhibitor, both cholesterol and triglycerides are effectively reduced, and HDL-cholesterol levels are increased. It is unfortunate that this combination is associated with an increased risk for severe myopathy, and patients who are treated with this combination must be monitored carefully.

Finally, probucol is an LDL-lowering drug of moderate effectiveness and a relative lack of side effects. To date, probucol has not been shown to reduce risk for CHD, and therefore, it does not appear to be a drug of first choice for treatment of hypercholesterolemia. However, the drug has the interesting property of preventing oxidation of LDL, which is a putative atherogenic mechanism. Thus, future studies may reveal that probucol has the ability to prevent CHD beyond its effects on LDL cholesterol levels. Still, until this beneficial effect has been demonstrated through clinical trials, the use of probucol for its antioxidant properties cannot be advocated.

REFERENCES

1. Expert Panel: Report of the National Cholesterol Education Program. Expert Panel on detection, evaluation, and treatment of high blood cholesterol in adults. National Heart, Lung, and Blood Institute. *Arch Intern Med* 1988;148:36.

2. Grundy SM: Cholesterol metabolism in man. *West J Med* 1978;128:13.

3. Grundy SM, Ahrens EH Jr: An evaluation of the relative merits of two methods for measuring the balance of sterols in man: Isotopic balance versus chromatographic analysis. *J Clin Invest* 1966;9:1503.

4. Grundy SM, Ahrens EH Jr: Measurements of cholesterol turnover, synthesis and absorption in man, carried out by isotope kinetic and sterol balance methods. *J Lipid Res* 1969;10:91.

5. Grundy SM, Metzger AL: A physiological method for estimation of hepatic secretion of biliary lipids in man. *Gastroenterology* 1972;62:1200.

6. Hofmann AF, Borgstrom B: The intraluminal phase of fat digestion in man—The lipid content of the micellar and oil phases of intestinal content obtained during fat digestion and absorption. *J Clin Invest* 1964;43:247.

7. Kane JP, Hardman DA, Paulus HE: Heterogeneity of apolipoprotein B: isolation of a new species from human chylomicrons. *Proc Natl Acad Sci USA* 1980;77:2465.

8. La Rosa JC, Levy RI, Herbert P, Lox SE, Fredrickson DS: A specific apoprotein activator for lipoprotein lipase. *Biochim Piophys Res Commun* 1955;215:15.

9. Mahley RW: Apolipoprotein E: cholesterol transport protein with expanding role in cell. biology. *Science* 1988;240:622.

10. Havel RJ, Goldstein JL, Brown MS: Lipoproteins and lipid transport. In: Bondy PK, Rosenberg LE, eds. *Metabolic Control and Disease* Philadelphia, Pa: WB Saunders; 1980.

11. Spady DK, Bilheimer DW, Dietschy JM: Rates of receptor-dependent and independent low-density lipoprotein uptake in the hamster. *Proc Natl Acad Sci USA* 1983;80:3499.

12. Bilheimer DW, Goldstein JL, Grundy SM, et al: Liver transplantation to provide low-density-lipoprotein receptors and lower plasma cholesterol in a child with homozygous familial hypercholesterolemia. *N Engl J Med* 1984;311:1658.

13. Brown MS, Goldstein JL: Receptor-mediated pathway for cholesterol homeostasis. *Science* 1986;232:34.

14. Brown MS, Goldstein JL: How LDL receptors influence cholesterol and atherosclerosis. *Scientific American* 1984;251(5):58.

15. Brown MS, Kovanen PT, Goldstein JL: Regulation of plasma cholesterol by lipoprotein receptors. *Science* 1981;212:628.

16. Grundy SM: Pathogenesis of hyperlipoproteinemia. *J Lipid Res* 1984;25:1611.

17. Hamilton RL, Williams MC, Fielding CJ, Havel RJ: Discoidal bilayer structure of nascent high density lipoproteins from perfused rat liver. *J Clin Invest* 1976;58:667.

18. Glomset JA: The plasma lecithin: Cholesterol acyltransferase reaction. *J Lipid Res* 1968;9:155.

19. Grundy SM, Vega GL: Fibric acids: Effects on lipids and lipoprotein metabolism. *Am J Med* 1987;83:9.

20. Helser CB, Swenson TL, Tall AR: Purification and characterization of a human plasma cholesterol ester transfer protein. *J Biol Chem* 1987;262:2275.

21. Grundy SM: Atherosclerosis: pathology, pathogenesis, and role of risk factors. *Disease-a-Month* 1983;29(9):1.

22. Steinberg D, Parthasarathy S, Carew TE, et al: Beyond cholesterol: modification of low-density lipoprotein that increase its atherogenicity. *N Eng J Med* 1989;320:915.

23. Havel RJ: Familial dysbetalipoproteinemia: New aspects of pathogenesis and diagnosis. *Med Clin North Am* 1982;66:441.

24. Mahley RW: Atherogenic hyperlipoproteinemia: The cellular and molecular biology of plasma lipoproteins altered by dietary fat and cholesterol. *Med Clin North Am* 1982;66:375.

25. Parthasarathy S, Barnett J, Fong LG: High density lipoprotein inhibits the oxidative modification of low density lipoprotein. *Biochem Biophys Acta* 1990;1044:275.

26. Khoo JC, Miller EA, McLoughlin P, et al: Prevention of low density lipoprotein aggregation by high density lipoprotein or apolipoprotein A-I. *J Lipid Res* 1990;31:645.

27. Meyers LH, Phillips NR, Havel RJ: Mathematical methods for estimation of the concentration of the major lipid components of human serum lipoproteins. *J Lab Clin Med* 1976;88:491.

28. Keys A: Coronary heart disease in seven countries. *Circulation* 1970;41(suppl 1):1.

29. Marmot MG, Syme SL, Kagan H, et al: Epidemiologic studies of coronary heart disease and stroke in Japanese men living in Japan, Hawaii, and California: prevalence of coronary and hypertensive heart disease and associated risk factors. *Am J Epidemiol* 1975;102:514.

30. Kannel WB, Castelli W, Gordon T, et al: Serum cholesterol, lipoproteins, and risk of coronary heart disease: the Framingham study. *Ann Intern Med* 1971;74:1.

31. Stamler J, Wentworth D, Neaton J: Is the relationship between serum cholesterol and risk of death from CHD continuous and graded? *JAMA* 1986;256:2823.

32. Anderson KM, Castelli WP, Levy D: Cholesterol and mortality. 30 years of follow-up from the Framingham study. *JAMA* 1987;257:2176.

33. Kannel WB, Castelli WP, Gordon T: Cholesterol in the prediction of atherosclerotic disease: new perspectives in the Framingham study. *Ann Intern Med* 1979;90:85.

34. Austin MA: Plasma triglyceride and coronary heart disease. *Arteriosclerosis and Thrombosis* 1991;11:2.

35. Castelli WP: The triglyceride issue: A view from Framingham. *Am Heart J* 1986;112:432.

36. Cordon T, Castelli WP, Hjortland MC, et al: High density lipoprotein as a protective factor against coronary heart disease: The Framingham study. *Am J Med* 1977;62:707.

37. Gordon DJ, Probstfeld JL, Garrison RJ, et al: High-density lipoprotein cholesterol and cardiovascular disease. Four prospective American series. *Circulation* 1989;79:8.

38. Coronary Drug Project Research Group: Clofibrate and niacin in coronary heart disease. *JAMA* 1975;231:360.

39. Canner PL, Berge KG, Wenger NK, et al: Fifteen year mortality in Coronary Drug Project patients: Long-term benefit with niacin. *J Am Coll Cardiol* 1986;8:1245.

40. Carlson LA, Rosenhamer G: Reduction of mortality in the Stockholm Ischaemic Heart Disease Secondary Prevention Study by combined treatment with clofibrate and nicotinic acid. *Acta Med Scand* 1988;223:405.

41. Levy RI, Brensike JF, Epstein SE, et al: The influence of changes in lipid values induced by cholestyramine and diet on progression of coronary artery disease: Results of the NHLBI Type II Coronary Intervention Study. *Circulation* 1984;69:325.

42. Blankenhom DH, Nessim SA, Johnson RL, et al: Beneficial effects of combined colestipol-niacin therapy on coronary atherosclerosis and coronary venous bypass grafts. *JAMA* 1987;257:3233.

43. Cashin-Hemphill L, Mack WJ, Pogoda JM, et al: Beneficial effects of colestipol-niacin on coronary atherosclerosis. *JAMA* 1990;264:3013.

44. Brown G, Albers JJ, Fisher LD, et al: Regression of coronary artery disease as a result of intensive lipid-lowering therapy in men with high levels of apolipoprotein B. *N Engl J Med* 1990;323:1289.

45. Kane JP, Malloy MJ, Ports TA, et al: Regression of coronary atherosclerosis during treatment of familial hypercholesterolemia with combined drug regimens. *JAMA* 1990;264:3007.

46. Hjermann I, Velve Byre K, Holme I, et al: Effect of diet and smoking intervention of the incidence of coronary heart disease. Report from the Oslo Study Group of a randomized trial in healthy men. *Lancet* 1981;2:1303.

47. Lipid Research Clinics Program: The Lipid Research Clinics Coronary Primary Prevention Trial results. I. Reduction in incidence of coronary heart disease. *JAMA* 1984;251:351.

48. Lipid Research Clinics Program: The Lipid Research Clinics Coronary Primary Prevention Trial Results. II. The relationship of reduction in incidence of coronary heart disease to cholesterol lowering. *JAMA* 1984;251:365.

49. Frick MH, Elo O, Haapa K, et al: Helsinki Heart Study: primary prevention trial with gemfibrozil in middle-aged men with dyslipidemia: safety of treatment, changes in risk factors, and incidence of coronary heart disease. *N Engl J Med* 1987:317:1237.

50. Manninen V, Elo MO, Frick MH, et al: Lipid alterations and decline in the incidence of coronary heart disease in the Helsinki Heart Study. *JAMA* 1988;260.

51. Committee of Principal Investigators: WHO cooperative trial on primary prevention of ischemic heart disease with clofibrate to lower serum cholesterol: Final mortality follow-up. *Lancet* 1984;2:600.

52. Grundy SM, Goodman DEW, Rifkind BM, Cleeman JI: The place of HDL in cholesterol management: A perspective from the National Cholesterol Education Program. *Arch Intern Med* 1989;149:505.

53. Coronary Risk Handbook: *Estimating Risk of Coronary Heart Disease in Daily Practice.* Dallas, Texas: The American Heart Association; 1973.

54. Grundy SM, Barrett-Connor E, Bierman EL, et al: The consensus development conference on the treatment of hypertriglyceridemia, National Institutes of Health. *JAMA* 1984;251:1196.

55. Grundy SM, Vega GL: Hypertriglyceridemia: causes and relation to coronary heart disease. *Seminars in Thrombosis and Hemostasis* 1988;14:149.

56. Miller A, Lees RS, McCluskey MA, et al: The natural history and surgical significance of hyperlipidemic abdominal crisis. *Ann Surg* 1979;190:401.

57. Goldstein JL, Brown MS: Familial hypercholesterolemia. In Stanbury JB, Wyngaarden JB, Fredrickson DS, Goldstein JL, Brown MS et al, eds: *The Metabolic Basis of Inherited Disease.* New York: McGraw-Hill;1983:672.

58. Vega GL, Grundy SM: In vivo evidence for reduced binding of low density lipoproteins to receptors as a cause of primary moderate hypercholesterolemia. *J Clin Invest* 1986;78:1410.

59. Innerarity TL, Weisgraber KH, Arnold KS, et al: Familial defective apolipoprotein B-100: low density lipoproteins with abnormal receptor binding. *Proc Natl Acad Sci USA* 1987;84:6919.

60. Weisgraber KH, Innerarity TL, Newhouse YM, et al: Familial defective apolipoprotein B-100: enhanced binding of monoclonal antibody MB47 to abnormal low density lipoproteins. *Proc Natl Acad Sci USA* 1988;85:9758.

61. Soria LF, Ludwig EH, Clarke HRG, Vega GL, Grundy SM, McCarthy BJ: Association between a specific apolipoprotein B mutation and familial defective apolipoprotein B-100. *Proc Natl Acad Sci USA* 1989;86:587.

62. Innerarity TL, Mahley RW, Weisgraber KH, et al: Familial defective apolipoprotein B-100: A mutation of apolipoprotein B that causes hypercholesterolemia. *J Lipid Res* 1990;31:1337.

63. Goldstein JL, Hazzard WR, Schrott HG, et al: Hyperlipidemia in coronary heart disease. I. Lipid levels in 500 survivors of myocardial infarction. *J Clin Invest* 1973;52:1533.

64. Goldstein JL, Schrott HG, Hazzard WR, et al: Hyperlipidemia in coronary heart disease. II. Genetic analysis of lipid levels in 176 families and delineation of a new inherited disorder, combined hyperlipidemia. *J Clin Invest* 1973;52:1544.

65. Hazzard WR, Goldstein JL, Schrott HG, et al: Hyperlipidemia in coronary heart disease. III. Lipoprotein phenotyping of 156 genetically defined survivors of myocardial infarction. *J Clin Invest* 1973;52:1569.

66. Uauy R, Vega GL, Grundy SM: Coinheritance of two mild defects in low density lipoprotein receptor function produces severe hypercholesterolemia. *J Clin Endocrinol Metab* 1991;72:179.

67. Fredrickson DS, Levy RI, Lees RS: Fat transport in lipoproteins—an integrated approach to mechanisms and disorders. *N Engl J Med* 1967;276:32.

Treatment of Hyperlipidemias

68. Nikkila EA: Familial lipoprotein lipase deficiency and related disorders of chylomicron metabolism. In: Stanbury JS, Wyngaarden BJ, Fredrickson DS, et al, eds. *The Metabolic Basis of Inherited Disease* 5th ed. New York, NY: McGraw-Hill; 1983:622.

69. Chait A, Albert JJ, Brunzell JD: Very low density lipoprotein overproduction in genetic forms of hypertriglyceridaemia. *Eur J Clin Invest* 1980;10:17.

70. Dunn FL, Grundy SM, Bilheimer DW, et al: Impaired catabolism of very low-density lipoprotein-triglyceride in a family with primary hypertriglyceridemia. *Metabolism* 1985;34:316.

71. Grundy SM, Chait A, Brunzell JD: Familial combined hyperlipidemia workshop. *Arteriosclerosis* 1987;7:203.

72. Kissebah AH, Alfarsi S, Evans DJ: Low density lipoprotein metabolism in familial combined hyperlipidemia: Mechanism of the multiple lipoprotein phenotypic expression. *Arteriosclerosis* 1984;4:614.

73. Katz LN, Stamler J: Experimental atherosclerosis. Publication No. 124 American lectures series. monograph. In: Thomas CC, ed. *Bannerstone Division of American Lectures in Metabolism* Springfield, Illinois, 1953.

74. Rudel LL, Parks JS, Bond MG: LDL heterogeneity and atherosclerosis in nonhuman primates. *Ann NY Acad Sci* 1985;454:248.

75. McGill HC Jr, McMahan CA, Kruski AW, Mott GE: Relationship of lipoprotein cholesterol concentrations to experimental atherosclerosis in baboons. *Arteriosclerosis* 1981;1:3.

76. Strong JP: Atherosclerosis in primates. Introduction and overview. *Primates Med* 1976;9:1.

77. Grundy SM, Barrett-Connor E, Rudel LL, Miettinen T, Spector AA: Workshop on the impact of dietary cholesterol on plasma lipoproteins and atherogenesis. *Arteriosclerosis* 1988;8:95.

78. Slater G, Mead J, Dhopeshwarkar G, Robinson S, Alfin-Slater RB: Plasma cholesterol and triglycerides in men with added eggs in the diet. *Nutr Reps Internat* 1976;14:249.

79. Porter MW, Yamanaka W, Carlson SD, Flynn MA: Effect of dietary egg on serum cholesterol and triglyceride of human males. *Am J Clin Nutr* 1977;30:490.

80. Flynn MA, Nolph GB, Flynn TC, Kahns R, Krause G: Effect of dietary egg on human serum cholesterol and triglyceride. *Am J Clin Nutr* 1979;32:1050.

81. Keys A, Anderson JT, Grande F: Serum cholesterol response to changes in the diet. II. The effect of cholesterol in the diet. *Metabolism* 1965;14:759.

82. Hegsted DM: Serum-cholesterol response to dietary cholesterol: A reevaluation *Am J Clin Nutr* 1986;44:299.

83. Mattson FH, Erickson BA, Kligman AM: Effect of dietary cholesterol on serum cholesterol in man. *Am J Clin Nutr* 1972;25:589.

84. Beynen AC, Katan MB: Reproducibility of the variations between humans in the response of serum cholesterol to cessation of egg consumption. *Atherosclerosis* 1985;57:19.

85. Katan MB, Beynen AC, DeVries JH, et al: Existence of consistent hypo- and hyperresponders to dietary cholesterol in man. *Am J Epidemiol* 1986;123:221.

86. Katan MB, Beynen AC: Characteristics of human hypo- and hyperresponders to dietary cholesterol. *Am J Epidemiol* 1987;125:387.

87. Zanni EE, Zannis VI, Blum CB, et al: Effect of egg cholesterol and dietary fats on plasma lipids, lipoproteins, and apoproteins of normal women consuming natural diets. *J Lipid Res* 1987;28:518.

88. Katan MB, Bums MAM, Glatz JFC, et al: Congruence of individual responsiveness to dietary cholesterol and to saturated fat in man. *J Lipid Res* 1988;29:883 .

89. Kovanen PT, Brown MS, Basu SK, et al: Saturation and suppression of hepatic lipoprotein receptors: A mechanism for the hypercholesterolemia of cholesterol-fed rabbits. *Proc Natl Acad Sci USA* 1981;78:1396.

90. Sorci-Thomas M, Wilson MD, Johnson FL, et al: Studies on the expression of genes encoding apolipoproteins B100 and B48 and the low density lipoprotein receptor in nonhuman primates. *J Biol Chem* 1989;264(15):9039.

91. Dawson PA, Hofmann SL, van der Westhuyzen DR, et al: Sterol-dependent repression of low density lipoprotein receptor promoter mediated by 16-base pair sequence adjacent to binding site for transcription factor Sp1. *J Biol Chem* 1988;263:3372.

92. Zilversmit DB: Atherogenesis: a postprandial phenomenon. *Circulation* 1979;60:473.

93. Quintao E, Grundy SM, Ahrens EH Jr: Effects of dietary cholesterol on the regulation of total body cholesterol in man. *J Lipid Res* 1971; 12:233.

94. Stamler J, Shekelle R: Dietary cholesterol and human coronary heart disease: the epidemiological evidence. *Arch Pathol Lab Med* 1988;112:1032.

95. Committee on Technological Options to Improve the Nutritional Attributes of Animal Products. Board on Agriculture. National Research Council Designing Foods. *Animal Product Options in the Marketplace* Washington, DC: National Academy Press; 1988.

96. Spady DK, Dietschy JM: Dietary saturated triglycerides suppress hepatic low density lipoprotein receptors in the hamster. *Proc Natl Acad Sci USA* 1985;82:4526.

97. Nicolosi RJ, Stucchi AF, Kowala MC, et al: Effect of dietary fat saturation and cholesterol on LDL composition and metabolism. *Arteriosclerosis* 1990;10:119.

98. Ahrens EH, Hirsch J, Insull W, et al: The influence of dietary fats on serum-lipid levels in man. *Lancet* 1957;1:943.

99. Keys A, Anderson JT, Grande F: Serum cholesterol response to changes in the diet. IV. Particular saturated fatty acids in the diet. *Metabolism* 1965;14:776.

100. Hegsted DM, McGandy RB, Myers ML, et al: Quantitative effects of dietary fat on serum cholesterol in man. *Am J Clin Nutr* 1965;17:281.

101. Grande F: Dog serum lipid responses to dietary fats differing in the chain length of the saturated fatty acids. *J Nutr* 1962;76:255.

102. Hashim SA, Arteaga A, van Itallie TB: Effect of a saturated medium-chain triglyceride on serum-lipids in man. *Lancet* 1960;1:1105.

103. Horlick L, Craig BM: Effect of long-chain polyunsaturated and saturated fatty acids on the serum lipids of man. *Lancet* 1957; 2:566.

104. Grande F, Anderson JT, Keys A: Comparison of effects of palmitic and stearic acids in the diet on serum cholesterol in man. *Am J Clin Nutr* 1970;23:1 184.

105. Bonanome A, Grundy SM: Effect of dietary stearic acid on plasma cholesterol and lipoprotein levels. *N Engl J Med* 1988;318:1244.

106. Wilson JD: The quantification of cholesterol excretion and degradation in the isotopic steady rate in the rat: The influence of dietary cholesterol. *J Lipid Res* 1964;5:409.

107. Grundy SM: Trans monounsaturated fatty acids and serum cholesterol levels *N Engl J Med* 1990;323:480.

108. Keys A:Seven Countries:*A Multivariate Analysis on Death and Coronary Heart Disease*. Cambridge, MA; Harvard University Press; 1980.

109. Ashley FW Jr, Kannel WB: Relation of weight change to changes in atherogenic traits: The Framingham Study. *J Chron Dis* 1974;27:103.

110. Kannel WB, Gordon T, Castelli WP: Obesity, lipids, and glucose intolerance: The Framingham Study. *Am J Clin Nutr* 1979;32:1238.

111. Garrison RJ, Wilson PW, Castelli WP, et al: Obesity and lipoprotein cholesterol in the Framingham offspring study. *Metabolism* 1980;29:1053.

112. Shekelle RB, Shryock AM, Paul O, et al: Diet, serum cholesterol, and death from coronary heart disease: The Western Electric Study. *N Engl J Med* 1981;304:65.

113. Stamler J: Overweight, hypertension, hypercholesterolemia and coronary heart disease. In: Mananni M, Lewis B, Contaldo F, eds. *Medical Complications of Obesity* London: Academic Press;1979:191.

114. Havel RJ: Familial dysbetalipoproteinemia: New aspects of pathogenesis and diagnosis. Med Clin North Am 1982;66:441.

115. Egusa G, Beltz WF, Grundy SM, Howard BV: Influence of obesity on the metabolism of apolipoprotein B in man. *J Clin Invest* 1985;76:596.

116. Kesaniemi YA, Grundy SM: Increased low density lipoprotein production associated with obesity. *Arteriosclerosis* 1983;3:170.

117. Wolf R, Grundy SM: Influence of weight reduction on plasma lipoproteins in obese patients. *Arteriosclerosis* 1983;3:160.

118. Mattson FH, Grundy SM: Comparison of effects of dietary saturated, monounsaturated, and polyunsaturated fatty acids on plasma lipids and lipoproteins in man. *J Lipid Res* 1985;26:194.

119. Mensink RP, Katan MB: Effect of a diet enriched with monounsaturated or polyunsaturated fatty acids on levels of low-density and high-density lipoprotein cholesterol in healthy women and men. *N Engl J Med* 1989;321:436.

120. Vega GL, Groszek E, Wolf R, et al: Influence of polyunsaturated fats on plasma lipoprotein composition apolipoprotein. *J Lipid Res* 1982;23:811.

121. Shepherd J, Packard CJ, Patsch JR: Effects of dietary polyunsaturated and saturated fat on the properties of high density lipoproteins and the metabolism of apolipoprotein A-I. *J Clin Invest* 1978;1582.

122. Jackson RL, Kashyap ML, Barnhart RL, et al: Influence of polyunsaturated and saturated fats on plasma lipids and lipoproteins in man. *Am J Clin Nutr* 1984;39:589.

123. Parthasarathy S, Khoo JC, Miller E, et al: Low density lipoprotein rich in oleic acid is protected against oxidative modification: Implications for dietary prevention of atherosclerosis. *Proc Natl Acad Sci USA* 1990;87:3894.

124. Berry EM, Eisenberg S, Haratz D, et al: Effects of diets rich in monounsaturated fatty acids on plasma lipoprotein—the Jerusalem Nutrition Study: high MUFAs vs. high PUFAs. *Am J Clin Nutr* 1991;53:889.

125. Committee on Diet and Health Food and Nutrition Board, Commission on Life Sciences, National Research Council: *Diet and Health: Implications for reducing chronic disease risk.* Washington, DC; National Academy Press; 1989.

126. Nestel PJ, Connor WE, Reardon MF, et al: Suppression by diets rich in fish oil of very low density lipoprotein production in man. *J Clin Invest* 1984;74:82.

127. Connor WE: Hypolipidemic effects of dietary omega-3 fatty acids in normal and hyperlipidemic humans: Effectiveness and mechanisms. In: Simopoulos AP, Kifer RR, Martin RE, eds. *Health Effects of Polyunsaturated Fatty Acids in Seafoods.* Orlando, Fl: Academic Press; 1986:173.

128. Grundy SM, Bilheimer D, Blackburn H, et al: Rationale of the diet-heart statement of the American Heart Association. Report of Nutrition Committee. *Circulation* 1982;65:839A.

129. Nestel PJ, Hirsch EZ: Triglyceride turnover after diets rich in carbohydrate or animal fat. *Asian Ann Med* 1965;14:265.

130. Quarfordt SH, Frank A, Shames DM, et al: Very low density lipoprotein triglyceride transport in type IV hyperlipoproteinemia and the effects of carbohydrate-rich diets. *J Clin Invest* 1970;49:2281.

131. Nestel PJ, Carroll KF, Havenstein N: Plasma triglyceride response to carbohydrates, fats and caloric intake. *Metabolism* 1970;19:1.

132. Fredrickson DS, Ono K, Davis LL: Lipolytic activity of post-heparin plasma in hyperglyceridemia. *J Lipid Res* 1963;4:24.

133. Jackson RL, Yates MT, McNerney CA, et al: Diet and HDL metabolism: High carbohydrate vs. high fat diets. *Adv Exp Med Biol* 1987;210:165.

134. Abbott WGH, Swinburn B, Ruotolo G, et al: Effect of a high-carbohydrate, low-saturated-fat diet on apolipoprotein B and triglyceride metabolism in Pima Indians. *J Clin Invest* 1990;86:642.

135. Grundy SM: Comparison of monounsaturated fatty acids and carbohydrates for lowering plasma cholesterol. *N Engl J Med* 1986;314:745.

136. Brussaard JH, Katan MB, Groot PHE, et al: Serum lipoproteins of healthy persons fed a low-fat diet or a polyunsaturated fat diet for three months: A comparison of two cholesterol-lowering diets. *Atherosclerosis* 1982;42:205.

137. Mensink RP, Katan MB: Effect of monounsaturated fatty acids versus complex carbohydrates on high-density lipoproteins in healthy men and women. *Lancet* 1987;1:122.

138. Kuusi T, Ehnholm C, Huttunen JK, et al: Concentration and composition of serum lipoproteins during a low-fat diet at two levels of polyunsaturated fat. *J Lipid Res* 1985;26:360.

139. Hjermann I, Enger SC, Helgeland A, et al: The effect of dietary changes on high density lipoprotein cholesterol. *Am J Med* 1979;66:105.

140. Jones DY, Judd JT, Taylor PR, *Campbell WS, Nair PP*: Influence of caloric contribution and saturation of dietary fat on plasma lipids in premenopausal women. *Am J Clin Nutr* 1987;45:1451.

141. Nestel PJ, Hirsh EZ: Mechanism of alcohol induced hypertriglyceridemia. *J Lab Clin Med* 1965;66:357.

142. Baraona, Lieber CS:Effects of ethanol on lipid metabolism. *J Lipid Res* 1975;20:289.

143. Nikkila EA: Influence of dietary fructose and sucrose on serum triglycerides in hypertriglyceridemia and diabetes. In: Sipple H, McNutt KW, eds. *Sugars in Nutrition* New York, NY: Academic Press; 1974.

144. Wolfe BM, Havel RJ, Marlis EB, et al: Effects of a 3-day fast and ethanol on splanchnic metabolism of FFA, amino acids, and carbohydrates in healthy young men. *J Clin Invest* 1976;57:329.

145. Grundy SM: Bile acid resins. Mechanisms of action. In: *Pharmacological Control of Hyperlipidemia* South America: JR Prous Science Publishers; 1986:3.

146. LaPorte RE, Cresanta JL, Kuller LH: The relation of alcohol to coronary heart disease and mortality. *Prev Med* 1980;9:22.

147. Endo A, Kuroda M, Tsujita Y: ML-236A, ML-236B, and ML-236C, new inhibitors of cholesterogenesis produced by Penicillium citrinum. *J Antibiot (Tokyo)* 1976;29:1346.

148. Endo A, Kuorda M, Tanzawa K: Competitive inhibition of 3-hydroxy-3-methylglutaryl coenzyme A reductase by ML-236A and ML-236B fungal metabolites, having hypocholesterolemic activity. *FEBS Lett* 1976:72:323.

149. Tsujita Y, Juroda M, Tanzawa K, et al: Hypolipidemic effects in dogs of ML-236B, a competitive inhibitor of 3-hydroxy-3-methylglutaryl coenzyme A reductase. *Atherosclerosis* 1979;32:307.

150. Shigematsu H, Hata Y, Yamamoto M, et al: Treatment of hypercholesterolemia with a HMG CoA reductase inhibitor (CS-500). I. Phase I study in normal subjects. *Geriatr Med (Japan)* 1979;17:564.

151. Yamamoto A, Sudo H, Endo A: Therapeutic effects of ML-236B in primary hypercholesterolemia. *Atherosclerosis* 1980;35:259.

152. Mabuchi H, Haba T, Tatami R, et al: Effects of an inhibitor of 3-hydroxy-3-methylglutaryl coenzyme A reductase on serum lipoproteins and ubiquinone-10 levels in patients with familial hypercholesterolemia. *N Engl J Med* 1981;305:478.

153. Alberts AW, Chen J, Kuron G, et al: Mevinolin: a highly potent competitive inhibitor of hydroxymethylglutaryl-coenzyme A reductase and a cholesterol-lowering agent. *Proc Natl Acad Sci USA* 1980;77:3957.

154. Kovanen PT, Bilheimer DW, Goldstein JL, et al: Regulatory role for hepatic low density lipoprotein receptors in vivo in the dog. *Proc Natl Acad Sci USA* 1981;78:1194.

155. Bilheimer DW, Grundy SM, Brown MS, Goldstein JL: Mevinolin and colestipol stimulate receptor-mediated clearance of low density lipoprotein from plasma in familial hypercholesterolemia heterozygotes. *Proc Natl Acad Sci USA* 1983;80:4124.

156. Bilheimer DW, Grundy SM, Brown MS, Goldstein JL: Mevinolin and colestipol stimulate receptor-mediated clearance of low density lipoprotein from plasma in familial hypercholesterolemia heterozygotes. *Proc Natl Acad Sci USA* 1983;80:4124.

157. Ginsberg HN, Le N-A, Short MP, et al: Suppression of apolipoprotein B production during treatment of cholesterol storage disease with lovastatin: Implications for regulation of apolipoprotein B synthesis *J Clin lnvest* 1987;80:1692.

158. Arad Y, Ramakrishnan R, Ginsberg HN: Lovastatin therapy reduces low density lipoprotein apo B levels in subjects with combined hyperlipidemia by reducing the production of apo B containing lipoproteins: Implications for the pathophysiology of apo B production. *J Lipid Res* 1990;31:567.

159. Uauy R, Vega GL, Grundy SM, et al: Lovastatin therapy in receptor-negative homozygous familial hypercholesterolemia: lack of effect on low-density lipoprotein concentrations or turnover. *J Pediatr* 1988; 1 13:387.

160. Bradford RH, Shear CL, Chremos AN, et al: Expanded clinical evaluation of lovastatin (EXCEL) study results. I. Efficacy in modifying plasma lipoproteins and adverse event profile in 8245 patients with moderate hypercholesterolemia. *Arch Intern Med* 1991;151:43.

161. Shepherd J, Packard CL: An overview of the effects of p-chlorophenoxyisobutyric acid derivatives on lipoprotein metabolism. In: Fears R, Prous JR, eds. *Pharmacological Control of Hyperlipidemia.* Barcelona, Spain: Science Publications; 1986:135.

162. Oliver MF, et al: Ischaemic heart disease: A secondary prevention trial using clofibrate. *Brit Med J* 1971;4:775.

163. Rodney O, Uhlendorf P, Maxwell RE: The hypolipidemic effect of gemfibrozil (CI-719) in laboratory animals. *Proc R Soc Med* 1976;69:6.

164. Boberg J, Boberg M, Gross R, et al: The effect of treatment with clofibrate on hepatic triglyceride and lipoprotein lipase activities of postheparin plasma in male patients with hyperlipoproteinemia. *Arteriosclerosis* 1977;267:499.

165. Taylor KG, Holdsworth G, Dalton DJ: Clofibrate increases lipoprotein lipase activity in adipose tissue of hypertriglyceridaemic patients. *Lancet* 1977;2:1106.

166. Nikkila EA, Huttunen JK, Ehnholm C: Effect of clofibrate on postheparin plasma triglyceride lipase activities in patients with hypertriglyceridemia. *Metabolism* 1977;26:179.

Treatment of Hyperlipidemias

167. Bernt J, Gaumert R, Still J: Mode of action of the lipid lowering agents clofibrate and BM 15.075 on cholesterol biosynthesis in rat liver. *Arteriosclerosis* 1978;30:147.

168. Schneider AG, Ditschuneit HH, Stang EF, et al: Regulation of 3-hydroxy-3-methylglutaryl coenzyme A reductase in freshly isolated human mononuclear cells by fenofibrate. In: Carlson LA, Olsson AG, eds. *Treatment of Hyperlipoproteinemia*. New York, NY: Raven Press; 1984:81.

169. Grundy SM, Ahrens EGJ, Salen G, et al: Mechanism of action of clofibrate on cholesterol metabolism in patients with hyperlipidemia. *J Lipid Res.*

170. von Bergmann K, Leiss O: Effect of short-term treatment with bezafibrate and fenofibrate on biliary lipid metabolism in patients with hyperlipoproteinaemia. *Eur J Clin Invest* 1984;14:150.

171. Palmer RH: Effects of fenofibrate on bile lipid composition. *Arteriosclerosis* 1985;5:631.

172. Shepherd J, Packard CJ: An overview of the effects of p-chlorophenoxy-isobutyric acid derivatives on lipoprotein metabolism. In: Fears R, ed. *Pharmacological Control of Hyperlipidaemia*. Barcelona, Spain: JR Prous Science Publishers; 1986:135.

173. Newton RS, Krause BR: Mechanisms of action of gemfibrozil: Comparison of studies in the rat to clinical efficacy. In: Fears R, ed. *Pharmacological Control of Hyperlipidaemia*. Barcelona, Spain: JR Prous Science Publishers; 1986:171.

174. Saku K, Gartside PS, Hynd BA, et al: Mechanism of action of gemfibrozil on lipoprotein metabolism. *J Clin Invest* 1985;75:1702.

175. Vega GL, Grundy SM: Gemfibrozil therapy in primary hypertriglyceridemia associated with coronary heart disease. *JAMA* 1985;253:2398.

176. Vega GL, Grundy SM: Primary hypertriglyceridemia with borderline high cholesterol and elevated apolipoprotein B concentrations. *JAMA* 1990;264:2759.

177. Vega GL, Grundy SM: Comparison of lovastatin and gemfibrozil in normolipidemic patients with hypoalphalipoproteinemia. *JAMA* 1989;262:3148.

178. Kesaniemi YA, Grundy SM: Influence of probucol on cholesterol and lipoprotein metabolism in man. *J Lipid Res* 1984;25:780.

179. Parthasarathy S, Young S, Witztum JL, et al: Probucol inhibits oxidative modification of low density lipoprotein. *J Clin Invest* 1986;77:641.

180. Jialal I, Vega GL, Grundy SM: Physiologic levels of ascorbate inhibit the oxidative modification of low density lipoprotein. *Atherosclerosis* 1990;82:185.

181. Jialal I, Grundy SM: Preservation of the endogenous antioxidants in low density lipoprotein by ascorbate but not probucol during oxidative modification. *J Clin Invest* 1991;87:597.

182. Kita T, Nagano Y, Yokode K: Probucol prevents the progression of atherosclerosis in Watanabe heritable hyperlipidemic rabbit, an animal model for familial hypercholesterolemia. *Proc Natl Acad Sci USA* 1987;84:5928.

183. Kane JP, Malloy MJ, Tun P, et al: Normalization of low-density-lipoprotein levels in heterozygous familial hypercholesterolemia with a combined drug regimen. *N Engl J Med* 1981;304:251.

184. Grundy SM, Vega GL, Bilheimer DW: Influence of combined therapy with mevinolin and interruption of bile-acid re-absorption on low density lipoproteins in heterozygous familial hypercholesterolemia. *Ann Intern Med* 1985;103:339.

185. Vega GL, Grundy SM: Comparison of lovastatin and gemfibrozil in normolipidemic patients with hypoalphalipoproteinemia. *JAMA* 1989;262:3148.

186. Grundy SM, Vega GL: Causes of high blood cholesterol. *Circulation* 1990;81:412.

187. Vega GL, Denke MA, Grundy SM: Metabolic basis of primary hypercholesterolemia. *Circulation* 1991;84:118.

188. Denke MA, Grundy SM: Hypercholesterolemia in the elderly: resolving the treatment dilemma. *Ann Intern Med* 1990;112:780.

189. Vega GL, Grundy SM: Management of primary mixed hyperlipidemia with lovastatin. *Arch Int Med* 1990;150:1313.

190. East C, Bilheimer DW, Grundy SM: Combination drug therapy for familial combined hyperlipidemia. *Ann Intern Med* 1988;109:25.

191. East C, Alivizatos PA, Grundy SM, et al: Rhabdomyolysis in patients receiving lovastatin after cardiac transplantation [letter]. *N Engl J Med* 1988;318:47.

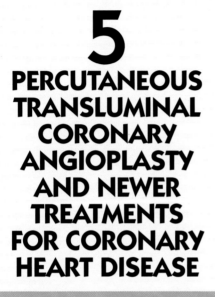

5

PERCUTANEOUS TRANSLUMINAL CORONARY ANGIOPLASTY AND NEWER TREATMENTS FOR CORONARY HEART DISEASE

DONALD S. BAIM, MD

Synopsis of Chapter Five

Percutaneous Transluminal
Coronary Angioplasty
History
Mechanisms
Technique
Indications
Success Rates
Complications
Restenosis

New Technologies
Stents
Atherectomy
Lasers

Treatment of Valvular Stenosis
Pulmonary Valvuloplasty
Mitral Valvuloplasty
• Technique
• Results of Clinical Trials
Aortic Valvuloplasty
• Technique
• Results of Clinical Trials

Other Interventional
Catheterization Techniques

Conclusions

PERCUTANEOUS TRANSLUMINAL CORONARY ANGIOPLASTY (PTCA)

Although coronary angiography came into widespread use during the 1960s and 1970s, it was limited to the purely **diagnostic** role of defining the location and severity of coronary lesions prior to surgical intervention—coronary artery bypass. Rapid and progressive growth of **interventional** techniques was seen during the late 1970s and the 1980s. Percutaneously inserted cardiac catheters, which were advanced transluminally into diseased segments of the coronary circulation, provided nonsurgical enlargement of the stenotic lumen.

By 1990, more than 250,000 such procedures were being performed each year in the United States, roughly equalling the annual number of coronary bypass surgeries.[1,2] Beginning with simple mechanical enlargement (balloon dilatation), this field now includes:
- The investigational use of implantable supports (stents).
- Devices to excise atherosclerotic plaque (atherectomy catheters).
- Ablative or photothermal laser systems.[3,4]

HISTORY

Dotter and Judkins originated the concept of catheter intervention in vascular disease. In 1964, they reported improvement in angiographic lumen diameter after passage of a guidewire and diagnostic catheter across an almost totally occluded peripheral arterial lesion.[5] Seizing upon this idea, they developed what came to be known as the "Dotter technique" in which a series of progressively larger concentric dilators were advanced over a guidewire until satisfactory enlargement of the stenotic lumen was established (Figure 5.1). While the developers immediately foresaw the potential extension of their technique into the renal, cerebral, and coronary circulations, many were skeptical. With this approach, local vascular injury was common at the entry site of the full-sized dilators, as was plaque trauma related to their passage across the target lesion. Because of these complications, the Dotter technique remained limited to the peripheral circulation, receiving greater use in Europe than in the United States.

In the mid-1970s, Andreas Gruentzig began working on balloon dilatation, a refinement of the Dotter technique in which a noncompliant balloon-tipped catheter was introduced uninflated, passed across the target lesion, and then inflated to a predetermined diameter in order to enlarge the stenotic lumen[6] (Figure 5.2). While others had explored this concept, Gruentzig was the first to produce a workable

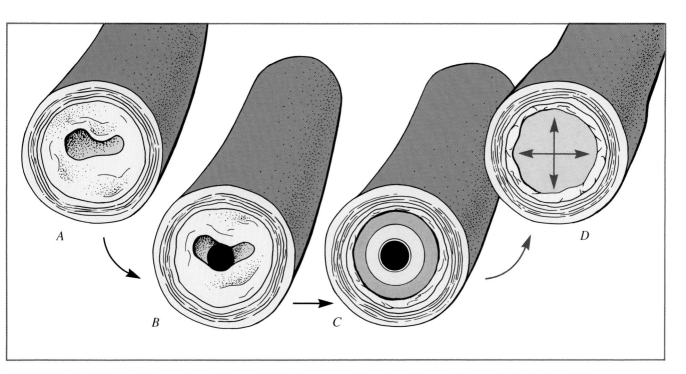

FIGURE 5.1 • The Dotter technique as it would be applied to the vessel displayed in cross-section:
- The stenotic vessel at baseline (A).
- The lesion crossed with a guidewire (B).
- Passage of two coaxial dilators over the guidewire (C).

- The enlarged lumen of the vessel after treatment (D).
Note that the original concept of this process involved compression of the plaque rather than enlargement of the vessel's outer diameter.

catheter system based on a relatively noncompliant PVC balloon. Following clinical use in peripheral and renal arterial disease and investigation in human coronary disease at the time of bypass surgery, he performed the first percutaneous transluminal coronary angioplasty (PTCA) on September 16, 1977[7] (Figure 5.3).

Early reports of success captured the interest of a number of investigators in the United States and Europe, who began attempting PTCA in carefully selected lesions. Ultimately, a voluntary registry of PTCA procedures under the sponsorship of the National Heart, Lung, and Blood Institute (NHLBI) was formed. With data on some 3,000 patients before it closed in 1981, this Registry played an important role in defining the indications, success, and complication rates of the new procedure, and helped set the stage for approval of the first angioplasty balloon catheters by the Federal Drug Administration (FDA) in 1983.[8]

The initial application of PTCA was confined to fewer than 1,000 cases/year worldwide in 1978-80, but it was clear that much of the limitation was caused by deficiencies of the original dilatation equipment (Figure 5.4A,B). The equipment's large deflated 1.5 mm diameter, lack of steering control, and limited pressure tolerance—6 atm or 90 psi—frequently prevented successful crossing and dilatation of even carefully se-

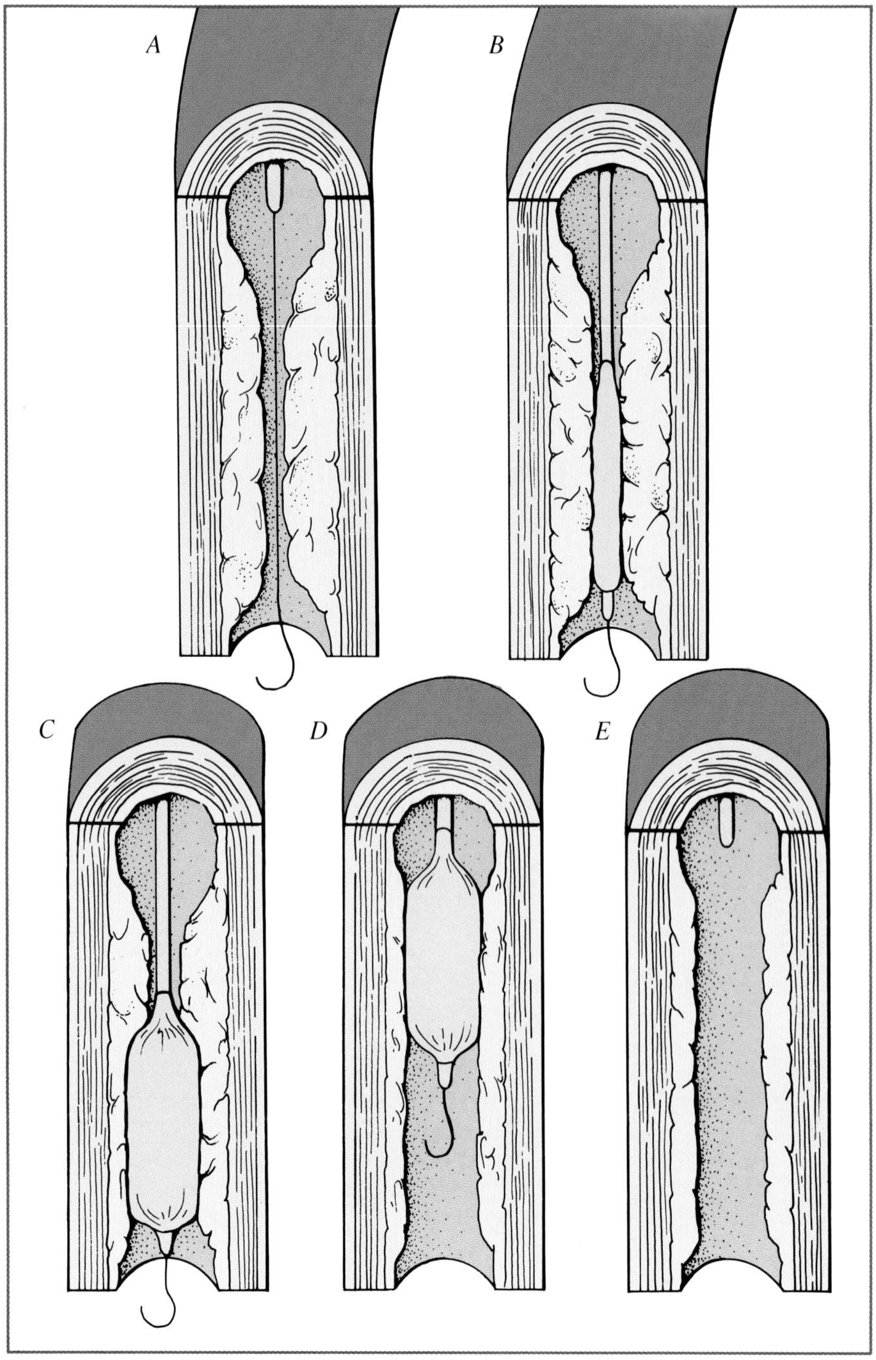

FIGURE 5.2 • The technique of balloon dilatation as proposed by Gruentzig for use in peripheral arteries:
• A guidewire is passed across the stenosis (A).
• This is followed by the deflated balloon catheter (B).
•The balloon catheter is inflated within the stenotic lumen (C,D).
• The lumen is enlarged after balloon removal (E).

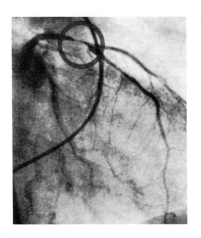 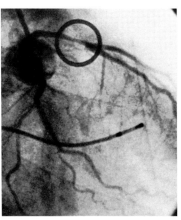 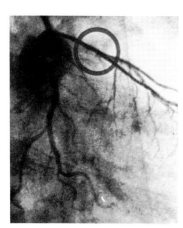

FIGURE 5.3 •
Angiograms from
the first patient to
undergo coronary
angioplasty per-
formed by Andreas
Gruentzig on
September 16,
1977—predilata-
tion (A), immediate
postdilatation (B),
and 1-month fol-
low-up study (C).
(Courtesy of USCI,
Division of CR Bard,
Inc, Billerica, MA)

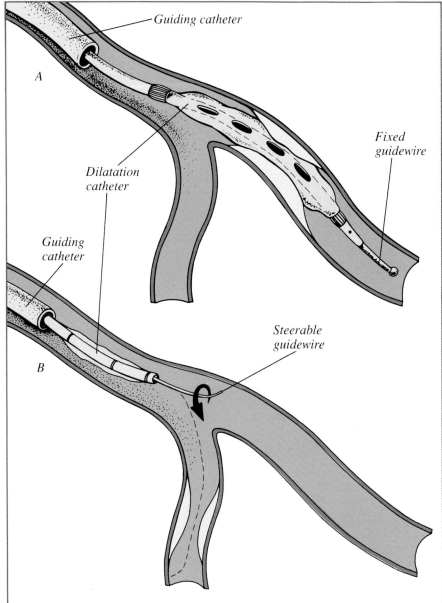

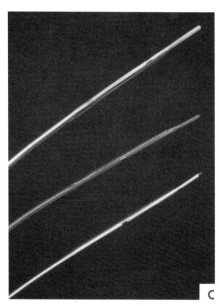

FIGURE 5.4 • Original coronary dilatation
balloon as used in the 1977–1981 PTCA
Registry. The design was marked by a large
deflated profile, a low rupture pressure, and
a fixed nonsteerable guidewire at its tip (A).
More recent designs include a balloon with
much lower deflated profile and higher rupture pressure, which travels over a fully
moveable and steerable guidewire that can
be precisely placed virtually anywhere
in the coronary circulation (B). Progressive
evolution in catheter design has led to ongoing improvement in both shaft size and
crossing profile. (C) Three 3.0 mm catheters
manufactured by Advanced Cardiovascular
Systems. The Simpson-Robert , introduced in
1983, uses a 0.018 inch guidewire and has a
4.3 F shaft diameter and a 0.055 inch crossing profile. The Hartzler ACX (1989) utilizes a
0.014 inch guidewire, and has a shaft diameter of 3.7F and a crossing profile of 0.035
inch. The TEN (1990) utilizes a 0.010 inch
guidewire and has a shaft diameter of 2.8F
with a crossing profile of 0.028 inch.

lected early PTCA candidates. A competitive effort by a handful of manufacturers led to the development of improved catheters, that currently have deflated diameters as small as 0.5 mm, are fully steerable, and can tolerate inflation pressures up to 20 atm or 300 psi[9,10] (Figure 5.4C). This ongoing refinement in equipment, coupled with the growing expertise of angioplasty operators[11] and acceptance of the procedure by both patients and the medical community, has made coronary angioplasty as accepted as bypass surgery for the performance of coronary revascularization[1,2] (Figure 5.5).

Despite the improvements that occurred in PTCA throughout the 1980s, the technique still faces four major limitations:
• Failure to cross some lesions, particularly chronic total occlusions.
• Failure to dilate other lesions—rigid calcified, or elastic eccentric stenoses.
• Abrupt closure due to local vessel trauma, which may necessitate emergency surgical revascularization.
• Late restenosis due to intimal proliferation at the dilatation site.

• • • • • • • • • • • • • • • •

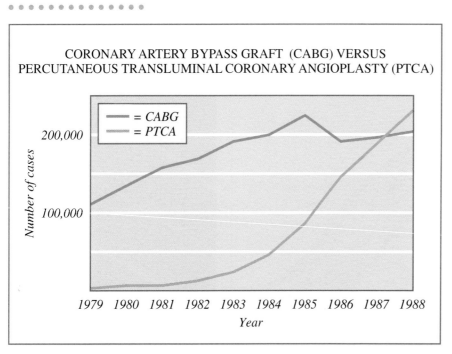

FIGURE 5.5 • Growth of percutaneous transluminal coronary angioplasty (PTCA) volume versus coronary after bypass graft (CABG) volume during the 1980's. Between 1979 and 1981, fewer than 1,000 PTCAs were performed each year. With the advent of improved equipment, PTCA volume grew progressively through the mid-1980's, equalling CABG volume at more than 200,000 cases/year in 1987.

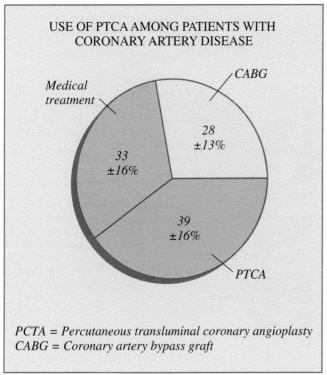

FIGURE 5.6 • Estimated use of medical treatment coronary after bypass graft and percutaneous transluminal coronary angioplasty among patients undergoing first time diagnostic coronary angiography in 1987. This supports the concept that PTCA was then supplying roughly half of the coronary revascularization being performed.

An effort over the last several years to address these residual limitations of conventional balloon angioplasty has resulted in the development and clinical investigation of nearly two dozen adjunctive devices for use in coronary intervention.[3,4] With further refinement, these devices may help to improve the predictability, success, and safety of PTCA, allowing it to play an even more important role in revascularization of patients with coronary heart disease (Figure 5.6).

MECHANISMS

Early statements by both Dotter and Gruentzig suggested that compression or redistribution of plaque along the vessel wall might account for much of the improvement in lumen diameter.[5,6] Others feared that distal embolization of disrupted plaque constituents might be an important adverse mechanism. Experiments in animal and cadaveric human arteries, however, failed to support either of these potentialities. They instead showed that balloon expansion within a stenotic vessel segment causes a cracking of the vessel wall that frequently extends through the plaque and into the underlying media, allowing expansion of both the inner and outer diameters of the treated segment[12,13] (Figure 5.7).

Full appreciation of this now widely accepted mechanism explains many of the observed consequences and limitations of PTCA. Applications of pressure insufficient to crack calcified or densely fibrotic plaque precludes effective dilatation. Even full balloon expansion does not prevent a nearly immediate loss of part of the expanded diameter due to elastic recoil of the vessel wall and/or local vasospasm. Similarly, "controlled injury" of the treated plaque accounts for the frequently hazy appearance and the presence of intimal filling defects on the immediate post-PTCA angiogram (Figure 5.8). More extensive ves-

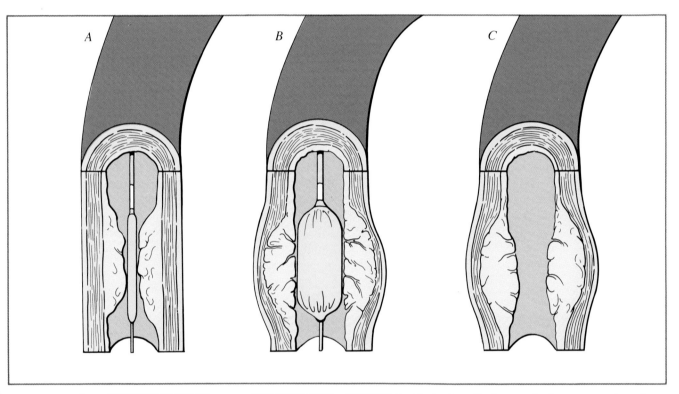

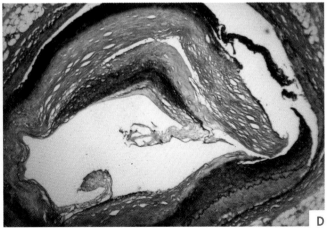

FIGURE 5.7 • Mechanism of balloon angioplasty as currently understood. Baseline appearance of stenotic segment :
• Deflated balloon passed across lesion (A).
• Balloon inflation cracks the atherosclerotic plaque and overdistends the surrounding media and adventitia (B).
• Due to partial elastic recoil of the vessel wall, however, the resulting lumen diameter is roughly 30% smaller than the size of the inflated balloon (C).
• Cross-section of a cadaver coronary artery subjected to balloon dilatation, showing clear cracking of the atherosclerotic plaque and surrounding media (D).

sel injury (dissection) accounts for most of the early occlusions that occur during the minutes or hours after PTCA.[14] Finally, creation of an irregular surface and exposure to the bloodstream of deep plaque and vessel wall constituents, particularly collagen, explains the rapid adhesion to the vessel wall of platelets and clotting proteins, with release of potent mitogens leading to the excessive local smooth muscle cell proliferation response that underlies late restenosis.[15]

Moreover, understanding the mechanism of balloon dilatation and how it underlies the observed limitations of the technique has fostered development of several new adjunctive technologies. These technologies strive to improve the acute lumen diameter by removing plaque or reducing elastic recoil, leaving behind a smoother vessel wall with less tendency to accumulate platelet-fibrin thrombus, and hopefully less proliferative tendency of the remaining smooth muscle cells.[4] At the same time, this understanding has guided the development of drug-based strategies that seek to block platelet adhesion and subsequent smooth muscle cell proliferation.[16–20]

TECHNIQUE

Coronary angioplasty relies on a guiding catheter to deliver the dilatation system to the ostium of the involved vessel. These catheters are inserted into the femoral artery under local anesthesia. Guiding catheters are similar in shape to those used for diagnostic angiography, but their internal lumen diameter is substantially larger—1.5 to 2.5 mm—to accommodate the angioplasty balloon. Patients are pretreated with antiplatelet agents—aspirin, 325 mg/d, and usually dipyridamole, 200 mg/d, for at least 24 hrs. Also, IV heparin, 10,000 to 15,000 U, is administered immediately after catheter insertion.[21]

Once the guiding catheter is engaged in the ostium, a flexible steerable guidewire—diameter 0.014 to 0.018 in or 0.3 to 0.5 mm—is advanced across the target stenosis and well into the distal vessel. Correct position is confirmed by contrast injection through the guiding catheter (refer to Figure 5.4). The guidewire serves as a rail along which the deflated balloon catheter can be advanced across the lesion, aided by the support of the guiding catheter. To obtain a smaller deflated diameter, specialized dilatation catheters have been developed in which the balloon is fused directly to a steerable guidewire and the whole dilatation system is advanced across the lesion as a unit.[10]

Generally, the balloon catheter is chosen for an inflated diameter—2.0 to 4.0 mm—that approximates the diameter of the uninvolved coronary segment on either side of the lesion.[22] Under fluoroscopic monitoring, the balloon is slowly inflated with liquid contrast material, using a special syringe-gauge combination that can monitor inflation pressures from 0 to 20 atm or 0 to 300 psi, until the balloon has expanded fully. Inflation may be maintained for one minute and repeated for 3 to 10 times until the desired luminal improvement is obtained. Improvement may be assessed by reducing the pressure gradient as measured between the guiding catheter and the tip of the deflated balloon. Successful procedures are generally associated with a residual gradient less than 15 mm Hg, or by satisfactory angiographic appearance—typical residual stenosis less than 30% to 40%. If improvement is inadequate, inflations can be repeated, often using longer inflation duration or a slightly larger diameter balloon. Flow through the dilated segment should be brisk, and angina, electrocardiographic changes, or hemodynamic abnormalities present during balloon inflation should resolve by the end of the procedure.

In most institutions, the vascular access sheaths are left in place either for 4 hrs (until the heparin wears off) or for 18 to 24 hrs with ongoing heparin infusion. Intravenous nitroglycerin may be administered overnight, and the aspirin/dipyridamole regimen continued. Patients can generally be discharged 24 hrs after sheath removal with a maximal exercise test scheduled within the next two weeks to evaluate the physiologic improvement produced by the PTCA.[23]

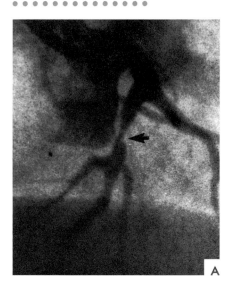 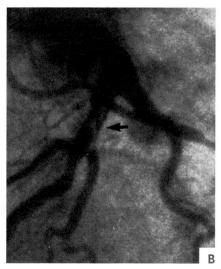 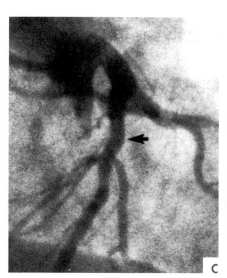

FIGURE 5.8 • Left anterior descending coronary angiograms show baseline stenosis (A), linear filling defects (arrow) corresponding to the presence of intimal flaps within the dilated segment immediately after PTCA (B), and resolution of filling defects with continued luminal patency at 6 weeks (C).

INDICATIONS

In the broadest sense, the indications for coronary angioplasty are a lesion or combination of lesions causing a clinical situation that makes revascularization desirable, and for which PTCA has an anticipated success and safety factor that compare favorably with the alternative medical and surgical treatment (Table 5.1).

The decision to perform an angioplasty must take into account not only the characteristics of the various coronary lesions (Table 5.2), but also the capabilities of the equipment and operator, the patient's overall condition—age, ventricular function, other medical problems, prior surgery, etc.—and the available data regarding the results of PTCA and alternative management options in that setting. In some situations, this may be very straightforward, while in others an optimal decision may require detailed discussion and film review by senior angioplasty operators and cardiac surgeons.[24]

In PTCA Registry I (1979–1981), limited equipment and operator capabilities led to the recommendation that PTCA be restricted to candidates for bypass surgery who had objective evidence of myocardial ischemia, and proximal, discrete, subtotal, noncalcified lesions of a single vessel. Such patients were estimated to comprise no more than 5% to 10% of the candidates for bypass surgery.[8] With progressive improvements in

---

TABLE 5.1 • CLINICAL INDICATIONS FOR PERCUTANEOUS TRANSLUMINAL CORONARY ANGIOPLASTY (PTCA)

Significant stenosis of one or more major epicardial arteries, which subtend at least a moderate-sized area of viable myocardium, in a patient who has:

• Recurrent ischemic episodes after myocardial infarction or major ventricular arrhythmia

• Angina which has not responded adequately to medical therapy

• Clear evidence of myocardial ischemia on resting, ambulatory, or exercise electrocardiography

• Objective evidence of myocardial ischemia which increases the overall risk of required noncardiac surgery.

Potential absolute or relative contraindications to PTCA

• High-risk anatomy, including significant left main disease in which vessel closure would likely result in hemodynamic collapse

• Severe, diffuse, and or extensive coronary artery disease better treated surgically

• Target lesion morphology (Type C) with anticipated success less than 60%, unless PTCA is the only reasonable treatment option

• No coronary stenosis greater than 50% diameter reduction

• No objective or compelling clinical evidence of myocardial ischemia

• Absence of on-site surgical back-up, qualified PTCA operators, or adequate radiographic imaging equipment

---

TABLE 5.2 • ANTICIPATED SUCCESS IN VARIOUS LESION MORPHOLOGIES

Type A Lesion—High: greater than 85% success with low risk	Type B Lesion—Moderate: 60% to 85% success with moderate risk	Type C Lesion—Low: less than 60% success and/or high risk
• Discrete (less than 10 mm long)	• Tubular (10 to 20 mm long)	• Diffuse (greater than 20 mm long)
• Concentric	• Eccentric	• Excessive tortuosity or angulation
• Readily accessible	• Moderate tortuosity	• Degenerated vein graft
• Nonangulated segment	• Moderate 45° to 90° angle	• Total occlusion greater than 3 months
• Smooth contour	• Irregular contour	
• Little or no calcification	• Moderate calcification	• Bifurcation with nonprotectable side branch
• Less than total occlusion	• Total occlusion less then 3 months	
• Not ostial	• Ostial location	
• No major branch involvement	• Treatable bifurcation lesion	
• Absence of thrombus	• Some thrombus present	

(Adapted from Ryan TJ, Klocke FJ, Reynolds WA, et al: *Circulation* 1990;81:2041 and the American Heart Association.)

---

equipment and technique, none of these criteria (except the absence of myocardial ischemia) necessarily contraindicates PTCA (refer to Table 5.2), although they still may influence the expected success and safety of the procedure.[11,24]

With the advent of steerable low profile catheter systems, angioplasty now accounts for half of all coronary revascularization (refer to Figure 5.6). Even very distal lesions are now accessible to PTCA (Figure 5.9), including stenoses that have developed in a native artery distal to the insertion of a surgical graft, or isolated stenoses in circumflex marginal or posterior descending branches of a patient with ongoing angina. Similarly, totally occluded vessels may usually be dilated successfully if the distal myocardium is viable but still ischemic due to inadequate collateral flow, particularly if the occlusion is less than several months old. Angioplasty of a chronic total occlusion (Figures 5.10, 5.11), however, carries a significantly lower success rate than that of conventional stenotic lesions— 60% to 70% versus 90%.[25] (Figures 5.12, 5.13).

• • • • • • • • • • • • • •

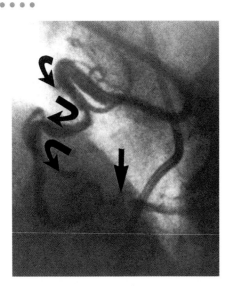

FIGURE 5.9 • Current PTCA equipment can now be used to attack even very distal lesions in markedly tortuous vessels.

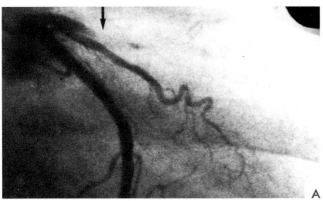

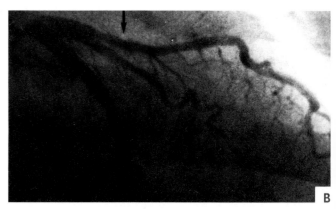

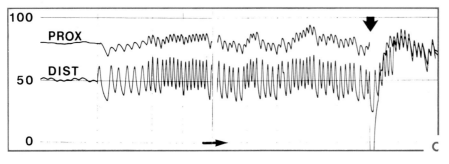

FIGURE 5.10 • Use of angioplasty to dilate a chronic total occlusion in the left anterior descending, shown before (A) and after PTCA (B). The pressure tracings show that prior to PTCA, collateral flow is able to provide a distal occluded pressure of roughly 50 mm Hg to the left anterior distal (LAD) territory; enough to maintain myocardial viability but not enough to support the myocardial demands during exercise. Following PTCA, LAD pressure is restored to parity with the aortic pressure (C).

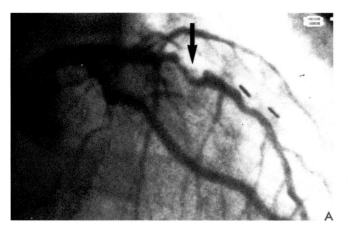

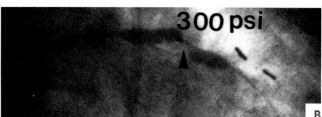

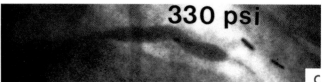

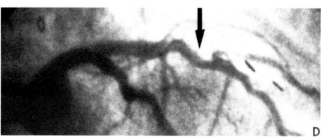

FIGURE 5.11 • The highly calcified lesion (arrow) in the left anterior distal (LAD) of this patient (A) resisted dilatation with a special high pressure balloon at 300 psi (B), but finally yielded at 330 psi or 22 atm (C) with an acceptable result (D). Such rigid lesions are relatively uncommon.

FIGURE 5.12 • Procedural success of coronary angioplasty by presentation and stenosis severity in 8,684 patients—19,615 lesions. (Reproduced with permission. Stone GW, Rutherford BD, McConahay, et al: *J Am Coll Cardiol* 1990;15:850.)

CORONARY ANGIOPLASTY SUCCESS

Presentation and stenosis severity	Procedural success rate (%)	n
Elective 75%-99%	96%	17,429
Acute myocardial infarction 75%-99%	95%	703
Acute myocardial infarction total occlusion	91%	512
Elective total occlusion	72%	971

Bifurcation lesions, those which involve a main vessel at the origin of a major branch, were initially avoided as PTCA targets because of the 14% to 20% risk that dilatation of the main vessel would lead to occlusion of the involved branch by the "snow-plow" effects (Figure 5.14). However, this risk can now be minimized by the use of either double-wire sequential dilatation or "kissing-balloon" simultaneous dilatation techniques[26] (Figure 5.15).

Discrete lesions less than 10 mm in length are the most favorable for dilatation, particularly if they are located in a relatively straight vessel segment and are concentric rather than eccentric, and free of heavy calcification. Longer lesions, 10 to 20 mm or greater than 20 mm, or those associated with lesions in the more proximal or distal portion of the same vessel may still be approached, although with less favorable short and longterm results. Patients with multivessel disease now constitute roughly half of all PTCA candidates, although they frequently undergo dilatation of just a single "culprit" lesion responsible for their current clinical syndrome.[27]

True multivessel dilatation has become increasingly common—accounting for an estimated one-quarter of current PTCA—with generally good results despite a higher complication rate than that seen in single-vessel procedures [28,29] (Tables 5.3, 5.4). Even lesions of the left main coronary artery can be dilated, particularly if either the left anterior descending or circumflex coronary arteries are protected by collaterals or a patent bypass graft. In general, however, unprotected left main lesions should not be approached by PTCA if the patient is an acceptable candidate for bypass surgery, since restenosis and cardiac events are common after such PTCA procedures.[30] At least two major trials are now in progress —the Emory Angioplasty Surgery Trial (EAST) and the Bypass Angioplasty Revascularization Investigation (BARI)—to compare the relative benefits of angioplasty and bypass surgery in patients with multivessel coronary disease approachable by either revascularization technique.

Patients with prior bypass graft surgery now account for 10% to 20% of PTCA procedures.[31] The target lesion may be in a native vessel—beyond a patent graft, in a vessel supplied by a totally occluded graft, or a new lesion that has developed after surgery—or in the bypass graft itself. Saphenous vein grafts may develop focal intimal hyperplasia—midgraft, distal or proximal anastomosis—within the first year after surgery, or more diffuse atherosclerotic narrowing thereafter.[32] Earlier lesions are easily treated by PTCA, but late lesions of greater than 1 year must be approached cautiously given the potential for distal embolization of friable plaque material. In either case, PTCA of vein graft lesions seems to carry a higher risk of subsequent restenosis than routine native vessel dilatation. Internal

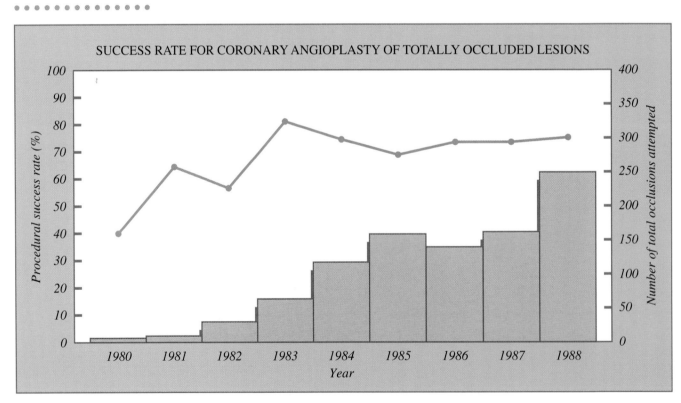

FIGURE 5.13 • Annual procedural success rate for coronary angioplasty of totally occluded lesions. (Reproduced with permission. Stone GW, Rutherford BD, McConahay, et al: *J Am Coll Cardiol* 1990;15:851.)

mammary arterial grafts are less prone to develop disease,[33] but it is not uncommon to see patients with earlier recurrent angina due to intimal proliferation within the distal anastomosis—a lesion that is readily treatable by PTCA.[34]

Whenever coronary angioplasty is performed in a patient with prior bypass surgery, it is necessary to keep in mind that emergency surgery to treat a PTCA complication may carry a higher risk due to the longer time required to open the chest, the potential for damaging other patent grafts, and the tendency for poorer left ventricular function in such patients.

The most common initial indication for PTCA was progressive stable angina, although a selection bias towards patients with angina of relatively short duration, less than 6 months, resulted in the inclusion of many patients with unstable syndrome as well.[8] Patients with unstable syndomes—new onset, progressive, or rest angina—now account for the majority of PT-

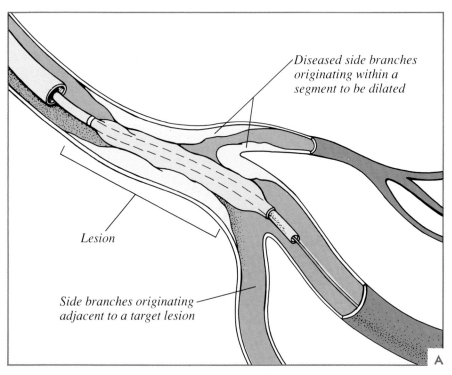

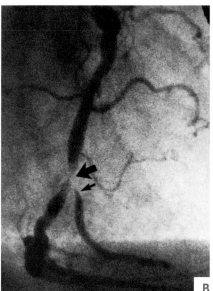

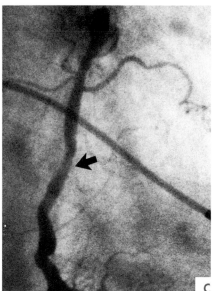

FIGURE 5.14 • Side branches that are diseased and originate within a segment to be dilated. These (arrow 1) have a 15% to 20% chance of being occluded by the "snow-plow" effect. Side-branches that originate adjacent to but not within a target lesion (arrow 2) have less than a 1% risk of occlusion (A). Right coronary angiogram shows severe mid-vessel stenosis (bold arrow) that involves a high-risk acute marginal branch (small arrow) (B). Following angioplasty of the right coronary artery lesion, the acute marginal branch is occluded (C).

Diseased side branches originating within a segment to be dilated

Lesion

Side branches originating adjacent to a target lesion

CA procedures. Results are generally excellent in this patient population, although unstable patients tend to have a slightly higher incidence of acute PTCA complications.[35] In patients whose unstable angina cannot be controlled medically, PTCA is indicated if the coronary anatomy is suitable. In patients who respond well to medical therapy, it is not clear if either PTCA or bypass surgery offer any additional benefits over continued drug therapy; this is one topic being investigated in the ongoing Thrombolysis In Myocardial Infarction-3 (TIMI-3) trial.

The optimal use of thrombolytic therapy and of coronary angioplasty in the patient with acute myocardial infarction has been the topic of several recent clinical trials. In experienced hands, primary angioplasty can reopen the infarct vessel within 4 to 6 hrs of the onset of symptoms in the majority of patients presenting.[36] Even patients treated with potent intravenous thrombolytic agents (rt-PA) may benefit from subsequent "salvage" angioplasty to open vessels refractory to thrombolysis, or angioplasty to treat the underlying lesions responsible for sub-

sequent myocardial ischemia. Routine angioplasty in the first hours after rt-PA infusion, however, carries a higher risk of both ischemic and hemorrhagic complications than it does at 18 to 48 hrs[37] (Table 5.5) Neither routine angioplasty strategy appears to improve survival or ventricular function when compared to a conservative strategy in which catheterization and angioplasty are reserved for patients with recurrent spontaneous or exercise-induced myocardial ischemia.[38]

SUCCESS RATES

In the initial PTCA Registry, successful angioplasty was defined as at least 20% reduction in diameter stenosis.[8] For the procedure to be considered successful by current standards, the postPTCA stenosis should be less than 50%, and there should be no major complication—death, myocardial infarction, or bypass surgery—prior to hospital discharge. Unsuccessful angioplasty may result from failure to cross the target lesion with the guidewire or dilatation catheter, failure to dilate the le-

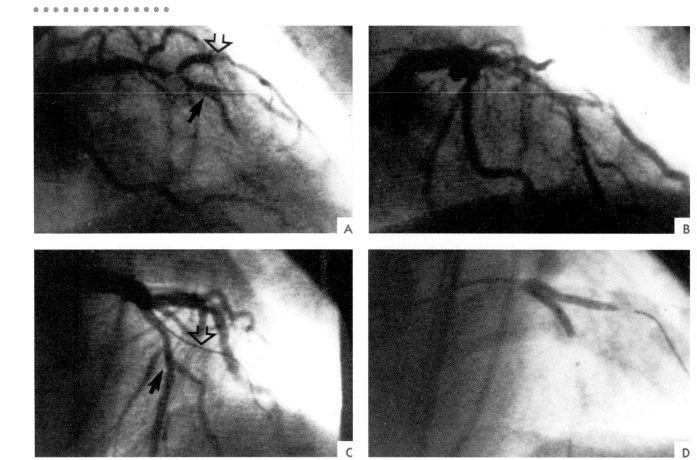

FIGURE 5.15 • When the jeopardized side branch is large, as in the case of this left anterior distal (LAD) (bold arrow) and diagonal (outline arrow), protection and/or dilatation of both vessels may be necessary. (A,B) The "double wire" technique involves placement of two angioplasty guidewires, one in the LAD and one in the diagonal branch, allowing angioplasty balloon to be alternately advanced down one or the other guidewire as needed. In this case, inflation of the balloon in the LAD has occluded the diagonal and vice versa. Accordingly, the "kissing balloon" technique (C) was used in which two balloon catheters were inflated simultaneously to produce a favorable result (D).

TABLE 5.3 COMPLICATIONS OF CORONARY ANGIOPLASTY BY NUMBER OF DISEASED VESSELS IN THE 1985–1986 COHORT —1,801 PATIENTS

| | Vessel disease[1] | | | | | | | | |
| | Single (n = 838) | | Double (n = 559) | | Triple (n = 367) | | Left main (n = 37) | | |
Complication	Number of patients	Per-cent	Number of patients	Per-cent	Number of patients	Per-cent	Number of patients	Per-cent	p value
Death	2	0.2	5	0.9	8	2.2	3	8.1	<0.001
Nonfatal myocardial infarction	29	3.5	29	5.2	19	5.2	1	2.7	Not significant
Emergency coronary artery bypass graft	24	2.9	22	3.9	16	4.4	1	2.7	Not significant
Death, myocardial infarction or emergency coronary artery bypass graft	46	5.5	45	8.1	34	9.3	4	10.8	<0.05
Spasm	15	1.8	4	0.7	4	1.1	0	0	Not significant
Occlusion	33	3.9	25	4.5	29	7.9	1	2.7	<0.01
Branch occlusion	13	1.6	15	2.7	9	2.5	1	2.7	Not significant
Dissection	33	3.9	35	6.3	16	4.4	2	5.4	Not significant
Ventricular fibrillation	9	1.1	4	0.7	6	1.6	2	5.4	Not significant
Prolonged angina	29	3.5	29	5.2	24	6.5	2	5.4	<0.05
Abrupt closure	18	2.1	9	1.6	11	3.0	1	2.7	Not significant

[1]Two tests for linear trend were used to compare the groups with single, double, and triple vessel disease because of the small number of patients with left main coronary artery disease.

(Reproduced with permission. Holmes DR Jr, Holubkov R, Vlietstra RE, et al: *J Am Coll Cardiol* 1988;12:1151.)

TABLE 5.4 • UNTOWARD EVENTS AND ELECTIVE BYPASS GRAFTING IN OLD- AND NEW-REGISTRY PATIENTS ACCORDING TO THE NUMBER OF DISEASE VESSELS

| | Single-vessel | | Double-vessel | | Triple-vessel | | Total | |
| | Percent | | | | | | | |
	Old (n = 863)	New (n = 839)	Old (n = 203)	New (n = 568)	Old (n = 89)	New (n = 395)	Old (n = 1,155)	New (n = 1,802)
Death	1.3[1]	0.2[1]	0.5	0.9	2.2	2.8	1.2	1.0
Nonfatal infarction	5.0	3.5	3.9	5.1	6.7	5.1	4.9	4.3
Coronary artery bypass graft	6.1[2]	2.9[2]	5.4	3.7	3.4	4.3	5.8	3.4
Emergency	19.5[3]	1.7[3]	27.6[3]	2.3[3]	16.9[3]	3.3[3]	20.7	2.2
Elective								

[1]p<0.05. [2]p<0.01. [3]p<0.001.   (Reproduced with permission. Detre K, Holubkov R, Kelsey S, et al: *N Engl J Med* 1988;318:269.)

sion due to rigidity or elasticity, or from the abrupt closure of an initially dilated segment.

Compared with the 65% success rate of 15 centers in PTCA Registry I (1979–1981), these same centers had an 85% success rate in Registry II (1985–1986).[29] This improved success was due to reductions in failure to cross and failure to dilate lesions, attributable largely to the introduction of lower profile, steerable equipment. Moreover, the success rate increased despite inclusion in Registry II of patients with more difficult anatomic situations.

COMPLICATIONS

As a percutaneous catheterization technique, PTCA has all of the risks associated with diagnostic coronary angiography

---

TABLE 5.5 • RESULTS FROM THE THROMBOLYSIS IN MYOCARDIAL INFARCTION (TIMI-IIA) TRIAL

	2 hr PTCA (n=195)	18-48 hr PTCA (n=194)	No PTCA (n=197)
Revascularization	158 (81%)	121 (62%)	55 (28%)
• PTCA	141 (72%)	107 (55%)	35 (17%)
• CABG after PTCA	15 (8%)	5 (3%)	5 (3%)
• CABG without PTCA	17 (10%)	14 (7%)	20 (10%)
Death[1]	15 (8%)	11 (6%)	17 (9%)
Re-infarction[1]	13 (7%)	8 (4%)	12 (6%)
LVEF (rest/exercise)[1]	49/52	48/53	50/52
Arterial patency[2]	119/152 (78%)	121/151 (80%)	142/168 (85%)
Transfusion (> 1 U with CABG)	27 (14%)	6 (3%)	4 (2%)

PTCA = Percutaneous transluminal coronary angioplasty

CABG = Coronary artery bypass graft

[1] Findings at 6-week follow-up

[2] Findings at discharge catheterization

(Reproduced with permission. Rogers WJ, Baim DS, Gore JM, et al: *Circulation* 1990;81:1457.)

TABLE 5.6 • COMPLICATIONS OF DIAGNOSTIC AND THERAPEUTIC CATHETERIZATION

	Total (n=2883)	Diagnostic (n=1609)	Percutaneous transluminal coronary angioplasty (PTCA) (n=993)	Percutaneous balloon valvuloplasty (n=199)
Allergic	0	0	0	0
Arrhythmic	16 (0.6%)	5 (0.3%)	6 (0.6%)	5 (2.5%)
Vasovagal	2 (0.06%)	1 (0.06%)	0	1 (0.5%)
Ischemic	12 (0.4%)	0	12 (1.2%)	0
Perforation	5 (0.2%)	0	0	5 (2.5%)
Embolic	4 (0.1%)	2 (0.1%)	1 (0.1%)	1 (0.5%)
Vascular	56 (1.9%)	26 (1.6%)	15 (1.5%)	15 (7.5%)
Death	8 (0.28%)	2 (0.12%)	3 (0.3%)	3 (1.5%)

(Reproduced with permission. Wyman RM, Safian RD, Portway V, et al: *J Am Coll Cardiol* 1988;12:1400.)

(Table 5.6).[39] In addition, some unique risks are associated with the plaque disruption that is part of the "controlled injury" underlying any balloon dilatation. Some intimal tearing is evident angiographically in most patients[14] (refer to Figure 5.8), and dissection alone may cause transient, frequently pleuritic chest discomfort in the absence of ischemia. In 5% of patients, frank abrupt closure of the dilated segment occurs due to a combination of dissection, coronary spasm, and thrombus formation[40] (Figure 5.16). Certain aspects of lesion morphology have been associated with a two-fold increased risk of abrupt closure events, and presence of a postPTCA dissection is associated with a five-fold increased risk of abrupt closure[41,42] (Tables 5.7, 5.8). About 80% of such reclosure events occur within 15 mins of the final balloon inflation, while the patient

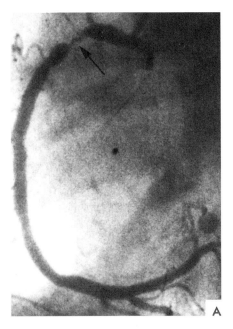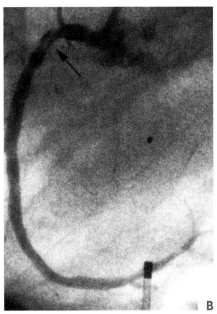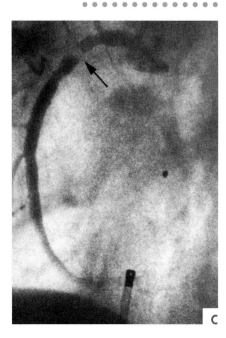

FIGURE 5.16 • Right coronary stenosis before (A) and immediately after (B) PTCA shows linear instal filling defect consistent with dissection. Within 15 minutes, the dissection became more severe (C), retarding antegrade flow in the dilated vessel and producing marked angina and ST-segment elevation in the inferior leads. In 1980, the only available option was referral of the patient to emergency bypass surgery, which was performed without evolution of a Q-wave myocardial infarction.

TABLE 5.7 • PREDICTOR OF ABRUPT CLOSURE

Preprocedure		
Clinical	**Angiographic**	**Procedural**
Female (1.66, 0.02)[1]	Branch point (1.87, 0.002)[21]	Tear or dissection (5.19, 0.001)[2]
Hypertension (1.48, 0.06)	Bend > 45 (2.03, 0.003)[2]	
Unstable (1.38, NS)	Length > 2 LD (1.80, 0.01)[1]	Gradient > 20 mm Hg (4.20, 0.001)
Hyperlipidemia (1.41, NS)	Eccentric (1.68, 0.05)	
Diabetes (1.41, NS)	Thrombus (1.68, 0.09)[1]	Stenosis > 35% (1.89, 0.01)[2]
	Other lesion 50% (2.05, 0.03)[1]	
	Multivessel disease (1.57, 0.07)	Prolonged heparin (2.70, 0.001)[2]

NS = Not significant

[1] Multivariate significance among preprocedural variables only

[2] Multivariate significance

(Reproduced with permission. Ellis SG, Roubin GS, King SB, et al: *Circulation* 1988;77:372.)

is still in the catheterization laboratory, with the remainder occurring within the next 24 hrs. Unless adequate collaterals are present, abrupt closure is marked by chest pain and ischemic EKG changes, which should prompt immediate angiographic restudy.

If restudy demonstrates vessel occlusion, it is usually possible to recross the affected segment and reestablish at least transient antegrade flow by redilatation[40] (Figures 5.17, 5.18). With prolonged balloon inflations at the site of obstruction, using a "perfusion" balloon to maintain antegrade flow during inflation, stable patency can be restored in more than half of abrupt closure lesions. Roughly 20% of patients will stabilize despite abrupt closure, as a result of collateral flow, prior infarction, or small size of the involved territory. These patients can be managed medically. The remaining patients, who account for roughly 2% of angioplasty attempts, have refractory vessel closure and active myocardial ischemia necessitating emergency bypass surgery. With a surgical team on standby, it should be possible to initiate cardiopulmonary bypass within one to two hours of vessel closure, but approximately half of

TABLE 5.8 • ANGIOGRAPHIC CHARACTERISTICS AND PREDICTORS OF ACUTE CLOSURE

	Percent closure group	Percent nonclosure group	Odds ratio	Univariate p value
Severity of disease				
Multivessel disease	23.6	16.4	1.57	.07
Percent stenosis ≥ 90%	9.3	9.0	1.08	Not Significant
Vessel dilated				
Other LAD	10.0	5.1	2.05	Not Significant
Ostial LAD	16.1	10.8	1.84	Not Significant
Proximal LCX	10.0	6.7	1.53	Not Significant
Proximal RCA	12.1	8.7	1.45	Not Significant
Proximal LAD	42.1	45.3	0.88	Not Significant
Other LCX	8.6	10.9	0.76	Not Significant
Other RCA	17.1	23.1	0.67	Not Significant
Morphology				
Branch point	51.8	36.4	1.87	.002
Bend point ≥ 45°	43.6	27.5	2.03	.003
Length ≥ 2 luminal diameters[1]	42.8	26.0	1.80	.01
Other stenosis ≥ 50%	22.8	12.6	2.05	.03
Eccentric	68.1	56.0	1.68	.05
Thrombus	14.2	8.9	1.68	.09
Calcification	24.2	19.7	1.30	Not Significant
Ulceration	9.1	5.7	1.66	Not Significant
Roughened lumen	24.6	18.2	1.43	Not Significant
Abrumpt proximal face	25.9	19.6	1.43	Not Significant
Distal ectasia	12.9	12.1	1.08	Not Significant
Diffuse disease	18.0	18.1	0.99	Not Significant
Active kink point	28.6	30.4	0.91	Not Significant
Healed dissection	2.8	3.4	0.83	Not Significant
Collaterals	7.3	11.4	0.61	Not Significant

[1]By the ≥ 50% stenosis definition.

(Reproduced with permission. Ellis SG, Roubin GS, King SB, et al: *Circulation* 1988;77:377 and the American Heart Association.)

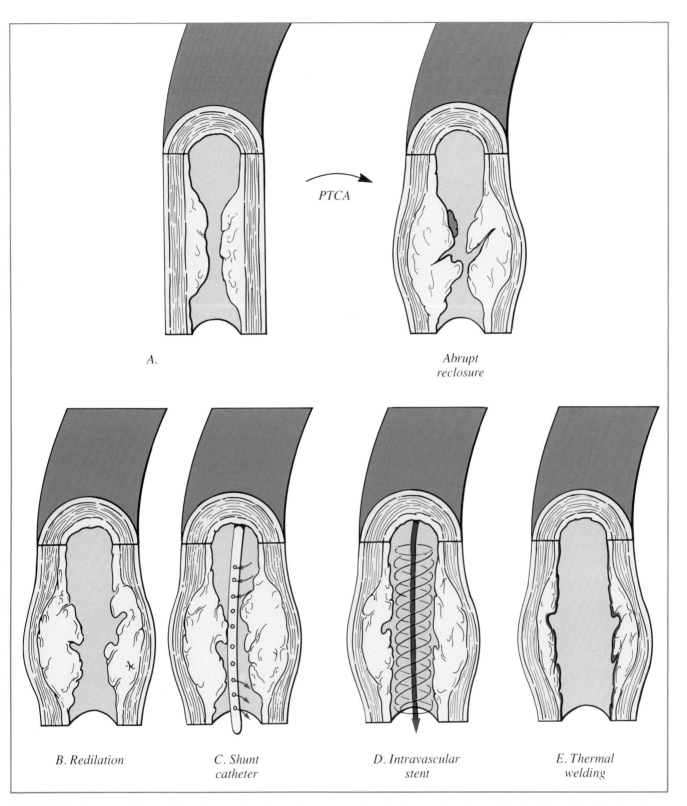

PTCA

A.

*Abrupt
reclosure*

B. Redilation

*C. Shunt
catheter*

*D. Intravascular
stent*

*E. Thermal
welding*

FIGURE 5.17 • The current view of abrupt closure implicates dissection with superimposed local thrombosis or spasm (A). The initial approach is now repeat dilatation (B), which re-establishes stable vessel patency in 40% to 50% of abrupt closures, thereby obviating emergency surgery. If patency cannot be restored and surgery is required, placement of a shunt or "bail-out" catheter (C) allows preservation of antegrade flow beyond the local dissection, thereby alleviating myocardial ischemia and reducing the probability of perioperative infarction. Two newer approaches include reversal of the abrupt closure by placement of an intravascular stent (D), or thermal welding with the laser balloon (E).

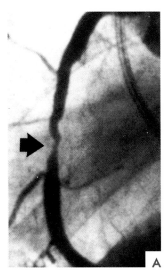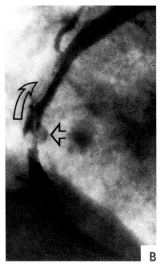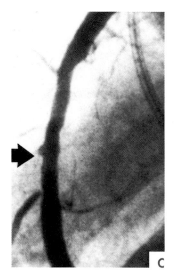

FIGURE 5.18 • Right coronary artery before attempted dilatation (A). Following initial attempts (B), there is marked dissection (open arrows) with restriction of distal flow. Repeat dilatation using prolonged 15 minute inflation of a 3.5 mm, rather than the initial 3.0 mm, balloon restored stable patency and averted the need for bypass surgery (C).

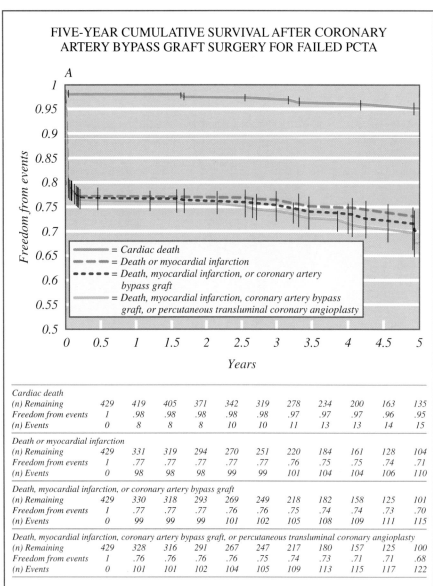

FIGURE 5.19 • Five-year cumulative survival in 430 patients who had failed elective percutaneous transluminal coronary angioplasty (PTCA) and underwent coronary artery bypass graft (CABG) surgery (A). Endpoints include cardiac survival (cardiac death); cardiac death and myocardial infarction—free survival (Death or MI); cardiac death–, myocardial infarction–, and CABG-free survival (Death, MI or CABG); and cardiac death–, myocardial infarction–, CABG–, and repeat PTCA-free survival (Death, MI, CABG or PTCA). (Reproduced with permission. Talley JD, Weintraub WS, Roubin GS, et al: *Circulation* 1990;82:1208.)

FIVE-YEAR CUMULATIVE SURVIVAL AFTER CORONARY ARTERY BYPASS GRAFT SURGERY FOR FAILED PCTA

Cardiac death											
(n) Remaining	429	419	405	371	342	319	278	234	200	163	135
Freedom from events	1	.98	.98	.98	.98	.98	.97	.97	.97	.96	.95
(n) Events	0	8	8	8	10	10	11	13	13	14	15

Death or myocardial infarction											
(n) Remaining	429	331	319	294	270	251	220	184	161	128	104
Freedom from events	1	.77	.77	.77	.77	.77	.76	.75	.75	.74	.71
(n) Events	0	98	98	98	99	99	101	104	104	106	110

Death, myocardial infarction, or coronary artery bypass graft											
(n) Remaining	429	330	318	293	269	249	218	182	158	125	101
Freedom from events	1	.77	.77	.77	.76	.76	.75	.74	.74	.73	.70
(n) Events	0	99	99	99	101	102	105	108	109	111	115

Death, myocardial infarction, coronary artery bypass graft, or percutaneous transluminal coronary angioplasty											
(n) Remaining	429	328	316	291	267	247	217	180	157	125	100
Freedom from events	1	.76	.76	.76	.76	.75	.74	.73	.71	.71	.68
(n) Events	0	101	101	102	104	105	109	113	115	117	122

such patients will sustain a transmural myocardial infarction and roughly 6% will die during hospitalization[43,44] (Figure 5.19).

Efforts to improve the safety of PTCA have centered on the prevention, reversal, or management of abrupt closure. When repeat dilatation fails to restore stable patency, a "bail-out" or perfusion balloon catheter can be placed to maintain perfusion of the distal vessel (Figure 5.20). This approach relieves ongoing ischemia, and is associated with a reduction in the incidence of infarction.[45] Active antegrade perfusion with arterial blood or oxygen transport medium—Fluosol—may have similar benefits, as may arterialized coronary sinus retroperfusion. The systemic circulation can be supported if necessary using intra-aortic counterpulsation or percutaneous cardiopulmonary support (CPS).[46,47] New technologies, such as the intracoronary stent and the laser balloon, promise to allow more reliable reversal of the abrupt closure phenomenon once they become generally available.

The 1985–1986 Registry reported only a slightly lower overall incidence of major complications—death (1.0%), nonfatal myocardial infarction (4.3%), or emergency bypass surgery (3.5%)—than the 1977–1981 Registry.[28] The most striking improvement in safety was for patients with single-vessel disease who had a mortality rate of 0.2%, compared to 0.9% for patients with double-vessel disease, and 2.2% for those with triple-vessel disease. Other high-risk subgroups, such as the elderly and patients with poor left ventricular function or acute infarction, may have substantially higher mortality rates when subjected to PTCA.[48]

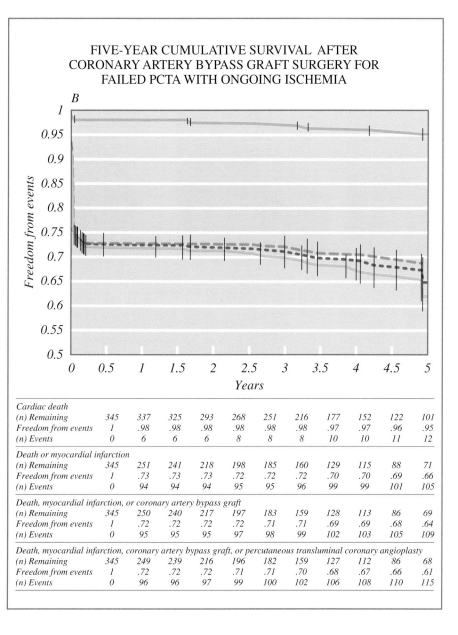

FIGURE 5.19 CONT'D • Five-year cumulative survival and event-free survival in 346 patients who had a failed elective percutaneous transluminal coronary angioplasty and coronary artery bypass graft surgery with ongoing myocardial ischemia. (B). End points include cardiac survival (Cardiac Death); cardiac death- and myocardial infarction-free survival (Death, MI or CABG); and cardiac death–, myocardial infarction–, CABG–, and repeat PTCA-free survival (Death, MI, CABG or PTCA). (Reproduced with permission. Talley JD, Weintraub WS, Roubin GS, et al: *Circulation* 1990;82:1208.)

FIVE-YEAR CUMULATIVE SURVIVAL AFTER CORONARY ARTERY BYPASS GRAFT SURGERY FOR FAILED PCTA WITH ONGOING ISCHEMIA

Cardiac death										
(n) Remaining	345	337	325	293	268	251	216	177	152	122	101
Freedom from events	1	.98	.98	.98	.98	.98	.98	.97	.97	.96	.95
(n) Events	0	6	6	6	8	8	8	10	10	11	12

Death or myocardial infarction										
(n) Remaining	345	251	241	218	198	185	160	129	115	88	71
Freedom from events	1	.73	.73	.73	.72	.72	.72	.70	.70	.69	.66
(n) Events	0	94	94	94	95	95	96	99	99	101	105

Death, myocardial infarction, or coronary artery bypass graft										
(n) Remaining	345	250	240	217	197	183	159	128	113	86	69
Freedom from events	1	.72	.72	.72	.72	.71	.71	.69	.69	.68	.64
(n) Events	0	95	95	95	97	98	99	102	103	105	109

Death, myocardial infarction, coronary artery bypass graft, or percutaneous transluminal coronary angioplasty										
(n) Remaining	345	249	239	216	196	182	159	127	112	86	68
Freedom from events	1	.72	.72	.72	.71	.71	.70	.68	.67	.66	.61
(n) Events	0	96	96	97	99	100	102	106	108	110	115

RESTENOSIS

When angioplasty is successful, angina is relieved and the exercise test is normalized. Within 6 months, roughly 20% to 25% of patients, however, will redevelop evidence of ischemia[49] (Figure 5.21). Repeat angiography in these patients usually shows recurrence or restenosis of a lesion at the site of prior dilatation. This problem seems to be even more common—greater than 40%—in certain clinical subgroups, such as male patients with unstable angina and severely stenotic lesions of the proximal left anterior descending coronary artery. If routine fol-

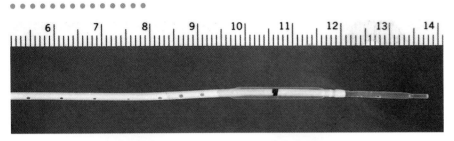

FIGURE 5.20 • Modified angioplasty balloon that allows antegrade perfusion during balloon inflation to reduce myocardial ischemia during the prolonged inflations commonly needed to reverse abrupt closure (Stack Perfusion Balloon, Advanced Cardiovascular Systems).

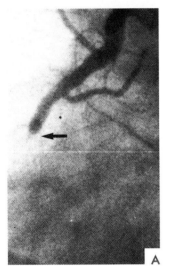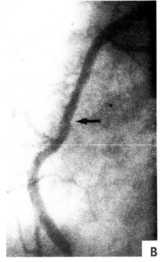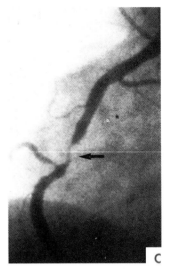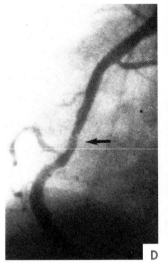

FIGURE 5.21 • Right coronary artery showing total occlusion before PTCA (A), and minimal residual stenosis after PTCA (B). Within 6 weeks, angina returned corresponding to restenosis of the dilated segment (C), treated by repeat dilatation (D).

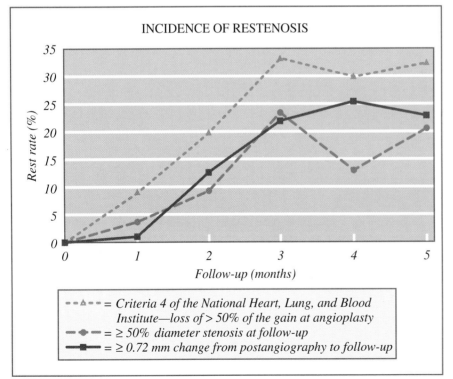

FIGURE 5.22 • Incidence of restenosis according to three criteria in the first 150 days after angioplasty derived from the patient group with 490 successfully dilated lesions. (Reproduced with permission. Beatt KJ, Surruys PW, Hugenholtz PG: *J Am Coll Cardiol* 1990;152:495.)

low-up angiography is performed between 4 and 6 months after successful PTCA, additional instances of angiographic restenosis may be evident in 10% to 15% of clinically asymptomatic patients. The exact incidence depends on the definition and measurement technique employed[50,51] (Figure 5.22, Table 5.9).

While part of the restenosis process undoubtedly represents the combined effect of elastic recoil, vasospasm,[52] dissection, and thrombus formation at the site of dilatation, both autopsy and atherectomy pathologic examination have established that local smooth muscle cell proliferation is

TABLE 5.9 • STUDIES ADDRESSING THE INCIDENCE OF CORONARY RESTENOSIS

Study	Patients		Interval (months) PTCA to follow-up	Restenosis criterion	Percent restenosis
	Total	Percent follow-up			
Meyer J, et al, 1983[1]	70	90	6	>85% area stenosis	20
Thorton MA, et al, 1984[2]	248	72	6-9	NHLBI 4	31
Holmes DR Jr, et al, 1984[3]	665	84	6.2	NHBLI 4	34
Kaltenback M, et al, 1985[4]	356	94	5.6	<20% diameter stenosis (mm) of pre-PTCA	12
Levin S, et al, 1985[5]	100	92	6	NHLBI 4	40
Corcos T, et al, 1985[6]	92	100	8.2	>70% diameter stenosis at follow-up	18.5
Leimgruber PP, et al, 1986[7]	1758	57	7		
				NHLBI 4	30
Bertrand ME, et al, 1986[8]	229	Not reported	7	NHLBI 4	32
Vandormael MG, et al, 1987[9]	129	62	7	≥ 20% reduction and ≥ 50% diameter stenosis	33

Studies addressing the timing and incidence of restenosis

Serruys PW, et al, 1988[10]	400	85	1	≥ 0.72 mm	0.9
			2	≥ 0.72 mm	12.45
			3	≥ 0.72 mm	22.6
			4	≥ 0.72 mm	25.5
Nobuyoshi M, et al, 1988[11]	185	81	24 hr	NHLBI 4	14.6
	229	100	1	NHLBI 4	12.7
	219	96	3	NHLBI 4	43.0
	149	65	6	NHLBI 4	49.4

NHLBI 4 = Criterion 4 of the National Heart, Lung, and Blood Institute—loss of ≥ 50% of gain

(Reproduced with permission. Beatt KJ, Surreys PW, Hugenholtz PG: *J Am Coll Cardiol* 1990;152:492.)

[1]Meyer J, Schmitz HJ, Kiesslich T, et al: Percutaneous transluminal coronary angioplasty in patients with stable and unstable angina pectoris: Analysis of early and late results. *Am Heart J* 1983;106:973.

[2]Thornton MA, Gruentzig AR, Hollman Y, et al: Coumadin and aspirin in the prevention of recurrence after transluminal coronary angioplasty: a randomized study. *Circulation* 1984;69:721.

[3]Holmes DK Jr, Vlietstra RE, Smith HC, et al: Restenosis after percutaneous transluminal coronary angioplasty: A report from the PTCA Registry of the National Heart, Lung, and Blood Institute. *Am J Cardiol* 1984;53:77C.

[4]Kaltenbach M, Kober G, Scherer D, et al: Recurrence rate after successful coronary angioplasty. *Eur Heart J* 1985;6:275.

[5]Levine S, Ewels CJ, Rosing DR, et al. Coronary angioplasty: clinical and angiographic follow-up. *Am J Cardiol* 1985;55:673.

[6]Corocos T, David PR, Val PG, et al: Failure of diltiazem to prevent restenosis after percutaneous transluminal coronary angioplasty. *Am Heart J* 1985;109:926.

[7]Leimgruber PP, Roubin GS, Hollman J, et al: Restenosis after successful coronary angioplasty in patients with single-vessel disease. *Circulation* 1986;73:710.

[8]Bertrand ME, LaBlanche JM, Thieuleux FA, et al: Comparative results of percutaneous transluminal coronary angioplasty in patients with dynamic versus fixed coronary stenosis. *J Am Coll Cardiol* 1986;8:504.

[9]Vandormael MG, Deligonul U, Kern MJ, et al: Multilesion coronary angioplasty: Clinical and angiographic follow-up. *J Am Coll Cardiol* 1987;10:246.

[10]Serruys PW, Luijten HE, Beatt KJ, et al: Incidence of restenosis after successful coronary angioplasty: A time-related phenomenon. *Circulation* 1988;77:361.

[11]Nobuyoshi M, Kimura T, Nosaka H, et al: Restenosis after successful percutaneous transluminal coronary angioplasty: Serial angiographic follow-up of 299 patients. *J Am Coll Cardiol* 1988;12:616.

the primary culprit in the genesis of the restenosis lesion[15] (Figure 5.23). Fortunately, restenotic lesions respond well to one or more repeat dilatations, although the chance of subsequent recurrence may rise to 50% or higher after a third dilatation of a particular lesion.[53,54]

There have been numerous attempts to develop strategies to decrease the incidence of restenosis after successful PTCA. While restenosis seems to be less common when the acute result shows little residual stenosis or gradient, efforts to alter the technical aspects of dilatation—balloon size or inflation duration—have failed to reduce restenosis.[22] Patients with poorly controlled vasopasm at the dilatation site have an up to 70% incidence of restenosis, but trials of prophylactic administration of calcium channel blockers in a general angioplasty population have been negative.

Based on the theory that early platelet adhesion to the dilated surface sets the stage for release of potent mitogens—PDGF—and subsequent smooth muscle cell proliferation, a variety of antiplatelet regimens have been evaluated.[22] Aspirin appears to reduce the incidence of thrombotic abrupt closure, but neither aspirin, coumadin, ticlopidine, nor ciprostene has demonstrated the ability to reduce subsequent restenosis.[16,18,21] Results with omega-3 fatty acid dietary supplements—fish oil—have been mixed.[55] A series of more potent antiplatelet and anti-thrombotic agents—IIb/IIIa antibodies, methylchloro-ketone, argatroban, hiruidin—are being considered for clinical testing based on promising animal studies.[19,20] Another line of treatment is based on decreasing smooth muscle cell proliferative responsiveness through the prolonged administration of corticosteroids, heparin or heparin-like substances, angiotensin converting enzyme inhibitors, or mevinolin, but an effective pharmacologic therapy has not yet been established.

NEW TECHNOLOGIES

Simple balloon dilatation has proven over the last 14 years to be a safe, effective, and versatile therapeutic modality. Encouraged by the broad acceptance of this technique, and in an effort to address some of its residual limitations, a number of physician-inventors have proposed alternative interventions for use in the coronary circulation[3,4] (Figure 5.24). Many of these innovations entered clinical testing only in 1988–1989, and most remain investigational. It is expected, however, that many of these new technologies will enter the clinical arena in the early 1990s.

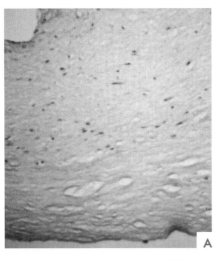
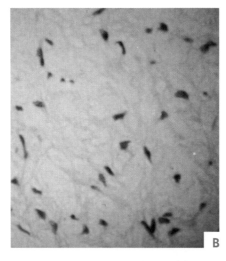
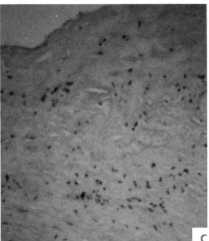
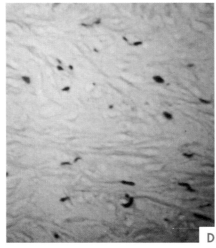

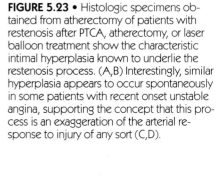

FIGURE 5.23 • Histologic specimens obtained from atherectomy of patients with restenosis after PTCA, atherectomy, or laser balloon treatment show the characteristic intimal hyperplasia known to underlie the restenosis process. (A,B) Interestingly, similar hyperplasia appears to occur spontaneously in some patients with recent onset unstable angina, supporting the concept that this process is an exaggeration of the arterial response to injury of any sort (C,D).

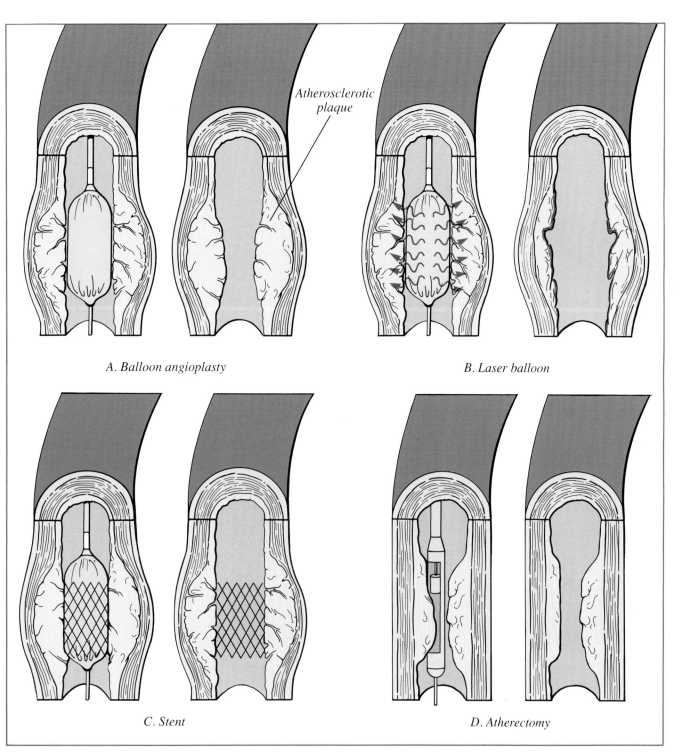

FIGURE 5.24 • Compared to conventional balloon angioplasty (A), both the laser balloon and stent (B,C) seek to provide a larger and smoother lumen by minimizing elastic recoil and sealing postdilata-tion cracking. In contrast, atherectomy seeks to provide luminal en-largement by smooth excision of obstructing plaque. Ablative lasers seek this same result via a different mechanism of plaque removal (D).

Atherosclerotic plaque

A. Balloon angioplasty

B. Laser balloon

C. Stent

D. Atherectomy

STENTS

After proposing the concept of mechanical angioplasty, Dotter foresaw that intravascular supports or stents might be deployed within the treated segments to maintain luminal patency.[56] Initial experiments with simple wire coils, thermally responsive nickel-titanium alloy showed that stenting was possible, but also identified three major problems of coronary endovascular prostheses:

- Successful deployment without migration.
- Prevention of luminal thrombosis.
- Formation of a thin but functional neo-intima over the stent material.

Little progress was made against these limitations until the late 1980s, when several new designs entered clinical testing[57] (Figures 5.25–5.27).

● ● ● ● ● ● ● ● ● ● ● ● ● ● ● ●

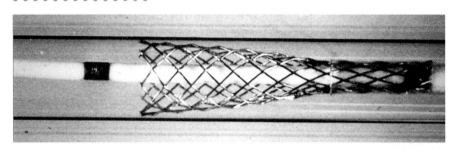

FIGURE 5.25 • Alternative stent designs now being tested in the coronary arteries. The self-expanding design (Medinvent) consists of a tubular mesh of 18 to 24 fine steel wires, which expands to its full size when freed of the restriction of a constraining membrane.

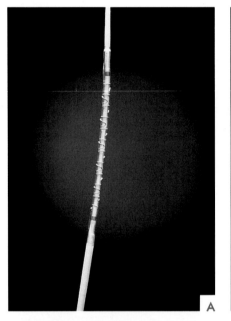

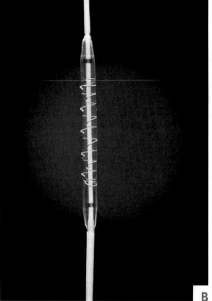

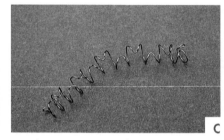

FIGURE 5.26 • Gianturco-Roubin Flex Stent preloaded on the expanded balloon delivery catheter (A). The inflated balloon delivery catheter showing the expansion of the Flex-Stent (B). The Flex-Stent alone (C). (Courtesy of Cook Cardiology, a division of Cook Inc, Bloomington, IN)

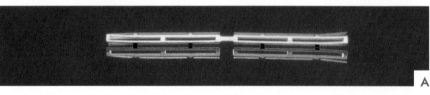

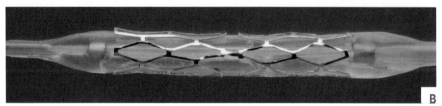

FIGURE 5.27 • A second balloon expandable design (Palmaz-Schatz, Johnson & Johnson Interventional Systems) consists of a slotted steel tube which is crimped onto an angioplasty balloon. Balloon inflation within the lesion enlarges and deploys the stent by turning each rectangular slot into a diamond-shaped aperture (A). To overcome delivery difficulties associated with the original rigid design, a more flexible "articulated" design is now used (B).

The self-expanding Medinvent design is a resilient mesh tube composed of 16 to 24 fine steel wires woven into a tubular braid of a predetermined diameter.[58] This braid is slipped onto a flexible delivery catheter, then compressed by a removable outer sheath. After being maneuvered into the target lesion, removal of the sheath allows the stent to expand spontaneously until it is constrained by the arterial wall.

The balloon-expandable design of Gianturco-Roubin is a serpiginous wire coil wound around a deflated delivery balloon.[59] Once advanced into position, balloon inflation expands the diameter of the coil to provide stent support. A second balloon-expandable design was put forward by Palmaz and later modified by Schatz[57] (refer to Figure 5.27). The latticed metal tube is crimped onto a deflated delivery balloon for advancement into the lesion. Inflation of the delivery balloon expands the diameter of the metallic tube as shown in Figure 5.27. Further enlargement is possible simply by inflation of a larger-diameter balloon within the stent. To maximize successful passage and minimize systemic stent embolization during withdrawal after an unsuccessful placement attempt, the delivery system for the Schatz-Palmaz stent was modified in early 1990 to include a 5F delivery sheath that covers the delivery balloon until it is correctly positioned.

All three designs are currently undergoing clinical investigation in the coronary circulation. This testing has shown that stenting improves acute luminal geometry, leaving a smooth lumen free of residual stenosis even in eccentric or irregular stenoses (Figure 5.28). Both the Sigwart and Gianturco-Roubin stents have demonstrated their ability to reverse abrupt closure due to extensive local dissection (Figure 5.29).

All designs are potentially thrombogenic,[60] mandating 1 to 3 months of coumadin anticoagulation therapy—prothrombin time 16 to 18 sec—in addition to antiplatelet therapy with aspirin and dipyridamole (Figure 5.30). This intensive pro-

• • • • • • • • • • • • • •

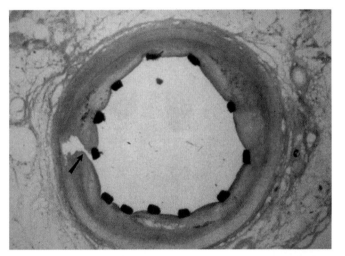

FIGURE 5.28 • Cross-section of a stented artery shows how the stent maintains the full diameter of the inflated balloon, and "tacks-up" dissections (arrow).

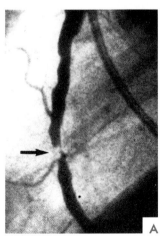
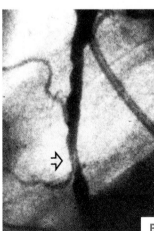
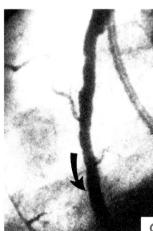

FIGURE 5.29 • Eccentric right coronary lesion shown before (A) and after (B) conventional PTCA has produced moderate localized dissection with residual stenosis. Following stent implantation (C) the dissection flap is no longer evident, and lumen diameter is increased to 3.5 mm.

gram of anticoagulation plus antiplatelet therapy has been associated with a greater incidence of local vascular complications following sheath removal, but apparently no unusual instances of bleeding at other sites[61,62] (Figure 5.31). With the Schatz-Palmaz design, this antithrombotic program has reduced the incidence of stent thrombosis to approximately 0.5%. By the end of the second month, the stent surface is colonized by fibroblasts and endothelial cells, which form a neo-intima 0.3–0.5 mm thick. In a typical 3 mm coronary artery, this neo-intimal hyperplasia results in mild 20% to 30% narrowing of the lumen within the stented segment (Figure 5.32), although 15% to 20% of patients will develop a more severe neo-intimal hyperplasia that can cause functional restenosis.[62] The stent, therefore, appears to be partially ef-

fective in reducing the 30% restenosis rate of conventional balloon dilatation—either by its ability to reduce the local proliferative response or due to the larger acute luminal result that allows better tolerance of the intimal proliferation that does occur. If additional refinements in stent design and surface coating can reduce thrombotic tendencies and local proliferative response, stenting is likely to play an important role in treating eccentric lesions, stabilizing abrupt closure, and treating restenosis.

ATHERECTOMY

While the goal of stenting is to enhance the mechanical dilatation produced by the balloon catheter, atherectomy seeks to enlarge the diseased lumen by physically removing the en-

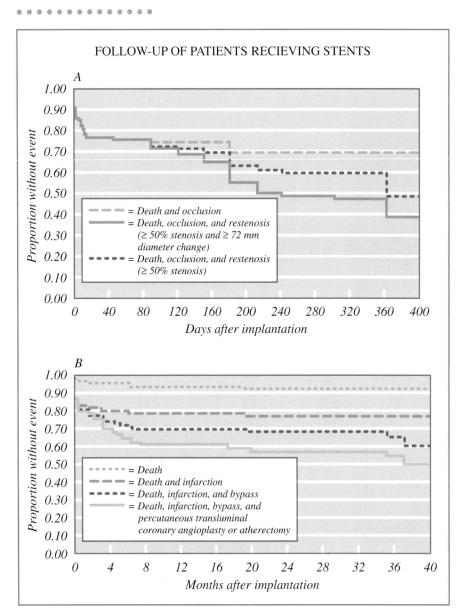

FIGURE 5.30 • Angiographic and clinical follow-up in 95 patients who received 105 Medinvent stents. Occlusion of the stent, cardiac death, and restenosis as determined by either or both of the criteria used —≥ 50% stenosis of the vessels and a change of ≥ 72 mm in the minimal luminal diameter—were considered angiographic end points (A). Death, myocardial infarction, bypass surgery, and PTCA or atherectomy were considered clinical end points (B). (Reproduced with permission. Surreys PW, Strauss BH, Beatt KJ, et al: *N Engl J Med* 1991;324:15.)

croaching plaque. Several designs have been proposed to meet this objective. The Directional AtheroCath makes use of a cylindrical steel housing with a 10 mm long oval window[63] that is pressed against the diseased vessel wall. Low-pressure inflation of a small balloon attached to the opposite side of the housing forces plaque to prolapse into the housing, where it is sliced off cleanly by advancement of a rotating cup-shaped cutter (Figure 5.33). The excised plaque is trapped safely in the device's nosecone, and can be removed for direct histologic examination.

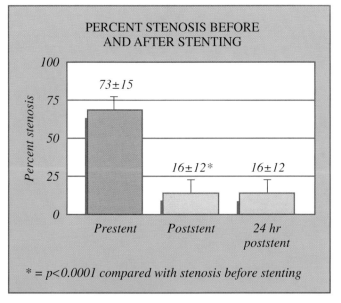

FIGURE 5.31 • Percent stenosis before, immediately after, and 24 hrs postsetting. (Reproduced with permission. Schatz RA, Baim DS, Leon M, et al: *Circulation* 1991;83:148.)

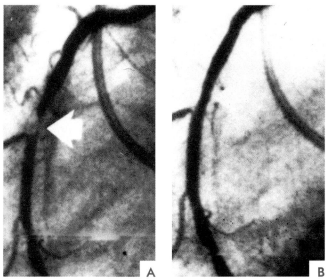
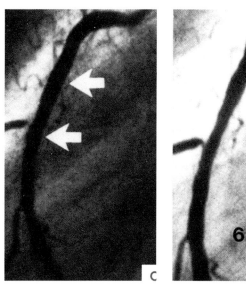

FIGURE 5.32 • An eccentric lesion in the mid-portion of the right coronary artery is shown before (A) and after (B) conventional balloon dilatation. Following placement of a single Palmaz-Schatz stent (C) further luminal enlargement is evident. Follow-up angiography at 6 months after stent implantation (D) shows mild 30% diameter reduction) due to 0.6 mm thick instal hyperplasia within the stent.

Trials of this concept in the peripheral circulation began in 1986, with extension to the coronary circulation in 1988, leading to Food and Drug Administration approval in mid-1990. Directional atherectomy is most effective in relatively short 10 mm lesions in proximal or midportions of noncalcified native vessels or vein grafts whose diameter is larger than 2.5 mm. In such cases, directional atherectomy provides a predictably large and angiographically smooth lumen, with overall safety comparable to that of conventional balloon dilatation,[64] and appears to be preferable to conventional balloon angioplasty in several anatomic settings (Figures 5.34–5.36).

Although vessel perforation is possible during aggressive cutting when the device is directed towards a nondiseased wall, the overall incidence of this complication was less then 0.7% in the first 1,000 coronary procedures. Since the amount of plaque removed is not sufficient to explain all of the improvement in angiographic lumen diameter, it seems likely that mechanical dilatation by the low pressure balloon also plays a contributory role.[65]

The end-cutting Transluminal Extraction Catheter (TEC) uses a rotating catheter whose tip is equipped with sharpened steel struts (Figure 5.37). Plaque cut free by these struts is as-

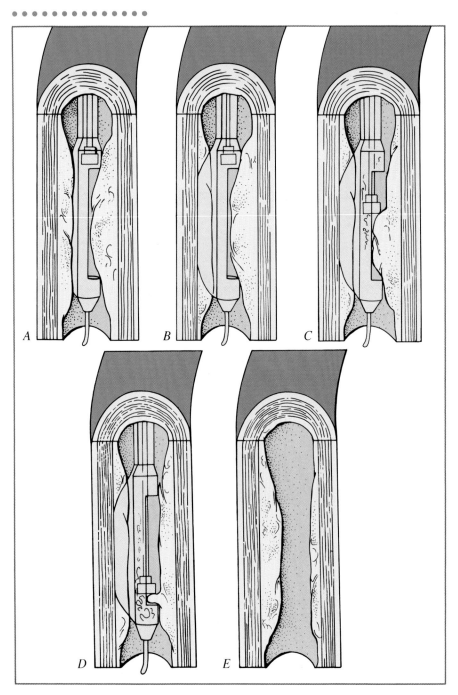

FIGURE 5.33 • Directional coronary atherectomy (Simpson AtheroCath, Devices for Vascular Intervention) (A) involves passage of the device across the lesion (B), and low-pressure inflation of the attached balloon (C) to press the housing window against the plaque. The cup-shaped cutter is spun at 2,000 rpm by a motor drive unit, as the cutter is advanced to cleanly excise any plaque protruding into the window (D). The excised plaque is trapped within the tip of the catheter during additional cuts in other orientations, with all plaque specimens then removed within the device (E).

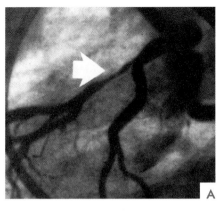 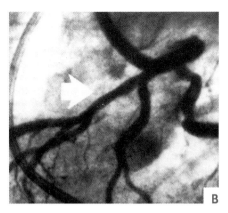

FIGURE 5.34 • Atherectomy procedure performed on an eccentric restenosis lesion in the left anterior distal (LAD). The lesion is shown before (A) and after (B) the procedure. Also shown are the atherectomy device and some of the retrieved specimens (C,D).

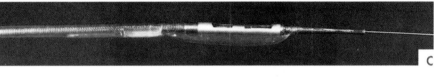

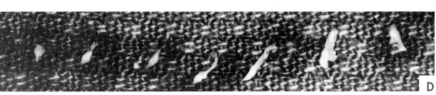

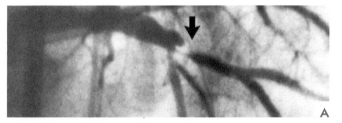 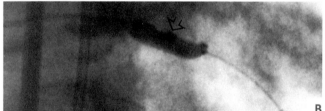

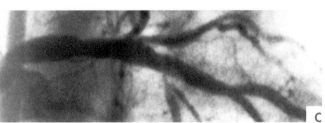

FIGURE 5.35 • Ideal lesions for coronary atherectomy rather than conventional angioplasty. This markedly eccentric left anterior descending (LAD) lesion (A) in a patient with unstable angina would be expected to dilate poorly with a conventional PTCA, but responded favorably to eight cuts with the AtheroCath (B,C).

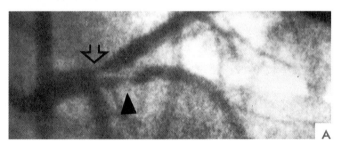 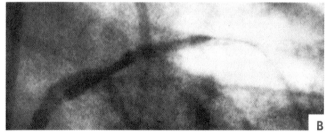

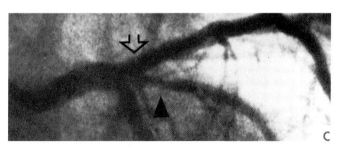

FIGURE 5.36 • Origin left anterior descending (LAD) lesions (A) tend to dilate poorly due to elasticity, but respond predictably to directional coronary atherectomy (B). A second lesion in the ramus branch was treated by conventional PTCA during the same procedure (C).

pirated back through the catheter lumen by application of suction during the cutting process. In contrast, the Rotablator (Figure 5.38) uses high-speed rotation of a metal burr studded with diamond chips that grinds plaque into small particles of approximately 25 microns. These will be able to pass through the distal microcirculation without causing vessel occlusion.[66] Both of these devices remain investigational, although several hundred coronary interventions have been performed with each.

LASERS

High power beams of coherent laser light have found numerous applications in industry and other medical fields—ophthal-mology, dermatology, surgery—making application to coronary interventions inevitable. One basic concept has been direct ablation or vaporization of plaque by laser energy, but a series of investigations using different wavelengths from ultraviolet to near infrared; modes—continuous wave versus pulsed energy; delivery systems—bare fibers, diffusing ball tips; and, more recently, multiple-fiber catheters have shown limited success.[67] Only the most recent multi-fiber catheters appear to have an acceptably low incidence of mechanical coronary perforation.[68,69] The use of short wavelengths, such as the 308 nm excimer, or longer wavelengths delivered in a pulsed mode seem to produce the greatest tissue ablation with the least surrounding thermal or acoustic (blast) injury[69] (Figures 5.39,

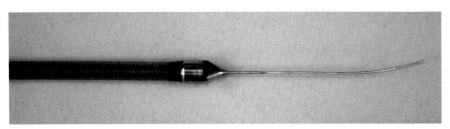

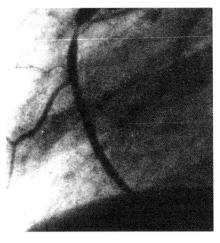 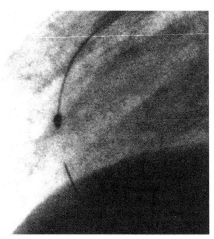 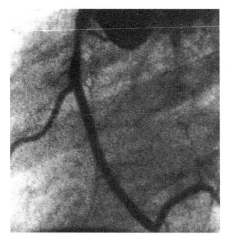

FIGURE 5.37 • Another atherectomy design is the Transluminal Extraction Catheter (IntraVascular Technologies), which consists of a pair of sharpened blades that form a cone at the tip of a rotating catheter. As the catheter is advanced through the diseased segment over a central guidewire, suction applied to the catheter lumen recovers a slurry of plaque fragments and blood.

FIGURE 5.38 • The Rotablator (Biophysics International) consists of a football-shaped metal tip whose leading surface is studded with abrasive diamond chips. The helical drive cable spins the device at up to 200,000 rpm as it advances across the target lesion over a central flexible guidewire. Since plaque is removed from the treated lesion, the Rotablator is technically an atherectomy device, although unlike other devices it allows the minute plaque fragments to pass into the distal myocardial microcirculation. Right coronary artery lesion shown (left to right) before, during, and after Rotablator therapy.

5.40). Such devices can treat even calcified or diffusely diseased vessels, but the small 1.6 mm diameter of the initial catheter systems made it difficult to treat more typical 2.5 to 3.5 mm coronary vessels without resort to post-laser balloon dilatation. Evaluation of late restenosis will therefore require follow-up angiography of patients who have undergone "stand-alone" treatment with the newer, larger diameter catheters. Attempts to use ablative lasers to cross chronic total occlusions have thus far been disappointing.[70]

Quite distinct from the ablative laser systems, some investigators have used laser light as a way of delivering high temperatures to diseased vessels. The Hot Tip consists of a metal cap placed over a bare laser fiber (Figure 5.41). The application of laser energy heats the metal tip to several hundred degrees, and appears to facilitate its passage through comparatively long, chronic total occlusions in the superficial femoral artery, but initial clinical trials in the coronary circulation have been much less successful (refer to Figure 5.41).

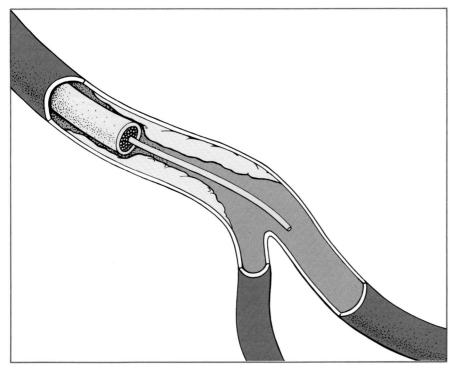

FIGURE 5.39 • The excimer ablative laser utilizes an over-the-wire design in which a ring of fibers carries excimer laser energy to the tip of the catheter.

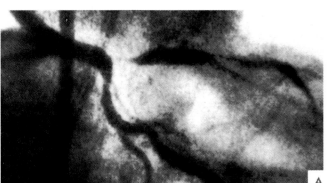

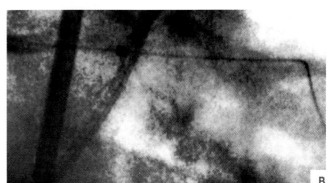

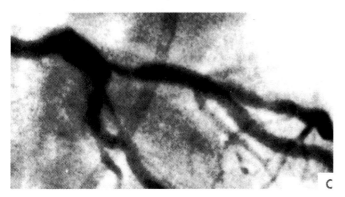

FIGURE 5.40 • A stenosis at the origin of the left anterior descending (LAD) before (A), during (B), and following (C) treatment with a 2.0 mm diameter catheter. The resulting lumen has a diameter equivalent to that of the excimer catheter, and would require subsequent balloon dilatation to reduce the residual stenosis below 50%. (Courtesy of Dr. Frank Litvack.)

Another laser-thermal device is the Spears Laser Angioplasty (LBA) catheter (Figure 5.42). This consists of an Nd:YAG-powered diffusing fiber positioned within an otherwise fairly conventional angioplasty balloon.[71] With the balloon inflated, laser energy radiates through the balloon and is absorbed by the surrounding vessel wall, which is heated to 80° to 90° C for 20 sec. It is then allowed to cool for 30 sec before balloon deflation, "casting" the treated vessel into the shape of the inflated balloon (Figure 5.43). It is proposed that this process decreases the tendency of the vessel to recoil after conventional balloon angioplasty, welds and smooths any surface irregularities, and favorably alters the local biologic reactivity of the vessel wall. Initial experience has demonstrated the ability of laser balloon angioplasty to reverse greater than 80% of otherwise refractory abrupt reclosure events following conventional balloon angioplasty, and to provide a consistent 2.4 mm diameter lumen following use of a 3.0 mm laser balloon angioplasty catheter (Figures 5.44, 5.45). Beneficial effects on the incidence of late restenosis have yet to be seen, and this device was withdrawn from active clinical investigation in late 1991.

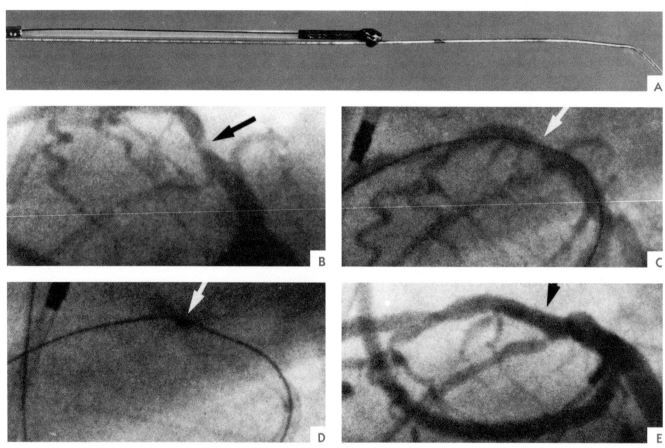

FIGURE 5.41 • The coronary Hot Tip consists of a sealed metal cap placed over the end of an optical fiber (A). Transmission of laser light heats the metal cap to several hundred degrees, possibly facilitating passage through severe stenoses. An eccentric lesion in the left anterior descending (arrow) is shown before (B), during hot tip treatment (C), after hot tip (D), and after subsequent balloon dilatation (E).

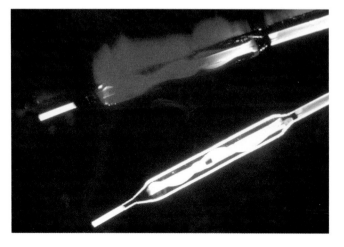

FIGURE 5.42 • The Spears LBA catheter (USCI) showing the diffusing fiber and the pattern of emitted light. While this system was initially called a "hot balloon," the balloon actually serves more as a transparent medium for transmission of Nd:YAG laser light to the vessel wall.

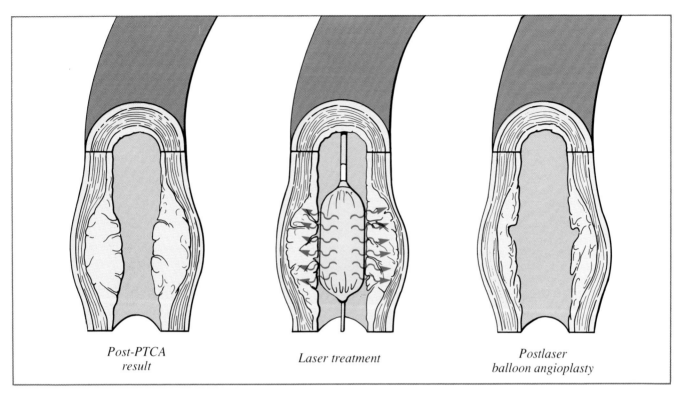

Post-PTCA
result

Laser treatment

Postlaser
balloon angioplasty

FIGURE 5.43 • The concept of Laser Balloon Angioplasty (LBA) involves treatment of the angioplasty site with simultaneous mechanical dilatation by low pressure balloon inflation and thermal heating via a laser diffusing fiber, in the hope that reduced vessel elasticity will provide a larger lumen with a smoother surface, free of the dissections seen after conventional PTCA.

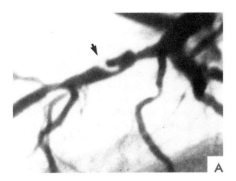
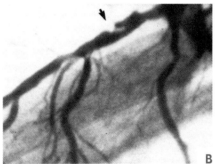
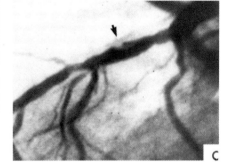

FIGURE 5.44 • A flap-like stenosis in the distal LAD artery (A) responds poorly to conventional angioplasty (B), but use of an identical size laser balloon angioplasty catheter molds the vessel into a more favorable configuration (C).

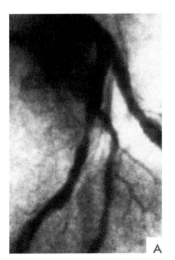
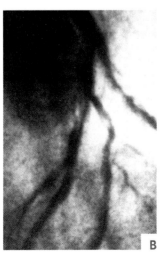
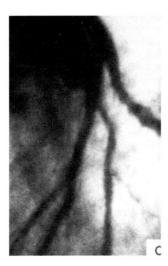

FIGURE 5.45 • This left anterior descending (LAD) lesion (A) manifested a severe dissection following conventional dilatation (B), which ultimately led to abrupt closure. Use of the laser balloon angioplasty led to stable vessel patency, avoiding emergency bypass surgery (C).

TREATMENT OF VALVULAR STENOSIS

PULMONARY VALVULOPLASTY

Pulmonary valvular stenosis, a relatively common congenital cardiac lesion, was traditionally corrected by surgical "valvuloplasty"—incision of fused commissures under direct vision. Beginning in 1982, pediatric cardiologists began using balloon dilatation catheters with inflated diameters 1 to 2 mm larger than the 20 to 25 mm annulus size to produce similar commisural splitting by way of a closed transluminal approach.[72]

This procedure has been quite successful, with a reduction of the pulmonic valve gradient to approximately one third of its baseline value. Given the high success rate and low incidence of complication, balloon valvuloplasty has essentially replaced open surgical repair for valvular pulmonic stenosis (Figures 5.46, 5.47). Application of balloon valvuloplasty for the treatment of congenital aortic stenosis has also been reported, with a 70% reduction in valve gradient and no significant increase in aortic regurgitation.[73]

MITRAL VALVULOPLASTY

In contrast to congenital pulmonic or aortic stenosis, it was believed that adult acquired rheumatic and/or calcific stenosis of the mitral or aortic valves might not be amendable to balloon valvuloplasty because of the:

- More rigid structure of such lesions.
- Potential for systemic embolization of valve debris.
- Potential for creating severe regurgitation.

However, in 1985, balloon valvuloplasty was first applied transseptally to young adult patients with acquired rheumatic mitral stenosis,[74] and the technique has become widely adapted as an alternative to surgical repair or replacement of stenotic mitral valves.[72]

Technique

After puncturing the intra-atrial septum with a needle and long sheath, a small balloon flotation catheter is advanced from the left atrium to the left ventricle. Although it was once common to then advance this catheter across the aortic valve into the descending aorta, a position near the apex of the left ventricle is easier to obtain and is adequate for most mitral valvuloplasty procedures (Figures 5.48–5.50). An exchange-length 260 cm

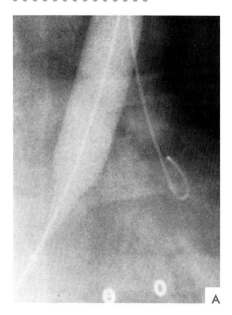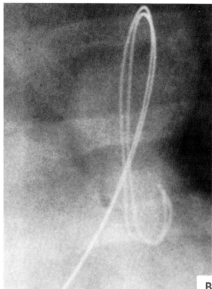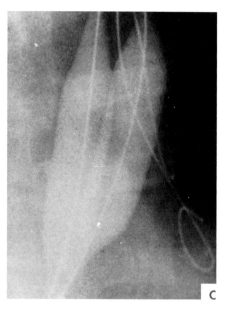

FIGURE 5.46 • Sequence of cineradiographs of pulmonary valvuloplasty. Anteroposterior projection of inflated balloon-dilatation catheter across the pulmonic value. The guidewire terminates in the left pulmonary artery. Radiopaque markers are used inside the annulus (A). A single balloon pulmonary valvuloplasty proved inadequate in the adult patient (B). A second guidewire was positioned in preparation for a double balloon valvuloplasty. The balloons are aligned and inflated simultaneously to perform a double balloon valvuloplasty. Each of the balloons is 5 cm in length (C). One is 20 mm while the other is 18 mm in diameter. (Reproduced with permission. Chatterjee K, Cheitlin MD, Karliner J, et al: *Cardiology. An Illustrated Text/Reference. Volume 2* New York, NY: Gower Medical Publishing; 1991:9.58.)

guidewire is then positioned through this catheter to allow removal of the balloon flotation catheter and advancement of a small 8 mm dilatation catheter for enlargement of the opening made in the intra-atrial septum. This step is required to facilitate passage of the larger 23 to 25 mm diameter valvuloplasty balloon through the intra-atrial septum and across the stenotic mitral valve. Inflation of this larger balloon results in separation of the fused commissures analogous to the earlier surgical technique of closed or open mitral commissurotomy. Subsequent variations of the technique have included the use of a sin-

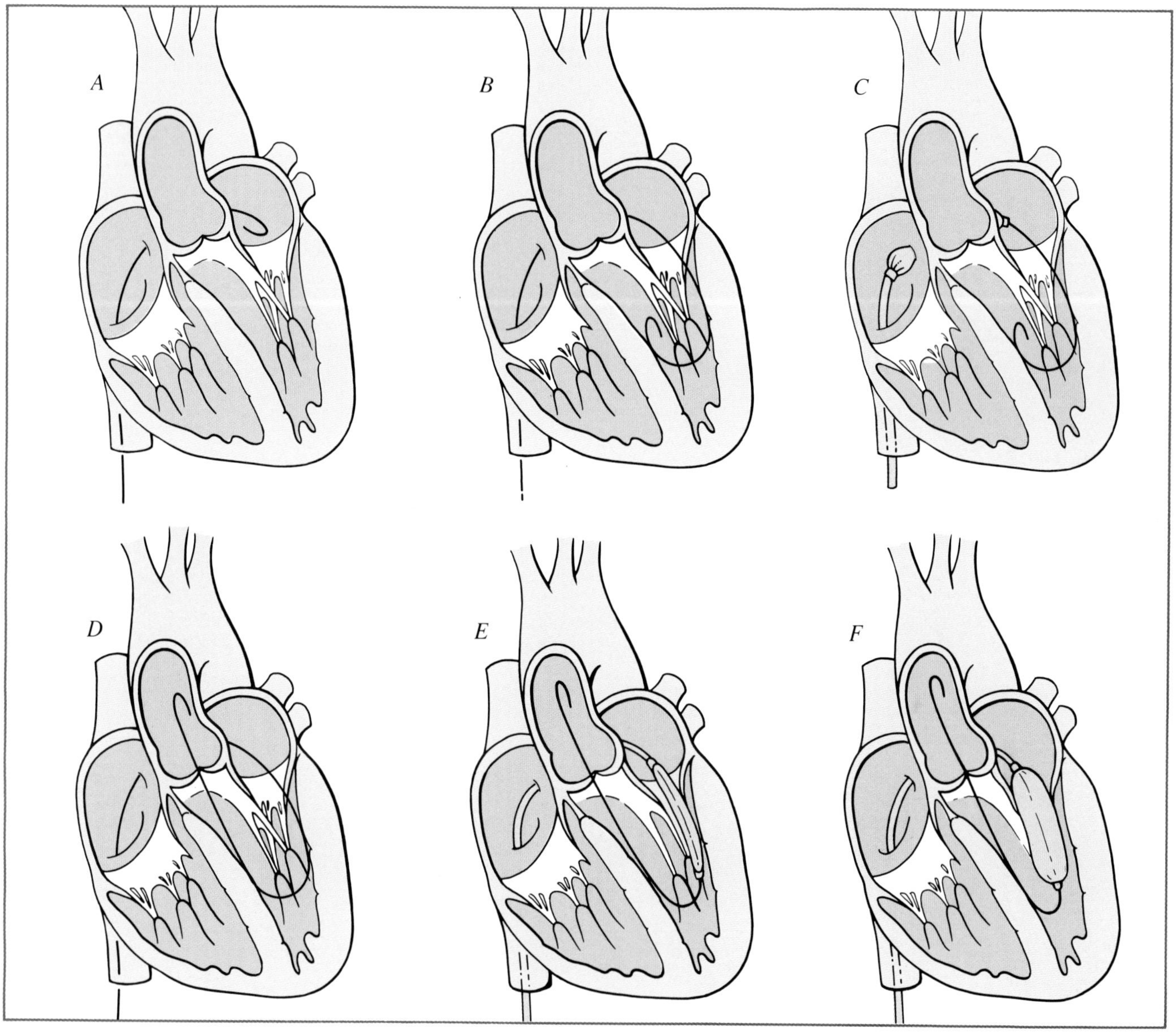

FIGURE 5.47 • Technique of balloon mitral valvuloplasty. The position of the guidewire in the left atrium after left atrial puncture using the Brockenbrough needle (A). The position of the guidewire after it is advanced into the left ventricle across the stenotic mitral valve (B). Inflation of a small (8 mm diameter) balloon catheter across the interatrial septum (C). Note that the guidewire may be advanced into the aorta in an antegrade fashion to provide greater stabilization (D). The valvuloplasty balloon is across the stenotic mitral valve (E). The appearance of the inflated balloon as the valvuloplasty is being performed (F). (Modified from Chatterjee K, Cheitlin MD, Karliner J, et al: *Cardiology. An Illustrated Text/Reference. Volume 2* New York, NY: Gower Medical Publishing; 1991:9.68.)

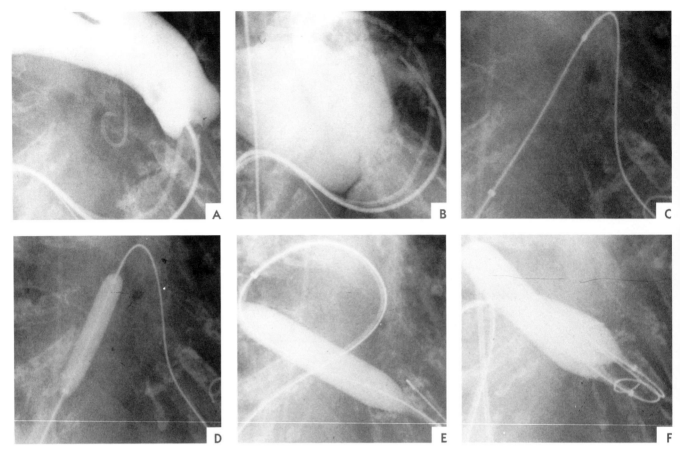

FIGURE 5.48 • Anteroposterior cineradiographs of mitral valvulo-plasty. A pulmonary angiogram, which may be performed at the be-ginning of the procedure to clarify the relationship of the left atrium and aortic root (A). Note the location of the pigtail catheter in the non-coronary cusp. Levophase left atrial filling and ventriculogram (B). The guidewire across the atrial septum with a small (8 mm) bal-loon catheter in place (C). Note the end markers of the balloon catheter. The atrial septum is dilated as the balloon is inflated (D). The end of an exchange-length J guidewire is in the left ventricle. The balloon-dilatation catheter is fully inflated (E). To enlarge the valve orifice further, two balloon-dilatation catheters are simultaneously in-flated across the stenotic mitral valve (F). (Reproduced with permis-sion. Chatterjee K, Cheitlin MD, Karliner J, et al: *Cardiology. An Illus-trated Text/Reference. Volume 2* New York, NY: Gower Medical Pub-lishing; 1991:9.69.)

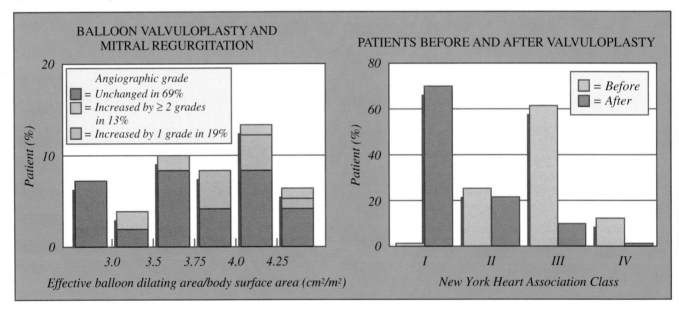

FIGURE 5.49 • Effect of balloon valvuloplasty on the development of mitral regurgitation in 48 patients who underwent left ventriculography before and after the procedure (A). The angiographic grade of regurgi-tation increased by ≥ 2 grades in 13%, by 1 grade in 19%, and was un-changed in 69%. There was no significant correlation—r = 0.17, p = not significant— between effective balloon dilating area normalized for body surface area and the change in grade of mitral regurgitation. Percent of patients in each New York Heart Association (NYHA) func-tional class before and after valvuloplasty among the 55 patients treat-ed only with this procedure. Mean functional class improved from 2.9 ± 0.1 to 1.4 ± 0.1 (B). (Reproduced with permission. Hermann HC, Kleaveland JP, Hill JA, et al: *J Am Coll Cardiol* 1990;15;1223.)

gle compliant dumbbell-shaped balloon,[75] or two smaller 12 to 18 mm balloon catheters, which can be advanced individually across the atrial septum and then inflated simultaneously within the mitral orifice.[72]

After these encouraging results in young adults with rheumatic mitral stenosis, similar procedures were attempted in adult patients with more rigid calcific lesions. Using this technique, it has been possible to achieve physiologically adequate enlargement of the mitral orifice area from 0.9 to 2.0 cm.[2] Overall procedural mortality is 1% to 2%, with cardiac perforation by the transseptal needle, guidewire, or dilatation catheter in approximately 1% of patients. In patients preselected by transesophageal echocardiography for absence of left atrial thrombus and pretreated with oral warfarin for 2 to 3 months before attenuated valvuloplasty, a significant increase in the degree of mitral regurgitation is uncommon, as are systemic emboli. Approximately 20% of patients show evidence of a small (less than 2:1) left-to-right shunt at the atrial level, owing to dilatation of the atrial septal puncture during passage of the valvuloplasty balloon. Approximately half of these shunts resolve spontaneously by the time of follow-up catheterization.[76] This minor complication should diminish as improved technology permits the production of valvuloplasty balloons with smaller collapsed profiles. Similarly, balloon catheters capable of more rapid inflation and deflation will be of value in minimizing the period of systemic arterial hypotension which invariably results from transient occlusion of left ventricular inflow during balloon inflation.

Results of Clinical Trials

Early 6- to 12-month follow-up studies have demonstrated preservation of the improved mitral orifice and similar physiologic improvements—fall in filling pressures and pulmonary vascular resistance—to those seen after surgical correction of mitral stenosis[74,77] (Figure 5.49). Both the early and late 1 year hemodynamic results can be predicted by an "echocardiographic score" in which four unfavorable features—poor leaflet mobility, valvular thickening, subvalvular thickening, and valvular calcification—are each assigned a value of 1 to 4. Patients with a cumulative score below 8 have a greater than 90% chance of good initial result—valve area greater than 1.5 cm[72] and only a 4% chance of significant restenosis at 1 year. In contrast, patients with a cumulative score of 8 to 16 have only a 50% chance of a good initial result and a 70% chance of restenosis at 1 year.[72] This pattern may relate to a greater contribution of separation of commissural fusion in patients with pliable leaflets versus a more limited benefit obtained by leaflet cracking and transient stretching of the mitral valve annulus in patients with more rigid valvular and subvalvular structures.

AORTIC VALVULOPLASTY

With evident success of balloon valvuloplasty in the treatment of acquired mitral stenosis, attention was then turned to dilatation of calcific aortic stenosis in the adult (Figure 5.50). This disorder is the principal indication for most of the approximately 20,000 aortic valve replacements performed each year in the United States. Narrowing of the valve orifice is due to a combination of an underlying congenital structural abnormality (a bicuspid aortic valve), commissural fusion, and stiffening of the leaflets by extensive calcium deposition. Postmortem and intraoperative balloon dilatations have demonstrated separation of fused commissures, increased leaflet pliability due to microfractures and macrofractures through the calcium deposits, and transient stretching of the aortic annulus.[79] These findings suggested that percutaneous aortic valvuloplasty might be possible in advanced aortic stenosis. By 1990 this procedure had been performed in more than 1,000 patients, principally using the retrograde approach.[72]

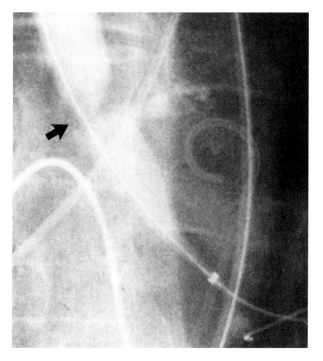

FIGURE 5.50 • Waist observed during aortic balloon valvuloplasty. Magnified anteroposterior view of aortic balloon valvuloplasty demonstrating a waist as the balloon is inflated. Calcification can be seen in the aortic annulus. A pigtail catheter is seen in the descending aorta and a bipolar pacing catheter is positioned in the right ventricular apex. (Reproduced with permission. Chatterjee K, Cheitlin MD, Karliner J, et al: *Cardiology. An Illustrated Text/Reference. Volume 2* New York, NY: Gower Medical Publishing; 1991:9.63.)

Technique

A conventional catheter is advanced retrogradely across the stenotic valve and into the left ventricle (Figures 5.51, 5.52). Through this catheter an exchange-length guidewire is then positioned in the left ventricular apex and used to advance balloon dilatation catheters—12, 15, 18, 20, and, occasionally, 23 mm in diameter—across the stenotic valve. The balloon is inflated several times using dilute liquid radiographic contrast material. Maintenance of the balloon within the aortic orifice during inflation is difficult because of a tendency for the balloon to be ejected by the force of left ventricular contraction but is facilitated by the use of catheters with 6 cm rather than 3 cm balloon segments. In patients with peripheral vascular disease, aortic balloon valvuloplasty can be performed using an antegrade or transseptal approach, similar to that used for mitral valvuloplasty.

Results of Clinical Trials

The magnitude of orifice improvement during aortic valvuloplasty, from 0.6 to 0.9 cm^2, peak gradient from 60 to 30 mm Hg, appears to be less than with mitral valvuloplasty, but is usually adequate to produce marked improvement in clinical sta-

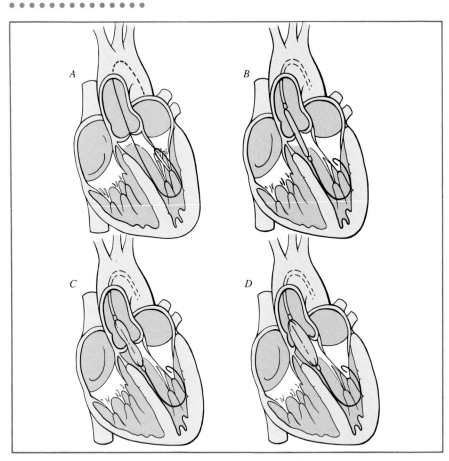

FIGURE 5.51 • Technique of aortic valvuloplasty by the femoral approach. The doublebend-guidewire across the stenotic aortic valve (A). The deflated balloon-dilatation catheter in position across the aortic valve (B). The balloon-dilatation catheter as it is filled with contrast. A noticeable "waist" is seen as the balloon is inflated across the stenotic aortic valve (C). The balloon-dilatation catheter when completely filled. The aortic orifice is dilated to the size of the balloon-dilatation catheter (D). (Modified from Chatterjee K, Cheitlin MD, Karliner J, et al: *Cardiology. An Illustrated Text/Reference.* Volume 2 New York, NY: Gower Medical Publishing; 1991:9.64.)

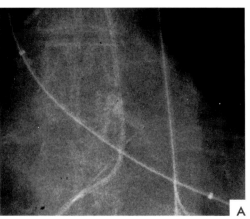
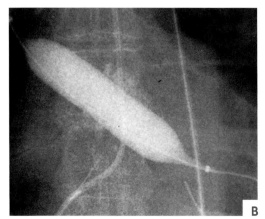

FIGURE 5.52 • Anteroposterior cineradiographs of aortic valvuloplasty. The guidewire and balloon-dilatation catheter in place across a calcified and stenotic aortic value (A). The balloon is inflated at 4 atm or 60 psi of pressure (B). A paceport Swan-Ganz catheter is shown in the pulmonary artery with the pacing wire in the right ventricular outflow tract. (Reproduced with permission Chatterjee K, Cheitlin MD, Karliner J, et al: *Cardiology. An Illustrated Text/Reference.* Volume 2 New York, NY: Gower Medical Publishing; 1991:9.64.)

tus, filling pressures, and left ventricular performance in patients with severe resting symptoms caused by critical aortic stenosis[80] (Figure 5.53). Procedural mortality is 5%, with other problems including systemic emboli (1.5%), worsened aortic regurgitation (1%), and vascular injury at the access site (5% to 10%). Balloon inflation seems to cause less hemodynamic compromise than seen during mitral dilatation because some left ventricular ejection can occur between the inflated balloon and the aortic commissures.

While aortic balloon valvuloplasty continues to play a role in the treatment of patients whose poor left ventricular function, advanced age, or other medical problems place them at high risk for surgical aortic valve replacement,[81,82] improvement in the orifice area is less than that usually obtained with a valve replacement, and an unacceptable high fraction of patients show evidence of poor long-term 24 month results by death (30% to 40%), repeat valvuloplasty (20%), or valve replacement (15% to 20%). Since the predominant effect is caused by leaflet cracking and annulus stretching, changes in technique, such as the use of larger diameter balloons, have increased the incidence of complications without providing better immediate or long-term results. Valve replacement is thus still preferred in patients with severe aortic stenosis who are candidates for surgery.

OTHER INTERVENTIONAL CATHETERIZATION TECHNIQUES

Some of the earliest applications of interventional cardiology were in patients with congenital heart disease. In 1966, Rashkind described passage of a balloon catheter through a pre-existing patent foramen ovale, followed by withdrawal of the inflated balloon to create a functional atrial septal defect in patients with transposition of the great arteries, tricuspid atresia, pulmonic atresia, mitral atresia, total anomalous pulmonary venous return, or single ventricle.[83] Sixteen years later Park and coworkers modified this technique by use of a catheter with a surgical blade, which can be deployed in the left atrium after transseptal puncture and then used to incise the atrial septum during withdrawal.[84] The resulting atrial septal defect can then be enlarged using a balloon catheter as described by Rashkind.

In addition to the creation or enlargement of vascular channels, pediatric cardiologists have developed devices for closing aberrant vascular channels. Rashkind developed a "double-disc" prosthesis that can be passed across an unwanted atrial septal defect, ventricular septal defect, or patent ductus arte-

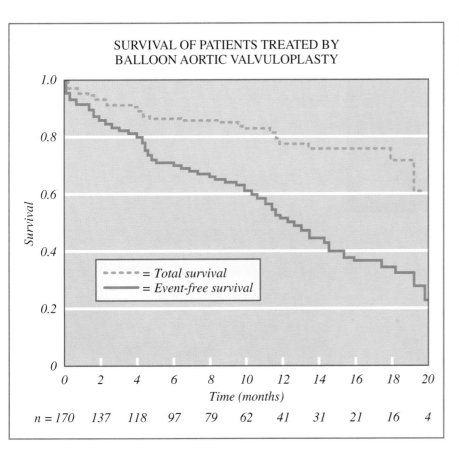

FIGURE 5.53 • Actuarial survival for patients treated by balloon aortic valvuloplasty. (Reproduced with permission. Safian RD, Berman AD, Diver DJ, et al: *N Engl J Med* 1988;319:128.)

riosus (Figures 5.54-5.56).[85–87] The first disc is deployed on the far side of the defect and held in place by three spring struts, as the remaining disc and struts are pulled back across the defect and deployed on its near side. The result is sealing of the defect between two layers of prosthetic material.

Methods have also been developed for preoperative closure of unwanted systemic-pulmonary collateral vessels in patients undergoing correction of tetralogy of Fallot, using preformed steel coils or detachable balloons embolized into the unwanted vessel through a catheter delivery system.[88,89] These approaches—similar to those used by vascular radiologists to treat arteriovenous malformations or actively bleeding vessels in other beds—lead to occlusion of the target vessel by local thrombosis.

CONCLUSIONS

The last 15 years have produced the rapid growth and evolution of catheter-based treatments for coronary artery disease. With refinements in conventional balloon angioplasty equipment and technique, up to half of current revascularization procedures are being performed by the percutaneous catheter rather than the surgical bypass approach. Success and safety of balloon angioplasty have proven to be excellent, but the procedure is still troubled by several limitations:

- Difficulty in crossing chronic total occlusions.
- Difficulty in dilating calcified, markedly eccentric, or diffusely diseased vessels.
- Difficulty in preventing or reliably reversing abrupt closure resulting from excessive vessel trauma.
- The inability to prevent the late (6 weeks to 6 months) restenosis of the dilated segment that occurs in roughly one third of patients due to excessive local tissue proliferation.

Some of these residual problems may yield to one or more of the new technologies—stents, atherectomy catheters, ablative or thermal laser devices—currently under investigation. Other devices to deal with chronic total occlusions or diffuse disease will follow. Control of restenosis, however, will require the concurrent use of potent pharmacologic agents to decrease platelet adhesion to the surface of the treated vessel, and the proliferative response of vascular smooth muscle. As effective solutions are developed, we are certain to see further growth of catheter-based therapeutics during the 1990s.

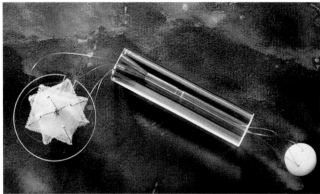

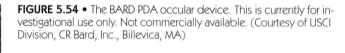

FIGURE 5.54 • The BARD PDA occular device. This is currently for investigational use only. Not commercially available. (Courtesy of USCI Division, CR Bard, Inc., Billevica, MA)

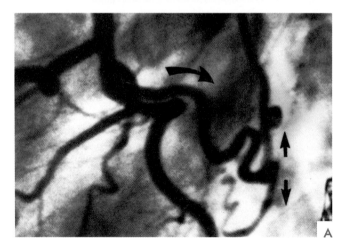
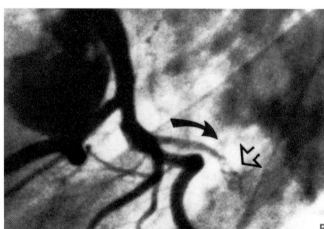

FIGURE 5.55 • Fistula from atrial branch of circumflex (curved arrow) to the pulmonary artery (A). This fistula has been closed by placement of an occlusion coil (open arrow) (B).

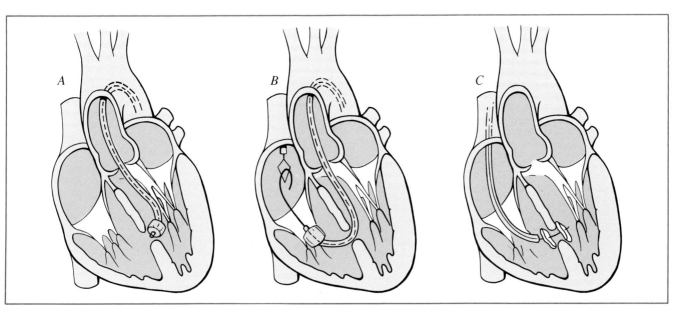

FIGURE 5.56 • Transcatheter muscular ventricular septal defect (VSD) closure. The 7F balloon end-hole catheter is passed retrograde onto the left ventricle (LV) and the inflated balloon "seats" in the VSD (A). The balloon and catheter are manipulated—with the use of partial balloon inflation—across the septum into the right heart. This is where a 400-cm guidewire is snared via a transvenous catheter (B). The wire is used to advance a venous long sheath and dialator across the VSD. The final outcome of the procedure is the placement of a double umbrella to straddle the defect (C). (Adapted from Lock JE, Block PC, McKay RG, et al: *Circulation* 1988;78:362.)

REFERENCES

1. Baim DS, Ignatius EJ: Use of percutaneous transluminal coronary angioplasty: Results of a current survey. *Am J Cardiol* 1988;61:3G.

2. Weintraub WS, Jones EL, King SB, et al: Changing use of coronary angioplasty and coronary bypass surgery in the treatment of chronic coronary artery disease. *Am J Cardiol* 1990;65:183.

3. Participants in the National Heart, Lung, and Blood Institute: Conference on the evaluation of emerging coronary revascularization technologies. Evaluation of emerging technologies for coronary revascularization. *Circulation* 1992;85:357.

4. Waller BF: "Crackers, breakers, stretchers, drillers, scrapers, shavers, burners, welders and melters"—The future treatment of atherosclerotic coronary artery disease—A clinical-morphologic assessment. *J Am Coll Cardiol* 1989;13:987.

5. Dotter CT, Judkins MP: Transluminal treatment of arteriosclerotic obstruction: description of a new technique and a preliminary report of its application. *Circulation* 1964;30:654.

6. Gruentzig A, Kumpe DA: Technique of percutaneous transluminal angioplasty with the Gruentzig balloon catheter. *Am J Radiol* 1979;132:547.

7. Gruentzig AR, Senning A, Siegenthaler WE: Nonoperative dilatation of coronary artery stenosis—Percutaneous transluminal coronary angioplasty. *N Engl J Med* 1979;301:61.

8. Kent KM, bentivoglio LG, Block PC, et al: Percutaneous transluminal coronary angioplasty: Report from the registry of the National Heart, Lung, and Blood Institute. *Am J Cardiol* 1982:49:2011.

9. Simpson JB, Baim DS, Robert EW, et al: A new catheter system for coronary angioplasty. *Am J Cardiol* 1982;49:1216.

10. Avedissian MG, Killeavy ES, Garcia JM, et al: Percutaneous transluminal coronary angioplasty: A review of current balloon dilatation systems. *Cathet Cardiovasc Diagn* 1989;18:263.

11. Ryan TJ, Klocke FJ, Reynolds WA, et al: Clinical competence in percutaneous transluminal coronary angioplasty—ACP/ACC/AHA Task Force on clinical privileges in Cardiology. *Circulation* 1990;81:2041.

12. Castaneda-Zuniga WR, Formanek A, Tadavarthy M, et al: The mechanism of balloon angioplasty. *Radiology* 1980;135:565.

13. Sanborn TA, Faxon DP, Haudenschild C, et al: The mechanism of transluminal angioplasty. Evidence for formation of aneurysms in experimental atherosclerosis. *Circulation* 1983;68:1136.

14. Black AJR, Namay DL, Niederman AL, et al: Tear or dissection after coronary angioplasty—Morphologic correlates of an ischemic complication. *Circulation* 1989;79:1035.

15. Liu MW, Roubin GS, King SB: Restenosis after coronary angioplasty: Potential biologic determinants and the role of intimal hyperplasia. *Circulation* 1989;79:1374.

16. Knudtson ML, Flintoft JD, Roth DL, et al: Effect of short-term prostacyclin administration on restenosis after percutaneous transluminal coronary angioplasty. *J Am Coll Cardiol* 1990;15:691.

17. Pepine CJ, Hirshfeld JW, MacDonald RG, et al: A controlled trial of corticosteroids to prevent restenosis after coronary angioplasty. *Circulation* 1990;81:1753.

18. Stone GW, Rutherford BD, McConahay DR, et al: A randomized trial of corticosteroids for the prevention of restenosis in 102 patients undergoing repeat coronary angioplasty. *Cathet Cardiovasc Diagn* 1989;18:227.

19. Jang IK, Gold HK, Ziskind AA, et al: Prevention of platelet-rich arterial thrombosis by selective thrombin inhibition (argatroban). *Circulation* 1990;81:219.

20. Heras M, Chesboro JH, Webster MWI, et al: Hirudin, heparin and placebo during deep arterial injury in the pig. *Circulation* 1990;82:1476.

21. Schwartz L, Bourassa MG, Lesperance J, et al: Aspirin and dipyridamole in the prevention of restenosis after percutaneous transluminal coronary angioplasty. *N Engl J Med* 1988;318:1714.

22. Roubin GS, Douglas JS, King SB, et al: Influence of balloon size on initial success, acute complications, and restenosis after percutaneous transluminal coronary angioplasty. A prospective randomized study. *Circulation* 1988;78:557.

23. Popma JJ, Dehmer GJ: Care of the patient after coronary angioplasty. *Ann Int Med* 1989;110:547.

24. Ryan TJ, Faxon DP, Gunnar RM, et al: Guidelines for percutaneous transluminal coronary angioplasty—A report of the ACC/AHA Task Force on assessment of diagnostic and therapeutic cardiovascular procedures. *J Am Coll Cardiol* 1988;12:529.

25. Stone GW, Rutherford BD, McConahay DR, et al: Procedural outcome of angioplasty for total coronary occlusion: An analysis of 971 lesions in 905 patients. *J Am Coll Cardiol* 1990;15:849.

26. Weinstein JS, Baim DS, Sipperly ME, et al: Salvage of branch vessels during bifurcation lesion angioplasty—Acute and long-term follow-up. *Cathet Cardiovasc Diagn* 1991;22:16.

27. Wohlgertner D, Cleman M, Highman HA, et al: Percutaneous transluminal angioplasty of the "culprit lesion" for the management of unstable angina pectoris in patients with multivessel coronary artery disease. *Am J Cardiol* 1986;58:460.

28. Holmes DR, Holubkov R, Vlietstra RE, et al: Comparison of complications during percutaneous transluminal coronary angioplasty from 1977 to 1981 and from 1985 to 1986. The NHLBI PTCA Registry. *J Am Coll Cardiol* 1988;12:1149.

29. Detre K, Holubkov R, Kelsey S, et al: Percutaneous transluminal coronary angioplasty in 1985–1986 and 1977–1981: The NHLBI Registry. *N Engl J Med* 1988;318:265.

30. O'Keefe JH, Hartzler GO, Rutherford BD, et al: Left main coronary angioplasty—Early and late results of 127 acute and elective procedures. *Am J Cardiol* 1989;54:144.

31. Cote G, Myler RK, Stertzer SH, et al: Percutaneous transluminal angioplasty of stenotic coronary artery bypass grafts: 5 years experience. *J Am Coll Cardiol* 1987;9:8.

32. Waller BF: Morphologic observations after percutaneous transluminal balloon angioplasty of early and late aortocoronary saphenous vein bypass grafts. *J Am Coll Cardiol* 1984;4:784.

33. Kuntz R, Baim D: Internal mammary angiography. *Cathet Cardiovasc Diagn* 1990;20:10.

34. Shimshak TM, Giogi LV, Johnson WL, et al: Application of percutaneous transluminal angioplasty to the internal mammary artery graft. *J Am Coll Cardiol* 1988;12:1205.

35. deFeyter PJ: Coronary angioplasty for unstable angina. *Am Heart J* 1989;118:860.

36. O'Keefe JH, Rutherford BD, McConahay DR, et al: Early results and long-term outcome of direct coronary angioplasty for acute myocardial infarction in 500 consecutive patients. *J Am Coll Cardiol* 1989;64:1221.

37. The TIMI Study Group: Comparison of invasive and conservative strategies following tissue plasminogen activator—Results of the Thrombolysis in Myocardial Infarction (TIMI) phase II trial. *N Engl J Med* 1989;320:618.

38. Baim DS, Diver DJ, Feit F, et al: Coronary angioplasty performed within the Thrombolysis in Myocardial Infarction (TIMI II) study. *Circulation* 1992;85:93.

39. Wyman RM, Safian RD, Portway V, et al: Current complications of diagnostic and therapeutic cardiac catheterization. *J Am Coll Cardiol* 1988;12:1400.

40. Sinclair IN, McCabe CH, Sipperly ME, et al: Predictors, therapeutic options and long-term outcome of abrupt reclosure. *Am J Cardiol* 1988;61:61G.

41. Ellis SG, Roubin GS, King SB, et al: Angiographic and clinical predictors of acute closure after native vessel coronary angioplasty. *Circulation* 1988;77:372.

42. Ellis SG, Vandormael MG, Cowley MJ, et al: Coronary morphologic and clinical determinants of procedural outcome with angioplasty for multivessel coronary artery disease. *Circulation* 1990;82:1193.

43. Detre KM, Holmes DR, Holubkov R, et al: Incidence and consequences of periprocedural occlusion: The 1985–86 National Heart, Lung, and Blood Institute's Percutaneous transluminal coronary angioplasty Registry. *Circulation* 1990;82:739.

44. Talley JD, Weintraub WS, Roubin GS, et al: Failed elective percutaneous transluminal coronary angioplasty requiring coronary artery bypass surgery: in-hospital and late clinical outcome at 5 years. *Circulation* 1990;82:1203.

45. Sundrum P, Harvey JR, Johnson RG, et al: Benefit of the perfusion catheter for emergency coronary artery grafting after failed percutaneous transluminal coronary angioplasty. *Am J Cardiol* 1989;63:282.

46. Kahn JE, Rutherford BD, McConahay DR, et al: Supported "high-risk" coronary angioplasty using intraaortic balloon counterpulsation. *J Am Coll Cardiol* 1990;15:1151.

47. Vogel RA, Shawl F, Tommaso C, et al: Initial report of the National Registry of Elective Cardiopulmonary Bypass Supported Coronary Angioplasty. *J Am Coll Cardiol* 1990;14:23.

48. Hartzler GO, Rutherford BD, McConahay GO, et al: "High-risk" percutaneous transluminal coronary angioplasty. *Am J Cardiol* 1988;61:33G.

49. Detre K, Holubkov R, Kelsey S, et al: One year follow-up results of the 1985–1986 National Heart, Lung, and Blood Institute's percutaneous transluminal coronary angioplasty registry. *Circulation* 1989;80:421.

50. Kuntz RE, Safian RD, Schmidt DA, et al: A novel approach to the analysis of restenosis following three new coronary interventions. *J Am Coll Cardiol* 1992. In press.

51. Nobuyoshi M, Kimura T, Nosaka H, et al: Restenosis after successful percutaneous transluminal coronary angioplasty: Serial angiographic follow-up of 220 patients. *J Am Coll Cardiol* 1988;12:616.

52. Fischell TA, Derby G, Tse TM, et al: Coronary artery vasoconstriction after percutaneous transluminal coronary angioplasty: A quantitative arteriographic analysis. *Circulation* 1988;78:1323.

53. Black AJR, Anderson HV, Roubin GS, et al: Repeat coronary angioplasty: Correlates of a second restenosis. *J Am Coll Cardiol* 1988;11:714.

54. Teirstein PS, Hoover CA, Ligon RW, et al: Repeat coronary angioplasty: Efficacy of a third angioplasty for a second restenosis. *J Am Coll Cardiol* 1989;13:291.

55. Reiss G, Sipperly ME, McCabe CH, et al: Randomized trial of fish oil for prevention of restenosis after coronary angioplasty. *Lancet* 1989;2:177.

56. Dotter CT: Transluminally placed coil-spring endarterial tube grafts: long-term patency in canine popliteal artery. *Invest Radiol* 1969;4:329.

57. Schatz, RA: A view of vascular stents. *Circulation* 1989;79:445.

58. Sigwart U, Puel J, Mirkovitch V, et al: Intravascular stents to prevent occlusion and restenosis after transluminal angioplasty. *N Engl J Med* 1987;316:701.

59. Roubin GS, King SB, Douglas JS, et al: Intracoronary stenting during percutaneous transluminal coronary angioplasty. *Circulation* 1990;81:IV-92.

60. Serruys PW, Strauss BH, Beatt KJ, et al: Angiographic follow-up after placement of a self-expanding coronary-artery stent. *N Engl J Med* 1991;324:13.

61. Schatz RA, Baim DS, Leon M, et al: Clinical experience with the Palmaz-Schatz coronary stent. Initial results of a multicenter study. *Circulation* 1991;83:148.

62. Carrozza JP, Kuntz RE, Levine MJ, et al: Angiographic and clinical outcome of intracoronary stenting: Acute and long-term results from a large single-center experience. *J Am Coll Cardiol* 1992. In press.

63. Simpson JB, Selmon MR, Robertson GC, et al: Transluminal atherectomy for occlusive peripheral vascular disease. *Am J Cardiol* 1988;61:96G.

64. Safian RD, Gelbfish JS, Erny RE, et al: Coronary atherectomy: Clinical, angiographic and histologic findings and observations regarding mechanism. *Circulation* 1990;82:69.

65. Penny WF, Schmidt DA, Safian RD, et al: Insights into the mechanism of luminal improvement following directional coronary atherectomy. *Am J Cardiol* 1991;67:435.

66. Fourrier JL, Bertrand ME, Auth DC, et al: Percutaneous coronary rotational atherectomy in humans. Preliminary report. *J Am Coll Cardiol* 1989;14:1278.

67. Litvak F, Grunfest WS, Segalowitz J, et al: International cardiovascular therapy by laser and thermal angioplasty. *Circulation* 1990;81:IV-109.

68. Litvak F, Grundfest WS, Goldenberg T: Percutaneous excimer laser coronary angioplasty of aortocoronary saphenous vein grafts. *J Am Coll Cardiol* 1989;14:803.

69. Karsch KR, Haase KK, Voelker W, et al: Percutaneous excimer coronary angioplasty in patients with stable and unstable angina pectoris. *Circulation* 1990;81:1849.

70. Isner JM, Rosenfeld K, Losordo DW, et al: Excimer laser angioplasty—The greening of Sisyphus. *Circulation* 1990;81:2018.

71. Spears JR, Reyes VP, Wynne J, et al: Percutaneous coronary laser balloon angioplasty: initial results of a multicenter experience. *J Am Coll Cardiol* 1990;16:293.

72. Block PC, Palacios IF: Aortic and mitral balloon valvuloplasty: The United States experience. In: Topol EJ, ed. *Textbook of Interventional Cardiology* Philadelphia, PA: WB Saunders Co; 1990.

73. Rochini AP, Beekman RH, Shachar GB, et al: Balloon aortic valvuloplasty: Results of the valvuloplasty and angioplasty congenital anomalies registry. *Am J Cardiol* 1990;65:784.

74. Lock JE, Khalilullah M, Shrivastava S, et al: Percutaneous catheter commissurotomy in rheumatic mitral stenosis. *N Engl J Med* 1985;313:1515.

75. Nobuyoshi M, Hamasaki N, Kimura T, et al: Indications, complications, and short-term clinical outcome of percutaneous transvenous mitral commissurotomy. *Circulation* 1989;80:782.

76. Casale P, Block PC, O'Shea JP, et al: Atrial septal defect after percutaneous mitral balloon valvuloplasty: Immediate results and folow-up. *J Am Coll Cardiol* 1990:15:1300.

77. Hermann HC, Kleaveland JP, Hill JA, et al: The M-Heart Percutaneous Balloon Mitral Valvuloplasty Registry: Initial results and early follow-up. *J Am Coll Cardiol* 1990;15:1221.

78. Palacios IF, Block PC, Wilkins GT, et al: Follow-up of patients undergoing percutaneous mitral balloon valvotomy: Analysis of factors determining restenosis. *Circulation* 1989;79:573.

79. Letac B, Gerber LI, Koning R: Insights on the mechanism of balloon valvuloplasty in aortic stenosis. *Am J Cardiol* 1988;62:1241.

80. Kuntz RE, Tosteson ANA, Berman AD, et al: Predictors of event-free survival after balloon aortic valvuloplasty. *N Engl J Med* 1991;325:17.

81. Berland J, Squavin T, Lefebvre E, et al: Percutaneous balloon valvuloplasty in patients with severe aortic stenosis and low ejection fraction. *Circulation* 1989;79:1189.

82. Levine MJ, Berman AD, Safian RD, et al: Palliation of valvular aortic stenosis by balloon valvuloplasty as preparation for noncardiac surgery. *Am J Cardiol* 1988;62:1309.

83. Rashkind RJ: Transcatheter treatment of congenital heart disease. *Circulation* 1983;67:711.

84. Park SC, Neches WH, Mullins CE, et al: Blade atrial septostomy: Collaborative study. *Circulation* 1982;66:258.

85. Lock JE, Cockerham JT, Keane JF, et al: Transcatheter umbrella closure of congenital heart defects. *Circulation* 1987;75:593.

86. Lock JE, Block PC, McKay RG, et al: Transcatheter closure of ventricular septal defects. *Circulation* 1988;78:361.

87. Dyck JD, Benson LN, Smallhörn JF, et al: Catheter occlusion of the persistently patent ductus arteriosus. *Am J Cardiol* 1988;62:1089.

88. Gewillig M, Van Der Hauwaert L, Daenen W: Transcatheter occlusion of high-flow Blalock-Taussig shunts with a detachable balloon. *Am J Cardiol* 1990;65:1518.

89. Miranda AA, Hill JA, Micklo JP, et al: Balloon occlusion of an internal mammary artery to anterior interventricular vein fistula. *Am J Cardiol* 1990;65:257.

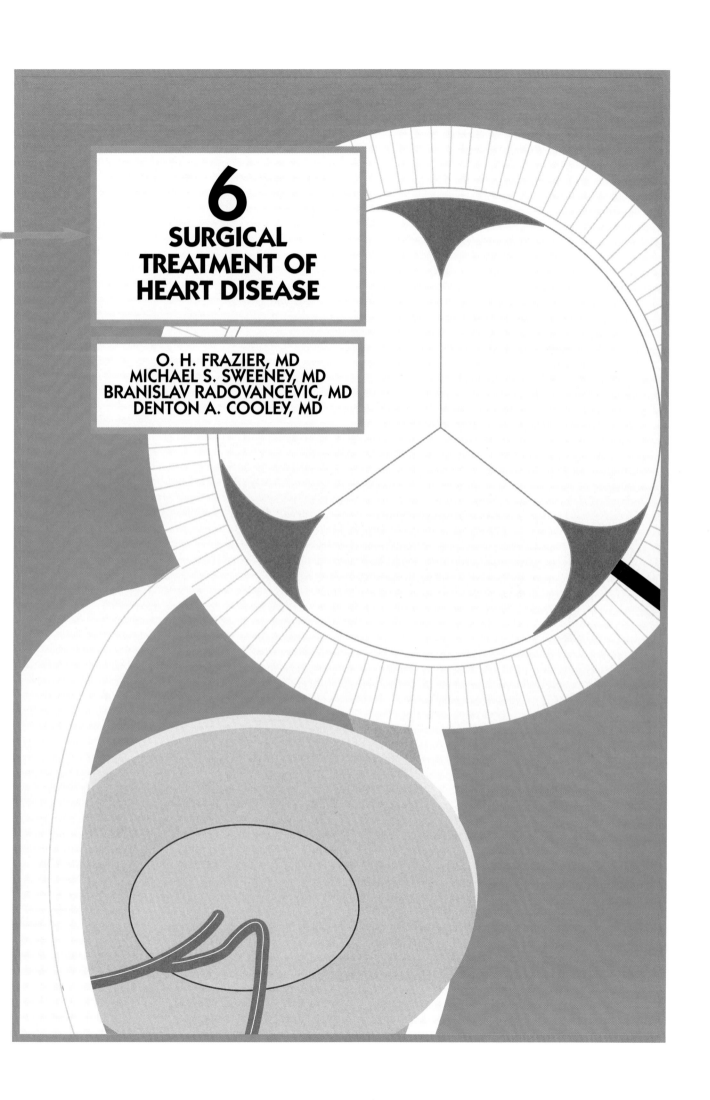

6
SURGICAL TREATMENT OF HEART DISEASE

O. H. FRAZIER, MD
MICHAEL S. SWEENEY, MD
BRANISLAV RADOVANCEVIC, MD
DENTON A. COOLEY, MD

Synopsis of Chapter Six

CORONARY ARTERY SURGERY

The goal of aortocoronary bypass surgery is to relieve myocardial ischemia and subsequent angina pectoris—in some instances, to avert early cardiac mortality. The indications for aortocoronary bypass surgery are, perhaps appropriately, not clear-cut and promise to be regularly modified for several years until the respective roles of percutaneous transluminal coronary angioplasty (PTCA), aortocoronary bypass surgery, and medical management can be precisely defined. Current indications for and methods of operation will be discussed herein, with the caveat that myocardial revascularization remains an art in evolution. Additionally, some emphasis will be given to the long-term results that might be expected from operative therapy.

INDICATIONS

During the 1970s, extensive information was collected regarding elective aortocoronary bypass surgery as a treatment for myocardial ischemia. This treatment strategy was hailed in some quarters, assailed in others, and ultimately raised enough concern that the American Medical Association (AMA) requested its Council on Scientific Affairs to appoint a group of expert consultants to review the issue. In 1979[1] the Council determined that although there were risks inherent in advising practitioners on the indications issue, aortocoronary bypass surgery seemed indicated for patients with angina and coronary artery disease in three clinical settings:

- Critical stenosis of the left main coronary artery.
- Triple-vessel coronary artery disease with moderate degrees of left ventricular dysfunction.
- Angina that was unresponsive to proper medical therapy.

Moreover, the panel noted nine other clinical settings in which aortocoronary bypass surgery might be indicated and suggested that these areas be further studied to determine whether the indications for bypass surgery should be expanded. These settings included:

- Unstable angina.
- Variant (Prinzmetal's) angina secondary to coronary spasm.
- Acute infarction (less than a few hrs old).
- Cardiogenic shock.
- Congestive heart failure.
- Sudden death syndrome.
- Recurrent ventricular arrhythmias.
- Ventricular tachycardia in association with ventricular aneurysm.
- Subsets of patients with coronary artery diseases anatomically distinct from those already included, with or without symptoms.

In the ensuing years, appropriate studies have been designed to further define the efficacy of aortocoronary bypass surgery in most of these areas.

With data collected on almost 25,000 patients from 15 different clinical centers, at a cost of $24 million, the Coronary Artery Surgery Study (CASS) is perhaps the largest single repository of information with regard to the treatment of coronary artery disease. At least 70 scientific articles have been published with CASS data, making it one of the most discussed, if not most informative, studies ever commissioned by the National Heart, Lung, and Blood Institute. CASS concentrated on two areas:

- As a registry of patients with coronary disease managed conventionally.
- As a randomized trial of medical versus surgical treatment for patients with mild angina. While a detailed analysis of the controversial CASS Randomized Trial is certainly beyond the scope of this chapter,[2–5] the CASS Registry studies have provided much insight into the continuing evolution of the role of aortocoronary bypass surgery in the treatment of coronary disease,[6] particularly in the nine areas targeted for further study by the Council on Scientific Affairs.

The severity of chronic angina is a potentially subjective symptom and, as such, is often not recognized in time for either medical or surgical therapy. However, Kaiser[7] has shown that this symptom can be an important predictor, since patients with severe angina and significant coronary disease, with either normal or abnormal left ventricular function, had significantly better outcomes after aortocoronary bypass surgery. Similar efficacy of aortocoronary bypass surgery for variant (Prinzmetal's) angina has not been demonstrated, and this condition is most often treated nonoperatively with antispasm agents.

Urgent aortocoronary bypass surgery for patients with acute myocardial infarctions, and even for patients with cardiogenic shock, has been attempted. The most remarkable studies of this type began in 1971 in Spokane, Washington, when a group of surgeons initiated attempts at early (within 24 hrs) operation upon complicated and uncomplicated acute myocardial infarctions.[8–10] Although the overall mortality rates resulting from this treatment strategy have been surprisingly good, recent reports from this group show a clear difference in mortality between early (6 hrs, 4% mortality) and later (8% to 9% mortality) surgery in those patients sustaining transmural infarctions. Additionally, the Spokane group has defined preexisting three-vessel disease as a higher risk condition for emergency aortocoronary bypass surgery, with at least a 10% mortality rate.[11] In many institutions, prompt initiation of thrombolytic therapy appears to result in early reperfusion of infarcted myocardium.[12,13] Although such therapy can be associated with reclosure,[14,15] the fact remains that the quickest and most practical way to initiate early reperfusion appears to be with thrombolysis rather than with emergency aortocoronary bypass surgery. When thrombolysis fails, or even if it succeeds, interventional therapies—PTCA or aortocoronary bypass surgery—may still be employed, and a variety of patient-specific and local institutional factors should be emphasized in the decisions regarding further treatment.[16]

Alderman[17] studied the benefits of surgical therapy in an elective, nonurgent setting for patients with severe ventricular dysfunction. While operative mortality figures were surprisingly low, 7% to 10% in this cohort, operative survival was not synonymous with freedom from symptoms. Aortocoronary bypass surgery most benefitted those patients whose primary symptom was angina, but surgery was neither more safe nor more helpful than medicine for those patients who suffered primarily from congestive heart failure.

Although resection of a ventricular aneurysm in conjunction with aortocoronary bypass surgery may relieve ventricular tachycardia, modern methods of cardiac electrophysiology have made this treatment philosophy seem simplistic. Currently, proper treatment for patients with recurrent ventricular arrhythmias or sudden death syndromes involves mapping both the character and location of the unwanted rhythm, followed by administration of antiarrhythmic medicines, surgical ablation with or without aortocoronary bypass surgery, or both. Surgically implantable defibrillators are also available and may be used more commonly in the coming years. While elective aortocoronary bypass surgery may benefit some patients with arrhythmias, it has not proved effective as a complete therapy and is not recommended for them.

The study of subsets of patients with known coronary disease, with or without symptoms, but anatomically distinct from that in the previously mentioned groups, remains the most interesting challenge. Moreover, the questions of if and when such patients should be treated with aortocoronary bypass surgery has been impacted by the widespread use of PTCA. While physicians are attempting to define the proper indications for aortocoronary bypass surgery, the true efficacy of PTCA, as well as how these two interventional treatment strategies can be combined to benefit patients, has yet to be established.[18,19] Currently, several large multicenter trials have begun to attempt to determine the relative successes of angioplasty and aortocoronary bypass surgery in terms of survival, event-free survival, and cost-effectiveness.

What are the indications for aortocoronary bypass surgery? At this time, aortocoronary bypass surgery seems appropriate for patients with significant left main coronary disease, triple-vessel disease with moderate ventricular dysfunction, and any angina that is unresponsive to medical therapy in patients who are not candidates for PTCA. Additionally, patients who have significant coronary disease with unstable or severe angina should be considered as operative candidates, even if ventricular function is normal. Acute myocardial infarctions can be treated by urgent aortocoronary bypass surgery but, because of time constraints, are more often treated with thrombolysis and PTCA when interventional therapy seems appropriate. Although the roles of PTCA and aortocoronary bypass surgery in nonurgent settings are not clearly defined, a harmonious relationship between the operators of both treatments is beneficial.

MYOCARDIAL PRESERVATION

Interestingly, hypothermia antedated cardioplegic solutions and even mechanical extracorporeal circulation as a functional means of protecting the heart and other organs during anoxic arrest. Bigelow's[20,21] experimental and clinical work in the late 1940s demonstrated the efficacy of hypothermic protection. In the early 1950s, closure of septal defects was accomplished with hypothermia and simple inflow occlusion.[22] John and Maly Gibbon[23] in Philadelphia in 1953, and later John Kirklin[24]

in Rochester, Minnesota, reported clinical successes with extracorporeal pumps and oxygenators. Almost simultaneously (1954) C. Walton Lillehei,[25] in Minneapolis, used cross-circulation between mother and child for successful "direct vision intracardiac surgery." Shumway[26] championed the addition of topical hypothermia in the 1960s. Although various methods of chemically induced arrest and protection had been attempted, none enjoyed widespread popularity until Gay and Ebert[27] revived the technique in the early 1970s. While some variations in techniques exist from center to center, currently the vast majority of adult cardiac procedures are accomplished by using cold chemical cardioplegic solutions in combination with both systemic and topical hypothermia.

Systemic hypothermia is classified as mild (more than 32° C), moderate (32 to 25° C), or deep (less than 25° C), with most procedures calling for moderate hypothermic levels achieved by perfusion cooling via the extracorporeal circuit. After 25 to 30 mins of global ischemia, the normothermic heart manifests severe metabolical, ultrastructural, and physiologic injuries, incapacitating its ability to sustain life.[28] Early pioneers of cardiac surgery quickly recognized that as temperature fell, oxygen consumption also decreased, and that adequate oxygen fortunately could be delivered to tissues in the hypothermic state. Although hypothermia shifts the oxyhemoglobin-dissociation curve to the left, this is counterbalanced by the marked increase in the plasma solubility of oxygen and carbon dioxide. Moreover, reduced metabolic demands during hypothermia allow for lower perfusion flows. Ellis[29] showed that with a low-flow of 40 cc/kg/min and a low-pressure of 60 mmHg, cardiopulmonary bypass did not result in cerebral dysfunction. Lower perfusion rates also enhance myocardial protection by reducing collateral venous return to the heart (Figure 6.1). These bronchial, pulmonary, and noncoronary collaterals can otherwise rewarm the heart during the arrest period, embarrassing myocardial protection and obscuring the operative field. Finally, systemic hypothermia and lower perfusion pressures add a "fail-safe" mechanism to routine cardiopulmonary bypass by generating lower arterial line pressures, making catastrophic line explosions less likely and allowing for a brief interruption of cardiopulmonary bypass should an accident occur or extra surgical exposure be required (Table 6.1).

When a surgeon cross-clamps the ascending aorta, the myocardium rapidly changes from its normal obligate aerobe state to an anaerobic state. Since myocardial oxygen reserves are depleted in less than 10 secs of global ischemic arrest, significant injury will occur unless the surgeon attempts to "protect" the vulnerable heart muscle with cardioplegic solutions.[30]

Cardioplegic solutions can generally be divided into two major groups:

- Crystalloid cardioplegic solutions.
- Blood cardioplegic solutions.

While a detailed review of the various permutations currently in use is beyond the scope of this chapter, the truth is that the formula for a perfect cardioplegic solution is still unknown. Moreover, the extrapolation of the considerable experimental work in this area to the operating room must be tempered with logic, reproducibility, and clinical relevance. Regardless of

the cardioplegic solution selected, current thinking dictates adherence to certain basic principles. The solution should:
- Produce a rapid cardiac arrest.
- Be cold, so as to "slow" the metabolic processes.
- Avoid the creation of intracellular edema.
- Provide buffering for the arrested, acidic tissues.

Cold (4–10° C) potassium, the most commonly used cardioplegic agent, induces rapid, diastolic arrest that, generally, can be sustained until it is washed out via noncoronary collateral flow during the arrest period, or coronary flow upon removal of the aortic cross-clamp. Concentrations between 15 and 30 mEq/L of potassium are used, and most centers employ intermittent (every 20 to 30 mins) reinfusions of the cardioplegic solution during the global arrest period to prevent washout and to combat rewarming. Rewarming of the heart during the arrest period, which is usually caused by noncoronary collateral flow, can be dangerous. Additionally, the higher temperatures in the operating room, surgical drapes, operating room lights, or some combination of these may also be involved. Rewarming can be minimized by employing systemic hypothermia via the heart-lung machine, by irrigating the pericardial contents with topical cold solutions, by lowering perfusion pressures to decrease noncoronary collateral flow, and by reinfusing cold cardioplegic solution intermittently. Myocardial temperatures of 10° C to 15° C are usually generated and sustained through these techniques.

Ischemic tissue commonly becomes edematous when it is reperfused, and such edema can seriously embarrass normal function if the tissue in question is cardiac muscle. Osmolar/oncotic agents—mannitol, glucose, albumin, dextran—are added to virtually all cardioplegic solutions to minimize fluid accumulation upon the return of coronary blood flow.[31] Although acidosis is a known consequence of ischemia, the ideal pH of cardioplegic solutions is yet to be determined.[32] Finding the solution to this problem may be difficult because the highly dynamic nature of myocardial ischemia created during elective cardiac surgical procedures greatly alters arrest times from day to day,

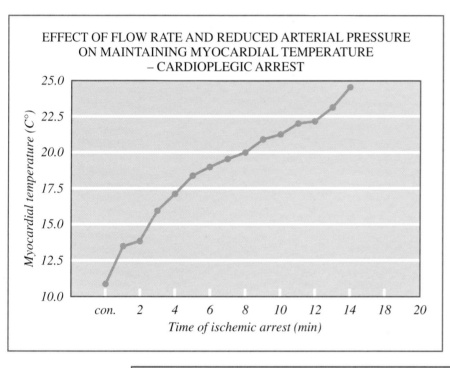

EFFECT OF FLOW RATE AND REDUCED ARTERIAL PRESSURE ON MAINTAINING MYOCARDIAL TEMPERATURE – CARDIOPLEGIC ARREST

Myocardial temperature (C°) — y-axis: 25.0, 22.5, 20.0, 17.5, 15.0, 12.5, 10.0

Time of ischemic arrest (min) — x-axis: con., 2, 4, 6, 8, 10, 12, 14, 18, 20

FIGURE 6.1 • The effect of maintaining flow rate less than 40 cc/kg and reduced arterial pressure less than 60 torr on sustaining the myocardial temperature below 20° C for 45 min of cardioplegic arrest. (Reproduced with permission. Ellis RJ, Wisniewski A, Potts R, et al: *J Thorac Cardiovasc Surg* 1983;79: 173.

TABLE 6.1 • HYPOTHERMIA "FAIL-SAFE"		
Temperature	Normal O$_2$ consumption (%)	Duration of anoxic circulatory arrest (min)
37° C	100	3–5
28° C	50	8–10
22° C	25	16–20
16° C	12	32–40
10° C	<10	64–80

case to case, and surgeon to surgeon. Hypothermia can alter other conditions as well. Rahn et al[33] have shown that pH rises .0134 units for each centigrade degree drop in temperature. Despite such vagaries, most cardioplegic solutions have buffering capacities that are thought to be appropriate for the times, temperatures, and surgeons that use them.

In recent years, some surgeons have used blood cardioplegia in their operating rooms. In theory, the red blood cells in the cardioplegic solution have the capacity to carry oxygen and deliver it in satisfactory amounts to the anoxic, hypothermic, arrested heart.[34] In practice, many centers have recognized no differences when blood cardioplegia is used in lieu of crystalloid solutions.[35] This may be due to the leftward shift of the oxyhemoglobin-dissociation curve that accompanies decreasing temperatures, for example the hypothermic conditions used in the operating room. Magovern et al.[36] demonstrated no effective benefits of blood cardioplegia in terms of tissue pO_2 at temperatures lower than 20° C. Since it appears that oxygen is efficiently released only at temperatures warmer than those employed in clinical cardiac surgery, the theoretical advantages of blood cardioplegia may be negated. Buckberg[37,38] and associates have recently suggested a scheme whereby warm (37° C) blood cardioplegia is infused initially ("warm induction"), followed by intermittent administration of cold (4°) cardioplegia to maintain hypothermia, and finally by infusion of warm cardioplegia ("hot shot") prior to removal of the aortic cross-clamp. Some surgeons have embraced this concept, but whether practical benefits are routinely derived remains to be seen.

Cardioplegia can be delivered through two possible routes—antegrade and retrograde. Antegrade delivery is usually accomplished through the aortic root by inserting a needle into the closed aorta proximal to an aortic cross-clamp, or it can be accomplished by directly cannulating a coronary os through an aortotomy incision. Potential disadvantages of antegrade delivery systems lie in these facts:

- The patient's native coronary artery disease may hinder even distribution of cardioplegia, since flow to the areas most affected by disease may be obstructed.
- Closed aortic root delivery requires a competent aortic valve to force the cardioplegic solution throughout the coronary artery tree.

In the latter case, many patients have some degree of aortic valvar incompetence, which leads to left ventricular distension when substantial volumes of cardioplegia are delivered in this fashion. Cardioplegia in the left ventricular chamber is not only useless for myocardial protection, it also distends the ventricle and increases left ventricular wall tension, both of which should be avoided if good protection is desired.

Retrograde delivery involves the infusion of cardioplegic solution through the coronary venous tree, via the coronary sinus. This can be accomplished either by directly cannulating the os of the coronary sinus or by creating a closed loop in the right atrium, causing solutions infused into the right atrium to exit via the coronary sinus (Figure 6.2). Proponents believe that retrograde

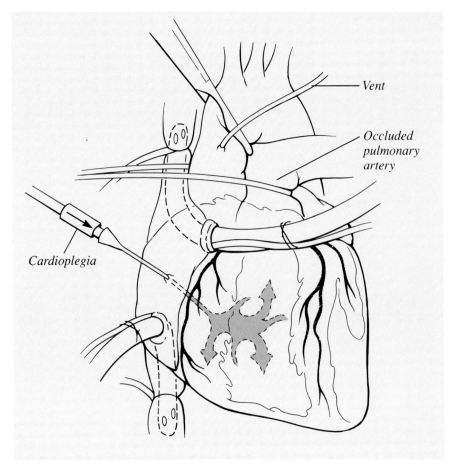

Cardioplegia

Vent

Occluded pulmonary artery

FIGURE 6.2 • Cannulation of the coronary sinus is achieved via a small puncture in the right atrial free wall. If needed, an atriotomy incision allows for placement of the cardioplegia line into the coronary sinus as under direct vision.

delivery systems generate better global distribution of cardioplegia and cooling than antegrade systems and that retrograde delivery may be the method of choice in patients with severe coronary artery disease.[39–41] Additionally, such systems may enhance the surgeon's vision during aortic valve surgery, since there are no needles or tubing lines directly within the aortotomy area. Detractors of retrograde systems point out that they may be more cumbersome and inexact, that delivery of the cardioplegic solution is slow since it must be given at lower pressures appropriate for veins, that injury to the coronary sinus is possible, and that individual variations in coronary sinus anatomy make uniform global protection less likely than originally thought (Figure 6.3).[42]

OPERATIVE PROCEDURE

Creative surgeons began to devise operative schemes for relief of angina pectoris near the turn of the century. In 1916, Jonnesco[43]

first employed cervical sympathectomy, hoping to interrupt the pain fibers to the heart. Although there were some successes reported with this technique, the recognition that the pain was due to a reduction in arterial blood flow to the heart muscle demanded new treatment strategies. In 1935, Beck[44] used epicardial abrasion to stimulate the development of intramyocardial collaterals, and in 1946, Vineberg[45] took this concept one step further by directly implanting the internal mammary artery into the left ventricular myocardium. Interestingly, both procedures achieved the stated goal of increasing the intramyocardial arterial circulation, although both the amount and durability of the increase were debated. Direct attacks upon the coronary arteries were initiated in 1957 by Bailey,[46] who advocated coronary endarterectomy. Because of the small size and fragility of the coronary arteries, endarterectomies were limited to larger, proximal segments of the vessels, thereby reducing the general utility of the procedure.

Favaloro,[47] in Cleveland, and Johnson,[48] in Milwaukee, were among the earliest to popularize direct anastomotic tech-

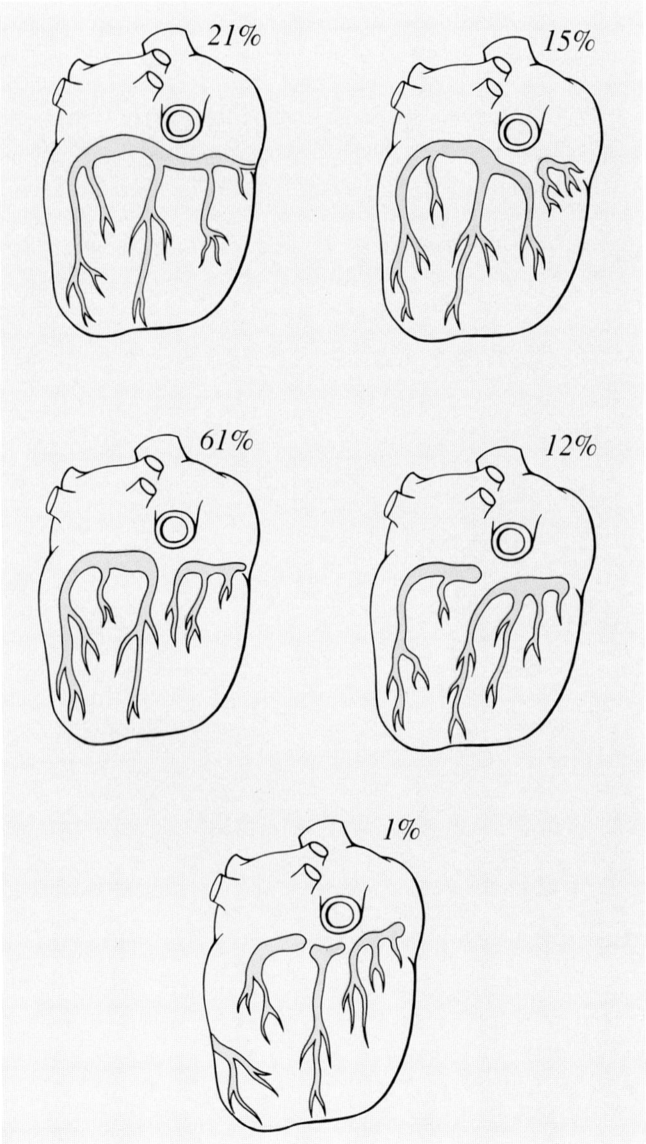

FIGURE 6.3 • Common coronary sinus anatomy patterns. The variety in this venous drainage system may create a less-than-uniform response to retrograde cardioplegia techniques. (Modified with permission. Ludinghausen M: Nomenclature and distribution pattern of cardiac veins in man. In: Mohl W, Faxon D, Wolner E, eds. *Clinics of CSI: Proceedings* New York, NY: Springer-Verlag; 1986:13.)

niques in which a segment of saphenous vein was interposed between the ascending aorta and a diseased coronary artery—aortocoronary bypass. These workers demonstrated that coronaries as small as 1 mm could be used in the procedure and that good long-term patency rates were achievable. More recently, the internal mammary artery has resurfaced as an efficacious tool, this time as a potentially superior bypass conduit when directly anastomosed to coronary arteries[49,50] (Figure 6.4). Today the majority of patients undergoing aortocoronary bypass surgery receive a combination of saphenous vein and internal mammary artery bypass grafts.

TECHNIQUE FOR AORTOCORONARY BYPASS

After systemic heparinization—approximately 3 mg/kg—is achieved, cardiopulmonary bypass is usually instituted by placing cannulas in the ascending aorta to return oxygenated blood from the extracorporeal circuit, and in the right atrium to shunt venous blood into the extracorporeal circuit. Right atrial cannulation is accomplished either via a single, large cannula or via two smaller cannulas that traverse the atrium to lie directly in the superior and inferior venae cavae. Once cannulation is completed, cardiopulmonary bypass is initiated, and some measure of systemic cooling is achieved through the heat exchanger in the bypass circuit. In general, temperatures of 28° C to 30° C are employed, although this may vary from case to case or surgeon to surgeon. When a longer pump run is anticipated, lower temperatures are often indicated. Moreover, the level of induced systemic hypothermia may influence the flow and pressure levels in the pump circuit. For instance, at 28° C, flow rates of 3.0 to 3.5 L/min/m^2

are possible in most adults. At lower temperatures, flow rates of 2.0 to 2.5 L/min/m^2, or even less, can be safely employed.

Once hypothermia has been induced and extracorporeal circulation has been instituted, the ascending aorta is cross-clamped and cardioplegic solution is delivered to arrest the cardiac muscle and to "protect" it. Many surgeons "vent" or decompress the left ventricle during the arrest period, either through the aortic root or, transatrially, through the right superior pulmonary vein.

In the final analysis, the selection of a particular artery or arteries requiring bypass grafting depends largely upon the experience and expertise of the surgeon.[51] Every major or secondary coronary artery in which the luminal diameter is occluded by more than 50% should be considered for bypass grafting. If these vessels are too small (less than 1 mm in diameter), have poor runoff, or are not functionally important (the vessel is not a significant source of blood for the respective region of myocardium), the time used in creating an anastomosis may be superfluous, dangerous, or both. Moreover, if an adjacent epicardial vessel has already been bypassed, the artery may often safely be ignored. Most patients undergoing aortocoronary bypass surgery will require three or more grafts, with the average ranging from 3.3 to 3.7.[51,52]

Anatomic considerations are important, and proper surgical treatment must be based upon a working knowledge of the functional aspects of coronary anatomy. When the right coronary artery system is dominant (greater than 80% of patients), the posterior aspects of the right and left ventricles, as well as a large portion of the interventricular system, are supplied by the right coronary flow. In this setting, the optimal site for a distal anastomosis is at or just above the crux—the point where the

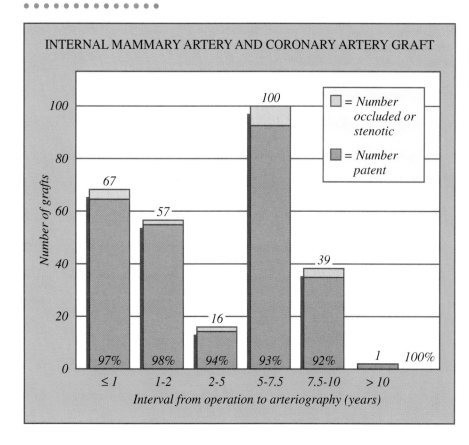

FIGURE 6.4 • Relationship of internal mammary artery to coronary artery graft status to postoperative interval. Even more than 7.5 years after operation, over 90% of grafts were patent. (Reproduced with permission. Lytle BW, Loop FD, Cosgrove DM, et al: *J Thorac Cardiovasc Surg* 1985;84:248.)

right coronary bifurcates into posterior descending and posterior ventricular branches. A direct anastomosis to the posterior descending branch or, less commonly, the posterior ventricular branch, may be required if the crux area is too diseased. If all three vessels are severely diseased, a coronary endarterectomy is usually indicated[53] (Figure 6.5). Patients with dominant left

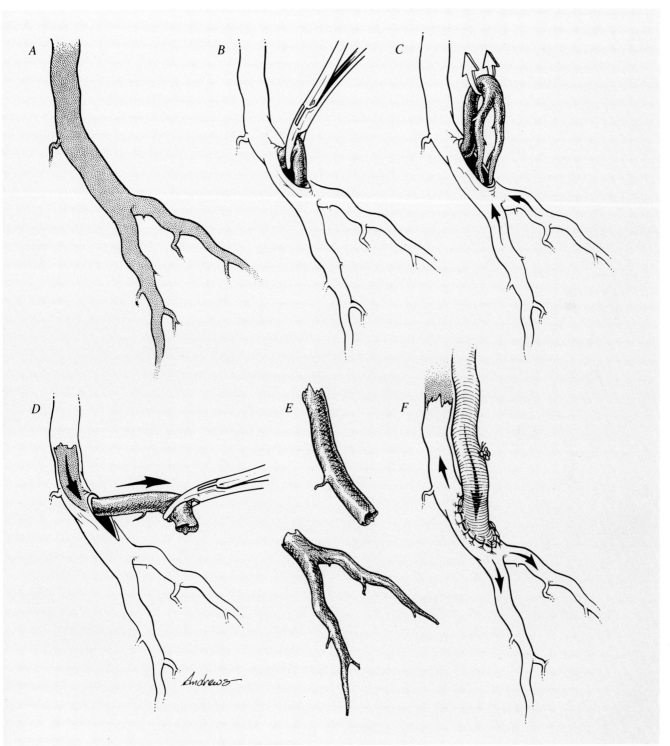

FIGURE 6.5 • Technique for performing right coronary artery endarterectomy. The occluded right coronary artery (A). Just above the crux, the incision is made and the core is brought out through the incision. Gentle traction is exerted on the distal portion while the artery is peeled back (B). Complete endarterectomy results when all the distal branches are free of plaquing. The distal vessels are individually cleared. The proximal portion is then removed by gentle traction until it breaks free from the proximal area. It is not important to obtain a clearly feathered proximal portion (C,D). When the distal specimen and small branches have feathered ends, the specimen is considered satisfactory (E). To assure flow in both directions, the vein graft is placed to the arteriotomy (F). (Modified from Cooley DA: *Techniques in Cardiac Surgery* Philadelphia, Pa: WB Saunders; 1982.)

coronary artery systems—the posterior left ventricle and interventricular septum are supplied via the left circumflex system—can rarely benefit from bypasses to the right coronary. Indeed, most of these patients have atrophic right coronary systems. In a few patients, the right and left coronary systems are balanced, and posterior descending arteries arise from both left and right coronary trees.

The preferred site for anastomosis in the left anterior descending coronary artery is just distal to the most significant obstruction. Generally, this region begins about one half to two thirds of the way down the course of the vessel, where it lies upon or close to the epicardial surface of the heart. Significantly diseased diagonal branches of the left anterior descending artery are also amenable to bypass grafting, but good judgment must be used to ensure that these vessels are of adequate size and of functional importance. The circumflex coronary system is revascularized by grafting the obtuse marginal branches. The circumflex artery proper, which lies in the atrioventricular groove, is not usually bypassed, because surgical exposure is difficult. In addition, when the heart is refilled and active, the bypass graft may be compressed between the heart and spine. The ramus medialis, when present, originates near the bifurcation of the left main coronary artery. This vessel is often bypassed because it is usually of good size and has functional impact (Figure 6.6).

Proximal anastomoses are created on the ascending aorta after measuring the length of each vein graft. The normal size of the filled, beating heart should be considered in sizing these vein grafts. Moreover, most vein grafts undergo some contraction with time. The anastomoses may be performed with the aorta cross-clamped or with a partially occluding aortic clamp that allows for some myocardial reperfusion through native coronaries after the aortic cross-clamp has been removed. Some attention should be given to evacuating air from the ascending aorta, the vein grafts, or both.

The greater saphenous vein is generally preferred for aorto-coronary bypass surgery, but when it has been previously removed or damaged, the lesser saphenous vein in the posterior calf, or arm cephalic or basilic veins may be used. Additionally, multiple sequential anastomoses using right and left internal mammary arteries can be performed. The use of prosthetic materials has been described, but current results are poor, and such practices should be considered experimental. Handling the bypass grafts gently is very important, as is avoiding trauma during their removal (Figure 6.7). Side branches should be ligated expertly to prevent the grafts from becoming kinked or distorted and, thus, to avoid compromising luminal flow. The grafts are commonly distended with some solution during this ligation process, although care must be taken to avoid the over-distension that leads to intimal damage.[54]

• • • • • • • • • • • • • • • •

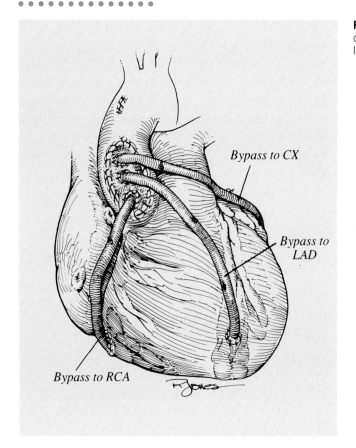

FIGURE 6.6 • Bypass grafts placed to the circumflex, left anterior descending, and right coronary arteries. (Courtesy of the Texas Heart Institute.)

Bypass to CX

Bypass to LAD

Bypass to RCA

Many surgeons[55,56] now consider the internal mammary artery to be an ideal conduit for bypassing diseased coronary arteries because of the following factors:

- The artery, with its associated vein and lymphatics, is encompassed in a living pedicle of muscle and tissue.
- The adventitial blood supply to the artery is intact.
- The diameter of the internal mammary more closely approximates that of the adult coronary arteries.

- An internal mammary-coronary anastomosis provides a match of arterial to arterial endothelium.
- No proximal anastomosis is required.

Despite such advantages, clinical settings may exist in which using an internal mammary artery bypass graft is unwise. For instance, patients with severe chronic obstructive pulmonary disease may have expansive lungs that place too much stress on

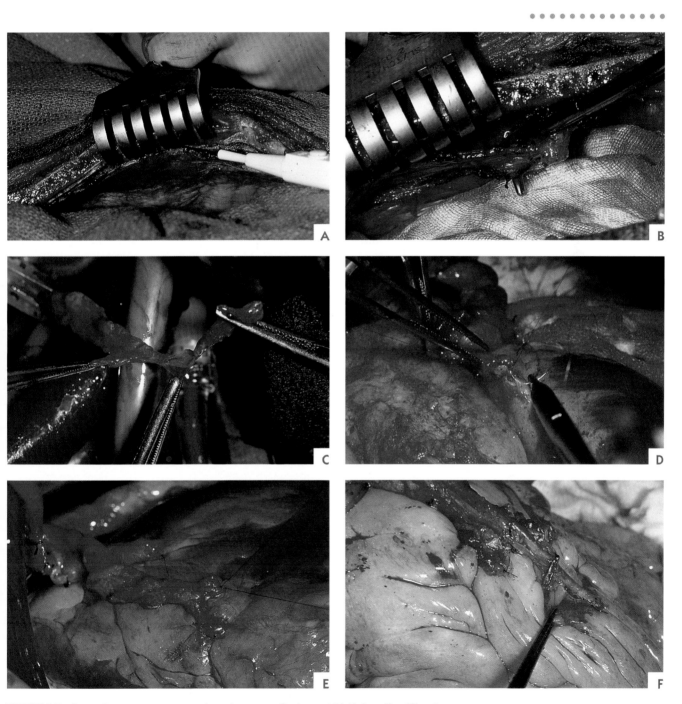

FIGURE 6.7 • Internal mammary artery used as a bypass graft—harvest (A,B), handling (C), suture anastomosis (D,E), and complete anastomosis (F). (Courtesy of the Texas Heart Institute.)

the internal mammary artery pedicle during inhalation. Also important, the flow through the internal mammary should be gauged, either formally or informally, prior to grafting to avoid using a diseased artery. The intercostal arteries must also be divided from the internal mammary artery lest a "steal" phenomenon occur, resulting in decreased flow to the coronary artery. The process of harvesting the internal mammary artery may produce a vasospasm that can severely limit flow to the bypassed vessel. Finally, harvesting the internal mammary pedicle may diminish the blood supply to the ipsilateral half of the divided sternum. Although there is no readily apparent increase in sternal wound complications following the harvest of one internal mammary artery, using both of them may cause such problems and is controversial.[57]

CLINICAL RESULTS

In operative survivors, the clinical results of myocardial revascularization are directly related to graft patency. This is true regardless of whether the yardstick used to measure "results" is relief of angina, survival, reoperation, or cardiac events. Despite this fact, identifying the true preoperative and intraoperative predictors of graft patency has been difficult. Specific factors once thought to influence graft patency, but now known to have no independent predictive value, include left ventricular end-diastolic pressure, global left ventricular function, duration of angina, and cigarette smoking.[58] Moreover, Sharma et al.[59] found that even the preoperative assessment of recipient coronary vessels and their proximal stenosis had no bearing on graft patency at one year. However, preoperative assessment of the left ventricular regional wall motion correlated well with one-year patency, in that grafts to normal or hypokinetic regions did much better than those to dyskinetic or akinetic regions—83% versus 45% patency. The relationship of the progression of atherosclerosis and graft patency to serum lipids has been examined,[60] but whether serum lipid levels are independent predictors of graft survival remains to be seen.

Much of this information is problematic, especially when viewed in the context of the most fundamental issue of all: What is the real quality of the distal vessel and the runoff in its particular myocardial bed? A direct measurement of the capacitance of a given recipient coronary bed is difficult and impractical in the everyday clinical setting, yet this information can be reliably inferred by direct intraoperative calibration of both the internal diameter of the recipient coronary artery and the graft flow rate. Flow rates above 100 mL/min have been associated with significantly higher patency rates than those below 50 mL/min—93% versus 56% patency.[61] Similarly, the vessels with the largest internal diameters have the best patency rates. Thus, optimal results will be gained by bypassing large vessels with greater than 2.0 mm internal diameter and high flow capacities greater than 100 mL/min. This information, although quite handy, unfortunately does not address a certain percentage of recipient vessels in the 1.0 to 2.0 mm size range with flow capacities of 60 to 90 mL/min that are bypassed because they are the best vessels available.

The type of bypass conduit, vein or internal mammary artery, also influences graft patency. The short- and long-term patency rates of saphenous vein coronary grafts have been evaluated at the Montreal Heart Institute using repeat angiography.[62–64] After one month, 8% of vein grafts in 94 patients were occluded, and at one year another 8% of the surviving grafts had occluded. This experience mirrors that of other centers. In general, these reports indicate that approximately 10% of saphenous vein bypass grafts occluded in the first postoperative month, and an additional 10% occluded between the first month and one year after surgery. From there, the attrition rate remained stable at about 1 to 2% per year until the sixth postoperative year. During the 6- to 10-year postoperative period, the graft failure rate increased to 5% per year, so that 10- to 12-year vein graft patency was 63% to 66%.[63] In fairness, many of these patients were operated upon prior to the time when careful treatment with antiplatelet agents became routine. Additionally, important technical advances in cardiovascular surgery have been developed within the last decade, so the long-term incidence of graft patency reported at over 10 years would probably not be influenced by current technical advantages.

Chesebro and Fuster[65,66] from the Mayo Clinic studied the influence of aspirin and dipyridamole upon early and one-year vein graft patencies. They concluded that administering dipyridamole for 48 hrs preoperatively, then aspirin and dipyridamole postoperatively, improved vein-graft patency regardless of the size of the bypassed vessel. In particular, repeat angiograms one month after aortocoronary bypass surgery showed overall patency rates of 97% in the treated group versus 80% in the nontreated group, and one year following surgery the difference was 89% versus 75%, respectively. Although debate about the efficacy of dipyridamole continues, most centers now routinely employ some form of antiplatelet therapy—aspirin alone, aspirin plus dipyridamole, or sulfinpyrazone—in hope of improving graft patency in the first postoperative years.[67]

While the progression of atherosclerosis in nonbypassed coronaries accounts for a majority of the reoperations within the initial five to six postoperative years, atherosclerosis developing in the vein graft itself becomes the major factor in later years. Whether antiplatelet medications or antilipid manipulations may alter this trend is unknown.

The internal mammary artery has been shown to be associated with improved bypass patency rates when compared with saphenous vein grafts. In one large study, the occlusion rate for internal mammary artery grafts was one half of that for vein grafts at one year, and in the ensuing 10 years only one (5%) new occlusion occurred in the internal mammary artery group, as opposed to 30 (31%) new occlusions among the vein graft group.[68,69] Additionally, Cosgrove, Loop, et al[70,71] have demonstrated improved patency, fewer late cardiac events, and increased long-term (10-year) survival when comparing internal mammary artery-grafted patients to those with vein grafts—87% versus 76%, p < 0.0001.

SURGERY FOR VALVULAR HEART DISEASE

In the 19th century, surgeons were challenged by the possibility of direct surgery on the human heart, despite the admonitions of surgical authorities such as Billroth[72] and Paget.[73] The surgical correction of valvular stenosis was first forecast by Samways[74] when he wrote that "with the progress of cardiac surgery, some of the severest cases of mitral stenosis will be relieved by slightly notching the mitral valve." In 1902, Sir Thomas Lauder Brunton[75] recorded the ease with which he was able to open a stenosed mitral valve in cadavers. Although criticism followed both of these reports, in 1914 Tuffier[76] reported the first "successful" aortic valvotomy when he invaginated the ascending aortic wall with his finger, but the effect was probably minimal.

The first direct attack on valvular disease came in 1923, when Cutler and Levine[77] introduced a special punch into the mitral valve of an 11-year-old girl in order to excise diseased mitral tissue. Although the procedure was completed successfully and the patient survived for more than four years, significant mitral regurgitation resulted. Two years later, Henry Souttar[78] performed the first finger-fracture valvuloplasty in a young woman who survived for seven years. Although there is some question regarding the true nature of the mitral lesion in this case, the technique of digital dissection through the left atrial appendage was later to become standard for closed repair of mitral stenosis. During this period of time, JH Powers, one of Cutler's surgical residents, demonstrated conclusively in laboratory animals the disastrous implications of mitral regurgitation superimposed on existing mitral stenosis.[79] This report, in addition to Cutler's discouraging results, caused surgeons to discontinue direct operations on the valves.

During World War II, cardiac trauma provided a major stimulus for the development of modern cardiac surgery. Dwight Harken, a captain in the United States Army Medical Corps in England, devised numerous ingenious techniques for removing foreign bodies from the heart and blood vessels. Harken applied these techniques to 134 wounded soldiers, all of whom survived with normal hearts.[80] His success in this endeavor demonstrated the heart's astonishing recuperative powers and helped establish cardiac surgery as a serious discipline.

In the late 1940s, three pioneers in cardiac surgery, Charles Bailey[81] and Dwight Harken[82] in the United States and Lord Brock[83] in England, reported their successes in mitral valve procedures, mitral commissurotomy, valvuloplasty, and valvotomy. Subsequently, Bailey followed Smithy's[84] lead and developed a technique for dilating the calcified, stenotic aortic valve with an instrument introduced through the apex of the left ventricle, but his results were often less than satisfactory. Working independently in London, Brock and Holmes developed a variety of cutting and dilating instruments with which they successfully relieved pulmonic stenosis. The valvotomy instruments were introduced transventricularly, with satisfactory results.

Although these "blind" cardiac procedures were ingenious and soon became routine, they dramatically revealed the need for direct-vision techniques. These were developed in 1953, when Gibbon[85] first used his technique of total cardiopulmonary bypass. Other investigators followed, and by 1955, the open heart era had begun. Acquired valvular disease became amenable to surgical correction. Some of the closed techniques such as mitral valvotomy were performed under direct vision, with improved results. At first, surgeons attacked aortic and mitral stenosis by debriding the calcium deposits and salvaging the natural valve. In most cases, however, particularly those involving the aortic valve, it became obvious that a prosthesis for total valve replacement was necessary.

Credit for developing valvular prostheses belongs to many investigators of that era, with the support and input of engineers and industry. In 1960, Harken[86] reported survival in two of seven patients in whom he had implanted a ball valve in the subcoronary position for severe aortic insufficiency. The next year Albert Starr and M.L. Edwards[87] described their ball-valve prosthesis. Whereas others had labored to create a prosthesis that imitated the anatomy of the human valve, these investigators seized upon an old principle using a caged-ball design. This valve was responsible for bringing valvular prostheses to clinical use. Other early investigators followed this lead, including Hufnagel, Smeloff, Wada, Braunwald, Cooley, Magovern, Kay, Beall, Barnard, Bjork, and Lillehei (Figures 6.8–6.13).

• • • • • • • • • • • • • •

FIGURE 6.8 • Starr-Edwards noncloth-covered aortic ball valve used during the mid-1960s. Development of the Starr-Edwards valve began in the 1950s.

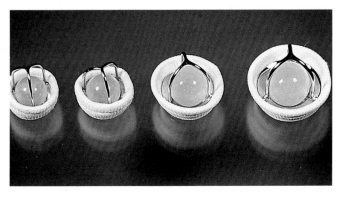

In 1968, Carpentier[88] introduced the use of a glutaraldehyde-treated porcine xenograft (Figure 6.14). The concept of bioprostheses evolved as Carpentier described crosslinkage of collagen fibers of porcine aortic valves with buffered glutaraldehyde. He used an asymmetric stent to support the muscular portion of the right cusp. Other investigators looked at other forms of tissue for valves, including autologous fascia lata, which did not prove to be successful. Discouraged by the poor results with fascia lata prostheses, Ross[89] resumed his work on aortic valve homografts, which he had begun in 1962, when he and Sir Barratt-Boyes[90] independently performed the first successful orthotopic implantations of a homograft valve. In the 1960s, Hancock[91] left Edwards Laboratories and his work with mechanical valves to design a new porcine valve

xenograft (Figure 6.15). Ionescu[92] further simplified the process of making a bioprosthesis. He fashioned a valve from readily available bovine pericardium (Figure 6.16). By using bovine pericardial tissue, Ionescu could make valves in any size desired, circumventing the problem of small aortic valve xenografts.

Today much experience has been gained with both mechanical and bioprosthetic valves. Both types of valves have advantages and disadvantages. Bioprostheses are not as durable as mechanical valves and are associated with more complications, especially calcification. We now prefer mechanical valves in most situations.[93] Although the older mechanical valves were beset with material failures, today's valves are much more durable. Many designs are made with pyrolytic carbon, which has proved to be very durable. These

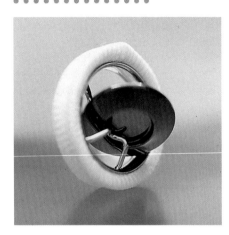

FIGURE 6.9 • Bjork-Shiley tilting disc valve used in the 1970s. The pyrolytic carbon disc is suspended in a Stellite cage.

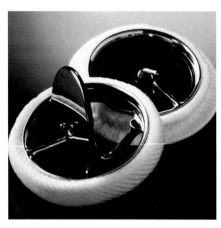

FIGURE 6.10 • The Medtronic-Hall tilting disc valve. The valve has a central perforation that allows the pivoting action of the disc to move more centrally. A guiding rod is inserted through the opening in the middle of the disc. (Crawford FA: *Current Heart Valve Prostheses, Cardiac Surgery: State of the Art Reviews* Philadelphia Pa: Hanley and Belfus; 1987.)

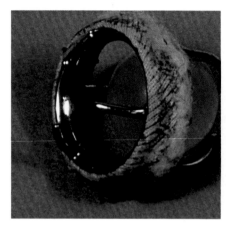

FIGURE 6.11 • Smeloff-Cutter full-orifice caged-ball valve. The valve, used in the 1970s, evolved from work performed in the early 1960s.

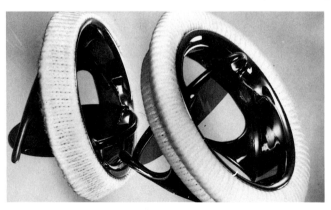

FIGURE 6.12 • Lillehei-Kaster mitral (right) and aortic (left) valves. The pivoting disc valve was introduced clinically in 1970. The valve consists of a pivoting disc suspended in a titanium housing encircled by a knitted Teflon fabric sewing ring. (Courtesy of C. Walter Lillehei, MD.)

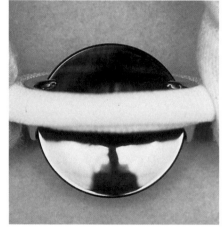

FIGURE 6.13 • Omniscience valve. The Omniscience valve prosthesis was developed as a second generation Lillehei-Kaster valve. This design was modified in 1977. At this time, the convex-concave disc was made smaller, the inner to outer diameter ratio was increased, and the struts were replaced with two rounded elevations.

new valves have wider openings, resulting in minimal regurgitation (Figure 6.17). The only disadvantage of these new mechanical valves is the need for anticoagulation to prevent thromboembolism.

Whenever possible, we repair rather than replace diseased mitral valves. For mitral stenosis, we still use an open valvotomy and have obtained good results. Repair is also generally indicated for mitral regurgitation, which results from either ischemic or degenerative disease and may cause the valve to prolapse. Correction, in these instances, can be accomplished by manipulation or partial excision of the prolapsed leaflet. Annular rings can be used to reinforce the annulus and prevent recurrence. When calcification is present, a mitral valve replacement may be indicated.

When the aortic valve is diseased, it usually needs to be replaced. Some surgeons, however, most notably Duran[94] and Cosgrove, attempt a conservative repair for rheumatic aortic insufficiency. Several surgeons have tried to debride calcified valves by using ultrasound. Recent results, however, have shown an early occurrence of severe and progressive aortic insufficiency after use of this technique.[95–97]

Other attempts to repair diseased valves have been made by interventional cardiologists. The double balloon technique has been used for both mitral and aortic valvotomy with varying degrees of success. This technique has been more successful with the mitral valve than with the aortic valve, although both procedures are associated with complications such as rupture of the annulus, regurgitation, and creation of an atrial septal defect.

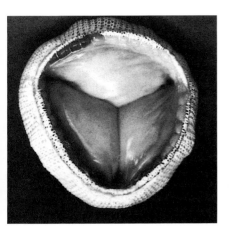
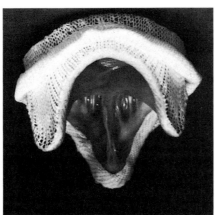
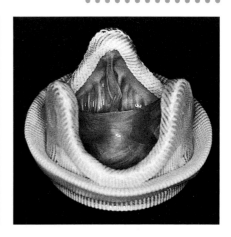

FIGURE 6.14 • Carpentier-Edwards porcine xenograft valve, circa 1976. The valve was preserved with glutaraldehyde.

FIGURE 6.15 • Hancock porcine xenograft valve, circa 1984.

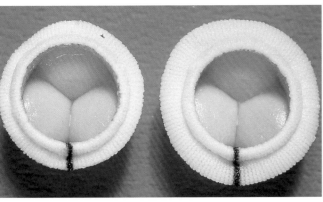
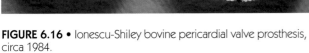
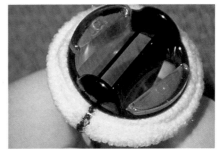

FIGURE 6.17 • St. Jude Medical mechanical valve. The valve was conceived in the 1960s, developed during the mid-1970s, and first implanted clinically in 1977. The valve is machined from graphite and coated with pyrolytic carbon. It has a Dacron sewing ring.

FIGURE 6.16 • Ionescu-Shiley bovine pericardial valve prosthesis, circa 1984.

Often, relief is only temporary. Complications associated with aortic valvotomy are even more severe, and relief is also only temporary. Because of the possibility that severe aortic insufficiency may occur and the generally poor results, our interventional cardiologists no longer perform balloon dilatation of the aortic valve. Children appear to do better than adults, however, and pediatric cardiologists are still using balloon dilatation for palliative treatment of congenital aortic stenosis, although results are variable and unpredictable.[98]

The surgical treatment of valvular disease has advanced far beyond its early beginnings. There has been constant progress toward improvement of valvular prostheses and techniques of repair, and hemodilution has simplified and improved cardiopulmonary bypass. Valve surgery is now an important part of most cardiac programs. Among the 3,000 open cardiac procedures performed annually at the Texas Heart Institute, approximately 20% involve valves. This chapter will describe the indications for operation and the surgical techniques we use to repair and replace diseased heart valves.

INDICATIONS FOR OPERATION

AORTIC STENOSIS

Most instances of aortic valve stenosis are congenital in origin. A large percentage of stenoses that are not diagnosed until adulthood show the anomalous changes, in addition to acquired calcific deposits, that often result from rheumatic fever. Congenital aortic stenosis occurs in approximately 3% of infants born with congenital heart disease.[99] The lesion may occur in many degrees of severity and valve deformity.[100,101] In some patients, the valve shows almost no leaflet development and is represented only by verrucous vestiges without sinuses of Valsalva. In other instances, a well-developed bicuspid arrangement may be present with sinuses of Valsalva.

When the stenosis is severe at birth, symptoms become evident immediately, as there is early onset of left ventricular failure and pulmonary edema. Infants with aortic stenosis often have associated anomalies, including coarctation, patent ductus arteriosus, or septal defects. The left ventricular strain may result in septal ischemia and frank infarction, further complicating the clinical picture. Some patients with a modest level of left ventricular hypertension have syncopal attacks, cardiac arrhythmias, and chest pain, particularly on exertion. Sudden death is not uncommon in such patients and is probably a result of left ventricular fibrillation. Poststenotic dilatation of the ascending aorta is another secondary effect. Ejection click, a systolic crescendo-decrescendo murmur, and aortic regurgitation may also be present.

Therefore, two syndromes seem to be evident in instances of aortic valve stenosis:

- Severe left ventricular failure during the first year of life.
- A milder degree of left ventricular failure appears late in childhood or even in early adolescence.

There may be a period during early childhood when patients are even free of symptoms. The small and fixed orifice may be adequate for cardiac output during the first 2 to 5 years of life, but because it does not increase in size, it cannot accommodate the output needed during late childhood or adolescence.

Physicians are increasingly turning to transthoracic echocardiography to diagnose aortic stenosis. Echocardiograms can show changes in valvular structure, such as thickening and calcification of the valve leaflets, as well as valve gradients. Transesophageal echocardiography (TEE), which is now a standard method used to evaluate prosthetic valves, is also used to diagnose endocarditis in native valves (Figure 6.18). Transesophageal echocardiography can detect abscesses of the aortic root and is useful in diagnosis when transthoracic echocardiography gives inadequate results (approximately 10% of patients). It is especially useful in diagnosing perivalvular leaks. Our cardiologists still occasionally perform catheterization and angiography to measure the pressure gradient across the valve and to evaluate the extent of stenosis and left ventricular function. Although we sometimes perform diagnostic exercise studies, we do so very cautiously in patients with a history of syncope.

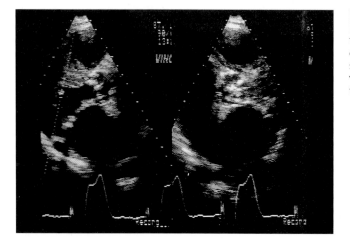

FIGURE 6.18 • Two-dimensional echocardiographic parasternal long axis view (left side) in a patient with severe aortic stenosis, illustrating a heavily calcified aortic valve with severely restricted leaflet excursion. Parasternal short axis view (right side) in the same patient showing severely calcified aortic valve. (LV, left ventricle; AV, aortic valve; AoR, aortic root; LA, left atrium; RA, right atrium.) (Courtesy of the Texas Heart Institute.)

Surgical treatment of aortic stenosis may become an acute emergency in infants, whereas in late childhood or adolescence elective operation may be performed under more optimal conditions. The risk of operation is much higher in infants and is probably related to the incidence of associated myocardial ischemia and infarction in that group.

AORTIC INCOMPETENCE

Aortic incompetence has a variety of causes, but the most common are rheumatic valve disease, bacterial endocarditis, a congenitally bicuspid or unicuspid valve, and annuloaortic ectasia. Patients with aortic incompetence generally have pulmonary venous hypertension. Patients with aortic incompetence should be evaluated for coronary artery disease, as the two often coexist. Mitral stenosis may also be present.

Aortic incompetence is diagnosed in much the same manner as aortic stenosis. The degree of aortic incompetence can be determined from cineangiography with contrast injection of the aortic root in the right anterior oblique position. Generally, we also perform coronary arteriography in patients over 40.

ANNULOAORTIC ECTASIA

We first applied the name annuloaortic ectasia to a characteristic lesion that had cystic medionecrosis confined to the aortic annular region.[102] The enlarged annulus on angiography has the appearance of a Florence flask, such as is used in the chemistry laboratory. In the classic case, aortic incompetence is produced by stretching the aortic valve leaflets and displacing the commissures. The coronary orifices are also displaced upward, making the standard valve replacement unsatisfactory.

Indications for operation in patients with aortic disease depend mostly upon the pressure flow gradient across the left ventricular outflow tract. In general, when the gradient exceeds 50 mmHg, operative correction is indicated.

MITRAL STENOSIS AND REGURGITATION

Lesions of the mitral valve may be either stenotic, regurgitant, or a combination of both. Acquired mitral stenosis is most often caused by acute rheumatic fever and chronic rheumatic valvulitis. Other factors, however, may cause mitral stenosis, including bacterial endocarditis, congenital prolapse, myxoid degeneration, rupture of the chordae tendineae, and myocardial ischemia, all of which result in incompetence and annular dilatation. Congenital lesions of the mitral valve can also be stenotic or regurgitant. Such lesions are often related to cystic medionecrosis, congenital clefts, or other rare conditions.

Mitral disease is generally diagnosed noninvasively by transthoracic echocardiography. Indications for using transesophageal echocardiography for diagnosis are the same as for the aortic valve. We are, however, using transesophageal echocardiography more often to diagnose mitral disease than to diagnose aortic disease.

Mitral Stenosis

About half of the patients with mitral stenosis have a history of rheumatic fever. Generally, patients have symptoms of dyspnea, orthopnea, and easy fatigability. They may also have dysphasia if the esophagus is obstructed in any way by the left atrium.

Although the cardiac silhouette may be normal on chest roentgenogram, there often is left atrial enlargement, including a prominent left atrial appendage and posterior displacement of the left atrium in the lateral projection. The left main stem bronchus may be elevated. Pulmonary venous hypertension may cause additional problems.

Cardiac catheterization is often still performed to determine the diastolic gradient across the mitral valve prior to operation. Based on this information, the physiologic severity of the stenosis can be determined, and a better guess as to the degree of repair necessary can be made.

The prognosis for patients with untreated mitral stenosis who progress to NYHA class III or IV is not good. In one analysis,[103] the only patients with a relatively good prognosis were those in NYHA class II with sinus rhythm. Patients in class III often develop atrial fibrillation, which severely limits their prognosis. Most patients die from complications of their disease,[104] most commonly congestive heart failure, 62%; thromboembolic complications, 22%; and infectious endocarditis, 8%. Over half of the patients older than 40 years and with episodes of atrial fibrillation experience systemic emboli.[104,105] Most emboli are cerebral,[104] causing death in 50% of patients.

Once patients with mitral stenosis develop symptoms, surgery should be considered. Certainly patients in class III or IV who have experienced onset of atrial fibrillation, increasing pulmonary hypertension, an episode of systemic embolization, or infective endocarditis should be operated upon. Any patient over the age of 40 whose lifestyle is limited or whose valve area is severely reduced, even though he/she may be in class II, should be considered for surgery.

Mitral Regurgitation

As in mitral stenosis, rheumatic fever causes most cases of mitral regurgitation. The other two most common causes are mitral valve prolapse and ischemic heart disease. Mitral valve prolapse, which is present in 3 to 4% of the population, may also cause mitral regurgitation. In approximately 5% of patients,[104] mitral regurgitation becomes significant, generally a result of myxomatous degeneration, and requires surgery. Patients with mitral regurgitation resulting from ischemic heart disease have a poor prognosis when there is severe ventricular dysfunction, usually an ejection fraction of less than 20%. Untreated, patients will eventually die from congestive heart failure and pulmonary edema.

In mitral regurgitation, the valve leaflets often become short and rigid. The chordae tendineae also become shortened and fibrotic. Fusion of the commissures precludes closure, allowing calcification to attack the leaflets. Calcification occurs most often in the presence of hypertension, which may result from diabetes, and aortic stenosis. The calcium can be localized to the annulus or move onto the ventricular myocardium and the subvalvular region. When it invades the myocardium, the coronary arteries and conduction system in the area may be affected.

The physical signs of mitral regurgitation are similar to those found in patients with mitral stenosis. Diagnosis of mitral regurgitation can be made definitively by cardiac catheterization, but noninvasive methods are extremely useful. A chest roentgenogram will show left atrial enlargement in chronic cases and dilatation of the left ventricle as a result of volume overload. Right ventricular enlargement is also common.

Patients with mitral regurgitation should be followed closely. Operation is recommended for patients whose symptoms progress to NYHA class III or IV and for any patient whose lifestyle is compromised by his symptoms. Many patients with mild regurgitation—those in class I or II—may remain stable for years before surgery is necessary. Even patients with mild symptoms, however, should be considered for surgery if they experience increasing pulmonary hypertension or atrial fibrillation. Emergency valve replacement should be done in patients with infective endocarditis who do not respond to antibiotic therapy and as a result develop pulmonary or systemic emboli, annular abscess, or hemodynamic deterioration. If antibiotic therapy is successful, operation can be performed on an elective basis.

TRICUSPID VALVE DISEASE

The tricuspid valve may be affected by both congenital and acquired disease. Surgical treatment depends on the etiology and pathological findings. Congenital lesions are usually due to stenosis or complete atresia, and such lesions are generally associated with a large right-to-left shunt through a foramen ovale. In acquired lesions, the annulus in the area of the septal leaflet, the valve leaflets, and the chordae are generally normal. Acquired disease is often caused by mitral valve disease, pulmonary hypertension, and congenital heart disease, especially ventricular septal defect, atrioventricular canal, and cor pulmonale. Cardiac tumors may also affect the tricuspid valve. Valve incompetence results.

The pathologic changes associated with tricuspid valve disease resemble those described for the mitral valve and include thickening and fusion of the leaflets and chordae. The valve becomes stenotic. The patient most likely develops significant right atrial hypertension in the presence of both stenotic and regurgitant valves. Symptoms are related mostly to the presence of systemic venous hypertension. Although isolated tricuspid valve disease may not be an indication for operation, especially in the presence of normal pulmonary artery pressure, when patients have coexisting disease of the mitral valve, pulmonary hypertension, or right ventricular failure, the patient's condition will deteriorate to the point that operation is indicated.

Acquired lesions of the tricuspid valve may be either primary or secondary. Tricuspid stenosis generally results from rheumatic disease and most often the mitral valve is also involved. Both tricuspid stenosis and regurgitation may cause systemic venous hypertension. Hepatic congestion is common. As a result, patients often experience fatigue and weakness with associated fluid retention and edema. Dyspnea is common and liver or renal failure can result. When tricuspid valve disease is combined with mitral valve disease and when

pulmonary hypertension and right ventricular failure are present, an operation will usually be necessary.

Transthoracic echocardiography is also used to diagnose disease of the tricuspid valve. Doppler ultrasonic measurements of valve flow profiles have been used to diagnose tricuspid disease. If disease is suspected, the tricuspid valve can be palpated during a procedure on the mitral valve.

OPERATIVE STRATEGY

AORTIC VALVE REPLACEMENT

The standard operation for correcting aortic valve lesions is performed through a median sternotomy incision.[106] In order to prevent complications associated with disruption of the brachial plexus, the surgeon must be careful not to open the sternum too widely, and the anesthesia staff must not hyperextend the shoulders. A midline incision is made in the pericardium.

Heparin, 3 mg/kg, is administered, and cannulation is begun by placing the cannula in the ascending aorta first. Sutures should be carefully inserted into the adventitia of the aortic wall to prevent perforation into the lumen. A single, large-bore 52F, right atrial cannula with multiple perforations is used for venous outflow. The tip of the catheter is placed into the orifice of the inferior vena cava so that some of the perforations are in the right atrium. In patients in whom mitral procedures are performed concomitantly or in any mitral procedure, we usually cannulate the superior and inferior venae cavae separately, because traction on the atrium will sometimes occlude the single-bore catheters. After cardiopulmonary bypass is initiated, the ascending aorta is cross-clamped, and hypothermic cardiac arrest is induced by injecting 500 cc of cold, lactated Ringer's solution (5% dextrose) containing 20 mEq of potassium chloride—an equivalent amount of potassium and calcium chloride—into the ascending aorta. If left ventricular hypertrophy is present, propranolol, approximately 1 mg in the normal adult patient, is routinely added to the cardioplegic solution. An insulating pad is placed behind the left ventricle to retard premature rewarming of the heart from surrounding normothermic mediastinal tissue during the procedure. A sump drain is placed into the left atrium through an atriotomy dorsal to the right interatrial groove and near the orifice of the right superior pulmonary vein.

With the heart arrested and most of the blood out of the left side, an aortotomy is done to expose the aortic valve and determine the extent of the pathological change and the best means of valve replacement (Figure 6.19A,B). After assessing the extent of disease, the aortic leaflets are removed (Figure 6.19C). Direct vision is enhanced by a Luxtec headlight (Luxtec Corporation, Box 225, Technology Park, Route 20, Sturbridge, Maine 01566-0225). Removal of the calcified valve leaflets must be done cautiously, taking care not to remove too much at the first excision. An overly aggressive removal could disrupt the continuity of the annulus and the sinus of Valsalva and result in uncontrollable hemorrhage. Valve implantation under such circumstances would be very difficult. While residual calcium is being debrided, a sponge is placed down into the left ventricle to catch any calcium fragments. Before the valve is removed, traction sutures are placed at each of the 3 commissural points to elevate and facilitate exposure of the annulus (Figure 6.19D).

Interrupted 2-0 mattress sutures with Dacron felt pledgets for reinforcement are used in the valve replacement. Some surgeons place the sutures, then secure them to a placement device, and finally put them separately into the valve sewing ring—an approach that is unnecessary and time consuming. The approach we use is much simpler. Generally, we begin at the commissure between the left and right coronary leaflets, although starting at this location is primarily a result of surgeon's preference. Blue and white sutures are placed alternately in the three annular areas, and the pledgets are positioned above the annulus (Figure 6.19E). The mattress sutures are passed through the sewing ring of the prosthetic valve. Alternating sutures is especially advantageous when the cavity is deep. Because the atrioventricular conduction bundle, which lies just beneath the membranous interventricular septum, is vulnerable to injury in the noncoronary cusp region, sutures must be placed carefully to avoid causing heart block.

The prosthesis is lowered into the annulus, and the sutures are tied by using 4 or 5 half-hitch knots on each suture (Figure 6.19F). Proper placement of the valve should be tested by opening the valve leaflets to see whether any obstruction exists (Figure 6.19G). A more optimal way has not been found. Once the valve is in place, the aortotomy is closed with 4-0 or 3-0 polypropylene sutures (Figure 6.19H).

The insulating pad is then removed, and the anesthesiologist puts pressure on the lungs to eliminate most of the air from the left atrium and pulmonary vein. Air is removed from the ascending aorta by suction and later from the apex of the ventricle by 19-gauge needle aspiration.

Moderately hypothermic body temperature of 30° C and cardiac hypothermia are used routinely for aortic valve replacement procedures. The period of cardiopulmonary bypass is usually less than one hour. The bubble oxygenator is used for oxygenation in patients undergoing aortic valve replacement; however, if a longer operative time is likely to occur, the membrane oxygenator should be considered. If atrial fibrillation should occur, countershock can be used to restore the heart to regular rhythm. At the end of the operation, venous line blood that remains in the pump is returned to the patient in the operating room. Any additional blood remaining can be retained to be given in the intensive care unit. This simple method decreases the need for transfusion.

After cardiopulmonary bypass is discontinued, the aspirating needle is removed from the ascending aorta. Sutures should be placed into the adventitia and should not penetrate the lumen of the aorta. The atrial catheter is then removed. The aortic cannula is removed next and a purse-string suture placed—again, only into the adventitia. Protamine sulfate, 4.5 mg/kg, is given to counteract the heparin. All suture lines should be examined carefully to ensure that bleeding is not occurring at any location.

Temporary pacing wires are placed in most patients who undergo aortic valve replacement as a safeguard against heart block or other arrhythmias that can occur in the early postoperative period. The wires usually remain for 4 to 5 days. A mediastinal chest tube is inserted, then removed approximately 48 hours after the operation. Extrapericardial mediastinal tissue is placed over the aorta to protect against dense adhesions in the event of a future sternotomy. The sternum is approximated using heavy-gauge sternal wires twisted evenly. The subcutaneous tissue is closed in a single layer with nonabsorbable sutures. Avoid trapping wires within a suture.

Operative Risk

The operative risk in aortic valve replacement has decreased progressively since the operation was first performed. In most institutions, the risk of early mortality in isolated aortic valve replacement is approximately 2%.[107] The risk primarily depends upon the condition of the left ventricle. If it is large, dilated, and dyskinetic, the risk is higher. If the valve is severely calcified, the risk increases.[108] Concomitant coronary artery disease also raises the risk. Although a coronary artery bypass procedure may improve the long-term results, the procedure also increases the immediate risk.[109]

ANNULOAORTIC ECTASIA

We approach surgical management of annuloaortic ectasia selectively, based upon findings at operation. Replacement of the incompetent aortic valve is certainly necessary, and the coronary ostia must also be reimplanted to maintain myocardial circulation. The conventional or conservative method of repair employs a supracoronary graft to replace the aneurysm and a standard valve replacement.[110,111] We use this technique for patients who do not have disease of the sinus portion of the aortic root, which would necessitate composite graft replacement. Because patients with annuloaortic ectasia, however, demonstrate a degenerative process in their aortic wall, operative techniques using supracoronary anastomosis can be hampered when a tongue of possibly abnormal proximal wall is left behind. This tissue has the potential for aneurysm formation,[112–114] dissection,[115] or parivalvular leakage.[116,117] In 1968, Bentall and DeBono[118] described a technique that overcame this limitation by employing a conduit composed of a fabric graft and a valve. The Bentall technique is applicable if the coronary ostia are 2.0 cm or more above the aortic annulus; otherwise, the repair is made above the ostia using a separate fabric graft and prosthetic valve.

In addition, we use the inclusion technique, first introduced by Creech[119] in 1966 and, recently, routine construction of a perigraft to right atrial fistula, a technique originally described by Cabrol.[120] Complete aortic root replacement with a composite graft has a number of advantages over the conventional operation when there is disease involving the aortic annulus and sinuses of Valsalva. All diseased tissue is excluded from the circulation, and, as a result, late reoperation on the aorta and heart to replace the diseased and unresected valve can be avoided. Technically, the operation is simple to perform. By using the inclusion technique with creation of the

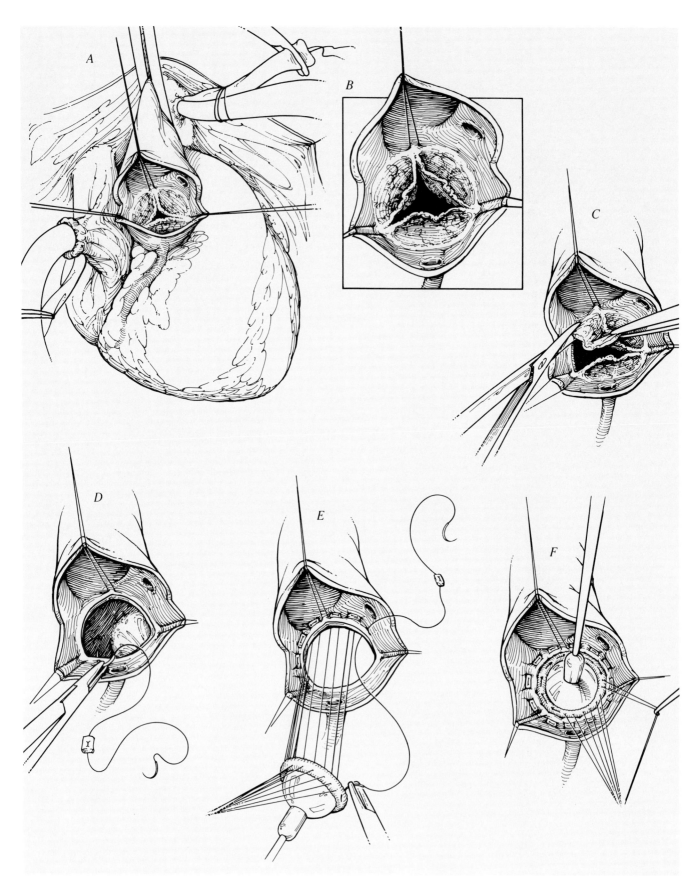

FIGURE 6.19 • Technique of aortic valve replacement. An aortotomy exposes the aortic valve to determine the extent of pathologic change and the best means of valve replacement (A,B). The aortic leaflets are removed (C). Before the valve is removed, traction sutures are placed at each of the three commissural points to elevate and facilitate exposure of the annulus (D). Blue and white sutures are placed alternately in the three annular areas, and the pledgets are positioned above the annulus (E). The prosthesis is lowered into the annulus and the sutures are tied by using 4 or 5 half-hitch knots on each suture (F).

perigraft to right atrial fistula, bleeding complications are minimized, as is late false aneurysm formation at the sites of coronary artery reimplantation. Compression of the neo-aorta by the formation of hematoma in the supravalvular position is also minimized.

Much of our technique has been described previously.[106] Recently, we have used the femoral artery almost exclusively for return of oxygenated blood. The femoral artery, in most cases, allows full access to the ascending aorta, the transverse arch, and the brachiocephalic vessels. We use moderate systemic hypothermia (30° C), unless we are repairing a type A dissection or an aneurysm that extends into the transverse arch, at which time we use profound hypothermia (20°–22° C) with the open technique that we have described previously.[121]

We bake the valved prosthesis in autologous serum[122] before we sew it to the annulus with a continuous 2-0 polypropylene suture. The coronary ostia are reimplanted using continuous 4-0 polypropylene sutures into holes made by hand-held cautery in the side of the composite graft. Care should be taken to place the sutures in the aorta around the coronary ostia, not in them. This may prevent false aneurysm formation.

To create the fistula from the perigraft space to the right atrium, we make a 2-cm slit in the medial aspect of the right atrial appendage. The proximal apex of the aortotomy is sewn to the slit to create the fistula. The remaining aorta is wrapped around the graft.

LEFT VENTRICULAR OUTFLOW TRACT OBSTRUCTION (LVOTO)

For children with severe left ventricular outflow tract obstruction (LVOTO), a technique of left ventricular outflow enlargement with aortic valve replacement known as the Rastan-Konno operation has been used in the past.[123,124] We seldom use this procedure today. Instead, we have found that we can implant a small 19-mm valve successfully and that this procedure will relieve the outflow obstruction in most instances.

A few patients with aortic stenosis cannot be managed successfully by conventional techniques. Included in this group are those with fibrous tunnel obstruction of the left ventricular outflow tract, hypoplasia of the aortic annulus, calcification of the ascending aorta, and tubular hypoplasia of the ascending aorta. Patients with recurrent aortic valve stenosis, after prior at-

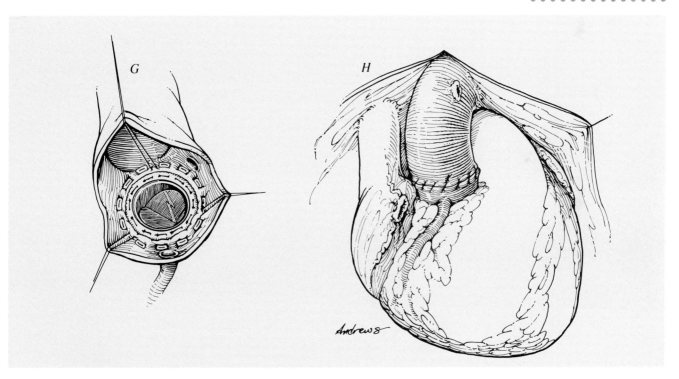

FIGURE 6.19 CONT'D • Proper placement of the valve is tested by opening the valve leaflets to see whether any obstruction exists (G). Once the valve is in place, the aortotomy is closed with 4-0 or 3-0 polypropylene sutures (H). (Modified from Cooley DA: *Techniques in Cardiac Surgery* Philadelphia, Pa: WB Saunders; 1984.)

tempts at aortic root repair or valvotomy, may also need radical outflow tract reconstruction with implantation of a left ventricular conduit, especially if infection has contributed to the failure of the previous procedure.

To implant a conduit, we use total cardiopulmonary bypass with cold potassium cardioplegia to effect a diastolic cardiac arrest. The left ventricular outflow tract, aortic valve, and ascending aorta are then examined to determine the feasibility of creating an apicoaortic shunt. We use a valved Dacron conduit with a St. Jude valve. An aperture is coned from the left ventricular apex. The connection at the apex of the ventricle should include a rigid device to ensure adequate opening into the conduit. The sewing ring is secured to the apex with mattress sutures and Teflon felt pledgets. The distal attachment of the graft may be placed into the supraceliac abdominal aorta, the ascending aorta, or the descending thoracic aorta. Our preference has been the abdominal aorta (Figure 6.20). When associated coronary insufficiency is present, revascularization using the internal mammary artery or reversed saphenous vein graft is performed. The vein graft is placed in the prosthesis distal to the valve.

In both children and adults, the shunt relieves signs and symptoms of left ventricular outflow tract obstruction. Analyses of postoperative angiograms (Figure 6.21) and pressure tracings in our patients show that the left ventricular aortic gradient has been corrected, ventricular function has been preserved or improved, and blood flow has been distributed normally through the coronary and systemic circulations.[125] Follow-up in our patients, now at 15 years for many, demonstrates that the procedure is well tolerated and does not hinder normal growth or exercise in children and young adults.

Because the conduit contains a valve, however, similar concerns regarding anticoagulation exist. Late calcification has occurred in some instances when bioprosthetic valves were used in the conduit. We also have seen a case of pseudoaneurysm at the conduit anastomosis.

Septoplasty Without Valve Replacement

A technique originally reported by Kirklin[101] and later by us[126] avoids the aortic valve and annulus and the use of a prosthetic valve replacement as in the Rastan Konno tech-

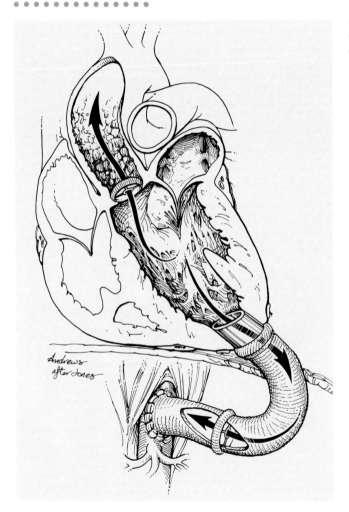

FIGURE 6.20 • Composite apico-aortic conduit, used in this instance to relieve ventricular hypertension resulting from a previously implanted small aortic prosthesis. (Modified from Cooley DA: *Techniques in Cardiac Surgery* Philadelphia, Pa: WB Saunders; 1984.)

nique. Operation is performed through a midline sternotomy incision. A vertical aortotomy incision is made just above the aortic valve, passing through the previous incision (Figure 6.22A). The aortic valve is inspected, and the outflow tract of the left ventricle is palpated, confirming the presence of severe diffuse stenosis.

An oblique incision is then made in the right ventricle below the level of the annulus of the pulmonary valve. After palpation of the left ventricular side of the ventricular septum, the septum is incised and the left ventricular cavity entered, carefully avoiding damage to the aortic valve (Figure 6.22B). Fibrous and muscular tissue is removed from the outflow tract. A woven Dacron patch is placed in the incision (Figure 6.22C). The right ventriculotomy is closed with a woven Dacron patch (Figure 6.22D). Final repair of the supravalvular stenosis with a pantaloon-shaped woven Dacron patch is shown in Figure 6.22E.

Exposure of the left ventricular cavity is excellent using this technique. The Dacron fabric patch provides total relief of the LVOTO without the need for excessive thinning of the septum. An additional patch is placed on the outflow area of the right ventricle because the septal patch conceivably could obstruct the right ventricular outflow. The surgeon should be careful not to injure the conduction system and the bundle branches of the common atrioventricular bundle of His.

MITRAL VALVE REPAIR AND REPLACEMENT

Surgical treatment of mitral valve lesions depends on the nature of the findings at cardiotomy. Although lesions of the mitral valve are usually repaired through commissurotomy or valvuloplasty, in certain instances, when there is advanced deterioration as a result of severe rheumatic valvulitis, replacement is necessary. In recent years, the approach to valve replacement for mitral stenosis has changed. It seems clear that chordal attachments to papillary muscles should be preserved to enhance ventricular function postoperatively. Thus, we try to remove only the anterior leaflet and preserve the posterior leaflet along with the chordal attachments, as these structures appear to have a direct effect on left ventricular function.[127-129]

· · · · · · · · · · · · · · ·

FIGURE 6.21 • Angiogram showing functioning left ventricular-aortic valved conduit used for relief of aortic stenosis in a 12-year-old patient.

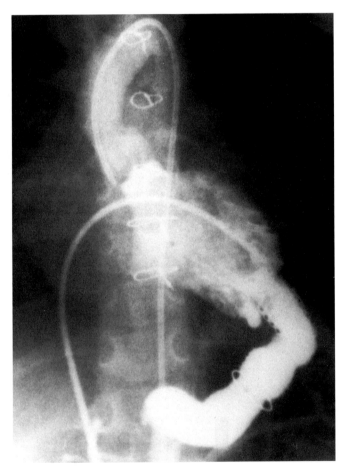

Mitral Stenosis

For most patients suffering from mitral stenosis, we perform a mitral commissurotomy (Figures 6.23, 6.24). In these cases, there is generally a slit-type of opening with fusion at both commissures. When there is fibrosis but no major cal-cification, opening the fused commissures produces an al-most normal, functioning valve. If the fibrosis extends down into the chordae tendineae and papillary muscles after the commissures are released, a subvalvular dissection is indi-cated. This involves separation of the fibrotic and fused

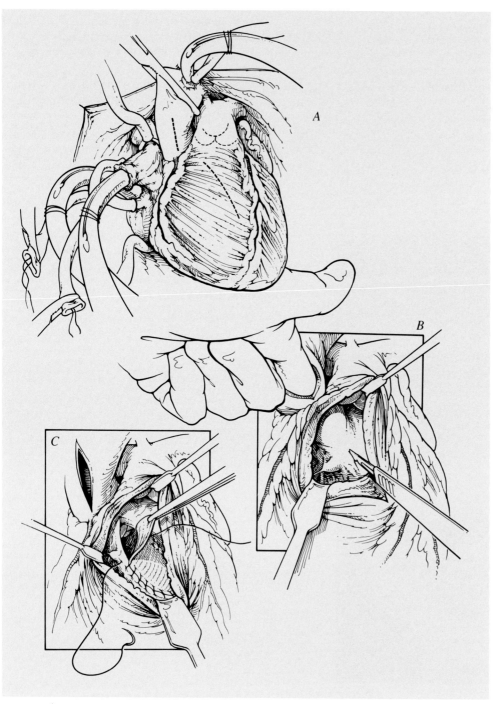

FIGURE 6.22 • Septoplasty without valve replacement. A vertical aortotomy incision is made just above the aortic valve, passing through the previous incision (A). The septum is incised and the left ventricular cavity entered, carefully avoiding damage to the aortic valve (B). A woven Dacron patch is placed in the incision, and fibrous and muscular tissue is removed from the outflow tract (C). (Modified from Cooley DA, Garrett JR: *Ann Thorac Surg* 1986;42:445.)

chordae tendineae and longitudinal splitting of the papillary muscles.

We use cardiopulmonary bypass for all commissurotomy procedures, even though the closed technique can be used with a transventricular dilator. We believe that direct vision is important to determine the extent of valvular disease and the type of repair that is necessary. The open technique permits careful removal of left atrial thrombi, which are frequently present. Using the open technique also enables the surgeon to divide the commissures more accurately. When extensive cal-

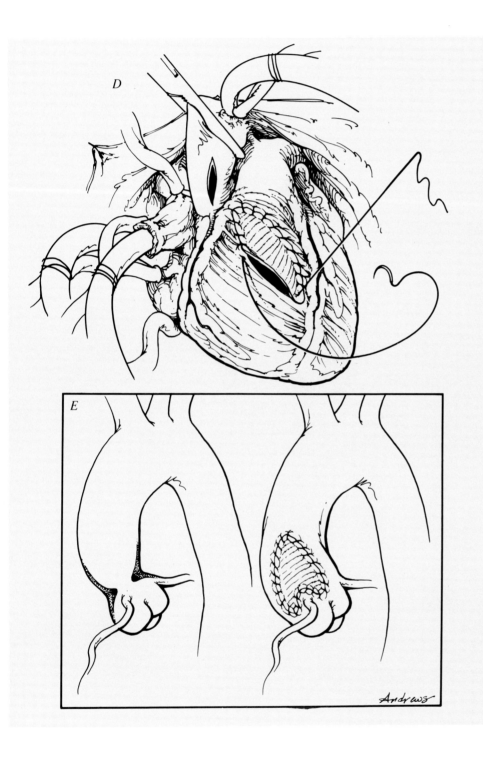

FIGURE 6.22 CONT'D • Right ventriculotomy is closed with a woven Dacron patch (D). Final repair of the supravalvular stenosis with a pantaloon-shaped woven Dacron patch (E). (Modified with permission. Cooley DA, Garrett JR: *Ann Thorac Surg* 1986;42:445.)

cification or severe fibrotic deformity is present, especially with subvalvular involvement, the valve should be replaced.

Mitral Regurgitation

Whenever possible, we repair rather than replace the mitral valve in instances of regurgitation. Valvuloplasty can be exe-cuted several ways. The technique we use most often is a valvuloplasty ring (Figures 6.25–6.27), although we occa-sionally perform annuloplasty by commissural plication (Fig-ure 6.28). The objective of both of these methods is to reduce the circumference of the mitral annulus. The anterior leaflet and the anterior mitral annulus should not be impaired by

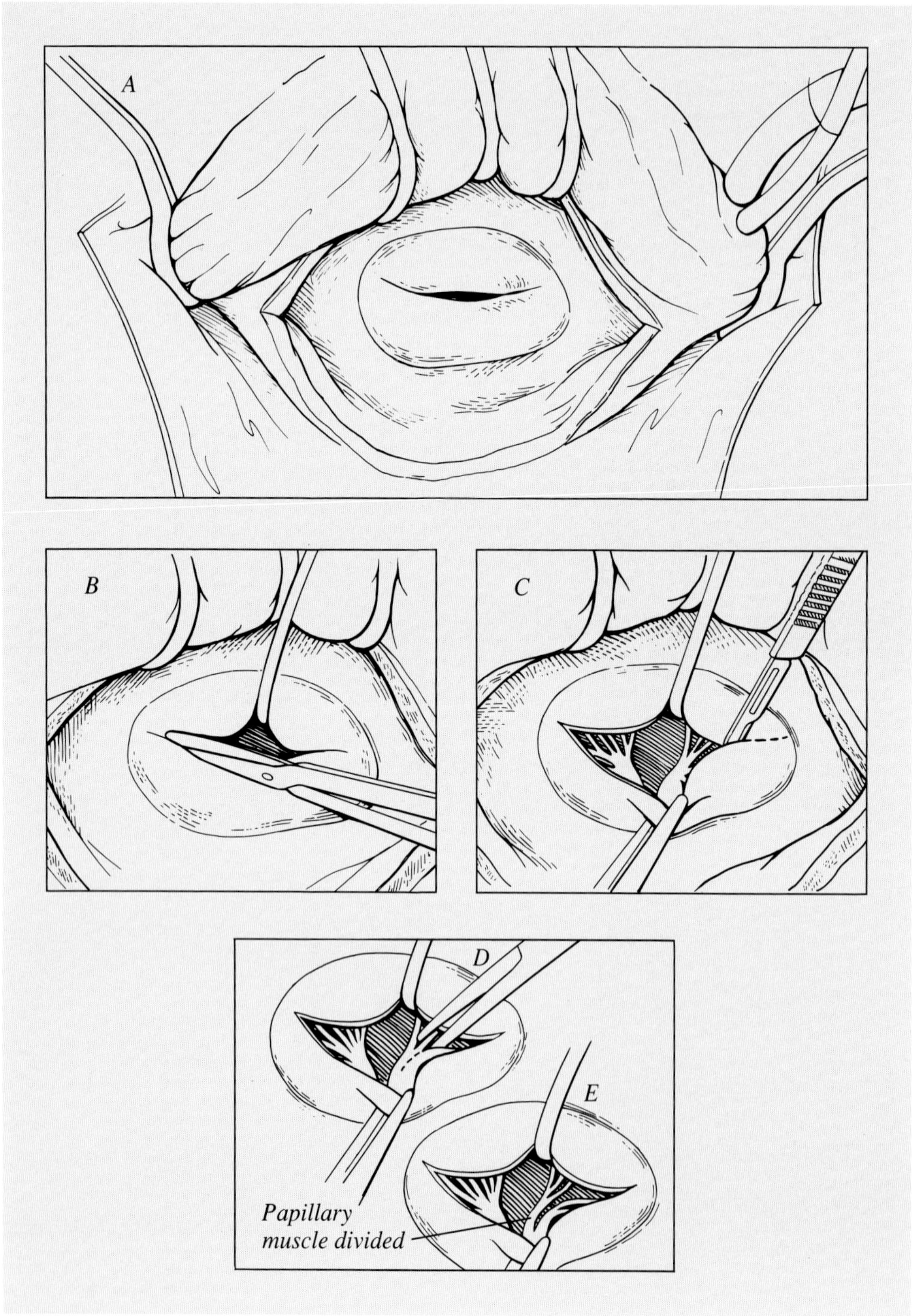

FIGURE 6.23 • Open mitral commissurotomy, performed to correct mitral stenosis. The fused commissures can be identified by a well-defined crease (A,B), and the valvotomy follows this line closely (C,D). Subvalvular mobilization of chordae tendineae and papillary muscles may be necessary, but these structures should not be de-tached from the leaflets (E). (Modified from Cooley DA: *Techniques in Cardiac Surgery* Philadelphia, PA: WB Saunders; 1984.)

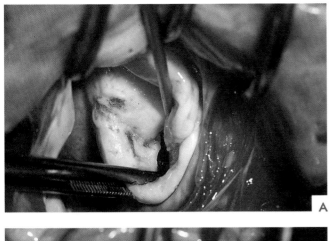

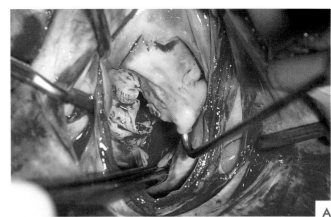

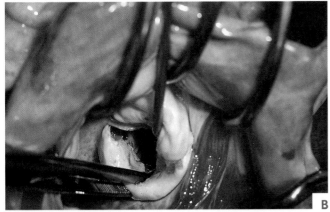

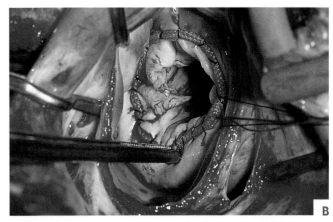

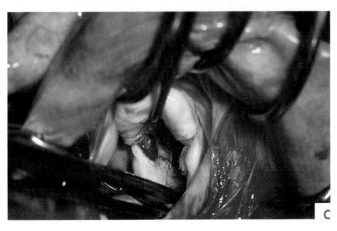

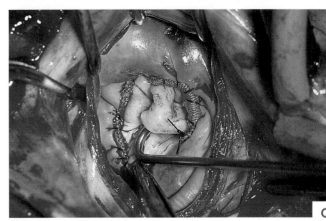

FIGURE 6.24 • Open mitral commissurotomy (A-C). (Courtesy of the Texas Heart Institute.)

FIGURE 6.25 • Mitral annuloplasty (A-C). (Courtesy of the Texas Heart Institute.)

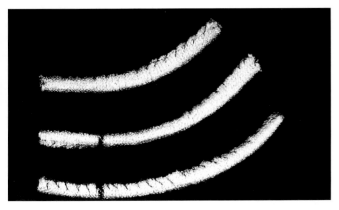

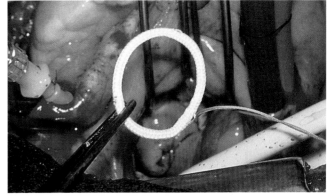

FIGURE 6.26 • Flexible C-rings.

FIGURE 6.27 • Annuloplasty ring.

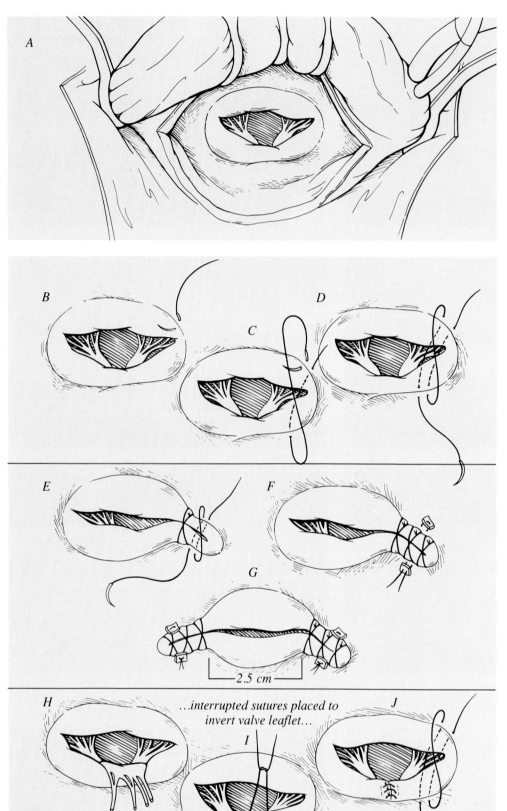

FIGURE 6.28 • Mitral annuloplasty by commissural plication. Incision reveals that the circumference of the mitral annulus needs to be reduced (A). Sutures are placed anteriorly at the commissure (B) and posteriorly in the annulus (C–E) The posterior leaflet is reduced (F) with the final length being 2.5 cm (G). In situations where the chordae are ruptured, interrupted sutures are placed to invert the valve leaflet (H,I) followed by annuloplasty (J). The length of the anterior annulus adjacent to the mitral leaflet should be preserved. It may be necessary to plicate the redundant scallop of the posterior annulus. (Modified from Cooley DA: *Techniques in Cardiac Surgery* Philadelphia, PA: WB Saunders; 1984.)

A

B

C

D

E

F

G

2.5 cm

H   ...interrupted sutures placed to invert valve leaflet...   J

I

When chordae are ruptured...   ...then annulplasty is performed

after Hvams

restrictive sutures. We also use the annuloplasty ring or collar prosthesis when a prolapsing valve is causing the regurgitation (Figures 6.29A,B). The ring allows us to attempt to correct the deformity by reducing the length of the posterior annulus, thus preventing prolapse of the posterior leaflet. If a partial rupture of the posterior leaflet has occurred, the flail scallop is ex-cised, the remaining leaflet is repaired (Figure 6.29C), and the annulus is reduced and supported by a circumferential fabric ring (Figures 6.29D, 6.30). When the anterior leaflet inter-feres with flow, the leaflet can be incised (Figure 6.31A) and tacked back to the side of the annulus (Figure 6.31B). This pro-cedure keeps the papillary muscle intact, giving it needed sup-

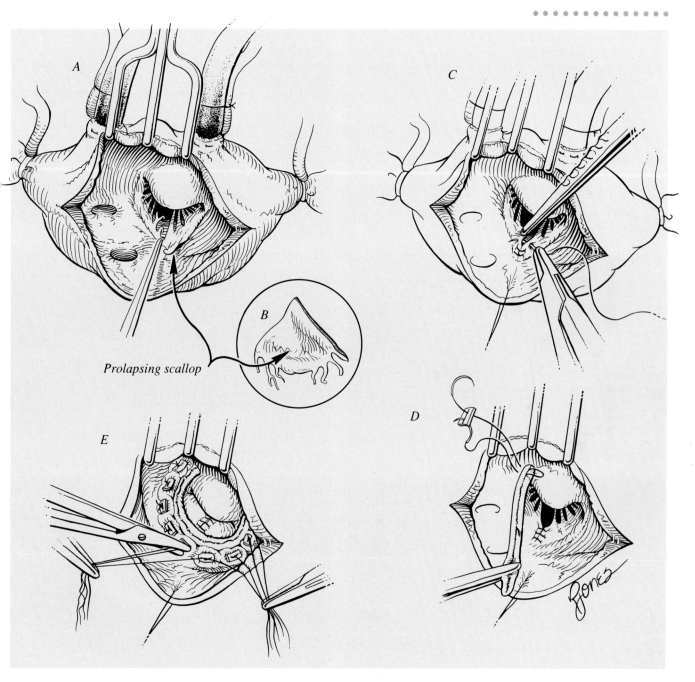

FIGURE 6.29 • Mitral annuloplasty with a flexible Dacron velour collar prosthesis (A-E). We now also use an annuloplasty ring. (Modified from Cooley DA: *Techniques in Cardiac Surgery.* Philadelphia, PA: WB Saunders; 1984.)

port. Mitral regurgitation frequently accompanies ischemic myocardial disease and generally responds to annular repair alone, as the leaflets are usually normal. Valvuloplasty does not require postoperative anticoagulation.

When mitral regurgitation is associated with ventricular aneurysm, we now use endoaneurysmorrhaphy to relieve the dysfunction[130] (Figure 6.32). We place an oval patch graft inside the left ventricle, which restores ventricular anatomy. By restoring the normal position of the papillary muscles, mitral dysfunction may be relieved. We have seen greatly improved functional results in our patients following repair of postinfarction ventricular aneurysm using this technique (Figures 6.33, 6.34).

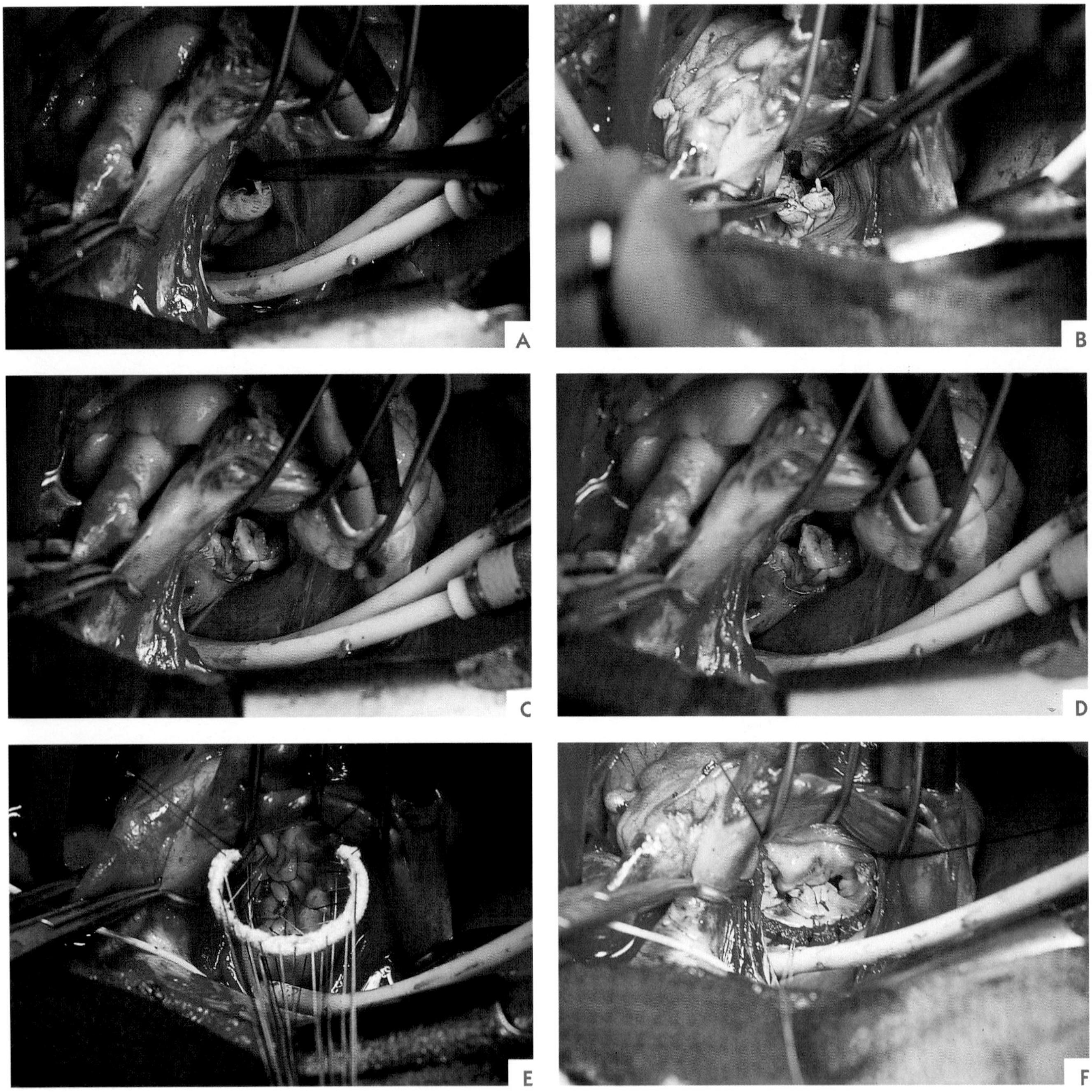

FIGURE 6.30 • Annuloplasty C-ring used to correct a "floppy" mitral valve (A-F). (Courtesy of the Texas Heart Institute.)

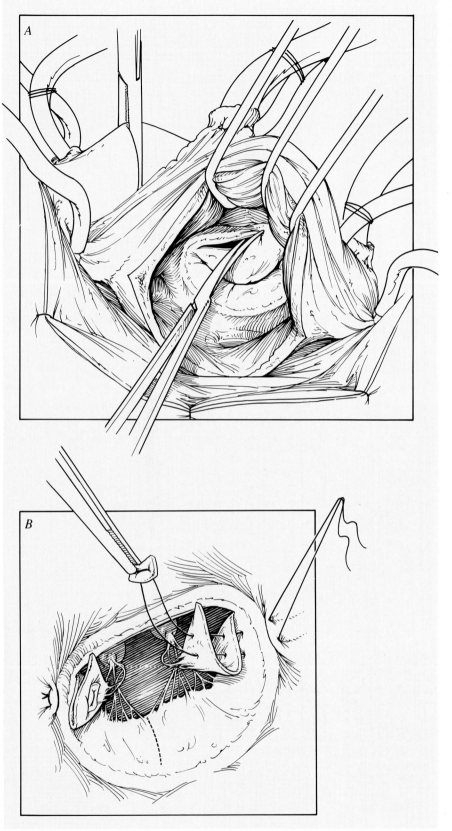

FIGURE 6.31 • Technique of mitral repair performed when the anterior leaflet interferes with flow. The leaflet is incised (A) and tacked back to the side of the annulus (B). (Modified from Cooley DA: Techniques in Cardiac Surgery. Philadelphia, Pa: WB Saunders; 1984.)

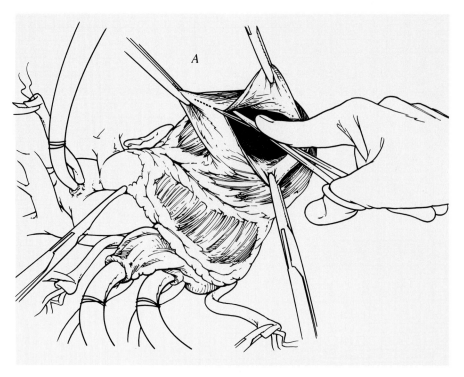

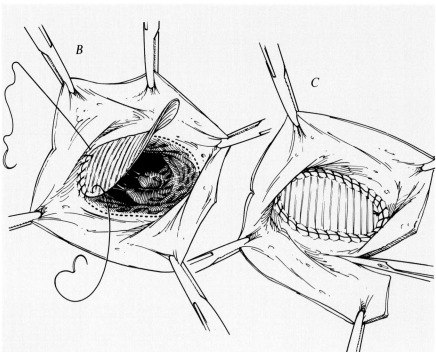

FIGURE 6.32 • Technique of left ventricular endoaneurysmorrhaphy used to restore shape, contour, and volume to the left ventricle (A-D). (Courtesy of the Texas Heart Institute.)

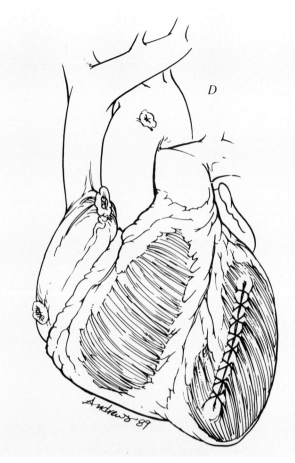

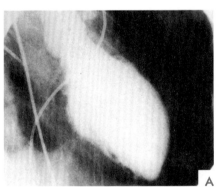
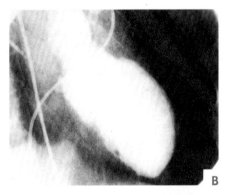

FIGURE 6.33 • Preoperative ventriculograms in the right anterior oblique view showing dilated cavity during diastole (A) and contraction at the base, with paradoxical dilatation at the aneurysmal apex (B).

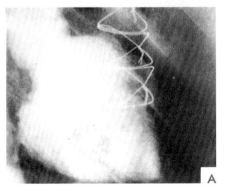
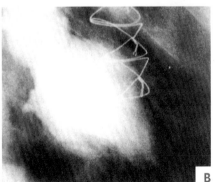

FIGURE 6.34 • Moderately magnified postoperative ventriculograms in right anterior oblique view made 8 days after operation. Diastolic view (A) with shortened cavity and systolic view (B) showing more effective ventricular ejection.

Mitral Valve Replacement

When the mitral valve cannot be repaired, replacement is indicated (Figure 6.35). For mitral valve procedures, we cannulate both venae cavae separately, since the atrial retractor can occlude a single cannula. In removing the mitral valve, the surgeon must be careful not to injure the posterior annulus. Annular rupture posteriorly may result from use of an oversized valve or excessive removal of tissue, which disrupts the integrity of the atrioventricular junction. Another important anatomical feature is the presence of the circumflex coronary artery along the posterior annulus of the mitral valve. This artery may be injured by deep placement of sutures during valve replacement or annuloplasty.

For a standard valve replacement, we use mattress sutures of 2-0 braided polyester, placing Teflon pledgets on top of the annulus. In some patients with a favorable annulus, a continuous suture of 2-0 polypropylene is used (Figure 6.36). We have not noted any difference in the instance of dehiscence in these suture techniques. Hemolysis is usually associated with perivalvular leak, and these patients may require reoperation for repair. Everting sutures of alternating color aid in separating the interrupted sutures before they are passed through the sewing ring of the prosthesis (Figure 6.37A–C). For mechanical valves, the mattress sutures can be placed around the entire circumference of the valve before lowering it into place (Figure 6.37B–D). We seldom use bioprosthetic valves. However, when they are used, the valve

must be lowered cautiously into place, because the struts can become entangled during implantation. In these instances, we attach the posterior sutures to the sewing ring and lower the valve into place before introducing the anterior suture line. This allows us to ascertain that none of the struts is encircled by a suture.

When the implantation is complete, we close the atriotomy incision with a continuous 3-0 polypropylene suture. After air is evacuated from the left side of the heart, the clamp is removed from the ascending aorta.

Intravalvular Implantation

When the mitral valve is intact, we occasionally use a technique we call in situ intravalvular implantation.[131] This technique preserves the anterior as well as posterior chordal and papillary mechanisms. In most instances, the anterior leaflet is split and tucked into the annulus to prevent obstruction to the valve prosthesis. As early as 1964, Lillehei and associates[128] recommended that preservation of these structures would enhance left ventricular function after operation. Carpentier[127] reported that valvuloplasty with preservation of chordal attachments carried a risk of 4% versus approximately 10% for standard valve replacement. We also have found that retaining the papillary muscles keeps the ventricle supported, thus maintaining ventricular tone (Figure 6.38).

To perform intravalvular implantation, the mitral valve is exposed, then inspected for ruptured chordae tendineae or papil-

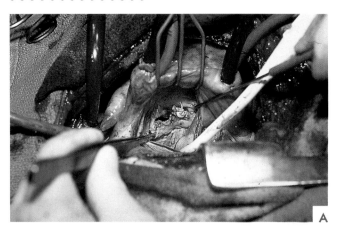

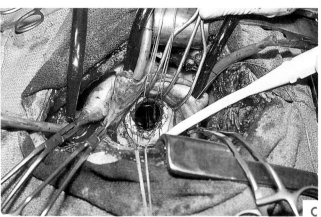

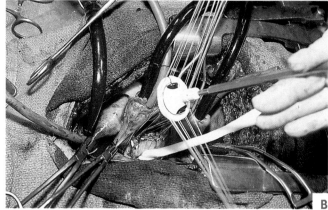

FIGURE 6.35 • Mitral valve replacement (A-C).

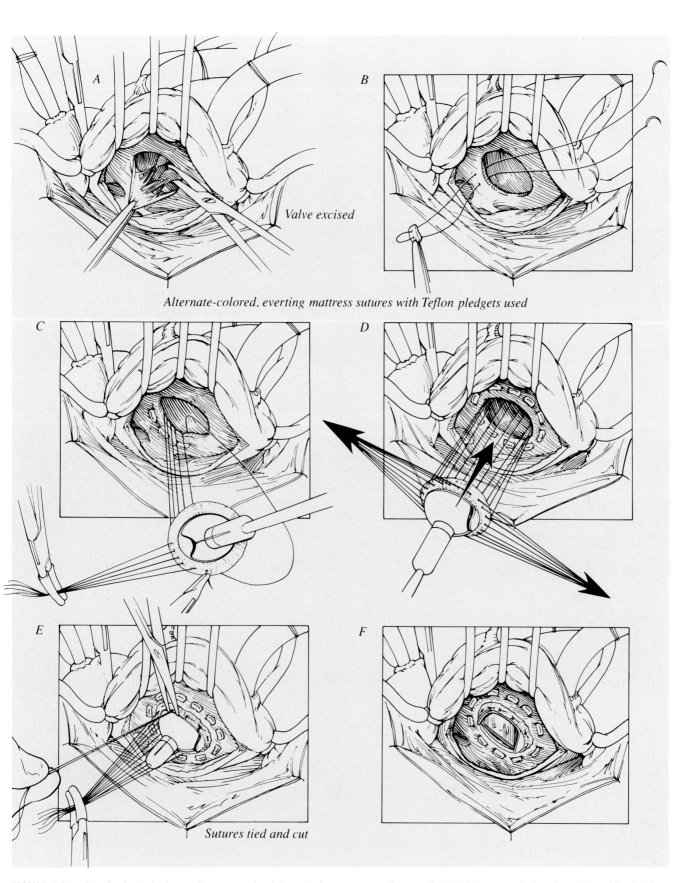

FIGURE 6.36 • Standard mitral valve replacement using interrupted mattress sutures. The mitral valve is excised (A,B). Alternate-colored, everting mattress sutures of 2-0 braided polyester with Teflon pledgets are then used (C,D). Sutures are tied and cut (E), and the holder is removed (F). (Modified from Cooley DA: *Techniques in Cardiac Surgery* Philadelphia, Pa: WB Saunders; 1984.)

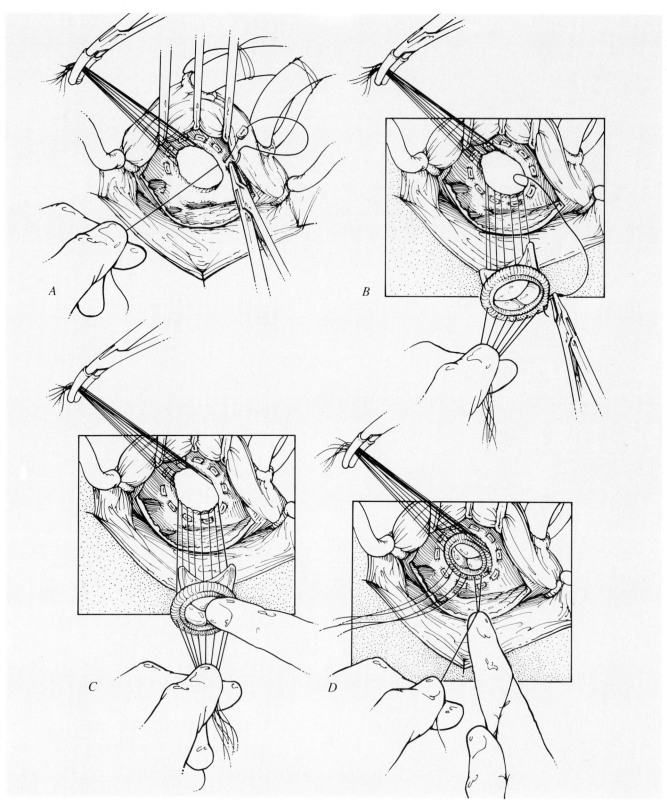

FIGURE 6.37 • Mitral valve replacement with a continuous suture of 2-0 polypropylene. We use this technique when the annulus is thickened, but not calcified. The diseased mitral valve (A). The valve is ex-cised (B,C). The superior and inferior rims are sutured (D). (Modified from Cooley DA: *Techniques in Cardiac Surgery.* Philadelphia, Pa: WB Saunders; 1984.)

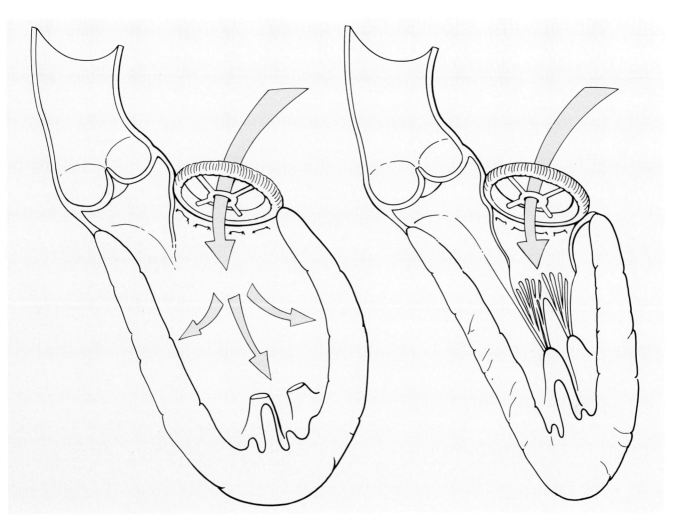

FIGURE 6.38 • Preservation of papillary muscles in mitral valve replacement lends tone post-operatively to the ventricle. (Modified from Cooley DA: *Techniques in Cardiac Surgery* Philadelphia, Pa: WB Saunders; 1984.)

lary muscles, which, if found, are excised or secured (Figure 6.39A). If the leaflets are intact and pliable and the chordae supple, we place a low-profile valve inside the annulus. The prosthesis is secured to the valve leaflet and annulus with interrupted mattress sutures and Teflon felt pledgets (Figure 6.39B). Before closing the atriotomy, the prosthesis should be inspected carefully to ensure that no underlying valve disease encroaches on the leaflets (Figure 6.39C). The ascending aortic clamp is released after air is evacuated from the cardiac chambers.

We always maintain as much of the valve as possible when we implant a prosthesis. When we cannot preserve both leaflets,

we remove the anterior leaflet and preserve the posterior leaflet, whenever possible (Figures 6.40, 6.41).

TRICUSPID VALVE REPAIR AND REPLACEMENT

Variations in cardiac anatomy and physiology determine the technique to be applied in the individual patient. Among the primary lesions of the tricuspid valve are rheumatic valvulitis, bacterial endocarditis, and traumatic rupture. Rheumatic valvulitis of the tricuspid valve, which may produce stenosis or regurgitation or both, may be relieved by a combination of valvuloplasty or valvotomy, or, if severe, valve replacement.

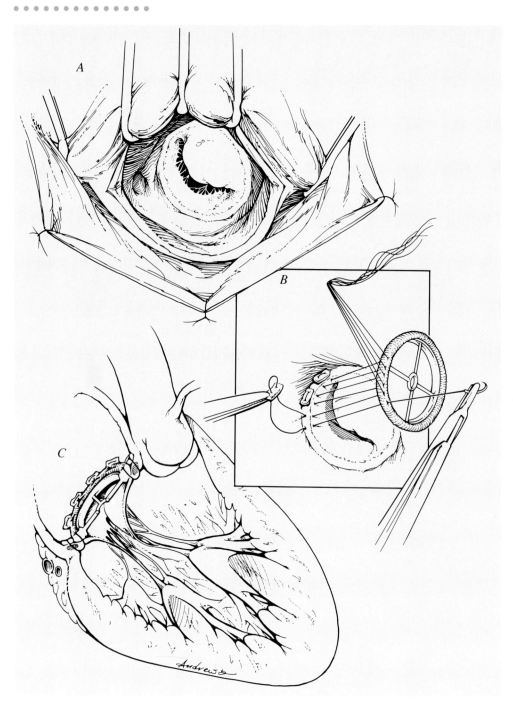

FIGURE 6.39 • Technique of intravalvular implantation of mitral valve prosthesis. The mitral valve is exposed and inspected for ruptured chordae tendineae or papillary muscles, which are excised or secured if found (A). The prosthesis is secured to the valve leaflet and annulus with interrupted mattress sutures and Teflon felt pledgets (B). The prosthesis needs to be inspected carefully, before closing the atriotomy, to ensure that no underlying valve disease encroaches on the leaflets (C). (Modified from Cooley DA, Ingram MT: *Tex Heart Inst J* 1987;14:188.)

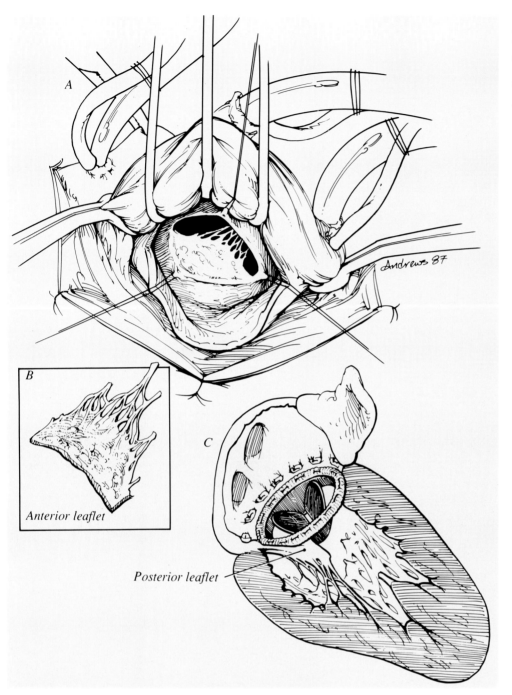

FIGURE 6.40 • Technique of mitral valve replacement (A–C). The anterior leaflet is removed (B), but the posterior leaflet is preserved (C). (Modified from Cooley DA: *Techniques in Cardiac Surgery* Philadelphia, Pa: WB Saunders; 1984.)

A

B

Anterior leaflet

C

Posterior leaflet

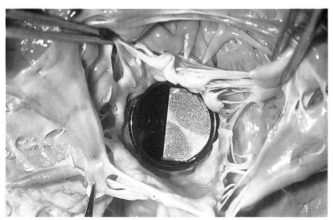

FIGURE 6.41 • Mechanical valve after intravalvular implantation. (Courtesy of the Texas Heart Institute.)

Secondary lesions of the tricuspid valve are probably most frequent. They accompany rheumatic valvulitis, which involves the mitral valve and, sometimes, the aortic valve as well. Under these conditions, pulmonary hypertension and increased pulmonary vascular resistance result in right ventricular strain, causing pulmonary and tricuspid valve insufficiency by secondary annular dilatation.

Treatment of secondary lesions requires careful judgment and experience by the surgeon. The most commonly applied repair is valvuloplasty, which is carried out in the presence of relatively normal leaflets by reducing the overall circumference of the tricuspid annulus (Figures 6.42–6.44). When the tricuspid leaflets have calcified or eroded from bacterial infection or ruptured chordae tendineae, valve replacement may be necessary. We use a low-profile mechanical valve for valve replacement.

POSTOPERATIVE MANAGEMENT

Postoperative management of patients undergoing valve surgery and, particularly, valve replacement depends upon knowledge of the potential complications.

THROMBOEMBOLISM

Thromboembolism, which has proven to be the most hazardous of all complications, primarily occurs after total valve replacement. Patients who have received mechanical valves should be given anticoagulants for the remainder of their lives. Although long-term anticoagulation is not necessary in patients with bioprostheses, we recommend anticoagulation for 6 to 8 weeks. In patients who have chronic

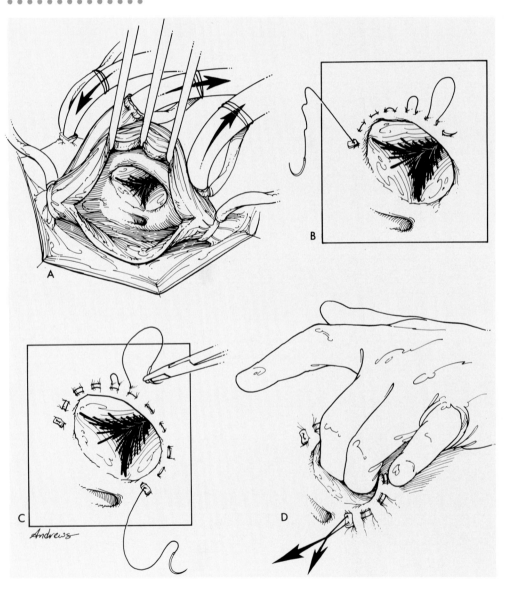

FIGURE 6.42 • Technique used to perform tricuspid valvuloplasty. Using the DeVega technique, an annular 2-0 polypropylene suture is inserted around the annulus (A,B). The posterior leaflet is left undisturbed to avoid injury to the atrioventricular (AV) node (C). The purse-string is drawn down by the assistant as the surgeon places his fingers into the orifice to ensure that the proper diameter is achieved (D). (Modified from Cooley DA, ed. *Techniques in Cardiac Surgery* Philadelphia, Pa: WB Saunders; 1984.)

atrial fibrillation or extensive left atrial dilatation and have received a bioprosthesis, anticoagulants should be prescribed indefinitely.

INFECTION

Infection is an unusual complication, but does occur in 2% to 3% of patients with implanted prostheses. When bacterial endocarditis is diagnosed, we advocate early surgical intervention and believe that surgery should be the treatment of choice for most cases (Figure 6.45). We also recognize that today cardi-

ologists are able to diagnose endocarditis more readily and specialists in infectious disease can manage many patients successfully with a wide range of antimicrobial agents. It appears that some patients with prosthetic valve endocarditis may be cured by intensive antibiotic therapy, but many patients are not and require surgical replacement of the infected valve. Prophylaxis against infection should always be considered when patients with valvular prostheses undergo dental procedures or operations on the lower genitourinary or gastrointestinal tracts.

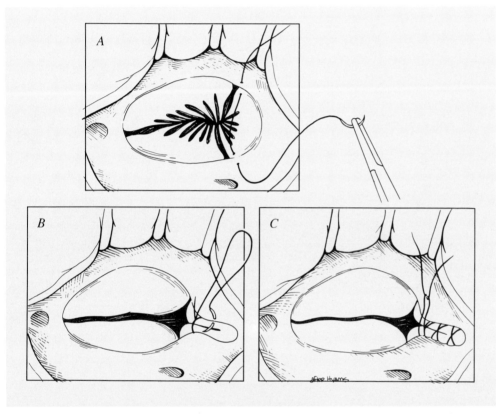

FIGURE 6.43 • Jerome Kay technique of obliteration of the lateral leaflet of the tricuspid valve (A–C). The entire lateral leaflet is obliterated (B) to form a bicuspid valve. (Modified from Cooley DA, ed: *Techniques in Cardiac Surgery* Philadelphia, Pa: WB Saunders; 1984.)

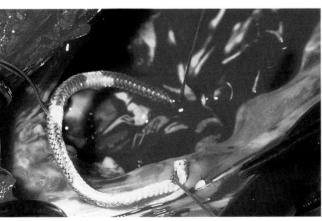

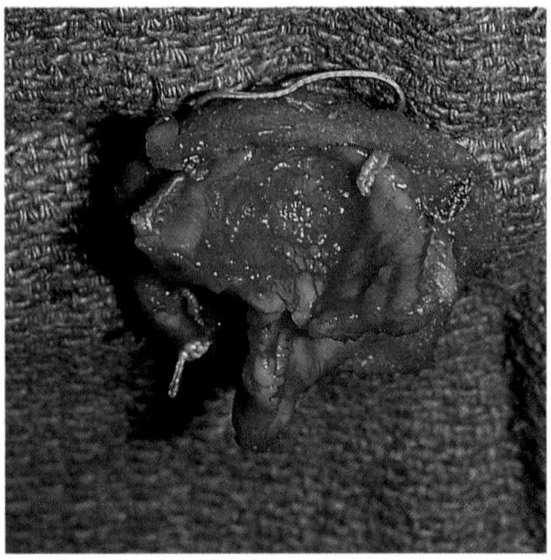

FIGURE 6.45 • Ionescu-Shiley valve, removed 3 months after operation. The patient had developed endocarditis. (Courtesy of the Texas Heart Institute.)

FIGURE 6.44 • Tricuspid annuloplasty. (Courtesy of the Texas Heart Institute.)

DEHISCENCE

Dehiscence is usually either a complication of infection or a technical or tissue failure that occurred during valve implantation. Often dehiscence can be corrected by a second open-heart procedure to resecure the valve with additional sutures.

MECHANICAL FAILURE

Since current mechanical prostheses are fabricated from extremely durable materials, mechanical failure seldom occurs. After 8 to 10 years, bioprosthetic valves tend to calcify (Figure 6.46) or stiffen and sometimes disrupt (Figure 6.47), particularly in adolescent or young adult patients and in those with severe renal insufficiency. When these complications occur, reoperation becomes necessary.

VALVE SELECTION

An ideal valve prosthesis must have the physiologic characteristics of unobstructed forward flow with prompt opening and closing. The valve should conform well to the anatomic position, without impinging upon adjacent structures. Valve materials should be biologically compatible. They should also have optimal mechanical properties and chemical stability and not be subject to degradation or absorption of body substances.

Excellent mechanical and bioprosthetic valves are currently available. Because of the problems associated with early calcification in bioprostheses, especially in young or adolescent patients, we prefer mechanical valves in most instances and reserve bioprostheses for patients over 70 years and women of childbearing age. Bioprostheses are preferred in patients in whom anticoagulation would impose a threat of hemorrhage or practical inconvenience. In determining valve size, it is better to err on the side of using a small rather than an oversized valve.

The valve prosthesis we generally choose is a St. Jude Medical bileaflet valve (St. Jude Medical, Inc., One Lillehei Plaza,

St. Paul, Minnesota 55117), which is made of pyrolytic carbon. The St. Jude valve was conceived in the 1960s and developed to its current form in the 1970s. It was first implanted clinically in 1977. The central leaflet of the valve opens to 85 degrees, providing a large effective orifice area with excellent hemodynamic function. Its low-profile design permits easy insertion, and its sewing ring is made of double-velour polyester Dacron, which helps to promote healing more solidly than other materials. The valve carries a very low incidence of complications, particularly thromboembolic complications—an important concern for all aortic valve replacement procedures.[132-134] Other currently available prostheses are also considered suitable, especially those that are constructed with pyrolytic carbon.

CONCLUSIONS AND FUTURE TRENDS

Many different techniques can be used to repair and replace diseased valves. We always carefully evaluate the patient before recommending any treatment. Whenever possible, we repair the valve. Repair, however, is usually not possible with the aortic valve. When valve replacement is necessary, we use the St. Jude Medical mechanical valve. Although imperfect when compared to a natural valve, the St. Jude valve provides superior hemodynamic function and is much safer than previous mechanical and bioprosthetic designs. Our experience with bioprosthetic valves was mostly with the Ionescu-Shiley, which we no longer use.

In comparison with the Ionescu-Shiley valve, the St. Jude valve is relatively resistant to infection, and its use has yielded greater freedom from adverse complications, including thromboembolism, as well as reduced early and late mortality.[133,134] Overall early mortality for St. Jude patients in our institution (7.8%) was significantly lower than that for the Ionescu-Shiley patients (9.3%) (p<0.05) in a recent study (unpublished data).

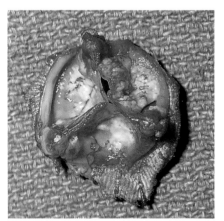

FIGURE 6.46 • Calcified Ionescu-Shiley mitral valve. (Courtesy of the Texas Heart Institute.)

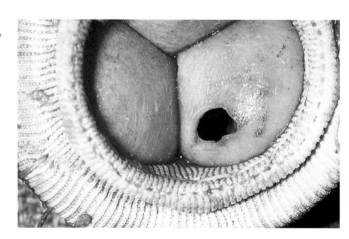

FIGURE 6.47 • Disrupted Ionescu-Shiley aortic valve, 4 years after implantation. There was no evidence of subacute bacterial endocarditis. (Courtesy of the Texas Heart Institute.)

As a group, our patients who receive St. Jude Valves are sicker, have more complex concomitant procedures, and have undergone more prior cardiac operations. Because a majority of Ionescu-Shiley patients receive anticoagulants, obviating a major benefit of a bioprosthetic valve, and given the proof that young patients are not necessarily at greater risk when low doses of anticoagulants are administered, the St. Jude valve may offer significant advantages over the Ionescu-Shiley valve. In our recent comparative study, we found a 0% incidence of anticoagulation complications in patients who had received the Ionescu-Shiley valve compared with a 0.2% incidence of thromboembolic complications in patients who received the St. Jude valve. With this low incidence in both groups, one of the proposed advantages of bioprosthetic valves appears to be diminished.

Although mechanical valves are more prone to early perivalvular leakage within 1 year,[135] late perivalvular leakage occurs more often in bioprosthetic valves, generally a result of commissural tears or calcification of the valve leaflets rather than dehiscence of the sewing ring.[136] Complications resulting from calcification are even more pronounced in young valve patients, with rare events having been described as early as 3 days postimplant.[137] For all of these reasons, we now prefer to use mechanical valves.

In the future, prosthetic cardiac valve development will herald the introduction of new device designs, as well as the improvement of existing ones. Alternatives to prosthetic devices, such as cryogenically preserved homograft valves,[138] will also undergo further scrutiny. Nonetheless, until greater experience with these substitute devices accrues, most patients requiring valve replacement in the near future can expect to receive mechanical or bioprosthetic valves that have already proved to be beneficial through careful experimental and clinical trials.

CIRCULATORY SUPPORT DEVICES

Numerous investigators have made important contributions to the research and development of mechanical devices to support or replace cardiac function[139–144] (Table 6.2). In 1969, Cooley[143] became the first surgeon to implant a total artificial heart in a patient who could not be weaned from cardiopulmonary bypass. The pneumatic, pulsatile device (Figure 6.48), developed by Liotta, successfully maintained circulation for 64 hrs until cardiac transplantation could be undertaken. Although the patient died of pneumonia shortly after the transplant, a result of less specific immunosuppressants at that time, the feasibility of providing total circulatory requirements with a mechanical device had been demonstrated. These first trials served as the impetus for continuing research on mechanical assist devices.

During the 1970s, Texas Heart Institute investigators participated in developing and testing an implantable, pneumatically powered left ventricular assist device (Figure 6.49),

TABLE 6.2 • MILESTONES IN MECHANICAL CIRCULATORY SUPPORT[1]

Investigator(s)	Accomplishment
Gibbon JH, 1937[2]	Roller pump for extracorporeal circulation
Gibbon JH, 1953[3]	First successful cardiopulmonary bypass
Stuckey JH, et al, 1957[4]	Use of cardiopulmonary bypass in massive myocardial infarction and cardiogenic shock
Liotta D, et al, 1963[5]	First clinical implantation of a pulsatile left ventricular assist device
Cooley DA, et al, 1969[6]	First staged cardiac transplant with total artificial heart
Turina MT, et al, 1978[7]	First successful clinical use of biventricular assist device
Norman JC, et al, 1978[8]	First use of a left ventricular assist device as a bridge to transplant

[1]Based on tables from Ghosh PK: Precedents and perspectives. In: Unger F, ed. *Assisted Circulation 3* New York, NY: Springer-Verlag; 1989:8.

[2]Gibbon JH: Artificial maintenance of circulation during experimental occlusion of the pulmonary artery. *Arch Surg* 1937;34:1105.

[3]Gibbon JH: Application of a mechanical heart and lung apparatus to cardiac surgery. *Minn Med* 1954;37:171.

[4]Stuckey JH, Newman MM, Dennis C, et al: The use of the heart-lung machine in selected cases of acute massive myocardial infarction. *Surg Forum* 1957;3:342.

[5]Liotta D, Hall CW, Walter SH, et al: Prolonged assisted circulation during and after cardiac and aortic surgery. Prolonged partial left ventricular bypass by means of intracorporeal circulation. *Am J Cardiol* 1963;12:399.

[6]Cooley DA, Liotta D, Hallman GL, et al: Orthotopic cardiac prosthesis for two-staged cardiac replacement *Am J Cardiol* 1969;24:723.

[7]Turina MT, Bosio R, Senning A: Paracorporeal artificial heart in postoperative heart failure. *Artif Organs* 1978;2:273.

[8]Norman JC, Cooley DA, Kahan BD, et al: Total support of the circulation of a patient with postcardiotomy stone heart syndrome by a partial artificial heart (ALVAD) for 5 days followed by heart and kidney transplantation. *Lancet* 1978;1:1125.

which functioned well in clinical trials. Survival was low, however, mainly because the patients had already experienced irreversible end-organ damage caused by poor perfusion.[145] In 1978, this left ventricular assist device was inserted into a postcardiotomy stone heart syndrome patient who required a bridge to transplant.[146] Despite the absence of both left and right ventricular function, the device successfully maintained circulation for 5 days, thus functioning as a total artificial heart. Although the patient died of septic complications after the actual transplant, this case demonstrated that left heart support is sufficient for temporarily maintaining circulation in a patient with normal pulmonary vascular resistance.

Two other total artificial hearts have been used as bridge-to-transplant devices at the Texas Heart Institute.[147] In 1981, one patient was successfully sustained to transplant with the Akutsu heart (Figure 6.50), which was developed and tested in the Institute laboratories. In 1986, a Jarvik-7 heart (Figure 6.51) was implanted in two patients, one of whom underwent transplantation and became a long-term survivor.

Researchers[148] from around the world are trying to develop devices that will overcome some of the problems associated with mechanical assist devices. Experimental devices with different types of blood-contacting surfaces and flow characteristics (for example, pulsatile versus nonpulsatile) are being studied to reduce the risk of thromboses. Development of devices that can be inserted without a major operative procedure or that have internal or transcutaneous power sources will help to overcome complications from infection. Reducing the size of the devices will allow treatment of patients with small body surface areas, including children. Eliminating bulky power sources will give patients greater mobility and return to normal activities.

Today the Texas Heart Institute is investigating several mechanical assist devices designed to treat a variety of heart conditions. Selection is based on whether cardiac dysfunction is reversible and on the extent of cardiac assistance necessary. Clinical experience has shown that instituting support before the onset of irreversible end-organ damage yields optimal results. Thus, any patient who becomes hemodynamically unstable is considered for a cardiac assist device (Table 6.3).

INTRAAORTIC BALLOON PUMP

Since the early 1960s,[149] intraaortic balloon pump (IABP) counterpulsation has proved beneficial for temporary circulatory augmentation (500 mL/min)[150] in patients who have re-

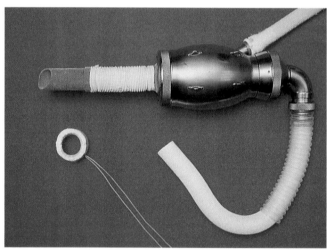

FIGURE 6.49 • The left ventricular assist device that was developed and tested at the Texas Heart Institute in the 1970s.

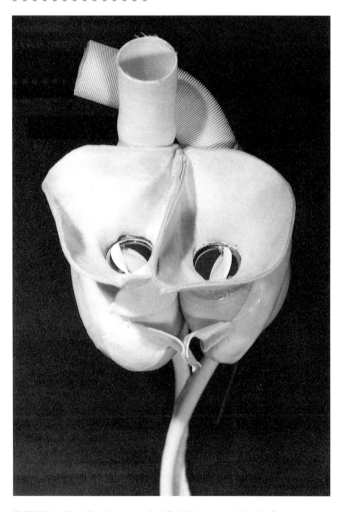

FIGURE 6.48 • The Liotta total artificial heart, used in the first staged cardiac transplant procedure.

versible left ventricular dysfunction. Whereas the effectiveness of IABP treatment has been attributed to result mostly from decreased afterload, we believe that increased perfusion of the myocardium resulting from diastolic augmentation plays a significant role. The IABP is a pneumatic, pulsatile device consisting of a special balloon catheter and a cable made of antithrombogenic, biocompatible materials. The indications for IABP support have been postcardiotomy or postinfarction cardiogenic shock unresponsive to treatment with maximal medical therapy, but experience has shown that left ventricular dysfunction resulting from other causes may also respond to this treatment (Table 6.4).[150–153] In addition, the IABP has been

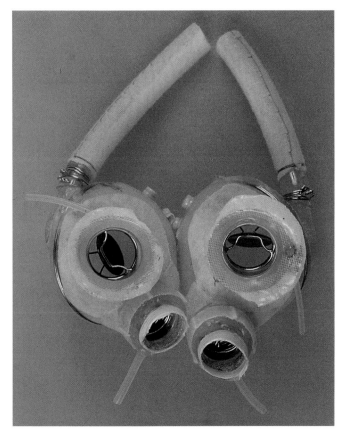

FIGURE 6.50 • The Akutsu total artificial heart.

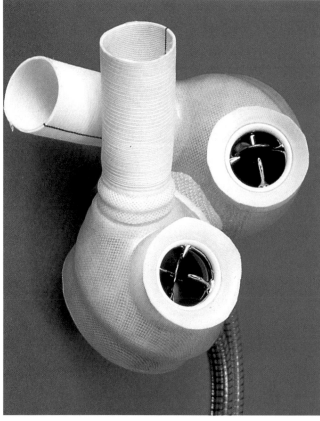

FIGURE 6.51 • The Jarvik-7 total artificial heart.

TABLE 6.3 • INDICATIONS FOR MECHANICAL CIRCULATORY SUPPORT
Progressive heart failure unresponsive to medical therapy
Signs of low perfusion
Increased blood urea nitrogen
Increased creatinine
Increased total bilirubin
Increased A-V0$_2$ difference
Decreased cardiac index
Refractory angina
Uncontrolled arrhythmias

TABLE 6.4 • INDICATIONS FOR INTRAAORTIC BALLOON PUMP SUPPORT	
Acute myocardial infarction or cardiogenic shock	Septic shock unresponsive to medical therapy
Rupture of the ventricular septum or papillary muscle	Intraoperative support for cardiac patients undergoing noncardiac surgery
Acute mitral regurgitation	
Postoperative low cardiac output syndrome	Cardiogenic shock resulting from cardiomyopathy
Unstable angina pectoris	Staged cardiac transplantation
Ventricular arrhythmias unresponsive to medical therapy	

(Reproduced with permission. Kantrowitz A: Intra-aortic balloon pumping: clinical aspects and prospects. In: Unger F, ed. *Assisted Circulation 3* New York, NY: Springer-Verlag; 1989:52.)

used to support patients with nonischemic cardiomyopathy who were waiting for a cardiac donor to become available.[154] Even though invasive monitoring lines are needed during IABP support, the risk of infection is low.[155]

The IABP is the simplest mechanical circulatory support device, and support can be easily instituted (Figure 6.52). Patient management involves monitoring hemodynamic status through a Swan-Ganz catheter. Antibiotics are given routinely for the first 48 hrs after insertion and continued when there is fever, high white blood count, or positive cultures. Renal, liver, and pulmonary function are also monitored. To prevent thrombo-embolic complications, patients are placed on low-molecular-weight dextran.

Based on the thousands of cases in which IABP support has been initiated, the risk of complications, such as thromboembolism, arterial occlusion, and aortic dissection, is relatively low. Moreover, the indications for the IABP should remain open to include any case of suspected heart failure that is hard to manage with inotropic support. Because of the increasing complexity of cardiac surgical procedures and the rising number of cardiac patients undergoing reoperation, we estimate that 5% could be helped by such support.

The only absolute contraindications to the IABP are severe aortic valve insufficiency, which would increase left ventricular afterload, and dissection of the aorta during balloon pumping, in which case support should be discontinued immediately.[153] Other relative contraindications include the presence of a prosthetic graft, although not all investigators agree,[153] and peripheral vascular disease, in which case a transthoracic approach may be taken.[155] Finally, the IABP would not provide enough assistance when myocardial function is profoundly compromised because it cannot replace cardiac function. In these instances, the patient should be considered to receive advanced support with a ventricular assist device.[150,152]

ADVANCED VENTRICULAR ASSISTANCE

EXTRACORPOREAL CENTRIFUGAL PUMP FOR LEFT OR RIGHT VENTRICULAR SUPPORT

The BioMedicus extracorporeal centrifugal pump (BioMedicus, Minneapolis, Minnesota) is one of the most frequently used ventricular assist devices[156,157] (Figure 6.53). Designed on the principle of a constrained vortex, the device consists of an acrylic cone house containing three magnetic cones that couple and rotate to produce unidirectional, nonpulsatile flows up to 10 L/min (Figure 6.54). Because the device contains no valves, there is minimal trauma to the blood elements, and full heparinization is not required.

Ready availability and the low risk of thrombosis have made the BioMedicus pump a suitable instrument for cardiopulmonary bypass instead of a roller pump. In addition, this pump can be used to provide short-term circulatory support in patients who cannot be weaned from cardiopulmonary bypass and in other circumstances of left ventricular failure, right ventricular failure, or failure of both ventricles[156,157]

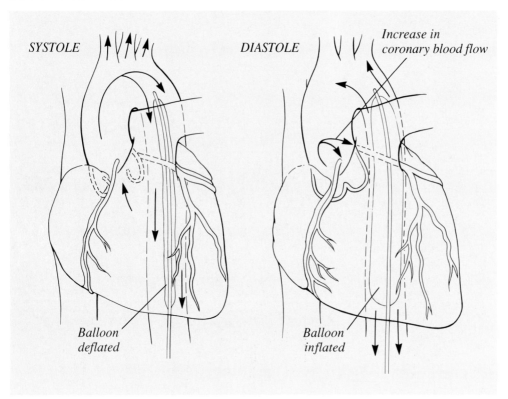

FIGURE 6.52 • Placement of the intraaortic balloon pump. After local anesthesia has been induced, the balloon is inserted percutaneously, through the common femoral artery, advanced to the descending thoracic aorta, distal to the left subclavian artery (Seldinger's technique). The drive cable, which is connected to an external portable console, provides pneumatic power to the balloon. Once the intra-aortic balloon is properly positioned, it is precisely timed to inflate during diastole and to deflate during systole, thus augmenting existing circulation by volume displacement. (Modified with permission. Frazier OH, Cooley DA: Use of cardiac assist devices as bridges to cardiac transplantation: Review of current status and report of the Texas Heart Institute's experience. In: Unger F, ed. *Assisted Circulation 3* New York, NY: Springer-Verlag; 1989:247.)

SYSTOLE

DIASTOLE

Increase in coronary blood flow

Balloon deflated

Balloon inflated

(Figures 6.55, 6.56 and Table 6.5). We have also used the BioMedicus pump after orthotopic cardiac transplantation in patients who experienced right ventricular failure, caused by increased pulmonary vascular resistance.[158]

In the case of combined left and right heart failure, two BioMedicus pumps can be used (refer to Figure 6.56). Alternatively, a BioMedicus pump can support the right ventricle, and a different type of device can support the left ventricle, depending on the patient's needs. Once right ventricular function

has been restored, the BioMedicus pump can be removed while left ventricular assistance is continued.

Unlike pulsatile assist devices in which the need for a compliance chamber creates additional problems concerning placement, the centrifugal force pump does not require this feature. Furthermore, device support can be instituted without cardiopulmonary bypass, although many patients are on bypass when the need for support arises. Another advantage of the BioMedicus pump is that it can be used to treat patients with small body

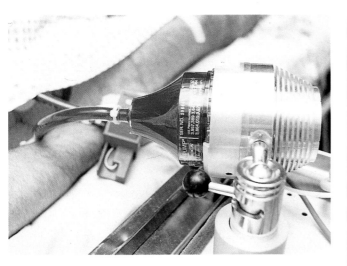

FIGURE 6.53 • The BioMedicus extracorporeal pump. (Courtesy of the Texas Heart Institute.)

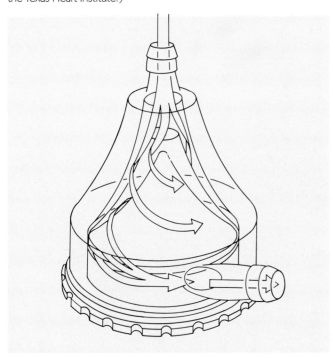

FIGURE 6.54 • The BioMedicus pump showing electromagnetic cones and unidirectional flow.

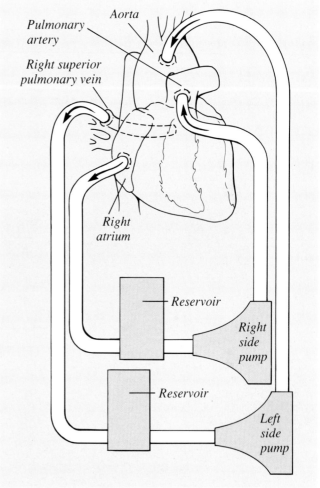

FIGURE 6.55 • Placement of BioMedicus cannulas for combined left and right ventricular assistance with two pumps. The cannulas would be placed in the same fashion to institute univentricular support of either ventricle. (Left side) After median sternotomy, the inflow cannula—a 36F, straight wire-reinforced cannula—is inserted into the right superior pulmonary vein. The outflow cannula—a 28F, straight wire-reinforced cannula—is inserted into the ascending aorta. (Right side) The inflow cannula is inserted into the right atrium, and the outflow cannula is inserted into the main pulmonary artery. After cannulation, the polyethylene tubes are secured with pledgeted 3-0 Tycron purse-string sutures. The pump is primed with the patient's own blood through the inflow cannula. After support has been instituted, the sternum is closed, and the tubes are exteriorized and secured with 2-0 Prolene sutures.

surface areas. We have used this pump as a bridge to cardiac transplantation in a pediatric patient.[159]

INTRAARTERIAL AXIAL-FLOW DEVICE FOR LEFT VENTRICULAR SUPPORT

The Hemopump® (Johnson & Johnson Interventional Systems, Rancho Cordova, California) is an intraarterial axial-flow device designed to support circulation temporarily in instances of reversible left ventricular failure (Table 6.6)[160,161] and is one of the simplest left ventricular assist systems (Figures 6.57, 6.58). The ability to institute support through peripheral insertion of the device eliminates the need for a major operative procedure, which can complicate the course of patients placed on various types of implantable left ventricular assist devices. Although the femoral approach is preferred (Figures 6.59, 6.60), the Hemopump can be inserted through the iliac artery or distal ab-

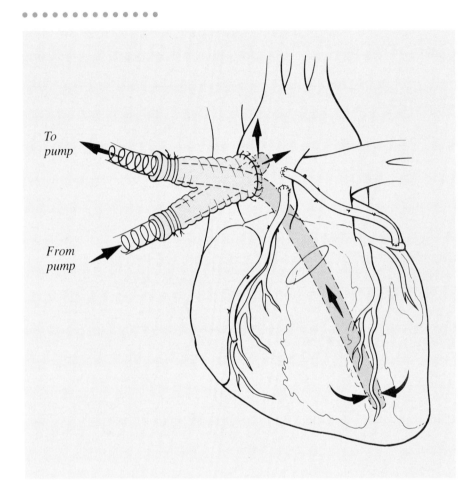

To pump

From pump

FIGURE 6.56 • Cannulation technique to treat intraoperative cardiogenic shock. An aortotomy is made in the ascending aorta while cardiopulmonary bypass is continued. The body of a woven Dacron bifurcation graft (22 x 11 mm) is anastomosed to the right lateral aspect of the aorta. The inflow cannula is inserted into the superior limb of the graft, then advanced across the aortic valve so that it rests in the left ventricle. The outflow cannula is placed in the inferior limb of the graft and directed toward the ascending aorta. The cannulas are secured by tying umbilical tape around the grafts, and the tubes are brought out the inferior aspect of the sternotomy. (Modified with permission. Duncan JM, Baldwin RT, Igo SR: *Ann Thorac Surg* 1991;52.)

TABLE 6.5 • INDICATIONS FOR USE OF THE BIOMEDICUS EXTRACORPOREAL PUMP
Cardiopulmonary bypass
Extracorporeal membrane oxygenation
Postcardiotomy cardiogenic shock
Acute myocardial infarction
Right ventricular failure
Cardiac allograft failure
Electromechanical disassociation

TABLE 6.6 • INDICATIONS FOR THE HEMOPUMP
Acute myocardial infarction
Failure to wean from cardiopulmonary bypass
Cardiac allograft rejection
Cardiac allograft dysfunction unrelated to rejection
Acute myocarditis
Cardiac sarcoidosis
Circulatory support during myocardial revascularization or percutaneous transluminal coronary angioplasty (PTCA) procedures

dominal aorta in patients with peripheral vascular disease or small-diameter femoral arteries.[162] The ascending aorta has also been used in patients who could not be weaned from cardiopulmonary bypass, but this method has been temporarily abandoned because cable fractures occurred during the Hemopump weaning process. Refinements being made to the cable will help to resolve this problem.

When activated, the Hemopump impeller screw, powered by the drive cable, rotates at speeds up to 25,000 rpm, drawing blood from the left ventricle and ejecting it into the aorta, creating unidirectional, nonpulsatile flows up to 4 L/min. The drive cable must be carefully monitored to prevent kinking or torsion, because bending can cause the cable to fracture. Finally, the speed of the pump controls the amount of flow and can be adjusted to meet the patient's requirements.

In cases where left ventricular function is severely depressed or when ventricular tachycardia or fibrillation occurs, no pulsation will be observed, but the device can maintain the blood pressure. Patient management includes afterload reduction to maintain mean arterial pressures around 50 mmHg, which facilitates flow and reduces stress on the rotating components. Because of the technical characteristics of the device, sys-temic heparinization is not required when it is operating at full speed. Administration of heparin is recommended, however, during the weaning process. As the myocardium recovers, pulsation resumes, and the patient is weaned from the device by progressively lowering the speed of rotation.

In our experience, the Hemopump has supported the circulation of patients with severe left ventricular dysfunction, allowing time for the myocardium to recover while helping to prevent severe end-organ damage.[161] No significant episodes of hemolysis or bleeding complications have been associated with use of the Hemopump, nor has limb ischemia related to the site of device insertion been a problem. The Hemopump does not appear to cause damage to the aortic valve.

Contraindications to Hemopump support include the presence of aortic valve stenosis or insufficiency, a mechanical aortic valve, a dissecting aortic aneurysm, or severe aortoiliac disease. The absence of cardiac function in cases of increased pulmonary vascular resistance contraindicates the use of any univentricular support system. However, the Hemopump can support both right and left ventricular function when pulmonary vascular resistance is low, allowing passive blood flow to the left side of the heart.

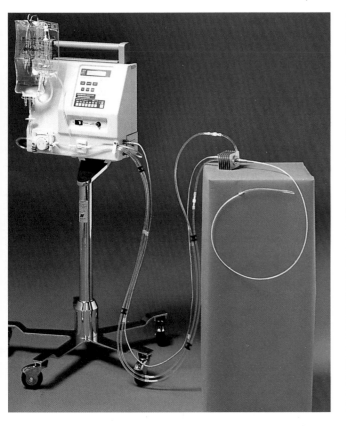

FIGURE 6.57 • The Hemopump system—the pump contained within the silicone cannula, the drive cable, and the portable electric console.

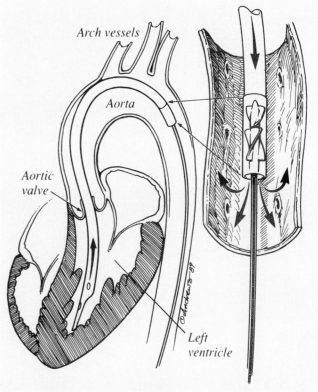

FIGURE 6.58 • Placement of the Hemopump assembly. The tip of the cannula rests within the left ventricle. The opposite end of the cannula, which contains the impeller screw, is positioned within the descending thoracic aorta, distal to the left subclavian artery. (Modified with permission. Duncan JM, Frazier OH, Radovancevic B, Velebit V: *Ann Thorac Surg* 1989;48:733.)

IMPLANTABLE DEVICE FOR LEFT VENTRICULAR SUPPORT

The HeartMate® (Thermo Cardiosystems, Inc., Woburn, Massachusetts) is an implantable, pneumatically activated left ventricular assist device that has a pulsatile pusher-plate pump (Figures 6.61–6.63). Producing flows up to 10 L/min, the pump provides adequate circulatory support. Patients supported for more than 1 month have improved to New York Heart Association functional class I status.[163,164] A percutaneous drive line connected to a control console provides power to the

• • • • • • • • • • • • • • •

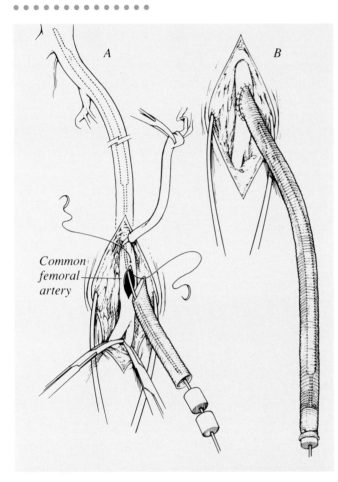

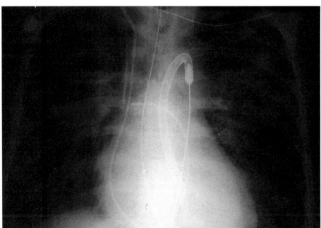

FIGURE 6.60 • Roentgenogram of the chest, showing correct placement of the Hemopump. (Courtesy of Texas Heart Institute.)

FIGURE 6.59 • Techniques for femoral insertion of the Hemopump. After heparinization, proximal and distal control of the femoral artery is achieved, then an arteriotomy is made. The pump can be advanced retrogradely into the artery, followed by end-to-side anastomosis of a 12-mm, low-porosity Dacron graft with continuous polypropylene sutures (A). Alternatively, the Dacron graft can be anastomosed to the arteriotomy first, then followed by retrograde advancement of the pump (B). If the patient is on cardiopulmonary bypass, the ventricle may need to be compressed manually to open the aortic valve, allowing the cannula to be advanced. Correct placement of the pump should be confirmed fluoroscopically, and adequate function confirmed through arterial pressure tracings. Silicone rubber plugs are then placed around the drive shaft at the end of the graft to prevent kinking or torsion during operation of the device. (Modified with permission. Duncan JM, Frazier OH, Radovancevic B, Velebit V: *Ann Thorac Surg* 1989;48:733.)

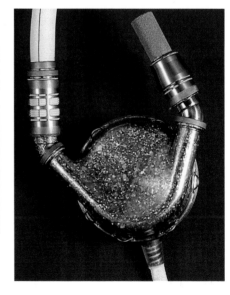

FIGURE 6.61 • The HeartMate left ventricular assist device. The housing is made of rigid titanium, and the conduits, which contain porcine valves, are made of low-porosity Dacron. (Courtesy of the Texas Heart Institute.)

pump. Currently, the device has been approved only for cardiac transplant candidates who experience profound left ventricular failure, unresponsive to maximal medical therapy and/or IABP support, as they await a donor heart. Since clinical trials began in 1986, more than 20 patients at the Texas Heart Institute have been successfully transplanted after HeartMate support. To date, the longest duration of support has exceeded 6 months. The favorable outcome can be attributed to several factors.

The HeartMate has textured blood-contacting surfaces, which distinguishes it from other currently available devices

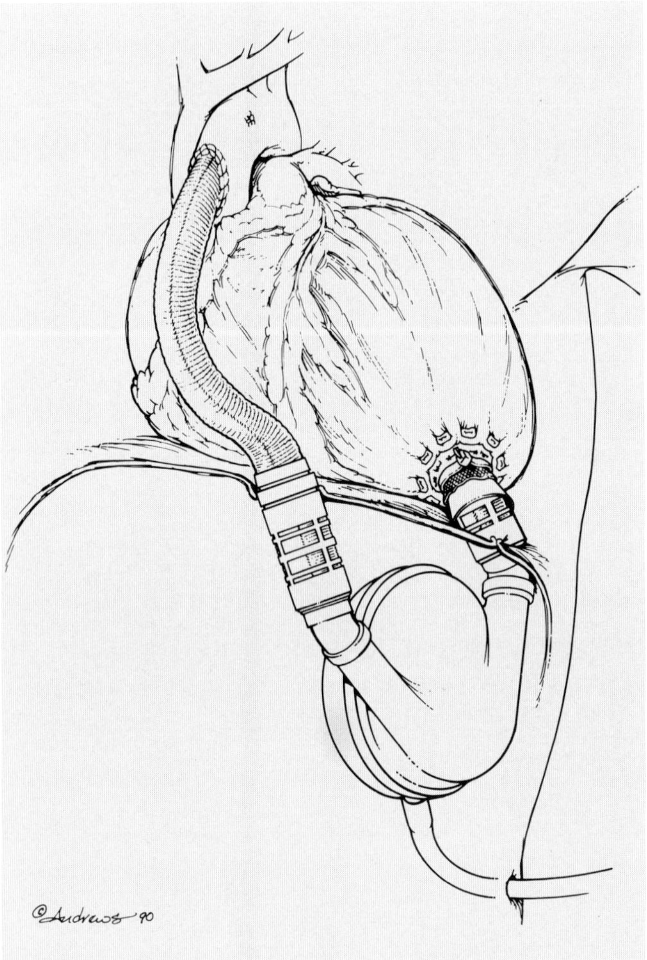

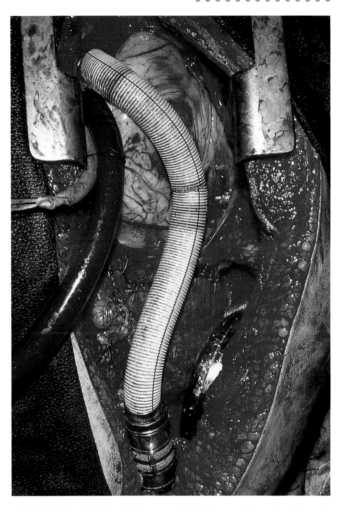

FIGURE 6.62 • Technique for implantation of the HeartMate left ventricular assist device. A midline chest incision is made and extended to the umbilicus. After cardiopulmonary bypass has been initiated, the left ventricular apex is cored, then reinforced with a Teflon ring. The pump is placed intraperitoneally in the left upper quadrant, and the inlet conduit is tunneled through the left hemidiaphragm. The outlet conduit is placed over the diaphragm, then anastomosed to the ascending aorta. The drive line exits the body from the lower left quadrant. After air has been vented from the system, pumping is initiated. (Modified with permission. Frazier OH, Radovancevic B: *Cardiac Surgery: State of the Art Reviews* 1990;4:335.)

FIGURE 6.63 • The HeartMate pump in the intraperitoneal cavity and the outlet conduit anastomosed to the ascending aorta. (Courtesy of the Texas Heart Institute.)

(Figures 6.64–6.66). Instead of deterring adhesion of blood elements, the textured surfaces of the pump promote deposition, so that a biologic blood interface forms. This pseudointimal lining reduces the risk of thromboembolic complications that have been associated with blood-biomaterial interfaces. Moreover, the need for anticoagulation with coumadin is eliminated, even during prolonged support (greater than 30 days). Patients are managed with antiplatelet therapy consisting of aspirin and dipyridamole.

Precise timing of implantation may also affect outcome. Our experience shows that support must be instituted before profound end-organ damage occurs.[164] In our early experience (1986), three of four patients treated with the HeartMate were successfully supported to the time of transplant, but they died

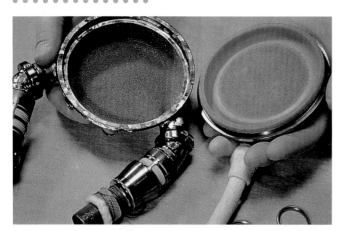

FIGURE 6.64 • Interior of the Heartmate left ventricular assist device. The fixed surfaces of the pump (left) are made of sintered titanium microspheres, and the moving components are covered with integrally textured polyurethane. The polyurethane surfaces promote adherence of blood elements to form a biologic lining. (Courtesy of the Texas Heart Institute.)

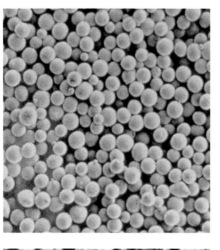
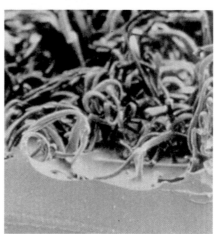

FIGURE 6.65 • Magnified view of the Heart-Mate surfaces. Sintered titanium microsphere surface for fixed components (50x) (left). Integrally textured polyurethane surface for flexing components (100x) (right). (Courtesy of Kurt A. Dasse, MD, and from Dasse KA, Chipman SD, Sherman CN, et al: *ASAIO Trans* 1987;33:418.)

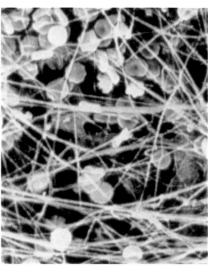
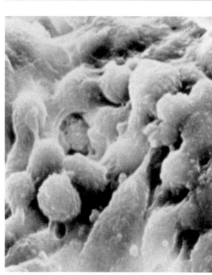

FIGURE 6.66 • Progression of pseudointimal development on the polyurethane surfaces of the HeartMate at 5, 19, and 41 days (1000x). (Courtesy of Kurt A. Dasse, MD, and from Dasse KA, Chipman SD, Sherman CN, et al: *ASAIO Trans* 1987; 33:418.)

soon afterward of multiorgan failure and sepsis. In our latter experience (1988), when support was instituted early, 12 patients were successfully supported to transplantation, and only one died—a result of an adverse reaction to OKT3. Moreover, once adequate perfusion was achieved, most patients were able to participate in rehabilitative exercise programs, further improving their clinical condition and making them optimal transplant candidates.

The HeartMate appears to cause minimal damage to blood cells, even when prolonged support is necessary. Infectious complications have also been minimal, occurring only at the drive line site; all have been resolved. At excision, the pump has been found to be encapsulated in a fibrous pocket, like that which forms around pacemakers.

Currently, an air-driven, electric HeartMate pump powered by a transcutaneous battery pack is undergoing clinical investigation. Should the device prove reliable, patients will be afforded even better mobility and, possibly, the opportunity to leave the hospital while receiving left ventricular support. These results may also have an impact on the development of permanently implantable ventricular assist devices, as well as total artificial hearts.

CARDIAC TRANSPLANTATION

During two decades of clinical experience, cardiac transplantation has evolved from a mostly experimental and newsworthy procedure to its present status as the only effective therapeutic alternative for patients with end-stage cardiac disease. This change has expanded the whole field of organ transplantation.

Cardiac transplantation has altered the prognosis of patients with end-stage cardiomyopathy, an ultimately fatal condition, and provided a rationale for expanding conventional approaches to treating these patients. Indications for aggressive procedures in a patient group normally excluded from these modalities have been implemented. For example, percutaneous transluminal coronary angioplasty (PTCA),[165] coronary artery bypass,[166,167] or left ventricular aneurysmectomy[168] have been successfully employed in patients with advanced disease.

In addition, the use of cardiac biopsy for detection of allograft rejection in transplant recipients has contributed to a better understanding of the evolution of myocarditis and the effect of various treatment interventions. It has also helped us gain a better perspective of the role in progressive heart failure of such diseases as sarcoidosis and amyloidosis.[169] Also, aggressive treatment needed for the types of infections seen in transplant patients has resulted in increased development of new drugs to combat opportunistic infections. Gancyclovir for the cytomegalovirus (CMV) infections and liposomal amphotericin B for aggressive, invasive aspergillosis have been used effectively in the transplant patient.[170]

Cardiac transplantation has offered an extended period of excellent quality of life to patients who were once facing imminent death. Although media interest surrounding cardiac transplantation has increased public awareness of the need for organ donation, the organ shortage persists, and only a limited number of patients can benefit from this procedure. However, the field of transplantation has made many major contributions to modern medicine, one of the most important being cardiac assist devices. Now used primarily as a bridge to transplantation, these devices may be perfected for permanent implantation in the near future.

HISTORY

Although changes in the medical practice frequently appear to be the result of sudden discoveries, they usually are the consequence of prolonged experimental work by dedicated individuals who, in many instances, do not live to see clinical application of their efforts. This is true for the field of cardiac transplantation. Its experimental history dates back to 1905 when Carrel and Guthrie performed the first heterotopic cardiac transplant.[171] Their development of the surgical technique and knowledge required to keep the transplanted heart beating—even if only for short periods—was the basis for subsequent developments in this field. Additional technical improvements in experimental transplantation were made by Mann and co-investigators in 1933,[172] leading to a better understanding of the transplanted heart's physiology and to the recognition that allograft survival depends less on surgical technique than on "biological factors."[172] In the early 1950s, Demikhov[173] performed the first orthotopic cardiac transplantation in a dog without the use of cardiopulmonary bypass and proved that the transplanted heart can completely support the circulation. With the introduction of cardiopulmonary bypass, Shumway and Lower perfected the basic orthotopic technique still used today in cardiac transplantation. Working through the mid-1950s and reporting in 1960,[174] they included mid-atrial resection and end-to-end aortic and pulmonary anastomosis in their procedure. Cass and Brock[175] reported a similar technique in 1959. Calne had demonstrated the efficacy of azathioprine in kidney transplantation, and Starzl and others[176] reported the synergistic effect of steroids with azathioprine. These immunological developments set the stage for the clinical phase of cardiac transplantation.

CONVENTIONAL IMMUNOSUPPRESSION: THE CLINICAL PHASE

After the first unsuccessful xenograft transplantation of the heart by Hardy in 1963,[177] clinical cardiac transplantation was officially begun in December 1967 by Barnard in South Africa.[178] During this first clinical phase of the late 1960s, impressive short-term results encouraged many centers to become involved with this fascinating procedure. Within a short period, however, most of these centers abandoned cardiac transplantation because of poor long-term results. Most recipients died within the first year after the procedure. Only a few centers continued with transplantation. Gradually results improved as immunosuppressive management was refined, and antilymphocyte preparations and endomyocardial biopsy were introduced.[179] These improvements were sufficient to increase the rate of one-year survival to 70%. Only after the introduction in the early 1980s of cyclosporin A (cyclosporine) as a primary immunosuppressive therapy, however, did cardiac transplantation appear feasible as a widely accepted procedure.

CYCLOSPORINE: THE CLINICAL PHASE

Borel discovered the immunosuppressive effects of the fungal metabolite cyclosporin A in 1976.[180–182] By 1980 it was already being used in clinical cardiac transplantation. The impact of this drug on development and acceptance of cardiac transplantation worldwide is difficult to overemphasize. Despite the difficulty in determining appropriate dosages for maintenance immunosuppression and despite the significant side effects—seizures, lymphomas, renal failure—associated with high doses of immunosuppressants, it became apparent that not only was survival improved with cyclosporine, but overall patient management improved therapeutic objectives. This was reflected in a much slower progression of the rejection episodes facilitating antirejection therapy.

Specific mechanisms of immunosuppression changed the pattern of infectious complications, preserving patients' ability to fight bacterial infections. Significant reduction or total withdrawal of maintenance steroid therapy also contributed to the control of infectious complications. Cyclosporine allowed for the change of donor and recipient contraindications as well, making cardiac transplantation available to a wider group of patients with end-stage cardiac disease[183–187] (Figure 6.67). All of this led to wide acceptance of cardiac transplantation. The number of centers performing cardiac transplantation increased worldwide from 17 in 1980 to 236 in the 1989 registry, and the number of cardiac transplants increased from less than 50 to approximately 2,500 worldwide.[188]

DONORS

Improvements in cardiac transplantation over the years actually contributed to the major limitation of this procedure—an increased shortage of donor hearts. Despite some restrictive criteria regarding placement of patients on the waiting list for cardiac transplantation, more than 1,700 people are registered at any given time in the United States. An average of only 4 to 5 donor hearts is available on a daily basis throughout the country. Considering this, it is obvious that an increase in mortality among these waiting patients will result.

THE CONCEPT OF BRAIN DEATH

Since Mollaret and Goulon[189] first described the concept of brain death in 1959, it has gained wide acceptance across the Western world. Technologic advances during the last 25 years have added to the increased number of patients with an irreversible absence of brain function. With the improvement of diagnosis by use of available clinical, electrophysiologic, and brain circulatory studies, there has been a wider acceptance of the concept of brain death among medical circles. Improved clinical results in cardiac transplantation, especially in the area of traumatic effects, have demonstrated the potential benefit of this procedure and emphasized the importance of the concept of brain death to the general population.[190]

Currently, major guidelines for determining brain death are those defined by the 1978 Uniform Brain Death Act.[191] A modification of this act, the Uniform Determination of Death Act, states that a patient with "irreversible cessation of all functions of entire brain, including the brain stem, is dead. A determination of death must be made in accordance with *accepted* medical standards."[192] Obviously, in both acts, there

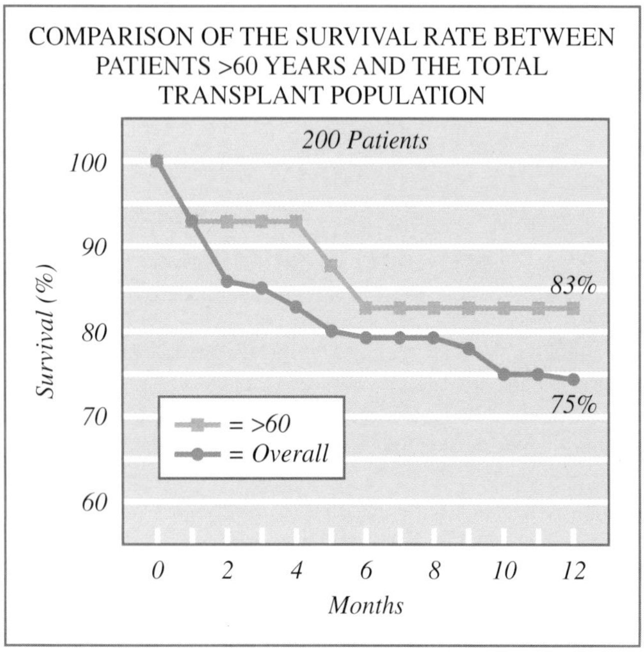

COMPARISON OF THE SURVIVAL RATE BETWEEN PATIENTS >60 YEARS AND THE TOTAL TRANSPLANT POPULATION

FIGURE 6.67 • One-year actuarial survival rate for the total transplant population compared with that of patients over 60 years of age. (Reproduced with permission. Frazier OH, Macris MP, Duncan JM, et al: *Ann Thorac Surg* 1988;45:129.)

are no strict definitions of the death criteria that can assist in the development of individual hospital policies referable to brain death. In the end, the decision process is a consequence of the physicians' clinical judgment, aided substantially by modern medical technology when appropriate—brain flow studies, electroencephalography, etc. Some of the most frequently used criteria are listed in Table 6.7.

CRITERIA FOR DONOR HEART ACCEPTANCE

During the early phase of transplantation, because of a much smaller discrepancy between the number of donors and recipients and the lack of experience with heart procurement, strict criteria were established for donor hearts (Table 6.8). With the introduction of cyclosporine and the virtual explosion of the use of cardiac transplantation, donor contraindications have become less stringent. In donor hearts from infected individuals or those with a history of cardiopulmonary resuscitation and cardiac arrest, high doses of inotropic agents had been successfully utilized with results comparable to those of "ideal" donors.[187,193] Based on this experience, it is conceivable that every organ donor should be assessed as a potential cardiac donor, and the decision for acceptance should not be based on donor heart function at the time of harvesting, but rather on the potential for the donor heart to *recover* full function. Even with the current extension of criteria to include donors not formerly utilized in transplantation, only 40% of the hearts taken from acceptable kidney donors are used. Disparity between organ banks may vary as much as 65% between procured kidneys and hearts.

All measures to optimize donor heart function, including optimal hydration, withdrawal of inotropic agents, and even the use of some newly introduced therapeutic options (T_3), can lead both to better perioperative survival and to an increased number of transplants performed.[194] In addition to pharmacologic methods of improving donor heart function, mechanical support of the inadequately functioning donor heart has been applied with limited success utilizing the intraaortic balloon pump (IABP), the BioMedicus pump, and, more recently, the Hemopump.[195,196] Improved organ preservation techniques that extend safe ischemic time allow for optimal matching of donors and recipients and can improve donor heart function after transplantation.

The results in transplant patients are similar for ABO-compatible and ABO-identical donors and recipients; however, ABO-identical blood groups are believed to promote equity for the transplant recipients, particularly those with O blood type.

TABLE 6.7 • DETERMINATION OF BRAIN DEATH		
Exclusion of other causes of the clinical picture simulating brain death	**Clinical criteria**	**Ancillary tests**
Body temperature > 95° F	Cerebral unresponsiveness, irreversible coma	• Isoelectric electroencephalogram (EEG)
Absence of drug intoxication or neuromuscular blocking agents	Brain stem unresponsiveness	• Absent cerebral blood flow by intracranial angiography or nuclear brain scan
Corrected metabolic abnormalities	• Fixed and dilated pupils, doll's eyes, negative caloric test, absent corneal reflex	
	• Absent gag and cough reflex, apnea—no respiratory efforts of the ventilator with $PaCO_2$ > 60 mmHg	
	• No posturing—spinal reflexes may be present	

TABLE 6.8 • HISTORICAL CONTRAINDICATIONS FOR USE OF CARDIAC DONORS		
Age >35, males; >40, females	High doses of inotropic medications (Dopamine >10 µg/kg/min)	Transferable disease—for example, human immunodeficiency virus (HIV)-positive donor
History of cardiac arrest, arrhythmias, cardiopulmonary resuscitation	Chest trauma	ABO incompatibility
Sepsis	Ischemic time > 4 hrs	

Crossmatching between donor and recipient lymphocytes is generally performed retrospectively. An exception would be those recipients who have a high serum reactivity, usually 5% to 10%, with random donor lymphocytes. Histocompatibility typing is performed retrospectively in most patients. Results obtained through retrospective studies of human lymphocyte antigen matching are controversial, and their benefit, even in the area of renal transplantation, has been recently questioned.[197–199]

RECIPIENT SELECTION

Patients with end-stage cardiac disease, regardless of its cause, can be considered as candidates for cardiac transplantation. Frequently, these are patients with either ischemic myocardial disease or idiopathic cardiomyopathy. A smaller number are patients with valvular disease, congenital cardiac disease, rare primary myocardial diseases like sarcoidosis and amyloidosis, infections (Chagas disease), or drug-induced myocardial destruction. It is generally accepted that patients should be in New York Heart Association (NYHA) class IV heart failure to proceed with cardiac transplantation, but patients in class III with an increased risk of sudden death (malignant arrhythmias) are also considered. Transplantation in patients in class II or in those who are at "high risk" for undergoing conventional cardiac surgery is usually not justified because of the lack of donors and the long-term complications of cardiac transplantation.

The contraindications for cardiac transplantation are still controversial, and some further changes can be expected based on results obtained during the last several years, especially regarding the long-term effects of recipient selection. Currently, whether a certain contraindication is absolute or relative depends mostly on the individual transplant center, with only a few exceptions (Table 6.9). Generally, patients with end-stage cardiac disease should be assessed individually in regard to the potential risks.

The introduction of cyclosporine played a major role in changing some of the absolute contraindications to transplantation. It is possible that further improvements in immunosuppressive therapy may make cardiac transplantation feasible for an even wider group of patients.

In the 1960s and 1970s, cardiac transplantation was performed in older patients, but experience showed that there were no survivors beyond two years in patients over the age of 50.[200] Since 1985, several centers have reported acceptable results with patients in older age groups. This underscores the fact that *physiologic* age is more important than *chronologic* age in patient selection.[185,201] A somewhat decreased tendency toward cardiac allograft rejection has been noted in this older group of patients. This may allow for a more rapid tapering of immunosuppressive therapy.[202]

Successful cardiac transplantation has been performed in patients with active infection, recent pulmonary infarction, and insulin-dependent diabetes mellitus.[183,184] In such cases, timing of transplantation is of paramount importance because rapid deterioration of cardiac function can preclude treatment of an acute infection or allow time for scarring of lung infarction.

An increased fixed pulmonary vascular resistance (PVR) of more than 6 Wood units is a contraindication for orthotopic transplantation, but does not preclude use of the heterotopic technique. All efforts to assess the real PVR level should be made, including use of prostaglandin E$_1$, inotropic agents, and oxygen. In patients with moderately increased PVR (4–6 Wood units), use of an oversized donor heart can prevent right ventricular failure.

MANAGEMENT OF PATIENTS AWAITING TRANSPLANTATION

Because the waiting period for a donor heart is progressively increasing, mortality for patients on the waiting list is approach-

TABLE 6.9 • CONTRAINDICATIONS FOR CARDIAC TRANSPLANTATION

Absolute	Relative
Active malignancy	Age
Hepatic cirrhosis	Insulin-dependent diabetes mellitus
Severe chronic obstructive lung disease	Active infection
Increased fixed pulmonary vascular resistance (orthotopic transplantation)	Recent pulmonary infarction
	Peripheral vascular disease
	Dysfunction of other organs
	Preexisting malignancy
	Drug or alcohol addiction, compliance history
	Mental illness

ing 40% in our experience. Proper management of patients awaiting transplantation, in many instances, can prevent death as well as improve posttransplantation results. Close follow-up of the patients is essential, and recurrent admission for heart failure, deterioration of either renal or hepatic function, and progressive cardiac cachexia are usually reason enough to institute either intravenous inotropic therapy or an intra-aortic balloon pump. Frequently, with the phasic but progressively declining nature of end-stage heart disease, it is possible to withdraw these modalities of treatment after the patient is stabilized. If these measures fail, advanced cardiac support by a left ventricular or biventricular assist device or a total artificial heart should be considered.

The history of the bridge-to-transplant approach has been almost as long as that of clinical cardiac transplantation. Clinical success has been obtained, however, only since the introduction of cyclosporine.[143,163,203] Today, comparable results in cardiac transplantation are obtained in patients with and without prior mechanical support.[204,205] Furthermore, in our own experience, the patients who have undergone successful mechanical circulatory support with an implantable device are the best group of transplant candidates because of a lack of end-organ dysfunction and the return to Class I NYHA status before transplantation.

SURGICAL TECHNIQUE

ORTHOTOPIC TECHNIQUE
Donor

Donor heart removal is only one aspect of multiorgan harvesting, and the technique is somewhat modified to facilitate lung and liver procurement. A median sternotomy is performed, followed by pericardial incision. Both the superior and inferior venae cavae are then dissected free up to pericardial reflections, and 2-0 silk sutures are placed around the superior vena cava. The heart and large vessels are carefully inspected at this point for both myocardial function and the presence of malformations. After the completion of other organ dissection, heparin (30,000 U) is given. Inflow occlusion is then obtained by ligation of the superior vena cava and transection of the inferior vena cava. After the placement of the aortic cross-clamp, cardioplegia is given and the left side of the heart is decompressed by opening the right superior pulmonary vein or the left atrial appendage. Topical cooling with 4° C normal saline solution is used for additional myocardial protection. Transection of the intrapericardial pulmonary veins is then performed, followed by transection of left and right pulmonary arteries just after bifurcation and transection of the aortic root at the level of the innominate artery. The donor heart is transferred to the basin with ice-cold saline solution, and openings of the pulmonary veins are connected to create a common left atrial opening. The pulmonary artery is incised at the bifurcation. The right atrium is opened, using an incision from the inferior vena cava toward the right atrial appendage. This should prevent injury to the sinoatrial node and atrioventricular conduction pathways. The heart is placed in two plastic bags containing ice-cold normal saline, the bags are placed in the ice chest, and transported.

Recipient

Under general endotracheal anesthesia, a median sternotomy is performed, and the pericardium is incised and retracted (Figures 6.68, 6.69). Heparin is given and, after the cannulation, cardiopulmonary bypass is started, and systemic hypothermia of 28–30° C is obtained. Tourniquets around the venae cavae are tightened, and the aorta is cross-clamped. The heart is excised at the mid-atrial level, just distal to both the aortic and pulmonary valves. The left atrial appendage is excised, and that point is used for the beginning of the left atrial anastomosis. First, the left lateral margin of the anastomosis is performed, followed by the septal inferior part, and completed with the second arm of the suture in the mid-part of the interatrial septum. The right atrial anastomosis is begun from the point of the recipient's excised right atrial appendage along the septum and is completed on the free atrial wall. Systemic rewarming is begun. The pulmonary artery anastomosis is performed by using a single-layer suture. Aortic anastomosis is also performed by using a single-layer suture. Aortic cross-clamp and caval tourniquets are released, and air is removed. If the heart does not resume a normal sinus rhythm, electrical conversion is performed. If the heart rate is slow, an Isuprel (isoproterenol hydrochloride) infusion is begun and titrated to maintain a heart rate of more than 100 beats/min. If there is no response to isoproterenol infusion, a temporary pacing wire is placed on the right ventricle and pacing is begun at the rate of 100 beats/min. The isoproterenol infusion is continued to maximally reduce pulmonary resistance of the pulmonary vasculature. The patient is gradually weaned from cardiopulmonary bypass. After the cannulae are removed, protamine is given to reverse heparin, and the operation is completed in the usual manner.

HETEROTOPIC TECHNIQUE
Donor

Most differences regarding donors in heterotopic and orthotopic procedures pertain to donor heart preparation rather than harvesting. To obtain a sufficient anastomotic opening of the right atria, the superior vena cava is dissected up to the level of the innominate vein, and the azygos vein is transected and ligated. The heart is excised in the same manner as for the orthotopic technique. The opening of the inferior vena cava is closed by using continuous double-layer 5-0 polypropylene sutures. Closure of the right superior and inferior pulmonary vein is then performed by using a double-layer 5-0 polypropylene suture. The left superior and inferior pulmonary veins are connected, extending the incision if necessary to provide an opening large enough for the left atrial anastomosis. The superior vena cava is double ligated, leaving the final incision for a right atrial anastomosis to be performed *in situ*.

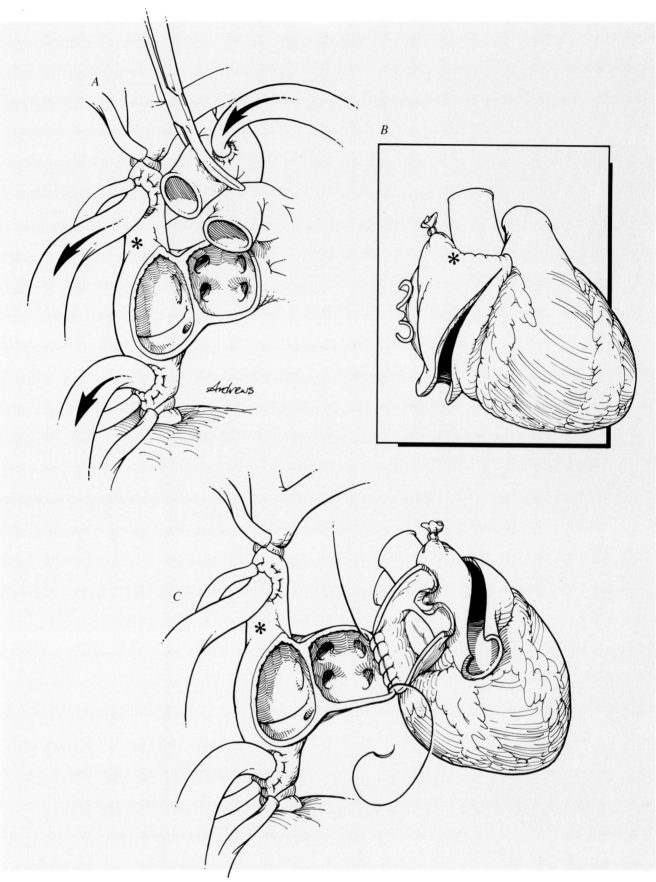

FIGURE 6.68 • The technical steps in cardiac transplantation. The asterisks denote the location of the sino-auricular nodes in the remnant of recipient heart and in the allograft. Care is taken to preserve sino-atrial (SA) to atrioventricular (AV) node continuity in the allograft to maintain a sinus conduction mechanism after implantation (A-G). (Modified from Cooley DA: *Techniques in Cardiac Surgery* Philadelphia, Pa: WB Saunders; 1984.)

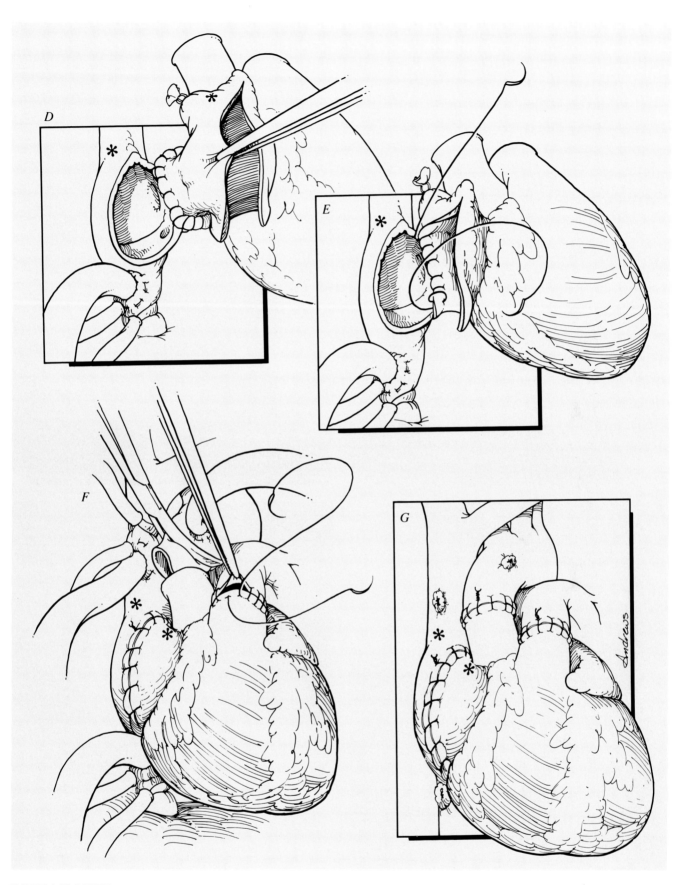

FIGURE 6.68 CONT'D

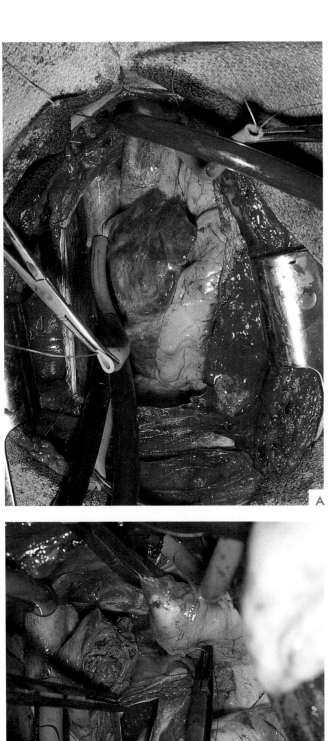

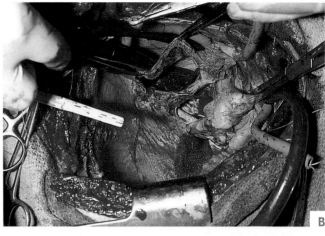

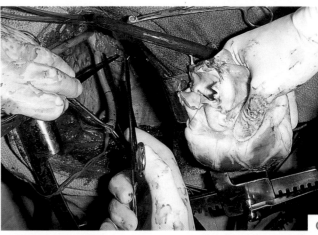

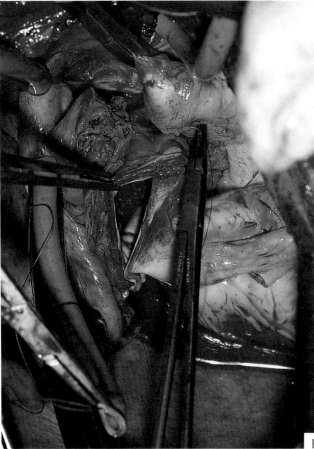

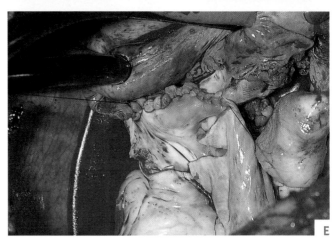

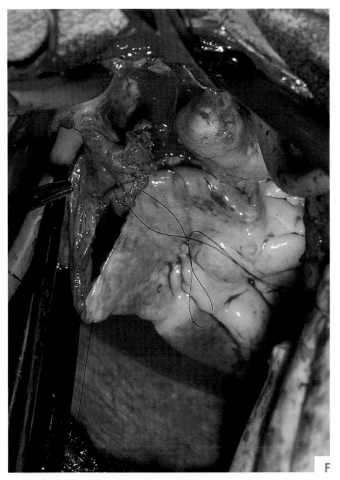

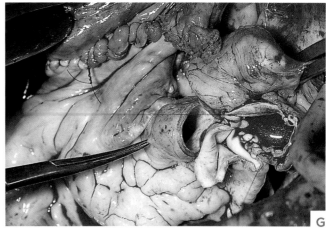

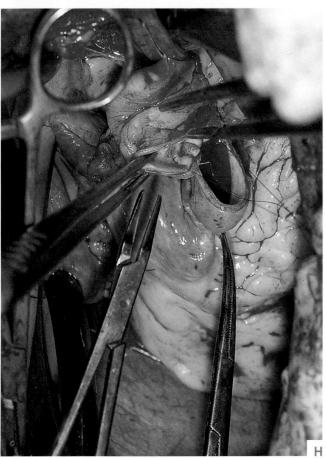

FIGURE 6.69 • Operative sequence of cardiac transplantation. An aortic cannula is placed in the ascending aorta at the base of the innominate artery. The superior and inferior venae cavae are cannulated via the right atrium, close to the atriocaval junction and as far posterior as possible to allow enough right atrial tissue to remain for the right atrial anastomosis (A). Cardiopulmonary bypass is started, tourniquets around the vena cava are tightened, and the aorta is cross-clamped. The native heart is excised at the atrioventricular junction of the right and left ventricles, just distal to the aortic and pulmonary valves (B). Remnants of both atria and great vessels are shown. The prepared donor heart is brought to the operative field. The point of the excised atrial appendage is the starting site for the left atrial anastomosis (C). After completion of the free atrial wall anastomosis, the septal portion of the left atrium is anastomosed (D). The right atrial anastomosis is begun at the point of the recipient's excised right atrial appendage and continued along the septum (E). The right atrial anastomosis is completed by suturing the free atrial wall (F). The pulmonary anastomosis is performed, end-to-end, with a continuous polypropylene suture, starting from the posterior pulmonary artery (G). The beginning of the aortic anastomosis, in which the donor and recipient aortas are joined end-to-end with single-layer suture (H). (Courtesy of the Texas Heart Institute.)

Recipient

The heterotopic technique was introduced several years after the initiation of clinical transplantation and was to be used only in selected cases. It is technically more demanding and has the potential for complications related to anatomic restrictions of the recipient heart[206] (Figure 6.70).

For heterotopic transplantation, the median sternotomy is performed in the usual manner, and the pericardium is opened to the left of the midline, then rectangularly to the right phrenic nerve, forming a flap for isolating the right lung. After heparinization, the aorta is cannulated proximal to the origin of the innominate artery. The superior vena cava is cannulated via the right atrial appendage and inferior vena cava at the atriocaval junction. Cardiopulmonary bypass is begun, and tourniquets are tightened around both venae cavae. The cross-clamp is placed on the ascending aorta. Cardioplegia and topical cooling are applied for maximal protection of the native heart. The left atrium is then opened between the right superior and inferior pulmonary veins. The maximal length of the incision should be ob-

tained to avoid any gradient over the anastomosis. The anastomosis is begun at the midpoint of the posterior parts of both atrial openings and completed by using a continuous running suture.

The recipient's right atrium is opened lateral to the atriocaval junction, with two thirds of the incision being on the superior vena cava. A diamond-shaped anastomosis is performed, allowing for a large interatrial opening. After making an incision on the greater curvature of the recipient aorta, an end-to-side aortic anastomosis is performed. The proper length of the donor aorta should be used to avoid kinking of the atrial anastomoses. The pulmonary anastomosis is assisted by using a 22-mm preclotted woven graft. An end-to-side anastomosis between the graft and the opening on the recipient pulmonary artery is performed, followed by the end-to-end anastomosis between the graft and the donor pulmonary artery. Before weaning, adequate function of both hearts is established. Pacing wires placed on both hearts are used for pacing and for direct separate monitoring of the respective electrocardiograms.

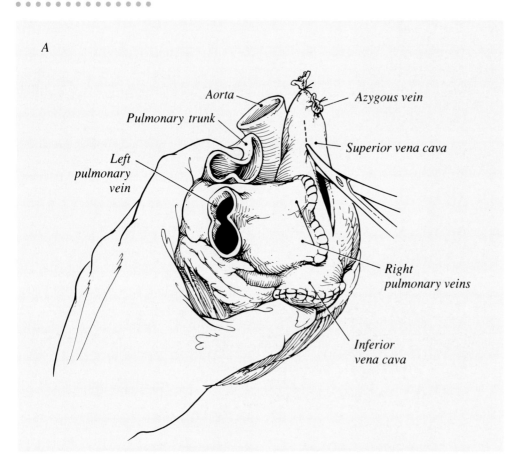

A

Aorta

Pulmonary trunk

Azygous vein

Superior vena cava

Left pulmonary vein

Right pulmonary veins

Inferior vena cava

FIGURE 6.70 • Donor heart preparation for heterotopic transplant. The openings of the right superior and inferior pulmonary veins and the inferior vena cava have been closed carefully. The right atrial incision is extended high up in the superior vena cava. The left superior and inferior pulmonary vein openings are connected by incising the bridge of tissue separating them (A). (Modified with permission. Frazier OH, Okereke OUJ, Cooley DA, et al: *Tex Heart Inst J* 1985;12:221.)

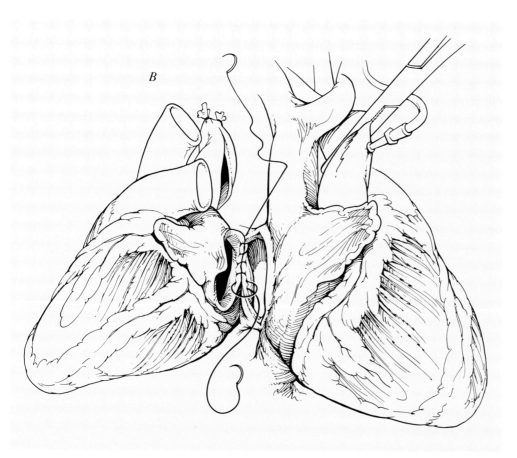

B

FIGURE 6.70 CONT'D • Anastomosis of the left atria. The opening in the donor left atrium may be extended to achieve a wider connection (B). (Modified with permission. Frazier OH, Okereke OUJ, Cooley DA, et al: *Tex Heart Inst J* 1985;12:221.)

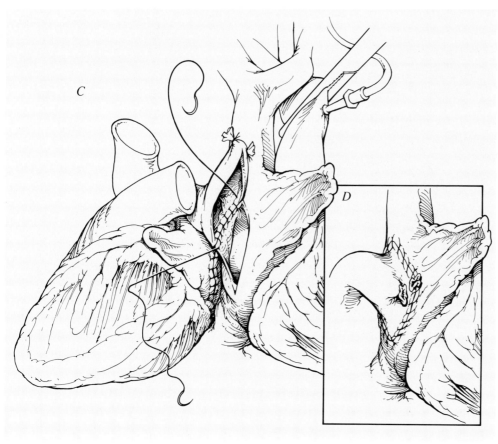

C

D

FIGURE 6.70 CONT'D • The right atrial anastomosis is started by suturing the inferior angle of the incision into the donor right atrium to the midpoint of the posterior edge in the native atrium (C). Completed right atrial anastomosis (D). (Modified with permission. Frazier OH, Okereke OUJ, Cooley DA, et al: *Tex Heart Inst J* 1985;12:221.)

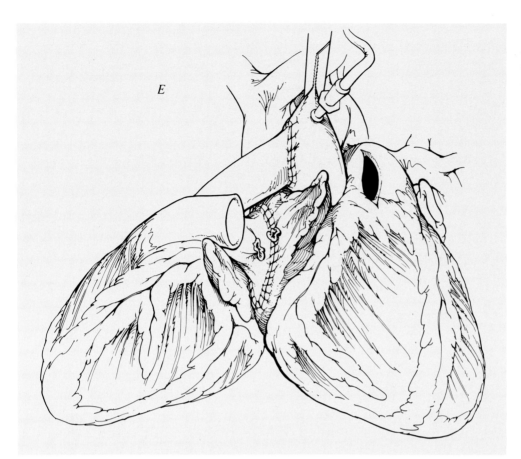

FIGURE 6.70 CONT'D • Anastomosis of the donor-heart aorta to the recipient ascending aorta (E). (Modified with permission. Frazier OH, Okereke OUJ, Cooley DA, et al: *Tex Heart Inst J* 1985;12:221.)

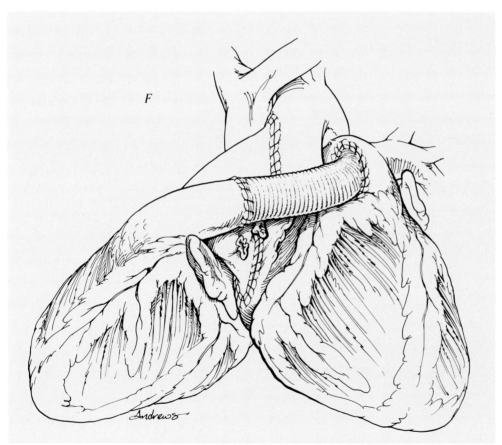

FIGURE 6.70 CONT'D • Completed heterotopic transplantation with interposed Dacron tube graft between the donor and recipient pulmonary arteries (F). (Modified with permission. Frazier OH, Okereke OUJ, Cooley DA, et al: *Tex Heart Inst J* 1985;12:221.)

EARLY POSTOPERATIVE MANAGEMENT

In general, postoperative management of cardiac transplant patients is similar to that for any postcardiac surgery patient. Postoperative complications that differ from those in general cardiac surgery include acute donor heart failure and side effects of immunosuppressive drugs. Donor heart failure may be caused by problems related to the:

- Recipient, as in the case of right ventricular failure due to pulmonary hypertension.
- Donor and procurement, causing depletion of myocardial energy stores.
- Immunologic reaction between donor and recipient, as in hyperacute rejection.

Despite all the previously mentioned measures for preoperative assessment, an acute increase in pulmonary resistance can occur at the time of weaning from cardiopulmonary bypass, thereby causing right ventricular failure. Overventilation of the patients, rapid and aggressive correction of acidosis, and the addition of isoproterenol infusion may prevent occurrence of this dangerous complication. Prostaglandin E_1 may reduce pulmonary pressures without significantly affecting the systemic circulation.[207]

Mechanical circulatory support can be used successfully in cases of right ventricular failure.[207] The other indication for use of mechanical circulatory support is in rare cases of biventricular failure, in which mechanical support can lead to complete recovery of the transiently nonfunctional donor heart.[208]

There are several complications in the early postoperative period related to the side effects of immunosuppressive drugs, especially cyclosporine. In the immediate postoperative period, renal dysfunction can be attributed to perioperative use of cyclosporine, but other factors may play a role in its development. These include preoperative renal dysfunction due to cardiac failure, cardiopulmonary bypass, and poor perioperative donor heart function. Arterial hypertension is frequently seen in the immediate postoperative period. This requires aggressive antihypertensive therapy since it may contribute to bleeding and seizures, well-recognized side effects of cyclosporine.[207–210]

IMMUNOSUPPRESSIVE THERAPY

The complexity of immunologic mechanisms leading to transplant rejection, difficulties in its diagnosis, and limited experience with specific immunosuppressive drugs influenced the development of many "immunosuppressive protocols," with ongoing discussions of their advantages and disadvantages. Since the immunosuppressive protocol is only a part of the complex therapy for end-stage cardiac disease, the differences are difficult to assess. Specific points of debate include the use or avoidance of monoclonal or polyclonal antilymphocytic preparations in the perioperative and initial postoperative periods, and the correct dosages and uses of cyclosporine and steroids.[211–213]

At the Texas Heart Institute, two major protocols are currently being utilized, and patients are assigned to a particular protocol based on their perioperative cardiac and end-organ functions. Preoperatively, all patients receive azathioprine, 2 mg/kg, and cyclosporine, 2 to 6 mg/kg, based on renal function as assessed by serum creatinine and creatinine clearance tests. Methylprednisolone, 500 mg, is given intraoperatively just before the release of the aortic cross-clamp. Postoperatively, methylprednisolone is continued and gradually tapered to 30 mg/d by day 11. Azathioprine is given at a dosage of 2 mg/kg/d and adjusted to maintain the patient's white cell count (5,000–7,000/ mL). Cyclosporine is begun at a dosage of 6 mg/kg/d. The dosage is adjusted according to the blood levels that are being maintained between 300–500 ng/mL, measured by whole blood monoclonal antibody (IncStar, Stillwater, Minnesota 55082). In patients with perioperative renal failure and/or hepatic dysfunction, a protocol that includes OKT3 monoclonal antibody is used to avoid additional nephrotoxic and hepatotoxic effects of cyclosporine. It is important to emphasize that since this is a very efficient and potent immunosuppressant drug, our approach is to minimize its use or "save" the drug for emergency situations, that is, at the time of advanced rejection episodes, and then restrict its use to one time to minimize the risk of posttransplant lymphoma.[214]

OKT3 is given daily at a dosage of 5 mg intravenously for 10 days. The effect of the drug is monitored daily by using CD3 levels and is considered efficient if the CD3 level is below 5% of that predicted. During therapy with OKT3, steroids are given at a dosage of 20 mg daily. On the sixth day of treatment with OKT3, azathioprine, 2 mg/kg/d, and cyclosporine, 5 mg/kg/d, are added to the immunosuppressive regimen. After the OKT3 therapy is completed, cyclosporine is increased to maintain blood levels between 350–500 ng/mL. At the same time, the steroid dosage is increased to 2 mg/kg/d and then tapered to 0.5 mg/kg/d by day 10 post-OKT3 therapy. This regimen evolved as a result of a high incidence of viral infections in the group of patients in which all drugs were given concomitantly from the first day of therapy. This approach to steroid therapy after the discontinuation of OKT3 significantly reduced the number of rebound rejections.

MAINTENANCE IMMUNOSUPPRESSION

Based on a very low incidence of late acute myocardial rejection episodes despite the gradual, significant reduction of both cyclosporine and prednisone dosages, the long-term efficiency of cyclosporine is acceptable.[215] Decreasing the cyclosporine dosage from an average of 6.5 mg/kg/d at 6 months posttransplant to 3.8 mg/kg/d at 5 years significantly reduced the incidence of some of the initially observed side effects, such as seizures and lymphomas. The positive effect of this approach is also noted in the stabilization of renal function after an initial deterioration that often is noted during the first 6 months.[216] Unfortunately, despite the dosage reduction, only the severity rather than the incidence of arterial hypertension decreases, and the majority of patients require multiple drug therapy for its control.

MYOCARDIAL REJECTION

DIAGNOSIS

Acute myocardial rejection is an immunologic phenomenon that occurs in majority of cardiac transplant patients with a declining frequency and severity during the posttransplant period. Since the introduction of cyclosporine, the clinical pattern of rejection includes a slower onset and progression of rejection episodes, with absent or minimal clinical signs of cardiac dysfunction. Advanced damage of the myocardium can occur before the signs of cardiac failure become obvious; thus routine surveillance is essential. A timely adjustment of the immunosuppressive therapy regimen, in most instances, can prevent irreversible myocardial damage. Based on their low sensitivity, clinical signs can be used only as an indication for endomyocardial biopsy rather than as an indicator for therapy. The exceptions are patients with obvious signs of cardiac failure, in whom treatment should be initiated, followed by histologic confirmation of severe rejection. Low-grade fever, arrhythmias or unexplained tachycardia, pericardial friction rub, and, rarely, chest discomfort should be suspected as early signs of a rejection episode.

TABLE 6.10 • STANDARDIZED CARDIAC BIOPSY GRADING

Grade	"New" nomenclature	"Old" nomenclature
0	No rejection	No rejection
1	A = Focal (perivascular or interstitial) infiltrate without necrosis	Mild rejection
	B = Diffuse but sparse infiltrate without necrosis	
2	One focus only with aggressive infiltration and/or focal myocyte damage	"Focal" moderate rejection
3	A = Multifocal aggressive infiltrates and/or myocyte damage	"Low" moderate rejection
	B = Diffuse inflammatory process with necrosis	"Borderline/severe"
4	Diffuse aggressive polymorphous ± infiltrate ± edema, ± hemorrhage, ± vasculitis, with necrosis	"Severe/acute" rejection

"Resolving" rejection denoted by a lesser grade.
"Resolved" rejection denoted by grade 0.

(Reproduced with permission. Billingham ME, Cary NRB, Hammond ME, et al: *J Heart Transplant* 1990;9:588.)

TABLE 6.11 • TEXAS HEART INSTITUTE'S EVALUATION OF CARDIAC ALLOGRAFT REJECTION BY ENDOMYOCARDIAL BIOPSY

0	No evidence of rejection
1–2	Perivascular aggregates of mononuclear cells
3	Perivascular aggregates of mononuclear cells with extension into the interstitium
4–8	Interstitial mononuclear cells with cardiac myocyte degeneration of increasing severity
9–10	Extensive cardiac myocyte degeneration, interstitial mononuclear cells and polymorphonuclear leukocytes

(Reproduced with permission. McAllister HA Jr, Schnee MJ, Radovancevic B, et al: *Tex Heart Inst J* 1986;13:1.)

Despite persistent trials to develop noninvasive methods for monitoring rejection, myocardial biopsy is still a standard method for diagnosing rejection. After almost 20 years of using endomyocardial biopsy to diagnose allograft rejection, and after the development of many grading systems for determining the severity of rejection, the first standardization of grading systems was introduced in August 1990 (Table 6.10).[217] As it gradually gains worldwide acceptance, this standardization should allow for better communication in the cardiac transplant community, as well as better understanding of the efficacy of antirejection therapy.

Since 1985 at our institution, the McAllister grading scale (Table 6.11) has been an excellent way to communicate not only the actual level of rejection, but also the direction and speed of change, which allows for appropriate adjustment of therapy.[218] A grading scale of 1 to 10 is used, and biopsies graded 5 or above are considered to indicate a rejection episode[219] (Figures 6.71, 6.72).

Although routine electrocardiographic findings do not correlate well with the onset of rejection under current immunosuppressive therapy protocols, specificity and sensitivity of intramyocardial electrocardiographic recordings taken during sleep do approach an acceptable range.[216,220] Under investigation are the whole array of hematologic and immunologic monitoring methods, including cytoimmunologic monitoring, interleukin-2, gamma interferon, and ß$_2$-microglobulin levels. In general, all of these tests either showed low correlation with endomyocardial biopsy findings or were unable to distinguish between rejection and infection.[221–226] Posttransplantation echocardiography, although extremely useful for assessing cardiac function, has not proved to be a substitute for endomyocardial biopsy. With the accumulation of more data, it appears feasible to use echocardiography to detect subtle changes in myocardial function.[227,228] This may may be helpful in adjusting antirejection therapy and assessing its effects. Some imaging techniques, like magnetic resonance imaging and indium-111 labeled antimyosin antibodies, are also under investigation for diagnosing rejection.[229,230] The initial results have been encouraging.

TREATMENT

Treatment options include methylprednisolone pulse, OKT3, increasing doses of oral cyclosporine, intravenous cyclosporine, methotrexate, and cyclophosphamide. For lower grades of re-

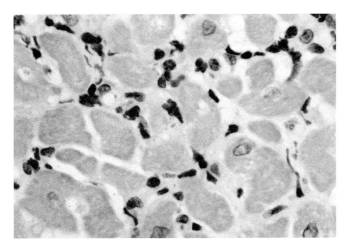

FIGURE 6.71 • Grade 3 rejection. Perivascular aggregates of mononuclear cells with extension into the myocardial interstitium but without evidence of significant cardiac myocyte degeneration. Hematoxylin-eosin stain. (Original magnification x 100) (Reproduced with permission. McAllister HA Jr: *J Heart Transplant* 1990;9:279.)

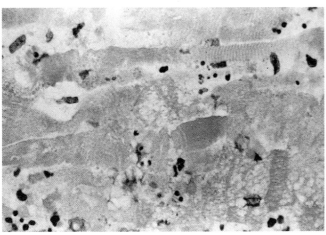

FIGURE 6.72 • Grade 10 rejection. Extensive cardiac myocyte degeneration associated with interstitial mononuclear cells and neutrophils. Hematoxylin-eosin stain. (Original magnification x 160) (Reproduced with permission. McAllister HA Jr: *J Heart Transplant* 1990;9:280.)

jection (5 and 6), our treatment of choice is either intravenous or oral cyclosporine because it reduces the risk of infectious complications[231] (Figure 6.73). OKT3 is the therapy of choice in patients with advanced rejection (grade greater than 7) and concomitant infection and for patients who have not responded to steroid pulse therapy. Simultaneous OKT3 and methylprednisolone pulse therapy is reserved for patients with clinical signs of cardiac failure, wherein only aggressive treatment can lead to a timely reversal of rejection. In patients with profound circulatory failure, mechanical support during treatment for rejection offers protection from end-organ failure.[207] Currently, the Hemopump (Nimbus, Inc., Rancho Cordova, California), which can be inserted with relative ease without the need for thoracotomy, is the device of choice in immunosuppressed patients at our center.[232]

INFECTIONS

In addition to rejection, infections are the major cause of morbidity and mortality in cardiac transplant recipients during the first year after transplantation.[233] Rejection prophylaxis and treatment are so closely related that adjustment of immunosuppressive therapy to treat one may lead to occurrence of the other. Therefore, an extremely careful adjustment of drugs should be made to prevent an erratic effect in the posttransplant period.

Bacterial infections occur primarily during the first month after transplantation, particularly in patients who have had central venous catheters and chest tubes placed for long periods. Nosocomial-acquired opportunistic infections, such as aspergillosis, Legionella pneumonia, and nocardiosis can be extremely dangerous during this period.[234] Viral infection caused by cytomegalovirus (CMV) or Epstein-Barr virus (EBV) usually occur after the first postoperative month and have been correlated with other complications in cardiac transplant recipients. With the broader application of OKT3 prophylaxis, the incidence of CMV had increased. However, after the introduction of gancyclovir therapy, the mortality from this infection significantly decreased. Avoidance of transplantation from a CMV-positive donor to a CMV-negative recipient and the use of CMV-negative blood products may further decrease the severity of this disease. Similarly, EBV infections had been associated with the occurrence of lymphoma in cardiac transplant recipients, and EBV matching may play a role in the avoidance of lymphomas in some patients.[235] With the introduction of sulfamethoxazole/trimethoprim prophylaxis during the first year after transplant, *Pneumocystis carinii* pneumonia has been practically eradicated from the clinical picture and now occurs

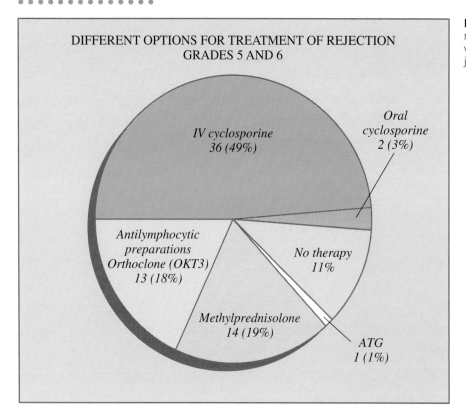

FIGURE 6.73 • Different options for treatment of rejection grades 5 and 6, which were based on individualization of each rejection episode.

only in patients with inadequate prophylaxis. We hope that further improvements in both prophylaxis and therapy of infections and more specific immunosuppressive therapy will decrease morbidity caused by infections.

CORONARY ARTERY DISEASE

Coronary artery disease is the most frequent cause of late death in cardiac transplant recipients.[236,237] There continues to be a high incidence of this complication despite changes in immunosuppressive therapy, use of antiplatelet agents, or use of lipid-controlling drugs. Immunologic injury—a type of rejection of the coronary vasculature—has been implicated as a major cause of this disease. Both humoral and cellular mechanisms have been described in conjunction with this complication. However, based on the present inability of immunosuppression to control this problem, humoral immunity may play a bigger role.

A correlation between coronary artery disease and CMV infections has been implied, but in our experience, CMV infections have not significantly influenced the development of this complication.[237,238] It is possible that some of the generally accepted risk factors, such as smoking and hypertension, may accelerate the development of posttransplant coronary artery disease. Until there is a better understanding of this process, use of antiplatelet agents, lipid-controlling drugs, and aggressive antihypertensive therapy with cessation of smoking are the only available measures to slow its progression.

In a selected subgroup of transplant recipients with eccentric coronary lesions, percutaneous transluminal coronary angioplasty and coronary artery bypass procedures have been performed[239–242] (Figure 6.74). Retransplantation can be considered in NYHA class IV patients. The survival for these retransplant patients, however, is somewhat decreased compared with patient survival after primary transplantation.[188,243]

PROGNOSIS

More than 85% of all cardiac transplants have been performed since 1985. Thus, it is still early to make any conclusions regarding actual long-term survival in these patients. With the growing experience in patient and donor selection, immunosuppressive therapy, diagnosis of rejection, and treatment and prophylaxis of infection, excellent one-year results have been obtained and are currently exceeding 80%.[188] Actually, results that exceed these values should raise the question of strict ad-

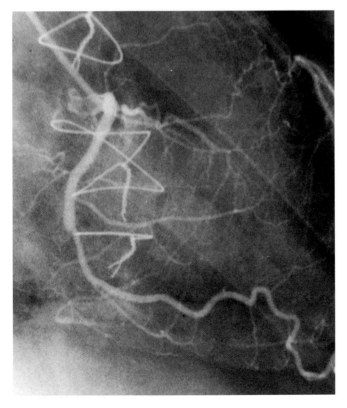

FIGURE 6.74 • Angiogram in a patient 18 months posttransplantation, revealing complete occlusion of the right coronary artery and left anterior descending (LAD) coronary artery, with retrograde filling of the LAD by the marginal branch. Good collateral circulation is shown. The patient successfully underwent coronary artery bypass several months later. Significant improvement was shown in left ventricular ejection fraction, which increased from 35% preoperatively to 56% after surgery. (Reproduced from Frazier OH, Vega JD, Duncan JM, et al: *J Heart Transplant* 1991. In press.)

herence to NYHA class IV patients and transplantation of patients who could be treated with conventional methods. Regarding long-term results, the nearly invariable occurrence of coronary atherosclerosis seems to be the most important limiting factor.[237,244–248] Better control of it may significantly decrease late mortality.

FUTURE TRENDS

It is realistic to expect an even faster increase in the number of patients being referred as potential candidates for cardiac transplantation. This, of course, aggravates the donor shortage problem. Two solutions to this problem are application of mechanical circulatory devices—total artificial hearts or left ventricular assist devices—and the use of xenografts. Experience gained in cardiac transplantation during the last ten years indicates that, with further improvements in management, there is no reason to believe that even the potential use of a mechanical heart will diminish the role of cardiac transplantation. Future improvements in cardiac transplantation are expected with the development of some new immunosuppressive medications, both in maintenance and antirejection therapy. Some of the newer medications, such as FK 506 and rapamycin, are undergoing initial trials as major immunosuppressants offering higher immunosuppressive effects in smaller doses with the promise of a significant decrease in side effects.[249,250] Areas of research include immunomodulation of the transplanted organs rather than immunosuppression of the recipient and xenotransplantation. Endomyocardial biopsy is still the best way to diagnose rejection, but improvements in noninvasive detection of rejection are expected, using immunologic markers and/or new imaging techniques such as magnetic resonance imaging and positron emission tomography.

Without minimizing its associated complications, cardiac transplantation appears to have become a routine procedure with excellent results in treating patients with end-stage cardiac disease. A better understanding of the immunologic factors involved in organ "acceptance" and the modification of such factors are the next steps in the continuing development of cardiac transplantation.

REFERENCES

1. Council on Scientific Affairs: Indications for aortocoronary bypass graft surgery, 1979. *JAMA* 1979;242:2709.

2. Braunwald E: Editorial retrospective: Effects of coronary-artery bypass grafting on survival, implications of the randomized Coronary Artery Surgery Study. *N Engl J Med* 1983;309:1181.

3. CASS Principal Investigators and their Associates: Coronary Artery Surgery Study (CASS): A randomized trial of coronary artery bypass surgery, comparability of entry characteristics and survival in randomized patients and nonrandomized patients meeting randomization criteria. *J Am Coll Cardiol* 1984;3:114.

4. CASS Principal Investigators and their Associates: Coronary Artery Surgery Study (CASS): A randomized trial of coronary artery bypass surgery, survival data. *Circulation* 1983;68:939.

5. CASS Principal Investigators and their Associates: Myocardial infarction and mortality in the Coronary Artery Surgery Study (CASS) randomized trial. *N Engl J Med* 1984;310:750.

6. Kennedy JW, Killip T, Fisher LD, et al: The clinical spectrum of coronary artery disease and its surgical and medical management, 1974–1979: The Coronary Artery Surgery Study. *Circulation* 1982;66(Suppl):3.

7. Kaiser GC, Davis KB, Fisher LD, et al: Survival following coronary artery bypass grafting in patients with severe angina pectoris (CASS): An observational study. *J Thorac Cardiovasc Surg* 1985;89:513.

8. Berg R, Selinger SL, Leonard JJ, et al: Immediate coronary artery bypass for acute evolving infarction. *J Thorac Cardiovasc Surg* 1981;81:492.

9. Selinger SL, Berg R, Leonard JJ, et al: Surgical treatment of acute evolving anterior myocardial infarction. *Circulation* 1981;64(Suppl II):II28.

10. Berg R, Selinger SL, Leonard JJ, et al: Acute evolving myocardial infarction: A surgical emergency. *J Thorac Cardiovasc Surg* 1984;88:902.

11. DeWood MA, Spores J, Berg R, et al: Acute myocardial infarction: A decade of experience with surgical reperfusion in 701 patients. *Circulation* 1983;68(Suppl II):II8.

12. Hillis LD, Borer J, Braunwald E, et al: High-dose intravenous streptokinase for acute myocardial infarction: Preliminary results of a multicenter trial. *J Am Coll Cardiol* 1985;6:957.

13. Serruys PW, Simmons ML, Suryapranta H, et al: Preservation of global and regional left ventricular function after early thrombolysis in acute myocardial infarction. *J Am Coll Cardiol* 1986;7:729.

14. Gold HK, Leinbach RC, Garabedian HD, et al: Acute coronary reocclusion after thrombolysis with recombinant human tissue-type plasminogen activator: Prevention by a maintenance infusion. *Circulation* 1986;73:347.

15. Topol EJ, Weiss JJ, Brinker JA, et al: Regional wall motion improvement after coronary thrombolysis with recombinant tissue plasminogen activator: Importance of coronary angioplasty. *J Am Coll Cardiol* 1985;6:426.

16. Sweeney MS, Lewis CTP, Murphy MC, et al: Cardiac surgical emergencies. *Critical Care Clinics* 1989;5:659.

17. Alderman EL, Fisher LD, Litwin P, et al: Results of coronary artery surgery in patients with poor left ventricular function (CASS). *Circulation* 1983;68:785.

18. Mata LA, Bosch X, David PR, et al: Clinical and angiographic assessment 6 months after double percutaneous coronary angioplasty. *J Am Coll Cardiol* 1985;5:446. Abstract.

19. Zaidi AR, Hollman JL, Galen K: Multivessel angioplasty, procedure, and follow-up trends. *Circulation* 1984;70(II):II266. Abstract.

20. Bigelow WG, Lindsay WK, Harrison RC, et al: Oxygen transport and utilization in dogs at low body temperatures. *Am J Physiol* 1950;160:125.

21. Bigelow WG, Lindsay WK, Greenwood WF: Hypothermia: Its possible role in cardiac surgery: An investigation of factors governing survival in dogs at low body temperatures. *Ann Surg* 1950;132:849.

22. Lewis FJ, Taufic M: Closure of atrial septal defects with the aid of hypothermia: Experimental accomplishments and the report of one successful case. *Surgery* 1953;33:52.

23. Gibbon JH Jr: Application of a mechanical heart and lung apparatus to cardiac surgery. *Minn Med* 1954;37:171.

24. Kirklin JW, DuShane JW, Patrick RT, et al: Intracardiac surgery with the aid of a mechanical pump-oxygenator system: Report of eight cases. *Proc Staff Meet Mayo Clin* 1955;30:201.

25. Lillehei CW, Cohen M, Warden HE, et al: The direct-vision intracardiac correction of congenital anomalies by controlled cross circulation: Results in thirty-two patients with ventricular septal defects, tetralogy of Fallot, and atrioventricularis communis defects. *Surgery* 1955;38:11.

26. Shumway NE, Lower RR, Stofer RC: Selective hypothermia of the heart in anoxic cardiac arrest. *Surg Gynecol Obstet* 1959;109:750.

27. Gay WA Jr, Ebert PA: Functional, metabolic, and morphologic effects of potassium-induced cardioplegia. *Surgery* 1973;74:284.

28. Hearse DJ, Braimbridge MV, Jynge P: *Protection of the Ischemic Myocardium: Cardioplegia* New York, NY: Raven Press; 1981.

29. Ellis RJ, Wisniewski A, Potts R, et al: Reduction of flow rate and arterial pressure at moderate hypothermia does not result in cerebral dysfunction. *J Thorac Cardiovasc Surg* 1983;79:173.

30. Feinberg H, Levitsky S: Biochemical rationale of cardioplegia. In: Engelman RM, Levitsky S, eds. *A Textbook of Clinical Cardioplegia* Mt Kisco, NY: Futura; 1982:131.

31. McGoon DC: The ongoing quest for ideal myocardial protection: A catalog of the recent English literature. *J Thorac Cardiovasc Surg* 1985;89:639.

32. Becker H, Vinten-Johansen J, Buckberg GD, et al: Myocardial damage caused by keeping pH 7.40 during systemic deep hypothermia. *J Thorac Cardiovasc Surg* 1981;82:810.

33. Rahn H, Reeves RB, Howell BJ: Hydrogen ion regulation, temperature, and evolution. *Am Rev Respir Dis* 1975;112:165.

34. Engelman RM, Rousou JH, Dobbs W, et al: The superiority of blood cardioplegia in myocardial preservation. *Circulation* 1980;62(Suppl I):I62.

35. Levine FH: Blood or crystalloid cardioplegia: An overview. In: Engelman RM, Levitsky S, eds. *A Textbook of Clinical Cardioplegia* Mt. Kisco, NY: Futura; 1982.

36. Magovern GJ, Flaherty JT, Gott VL, et al: Failure of blood cardioplegia to protect myocardium at lower temperatures. *Circulation* 1982;62(Suppl I):I60.

37. Rosenkranz ER, Buckberg GD, Laks H, et al: Warm induction of cardioplegia with glutamate-enriched blood in coronary patients with cardiogenic shock who are dependent on inotropic drugs and intra-aortic balloon support: Initial experience and operative strategy. *J Thorac Cardiovasc Surg* 1983;86:507.

38. Rosenkranz ER, Vinten-Johansen J, Buckberg GD, et al: Benefits of normothermic induction of blood cardioplegia in energy-depleted hearts, with maintenance of arrest by multidose cold blood cardioplegic infusions. *J Thorac Cardiovasc Surg* 1982;84:667.

39. Gundry SR, Kirsh MM: A comparison of retrograde cardioplegia versus antegrade cardioplegia in the presence of coronary artery obstruction. *Ann Thorac Surg* 1984;38:124.

40. Guiraudon GM, Campbell CS, McLellan DG, et al: Retrograde coronary sinus versus aortic root perfusion with cold cardioplegia: Randomized study of levels of cardiac enzymes in 40 patients. *Circulation* 1986;74(Suppl III):III105.

41. Bolling SF, Flaherty JT, Bulkley BH, et al: Improved myocardial preservation during global ischemia by continuous retrograde coronary sinus perfusion. *J Thorac Cardiovasc Surg* 1983;86:659.

42. Ludinghausen M: Nomenclature and distribution pattern of cardiac veins in man. In: Mohl W, Faxon D, Wolner E, eds. *Clinics of CSI: Proceedings* New York, NY: Springer-Verlag; 1986:13.

43. Jonnesco T: Angine de poitrine guerie par la resection du sympathique cervico-thoracique. *Bull Acad Med* 1920;84:93.

44. Beck CS: The development of a new blood supply to the heart by operation. *Ann Surg* 1935;102:801.

45. Vineberg AM: Development of an anastomosis between the coronary vessels and a transplanted internal mammary artery. *Can Med Assoc J* 1946;55:117.

46. Bailey CP, May A, Lemmon WM: Survival after coronary endarterectomy in man. *JAMA* 1957;164:641.

47. Favaloro RG: Direct myocardial revascularization. *Surg Clin North Am* 1971;51:1035.

48. Johnson WD, Flemma RJ, Lepley D Jr, et al: Extended treatment of severe coronary artery disease: A total surgical approach. *Ann Surg* 1969;170:460.

49. Loop FD, Cosgrove DM, Kramer JR, et al: Late clinical and arteriographic results in 500 coronary artery reoperations. *J Thorac Cardiovasc Surg* 1981;81:675.

50. Lytle BW, Loop FD, Cosgrove DM, et al: Long-term (5 to 12 years) serial studies of internal mammary artery and saphenous vein coronary bypass grafts. *J Thorac Cardiovasc Surg* 1985;84:248.

51. Cooley DA: Surgical treatment of coronary arteriosclerotic disease: Technique and results in 18,893 patients. *Ospedali d'Italia, Chirurgie* 1980;33:403.

52. Reul GJ Jr: New technique for surgical hemostasis of aorto-prosthetic anastomosis. *Cardiovascular Diseases, Bulletin of Texas Heart Institute* 1974;1:120.

53. Livesay JJ, Cooley DA, Hallman GL, et al: Early and late results of coronary endarterectomy: Analysis of 3,369 patients. *J Thorac Cardiovasc Surg* 1986;92:649.

54. Ramos JR, Berger K, Mansfield PB, et al: Histological fate and endothelial changes of distended and nondistended vein grafts. *Ann Surg* 1976;183:205.

55. Barner HB, Swartz MT, Mudd G, et al: Late patency of the internal mammary artery as a coronary bypass conduit. *Ann Thorac Surg* 1982;34:408.

56. Oschner JL: Institutional variations influencing results: Arterial versus venous graft. *Circulation* 1982;65(Suppl II):II81.

57. Cosgrove DM, Loop FD, Lytle BW, et al: Does mammary artery grafting increase surgical risk? *Circulation* 1985;72(Suppl II):II170.

58. Golfman S: Antiplatelet therapy in graft patency. *Cardiac Surgery: State of the Art Reviews* 1986;1:115.

59. Sharma GVRK, Khuri SF, Folland ED, et al: Prognosis for aortocoronary graft patency. *J Thorac Cardiovasc Surg* 1983;85:570.

60. Campeau L, Enjalbert M, Lesperance J, et al: The relation of risk factors to the development of atherosclerosis in saphenous-vein bypass grafts and the progression of disease in the native circulation: A study of 10 years after aortocoronary bypass surgery. *N Engl J Med* 1984;311:1329.

61. Sharma GVRK, Josa M: Factors influencing saphenous vein graft patency. *Cardiac Surgery: State of the Art Reviews* 1986;1:125.

62. Bourassa MG, Campeau L, Lesperance J, et al: Change in grafts and coronary arteries after saphenous vein aortocoronary bypass surgery: Results at repeat angiography. *Circulation* 1982;65(Suppl II):II90.

63. Campeau L, Enjalbert M, Lesperance J, et al: Atherosclerosis and late closure of aortocoronary saphenous vein grafts: Sequential angiographic studies at 2 weeks, 1 year, 5 to 7 years and 10 to 12 years after surgery. *Circulation* 1983;68(Suppl II):II1.

64. Grondin CM, Campeau L, Lesperance J, et al: Atherosclerotic changes in coronary vein grafts six years after operation: Angiographic aspects in 110 patients. *J Thorac Cardiovasc Surg* 1979;77:24.

65. Chesebro JH, Clements IP, Fuster V, et al: A platelet-inhibitor-drug trial in coronary-artery bypass operations: Benefit of perioperative dipyridamole and aspirin therapy on early postoperative vein graft patency. *N Engl J Med* 1982;307:73.

66. Chesebro JH, Fuster V, Elveback LR, et al: Effect of dipyridamole and aspirin on late vein-graft patency after coronary bypass operations. *N Engl J Med* 1984;310:209.

67. Hanson SR, Harker LA, Bjornsson TD: Effects of platelet-modifying drugs on arterial thromboembolism in baboons: aspirin potentiates the antithrombotic action of dipyridamole and sulfinpyrazone by mechanisms independent of platelet cyclooxygenase inhibition. *J Clin Invest* 1985;75:1591.

68. Grondin CM, Campeau L, Lesperance J, et al: Comparison of late changes in internal mammary and saphenous vein grafts in two consecutive series of patients 10 years after operation. *Circulation* 1984;70(Suppl I):I208.

69. Grondin CM, Lesperance J, Bourassa MG, et al: Coronary artery grafting with the saphenous vein or internal mammary artery: Comparison of late results in two consecutive series of patients. *Ann Thorac Surg* 1975;20:605.

70. Loop FD: CASS continued. *Circulation* 1985;72(Suppl II):II1.

71. Cosgrove DM, Loop FD, Lytle BW, et al: Determinants of 10 year survival after primary myocardial revascularization. *Ann Surg* 1985;202:480.

72. Billroth T, cited by Jeger E: *Die Chirurgie der Blutgefasse und des Herzens* Berlin, Germany: A. Hirschwald; 295: 1913.

73. McGoon DC: The dimensions of surgical progress in cardiac surgery. *Bull Am Coll Surg* 1982;67(11):15.

74. Samways DW: Cardiac peristalsis: Its nature and effects. *Lancet* 1898;1:927.

75. Brunton L: Preliminary note on the possibility of treating mitral stenosis by surgical methods. *Lancet* 1902;1:352.

76. Tuffier T: Etat Actuel de la Chirurgie Intrathoracique. *Trans Internat Cong Med* 1913, London, England: 1914, Sect VII, Surgery, pt 2, 249.

77. Cutler EC, Levine SA: Cardiotomy and valvulotomy for mitral stenosis: Observations and clinical notes concerning an operated case with recovery. *Boston Med Surg J* 1923;188:1023.

78. Souttar HS: Surgical treatment of mitral stenosis. *Br Med J* 1925;2:603.

79. Powers JH: Surgical treatment of mitral stenosis: Experimental study. *Arch Surg* 1932;25:555.

80. Harken DE: Management of retained foreign bodies in the heart and great vessels, European Theatre of Operations. In: *Surgery in World War II Vol 2. Thoracic Surgery* 353–95.

81. Bailey CP: The surgical treatment of mitral stenosis (mitral commissurotomy). *Dis Chest* 1949;15:377.

82. Harken DE, Ellis LB, Ware PF, et al: The surgical treatment of mitral stenosis. *N Engl J Med* 1948;239:801.

83. Baker C, Brock RC, Campbell M: Valvulotomy for mitral stenosis: Report of six successful cases. *Br Med J* 1950;1:1283.

84. Smithy HG: An approach to the surgical treatment of valvular disease of the heart. *Sixteenth Annual Assembly of the Southeastern Surgical Conference* Vol 14. Hollywood, FL: April 5-8; 1948.

85. Gibbon JH: Application of a mechanical heart and lung apparatus to cardiac surgery. *Minn Med* 1954;37:171.

86. Harken DE, Soroff HS, Taylor WJ, et al: Partial and complete prosthesis in aortic insufficiency. *J Thorac Cardiovasc Surg* 1960;40:744.

87. Starr A, Edwards ML: Mitral replacement: Clinical experience with a ball-valve prosthesis. *Ann Surg* 1961;154:726.

88. Carpentier A, Lemaigre G, Robert L, et al: Biological factors affecting long-term results of various heterografts. *J Thorac Cardiovasc Surg* 1969;58:467.

89. Ross DN: Homograft replacement of the aortic valve. *Lancet* 1962;2:487.

90. Barratt-Boyes BG: Homograft aortic valve replacement in aortic incompetence and stenosis. *Thorax* 1964;19:131.

91. Kaiser GA, Hancock WD, Lukban SB, et al: Clinical use of a new design stented xenograft heart valve prosthesis. *Surg Forum* 1969;20:137.

92. Ionescu MI, Pakrashi BC, Holden MP, et al: Results of aortic valve replacement with frame-supported fascia lata and pericardial grafts. *J Thorac Cardiovasc Surg* 1972;64:340.

93. Cooley DA, Duncan JM, Ott DA, et al: The Texas Heart Institute experience with the St. Jude Medical valve. In: D'Alessandro LC, ed. *Heart Surgery 1987* Rome, Italy: Casa Editrice Scientifica Internazionale; 1987: 289.

94. Duran CM, Alonso J, Gaite L, et al: Long-term results of conservative repair of rheumatic aortic valve insufficiency. *Eur J Cardiothorac Surg* 1988;2:217.

95. Freeman WE, Schaff HV, King RM, et al: Ultrasonic aortic valve decalcification: Doppler echocardiographic evaluation. *J Am Coll Cardiol* 1988;11:229A.

96. Brown AH, Davies PGH: Ultrasonic decalcification of calcified cardiac valves and annuli. *Br Med J* 1972;3:274.

97. Craver JM: Aortic valve debridement by ultrasonic surgical aspirator: A word of caution. *Ann Thorac Surg* 1990;49:746.

98. Mullins CE: Interventional techniques for congenital heart disease. In Cooley DA, ed. *How I Do It, Cardiac Surgery, State of the Art Reviews* Vol 4. Philadelphia, PA: Hanley and Belfus; 1990: 375.

99. Brown JW, Stevens LS, Holly S, et al: Surgical spectrum of aortic stenosis in children: A thirty-year experience with 257 children. *Ann Thorac Surg* 1988;45:393.

100. Ross J Jr, Braunwald E: Aortic stenosis. *Circulation* 1968;38(suppl V):V-61.

101. Kirklin JW, Barratt-Boyes BG: Aortic valve disease and congenital aortic stenosis. In *Cardiac Surgery*, New York, NY: John Wiley & Sons; 1986.

102. Ellis PR, Cooley DA, DeBakey ME: Clinical considerations and surgical treatment of annulo-aortic ectasia: Report of successful operation. *J Thorac Cardiovasc Surg* 1961;42:363.

103. Olesen KH: The natural history of 271 patients with mitral stenosis under medical treatment. *Br Heart J* 1962;24:349.

104. Rankin JS: Mitral and tricuspid valve disease. In Sabiston DC, *Textbook of Surgery*, Philadelphia, PA: WB Saunders Co; 1986.

105. Bannister RG: The risks of deferring valvotomy in patients with moderate mitral stenosis. *Lancet* 1960;2:329.

106. Cooley DA: *Techniques in Cardiac Surgery* 2nd ed. Philadelphia, PA: WB Saunders Co; 1984.

107. Craver JM, Weintraub WS, Jones EL, et al: Predictors of mortality, complications and length of stay in aortic valve replacement for aortic stenosis. *Circulation* 1988;78(Suppl I):I-85.

108. Cabrol C, Pavie A, Solis E, et al: Calcified aortic stenosis: Operative risk. *Eur Heart J* 1988;9(Suppl E):105.

109. Kay PH, Nunley D, Grunkemeier GL, et al: Ten-year survival following aortic valve replacement: A multivariate analysis of coronary bypass as a risk factor. *J Cardiovasc Surg* 1986;27(Torino):494.

110. Groves LK, Effler DB, Hawk WA, et al: Aortic insufficiency secondary to aneurysmal changes in the ascending aorta: Surgical management. *J Thorac Cardiovasc Surg* 1964;48:362.

111. Wheat MW Jr, Wilson JR, Bartley TD: Successful replacement of the entire ascending aorta and aortic valve. *JAMA* 1964;188:717.

112. Cabrol C, Pavie A, Gandjbakhch I, et al: Complete replacement of the ascending aorta with reimplantation of the coronary arteries: New surgical approach. *J Thorac Cardiovasc Surg* 1981;81:309.

113. Mayer JE Jr, Lindsay WG, Wang YT, et al: Composite replacement of the aortic valve and ascending aorta. *J Thorac Cardiovasc Surg* 1978;76:816.

114. Kouchoukos NT, Karp RB, Blackstone EH, et al: Replacement of the ascending aorta and aortic valve with a composite graft. Results in eighty-six patients. *Ann Surg* 1980;192:403.

115. Grey DP, Ott DA, Cooley DA: Surgical treatment of aneurysm of the ascending aorta with aortic insufficiency: A selective approach. *J Thorac Cardiovasc Surg* 1983;86:864.

116. Miller DC, Stinson EB, Oyer PE, et al: Concomitant resection of ascending aortic aneurysm and replacement of the aortic valve. *J Thorac Cardiovasc Surg* 1980;79:388.

117. Davis Z, Pluth JR, Giuliani ER: The Marfan syndrome and cardiac surgery. *J Thorac Cardiovasc Surg* 1978;75:505.

118. Bentall H, DeBono A: A technique for complete replacement of the ascending aorta. *Thorax* 1968;23:338.

119. Creech O Jr: Endoaneurysmorrhaphy and treatment of aortic aneurysms. *Ann Surg* 1966;164:935.

120. Cabrol C, Gandjbakhc I, Pavie A: Surgical treatment of ascending aortic pathology. *J Cardiac Surg* 1988;3:167.

121. Livesay JJ, Cooley DA, Duncan JM, et al: Open aortic anastomosis: Improved results in the treatment of aneurysms of the aortic arch. *Circulation* 1982;66(Suppl I):I-122.

122. Cooley DA, Romagnoli A, Milam JD, et al: A method of preparing woven Dacron grafts to prevent interstitial hemorrhage. *Cardiovasc Dis Bull Tex Heart Inst* 1981;8:48.

123. Rastan H, Koncz J: Aortoventriculoplasty. *J Cardiovasc Surg* 1976;71:920.

124. Konno S, Imai Y, Iida Y, et al: A new method for prosthetic valve replacement in congenital aortic stenosis associated with hypoplasia of the aortic valve ring. *J Thorac Cardiovasc Surg* 1975;70:909.

125. Sweeney MS, Walker WE, Cooley DA, et al: Apico-aortic conduits for complex left ventricular outflow obstructions: 18-year experience. *Ann Thorac Surg* 1986;42:609.

126. Cooley DA, Garrett JR: Septoplasty for left ventricular outflow obstruction without aortic valve replacement: A new technique. *Ann Thorac Surg* 1986;42:445.

127. Carpentier A, Chauvaud S, Fabiani JN, et al: Reconstructive surgery of mitral valve incompetence: Ten-year appraisal. *J Thorac Cardiovasc Surg* 1980;79:338.

128. Lillehei CW, Levy MJ, Bonnabeau RC Jr: Mitral valve replacement with preservation of papillary muscles and chordae tendineae. *J Thorac Cardiovasc Surg* 1964;47:532.

129. Hansen DE, Cahill PD, Derby GC, et al: Relative contributions of the anterior and posterior mitral chordae tendineae to canine global left ventricular systolic function. *J Thorac Cardiovasc Surg* 1987;93:45.

130. Cooley DA: Ventricular endoaneurysmorrhaphy: Results of an improved method of repair. *Texas Heart Inst J* 1989;16:72.

131. Cooley DA: Intravalvular implantation of mitral valve prosthesis. *Tx Heart Inst J* 1987;14:188.

132. Duncan JM, Cooley DA, Reul GJ, et al: Durability and low thrombogenicity of the St. Jude Medical valve at 5-year follow-up. *Ann Thorac Surg* 1986;42:500.

133. Duncan JM, Cooley DA, Reul GJ, et al: Experience with the St. Jude Medical valve and the Ionescu-Shiley bovine pericardial valve at the Texas Heart Institute. In: Matloff JM, ed: *Cardiac Valve Replacement: Current Status* (Proc: Fourth International Symposium on the St. Jude Medical Valve, March 11–14, 1984) Boston: Martinus Nijhoff; 1985: 73.

134. Sweeney MS, Reul GJ Jr, Cooley DA, et al: Comparison of bioprosthetic and mechanical valve replacement for active endocarditis. *J Thorac Cardiovasc Surg* 1985;90:676.

135. Horstkotte D, Körfer R, Seipel L, et al: Late complications in patients with Björk-Shiley and St. Jude Medical heart valve replacement. *Circulation* 1983;68(Suppl II):II175.

136. Reul GJ, Cooley DA, Duncan JM, et al: Valve failure with the Ionescu-Shiley bovine pericardial bioprosthesis: Analysis of 2680 patients. *J Vasc Surg* 1985;2:192.

137. Ishihara T, Ferrans VJ, Jones M, et al: Calcific deposits developing in a bovine pericardial bioprosthetic valve 3 days after implantation. *Circulation* 1981;63:718.

138. Angell WW, Angell JD, Oury JH, et al: Long-term follow-up of viable frozen aortic homografts: A viable homograft valve bank. *J Thorac Cardiovasc Surg* 1987;93:815.

139. Gibbon JH: Artificial maintenance of circulation during experimental occlusion of the pulmonary artery. *Arch Surg* 1937;34:1105.

140. Gibbon JH: Application of a mechanical heart and lung apparatus to cardiac surgery. *Minn Med* 1954;37:171.

141. Stuckey JH, Newman MM, Dennis C, et al: The use of the heart-lung machine in selected cases of acute massive myocardial infarction. *Surg Forum* 1957;3:342.

142. Liotta D, Hall CW, Walter SH, et al: Prolonged assisted circulation during and after cardiac and aortic surgery. Prolonged partial left heart bypass by means of intracorporeal circulation. *Am J Cardiol* 1963;12:399.

143. Cooley DA, Liotta D, Hallman GL, et al: Orthotopic cardiac prosthesis for two staged cardiac replacement. *Am J Cardiol* 1969;24:723.

144. Turina MT, Bosio R, Senning A: Paracorporeal artificial heart in postoperative heart failure. *Artif Organs* 1978;2:273.

145. Norman JC, Duncan JM, Frazier OH, et al: Intracorporeal (abdominal) left ventricular assist devices or partial artificial hearts: A five-year clinical experience. *Arch Surg* 1981;116:1441.

146. Norman JC, Cooley DA, Kahan BD, et al: Total support of the circulation of a patient with postcardiotomy stone heart syndrome by a partial artificial heart (ALVAD) for 5 days followed by heart and kidney transplantation. *Lancet* 1978;1:1125.

147. Frazier OH, Cooley DA: Use of cardiac assist devices as bridges to cardiac transplantation: Review of current status and report of the Texas Heart Institute's experience. In: Unger F ed. *Assisted Circulation 3* New York, NY: Springer-Verlag; 1989: 247.

148. Unger F ed. *Assisted Circulation 3* New York, NY: Springer-Verlag; 1989.

149. Moulopoulos SC, Topaz S, Kolff WL, et al: Diastolic balloon pumping (with carbon dioxide) in the aorta — A mechanical assistance to the failing circulation. *Am Heart J* 1962;63:669.

150. Norman JC, Cooley DA, Igo SR, et al: Prognostic indices for survival during post-cardiotomy intraaortic balloon pumping: Methods of scoring (O - 16) and classification (A - C) with implications for left ventricular assist device utilization. *J Thorac Cardiovasc Surg* 1977;74:709.

151. Igo SR, Hibbs CW, Trono R, et al: Intraaortic balloon pumping: Theory and practice: Experience with 325 patients. *Artif Organs* 1978;2:249.

152. Norman JC: The role of assist devices in managing low cardiac output. *Cardiovascular Diseases, Bulletin of the Texas Heart Institute* 1981;8:119.

153. Kantrowitz A: Intraaortic balloon pumping: Clinical aspects and prospects. In: Unger F ed. *Assisted Circulation 3* New York, NY: Springer-Verlag; 1989: 52.

154. Peric M, Frazier OH, Duncan JM, et al: Intraaortic balloon pump as a bridge to transplantation. *J Heart Transplant* 1986;5:380.

155. Frazier OH, Creager GJ, Reece IJ, et al: Morbidity in balloon counterpulsation: Transfemoral versus transthoracic insertion. *ASAIO Trans* 1984;30:108.

156. Hoy FB, Stables C, Gomez RC, et al: Prolonged ventricular support using a centrifugal pump. *Can J Surg* 1989;32:342.

157. Dembitsky WP, Daily PO, Raney AA, et al: Temporary extracorporeal support of the right ventricle. *J Thorac Cardiovasc Surg* 1986;91:518.

158. Nakatani T, Radovancevic B, Frazier OH: Right heart assist for acute right ventricular failure after orthotopic heart transplantation. *ASAIO Trans* 1987;33:695.

159. Frazier OH, Bricker JT, Macris MP, et al: Use of a left ventricular assist device as a bridge to transplantation in a pediatric patient. *Tex Heart Inst J* 1989;16:46.

160. Frazier OH, Wampler RK, Duncan JM: First human use of the Hemopump, a catheter-mounted ventricular assist device. *Ann Thorac Surg* 1990;49:299.

161. Burnett CM, Vega JD, Radovancevic B, et al: Improved survival after Hemopump insertion in patients experiencing postcardiotomy cardiogenic shock during cardiopulmonary bypass. *ASAIO Trans* 1990;36:M626.

162. Duncan JM, Frazier OH, Radovancevic B, et al: Implantation techniques for the Hemopump. *Ann Thorac Surg* 1989;48:733.

163. McGee MG, Parnis SM, Nakatani T, et al: Extended clinical support with an implantable left ventricular assist device. *ASAIO Trans* 1989:35:614.

164. Frazier OH, Duncan JM, Radovancevic B, et al: Successful bridge to cardiac transplantation using a new left ventricular assist device. *J Heart Lung Transplant* 1992. In press.

165. Loisance D, Deleuze PH, Dubois-Rande JL, et al: Hemopump ventricular support for patients undergoing high-risk coronary angioplasty. *ASAIO Trans* 1990;36:1990.

166. Kron IL, Flanagan TL, Blackbourne LH, et al: Coronary revascularization rather than cardiac transplantation for chronic ischemic cardiomyopathy. *Ann Surg* 1989;210:348.

167. Luu M, Stevenson LW, Brunken RD, et al: Delayed recovery of revascularized myocardium after referral for cardiac transplantation. *Am Heart J* 1990;119:668.

168. Cooley DA: Ventricular endoaneurysmorrhaphy: A simplified repair for extensive postinfarction aneurysm. *J Cardiac Surg* 1989;4:200.

169. Hosenpud JD, Uretsky BF, Griffith BP, et al: Successful intermediate-term outcome for patients with cardiac amyloidosis undergoing heart transplantation: Results of a multicenter survey. *J Heart Transplant* 1990;9:346.

170. Radovancevic B, Frazier OH, Gentry LO, et al: Successful treatment of invasive aspergillosis in a heart transplant patient. *Tex Heart Inst J* 1985;12:233.

171. Carrel A, Guthrie CC: The transplantation of veins and organs. *Am Med* 1905;10:1101.

172. Mann FC, Priestly JT, Markowitz J, et al: Transplantation of the intact mammalian heart. *Arch Surg* 1933;26:219.

173. Demikhov VP: Experimental transplantation of vital organs. Authorized translation from the Russian by Haigh B. Consultants Bureau, New York, 1962.

174. Lower RR, Shumway NE: Studies on orthotopic homotransplantation of the canine heart. *Surg Forum* 1960:11:18.

175. Cass MH, Brock R: Heart excision and replacement. *Guy's Hosp Rep* 1959;108:285.

176. Starzl TE, Marchioro TL, Waddell WR: The reversal of rejection in human renal homografts with subsequent development of homograft tolerance. *Surg Gynecol Obstet* 1963;117:385.

177. Hardy JD, Chavez CM, Kurrus FD, et al: Heart transplantation in man: Developmental studies and report of a case. *JAMA* 1964;188:1132.

178. Barnard CN: A human cardiac transplantation: An interim report of a successful operation performed at Groote Schuur Hospital, Capetown. *S Afr Med J* 1967;41:1271.

179. Caves PK, Billingham ME, Stinson EB, et al: Serial transvenous biopsy of the transplanted human heart—improved management of acute rejection episodes. *Lancet* 1974;1:821.

180. Borel JF, Feurer C, Gubler HU, et al: Biological effects of cyclosporin A: A new antilymphocytic agent. *Agents and Actions* 1976;6:468.

181. Calne RY, White DJ, Rolles K, et al: Prolonged survival of pig orthotopic heart grafts treated with cyclosporin-A. *Lancet* 1978;1:1183.

182. Reitz BA, Bieber CP, Raney AA, et al: Orthotopic heart and combined heart and lung transplantation with cyclosporin A immune suppression. *Transplant Proc* 1981;13:393.

183. Gradinac S, Frazier OH, Van Buren CT, et al: Heart transplants in diabetic patients. *Circulation* 1988;78(Suppl 2):II-252. Abstract.

184. Frazier OH, Cooley DA, Okereke OUJ, et al: Cardiac transplantation in a patient with septicemia after prolonged intraaortic balloon pump support: Implications for staged transplantation. *Tex Heart Inst J* 1986;13:13.

185. Frazier OH, Macris MP, Duncan JM, et al: Cardiac transplantation in patients over 60 years of age. *Ann Thorac Surg* 1988;45:129.

186. Ladowski JS, Kormos RL, Uretsky BF, et al: Heart transplantation in diabetic recipients. *Transplantation* 1990;49:303.

187. Lammermeier DE, Sweeney MS, Haupt HE, et al: Use of potentially infected donor hearts for cardiac transplantation. *Ann Thorac Surg* 1990;50:222.

188. Kriett JM, Kaye MP: The Registry of the International Society for Heart Transplantation: Seventh official report—1990. *J Heart Transplant* 1990;9:323.

189. Mollaret P, Goulon M: Le coma depasse: Memoire preliminaire. *Rev Neurol* 1959;101:3.

190. A Gallup Survey: The US public's attitudes toward organ transplants/organ donation. *The Gallup Organization* April 1987.

191. Stuart FP, Veith FJ, Crawford RE: Brain death laws and patterns of consent to remove organs for transplantation from cadavers in the United States and 28 other countries. *Transplantation* 1981;31:238.

192. Report of the Medical Consultants on the Diagnosis of Death to the President's Commission for the Study of Ethical Problems in Medicine and Biomedical Behavioral Research: Guidelines for the determination of death. *JAMA* 1981;246:2184.

193. Mulvagh SL, Thornton B, Frazier OH, et al: The older cardiac transplant donor: Relation to graft function and recipient survival longer than 6 years. *Circulation* 1989;80(Suppl 3):III-126.

194. Novitsky D, Cooper DKC, Human PA, et al: Triiodothyronine therapy for heart donor and recipient. *J Heart Transplant* 1988;7:370.

195. Frazier OH, Macris MP, Wampler RK, et al: Treatment of cardiac allograft failure by use of an intraaortic axial flow pump. *J Heart Transplant* 1990;9:408.

196. Frazier OH, Nakatani T, Lammermeier DE, et al: Cardiac transplantation and mechanical circulatory assistance: The Texas Heart Institute experience. *J Japn Assoc Thorac Surg* 1989;37:1873.

197. Radovancevic B, Birovljev S, Vega JD, et al: Inverse relationship between HLA mismatch and development of coronary artery disease. *Transplant Proc* 1991;23:1144.

198. Opelz G, Schwarz V, Engelmann A, et al: Long-term impact of HLA matching on kidney graft survival in cyclosporine-treated recipients. *Transplant Proc* 1991;23:373.

199. Kahan BD, Van Buren CT, Flechner SM, et al: Cyclosporine immunosuppression mitigates immunologic risk factors in renal allotransplantation. *Transplant Proc* 1983;15(Suppl 1):2469.

200. Cooper DKC, Lanza RP, Boyd ST, et al: Factors influencing survival following heart transplantation. *Heart Transplant* 1983;3:86.

201. Olivari M, Antolick A, Kaye M, et al: Heart transplantation in the elderly. *J Heart Transplant* 1986;5:366.

202. Renlund DG, Gilbert EM, O'Connell JB, et al: Age-associated decline in cardiac allograft rejection. *Am J Med* 1987;83:391.

203. Oaks TE, Wisman CB, Pae WE, et al: Results of mechanical circulatory assistance before heart transplantation. *J Heart Transplant* 1989;8:113.

204. Pennington DG, McBride LR, Kanter KR, et al: Bridging to heart transplantation with circulatory support devices. *J Heart Transplant* 1989;8:116.

205. Farrar DJ, Lawson JH, Litwak P, et al: Thoratec VAD system as a bridge to heart transplantation. *J Heart Transplant* 1990;9:415.

206. Barnard CN, Losman JG: Left ventricular bypass. *S Afr Med J* 1975;49:303.

207. Radovancevic B, Nakatani T, Frazier OH, et al: Mechanical circulatory support for perioperative donor heart failure. *ASAIO Trans* 1989;35:539.

208. Thompson ME, Shapiro AP, Johnsen AM, et al: New onset of hypertension following cardiac transplantation: A preliminary report and analysis. *Transplant Proc* 1983;15(Suppl 1):2573.

209. Scherrer U, Vissing SF, Morgan BJ, et al: Cyclosporine-induced sympathetic activation and hypertension after heart transplantation. *N Engl J Med* 1990;323:693.

210. Hughes RL: Cyclosporine-related central nervous system toxicity in cardiac transplantation. *N Engl J Med* 1990;323:420.

211. Crandell BG, Gilbert EM, Renlund DG, et al: A randomized trial of the immunosuppressive efficacy of vincristine in cardiac transplantation. *Transplantation* 1990;50:34.

212. Ratkovec RM, Wray RB, Renlund DG, et al: Influence of corticosteroid-free maintenance immunosuppression on allograft coronary artery disease after cardiac transplantation. *J Thorac Cardiovasc Surg* 1990;100:6.

213. Kormos RL, Herlan DB, Armitage JM, et al: Monoclonal versus polyclonal antibody therapy for prophylaxis against rejection after heart transplantation. *J Heart Transplant* 1990;9:1.

214. Swinnen LJ, Costanzo Nordin MR, Fisher SG, et al: Increased incidence of lymphoproliferative disease after immunosuppression with the monoclonal antibody OKT3 in cardiac transplant recipients. *N Engl J Med* 1990;323:1723.

215. Radovancevic B, Birovljev S, Frazier OH, et al: Long-term follow-up of cyclosporine-treated cardiac transplant recipients. *Transplant Proc* 1990;22(3 Suppl 1):22.

216. Locke TJ, Karnik R, McGregor CG, et al: The value of the electrocardiogram in the diagnosis of acute rejection after orthotopic heart transplantation. *Transplant Int* 1989;2:143.

217. Billingham ME, Cary NRB, Hammond ME, et al: A working formulation for the standardization of nomenclature in the diagnosis of heart and lung rejection: Heart rejection study group. *J Heart Transplant* 1990;9:587.

218. McAllister HA, Schnee MJ, Radovancevic B, et al: System for grading cardiac allograft rejection. *Tex Heart Inst J* 1986;13:1.

219. Radovancevic B, Birovljev S, Frazier OH: Treating cardiac allograft rejection: Present approach—analysis of 100 consecutive patients. *J Heart Transplant* 1990;9:288.

220. Warnecke H, Schuler S, Goetze HJ, et al: Noninvasive monitoring of cardiac allograft rejection by intramyocardial electrocardiogram recordings. *Circulation* 1986;74(5 Pt 2):II-172.

221. Wijngaard PL, Gimpel JA, Schuurman HJ, et al: Monitoring rejection after heart transplantation: Cytoimmunological monitoring on blood cells and quantitative birefringence measurements on endomyocardial biopsy specimens. *J Clin Pathol* 1990;43:137.

222. Roodman ST, Miller LW, Tsai CC: Role of interleukin 2 receptors in immunologic monitoring following cardiac transplantation. *Transplantation* 1988;45:1050.

223. Fieguth HG, Haverich A, Hadam M, et al: Correlation of interleukin-2 receptor positive circulating lymphocytes and acute cardiac rejection. *Transplant Proc* 1989;21:2517.

224. Woloszczuk W, Schwarz M, Havel M, et al: Neopterin and interferon gamma serum levels in patients with heart and kidney transplants. *J Clin Chem Clin Biochem* 1986;24:729.

225. Rosenbaum RW, Kately J, Sanchez TV, et al: Beta-2-microglobulin: An early indicator of renal transplant survival and function. *ASAIO Trans* 1980;26:77.

226. May RM, Cooper DK, DuToit ED, et al: Cytoimmunologic monitoring after heart and heart-lung transplantation. *J Heart Transplant* 1990;9:133.

227. Amende I, Simon R, Seegers A, et al: Diastolic dysfunction during acute cardiac allograft rejection. *Circulation* 1990;81(2 Suppl):III-66.

228. St Goar FG, Gibbons R, Schnittger I, et al: Left ventricular diastolic function. Doppler echocardiographic changes soon after cardiac transplantation. *Circulation* 1990;82:872.

229. Doornbos J, Verwey H, Essed CE, et al: MR imaging in assessment of cardiac transplant rejection in humans. *J Comput Assist Tomogr* 1990;14:77.

230. Lee KJ, Wallis JW, Miller TR: The clinical role of radionuclide imaging in cardiac transplantation. *J Thorac Imaging* 1990;5:73.

231. Radovancevic B, Frazier OH: Treatment of moderate heart allograft rejection with cyclosporine. *J Heart Transplant* 1986;5:307.

Surgical Treatment of Heart Disease

232. Duncan JM, Frazier OH, Radovancevic B, et al: Implantation techniques for the Hemopump. *Ann Thorac Surg* 1989;48:733.

233. Gentry LO, Zeluff BJ: Diagnosis and treatment of infection in cardiac transplant recipients. *Surg Clin North Am* 1986;66:459.

234. Gentry LO, Zeluff BJ: Infection in the cardiac transplant patient. In: Rubin RH and Lowel SY, eds. *Clinical Approach To Infection In The Compromised Host* Plenum Publishing Corporation; 1987: 623.

235. Dummer JS, Bound LM, Singh G, et al: Epstein-Barr virus-induced lymphoma in a cardiac transplant recipient. *Am J Med* 1984;77:179.

236. Cooper DKC: Orthotopic and heterotopic transplantation of the heart: The Cape Town experience. *Ann R Coll Surg* 1984;66:228.

237. Radovancevic B, Poindexter S, Birovljev S, et al: Risk factors for development of accelerated coronary artery disease in cardiac transplant recipients. *Eur J Cardiothor Surg* 1990;4:309.

238. Grattan MT, Moreno-Cabral CT, Vaughn AS, et al: Cytomegalovirus infection is associated with cardiac allograft rejection and atherosclerosis. *JAMA* 1989;261:3561.

239. Hastillo A, Cowley MJ, Vetrovec G, et al: Serial coronary angioplasty for atherosclerosis following heart transplantation. *J Heart Transplant* 1985;4/2:192.

240. Copeland JG, Butman SM, Sethi G: Successful coronary artery bypass grafting for high-risk left main coronary artery atherosclerosis after cardiac transplantation. *Ann Thorac Surg* 1990;49:106.

241. Frazier OH, Vega JD, Duncan JM, et al: Coronary artery bypass two years after orthotopic cardiac transplantation: A case report. *J Heart Lung Transplant* 1991;10:1036.

242. Avedissian MG, Bush HS, Leachman DR, et al: Percutaneous transluminal coronary angioplasty after cardiac transplantation. *Tex Heart Inst J* 1989;16:288.

243. Gao SZ, Schroeder JS, Hunt S, et al: Retransplantation for severe accelerated coronary artery disease in heart transplant recipients. *Am J Cardiol* 1988;62:876.

244. Gao SZ, Schroeder J, Alderman EL, et al: Clinical and laboratory correlates of accelerated coronary artery disease in the cardiac transplant patient. *Circulation* 1987;76(Suppl 5):56.

245. Gao SZ, Alderman EL, Schroeder JS, et al: Accelerated coronary artery bypass grafting for high-risk left main coronary artery atherosclerosis after cardiac transplantation. *Ann Thorac Surg* 1990;49:106.

246. Olivari MT, Homans DC, Wilson RF, et al: Coronary artery disease in cardiac transplant patients receiving triple-drug immunosuppressive therapy. *Circulation* 1989;80(Suppl 3):111.

247. Billingham ME: Cardiac transplant atherosclerosis. *Transplant Proc* 1987;19(Suppl 5):19.

248. DeCampli WM, Johnson DE, Gao SZ, et al: Transplant coronary vascular disease: Histomorphometric properties and clinical correlations. *Curr Surg* 1988;45:477.

249. Armitage J, Fung J, Kormos R, et al: Preliminary experience with FK 506 in thoracic transplantation. *Proceedings of XIII International Congress of Transplantation Society* 1990: 143. Abstract.

250. Stepkowski S, Chen H, Daloze P, et al: Rapamycin: A potent immunosuppressive drug for heart, kidney and small bowel allografts. *Proceedings of XIII International Congress of Transplantation Society* 1990: 218. Abstract.

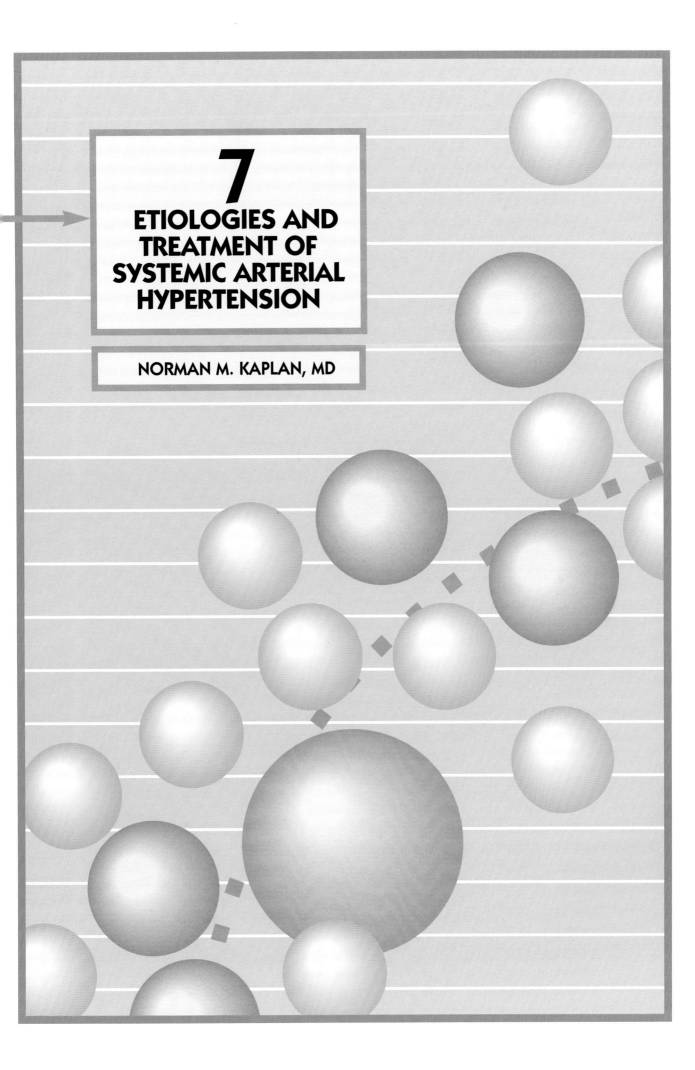

7

ETIOLOGIES AND TREATMENT OF SYSTEMIC ARTERIAL HYPERTENSION

NORMAN M. KAPLAN, MD

Synopsis of Chapter Seven

Diagnosis of Hypertension
Measurement of Blood Pressure
Criteria for Diagnosis
Evaluation of the Newly Diagnosed Patient
Assessment of Overall Cardiovascular Risk

Mechanisms of Hypertension
Primary Hypertension
Secondary Causes

General Principles of Therapy
Rationale for Therapy
Results of Clinical Trials
Guidelines for Treatment

Nondrug Therapy
Weight Reduction
Dietary Sodium Restriction
Potassium Supplementation
Magnesium Supplementation
Calcium Supplementation
Other Dietary Changes
Moderation of Alcohol
Isotonic Exercise
Relaxation Techniques

Antihypertensive Drug Therapy
General Guidelines
Diuretics
Adrenoceptor Blocking Drugs
Direct Vasodilators
Calcium-Entry Blockers
Angiotensin-Converting Enzyme (ACE) Inhibitors
Other Drugs

Special Considerations
Resistant Hypertension
The Elderly
Hypertension with Congestive Heart Failure
Hypertension with Ischemic Heart Disease
Regression of Left Ventricular Hypertrophy

Therapy for Hypertensive Crises

Future Directions for the Management of Hypertension

DIAGNOSIS OF HYPERTENSION

MEASUREMENT OF BLOOD PRESSURE

The measurement of blood pressure, as simple as it seems, is often done haphazardly and inadequately. Often, each measurement is done without adequate awareness of the many factors that can cause variation from one reading to another (Figure 7.1). For example, first readings tend to be elevated and readings taken by physicians tend to be higher than those taken by nurses, who are presumably less threatening to most patients. The problem may persist. Of almost 300 patients, repeatedly found to have diastolic pressures above 90 mm Hg over an average of 6 years when followed in the clinic, 21% were persistently normotensive when 24-hr ambulatory pressures were recorded by an automatic device while they performed their usual activities, including working in and traveling through Manhattan.[1] For obvious reasons, such hypertension is referred to as "office" or "white coat."

A proper sized cuff (Figure 7.2) is needed to preclude falsely high readings that may be noted when a cuff is too small for obese or muscular arms (Figure 7.3). In addition, the patient should have the torso and the arm supported to avoid the often significant rise in pressure that accompanies the isometric exertion without such support (Figure 7.4).

Because of progressively blunted baroreceptor reflexes with aging in older patients, there is the increased likelihood of postural falls in pressure. Those who have systolic elevations, usually secondary to atherosclerotic rigidity of the aorta and large arteries are more likely to have significant postural falls in pressure (Figure 7.5). Therefore, it is essential to repeat the supine measurement after one minute of quiet standing. If the upright reading is lower by 10 mm Hg or more, the patient should be kept standing for another minute or so, with support if needed to prevent falling, so as to identify the degree of postural fall. Obviously, therapy for the elderly should not be based only on seated or supine levels, which may neglect more marked drops in pressure that can lead to falls and syncope.

Out-of-the-office Readings

The existence of "white-coat" hypertension will never be recognized if only office readings are taken. Not only will that result in unnecessary labelling of some people as "hypertensive"—with all the psychological and economic consequences of having the diagnosis—but it will also lead to overtreatment of a number of patients with hypertension. The problem was nicely described in a study of 34 patients who had office readings above 95 mm Hg despite antihypertensive therapy.[2] At that time, the daytime out-of-the-office diastolic readings taken with an automatic ambulatory device were below an average of

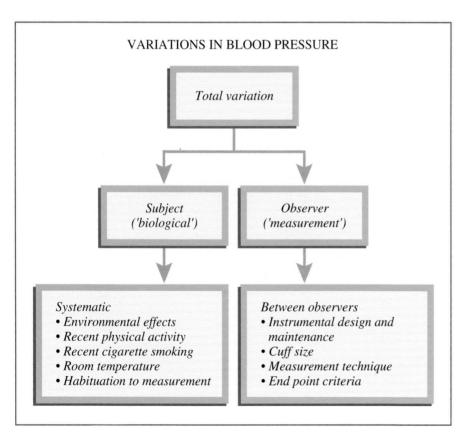

VARIATIONS IN BLOOD PRESSURE

FIGURE 7.1 • When blood pressure is measured in the same individual on two occasions the observed value may be different. The observed differences may be due to factors influencing blood pressure or to differences in measurement. (Reproduced with permission. Peart WS, Sever PS, Swales JD, et al: *Geigy Hypertension Illustrated. Measurement and Natural History.* New York, NY: Gower Medical Publishing; 1980:6.2.)

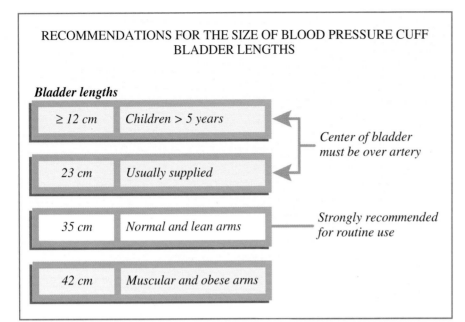

FIGURE 7.2 • Recommendations for the size of blood pressure cuff bladder lengths. (Reproduced with permission. Petrie JC, O'Brien ET, Littler WA, et al: *Br Med J* 1986;293:611.)

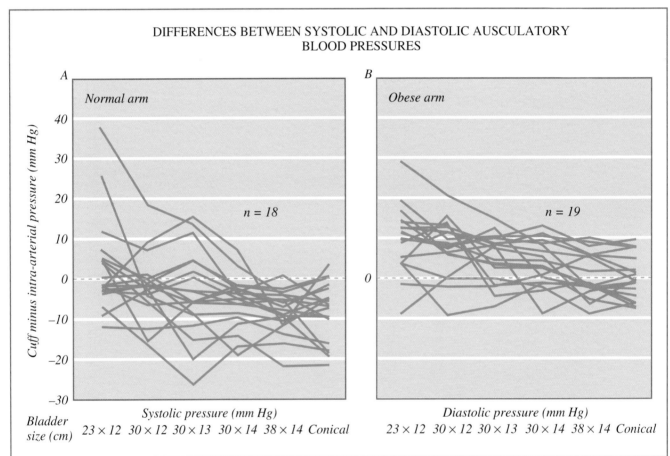

FIGURE 7.3 • Individual differences between systolic (A) and diastolic ausculatory (cuff) (B) blood pressures minus intra-arterial blood pressures in 19 subjects with obese arms (circumference greater than or equal to 34 cm) and 18 with normal sized arms. Six different cuffs with increasing bladder width are compared. Each measurement point represents the mean of three comparisons in one subject for one cuff. (Reproduced with permission. van Montfrans GA, van der Hoeven GMA, Karemaker JM, et al: *Br Med J* 1987;295:354.)

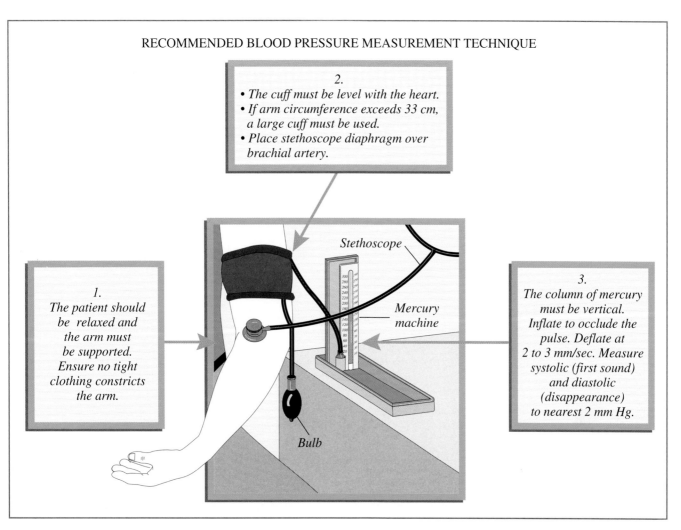

RECOMMENDED BLOOD PRESSURE MEASUREMENT TECHNIQUE

2.
• The cuff must be level with the heart.
• If arm circumference exceeds 33 cm, a large cuff must be used.
• Place stethoscope diaphragm over brachial artery.

1.
The patient should be relaxed and the arm must be supported. Ensure no tight clothing constricts the arm.

3.
The column of mercury must be vertical. Inflate to occlude the pulse. Deflate at 2 to 3 mm/sec. Measure systolic (first sound) and diastolic (disappearance) to nearest 2 mm Hg.

Stethoscope

Mercury machine

Bulb

FIGURE 7.4 • Technique of blood pressure measurement recommended by the British Hypertension Society. (Reproduced with permission. Gould BA, Hornung RS, Raftery EB: *J Hypertens* 1985; 3:293.)

FIGURE 7.5 • Relationship between basal supine systolic blood pressure and postural change in systolic blood pressure for old subjects—mean age = 87 ± 7 years. (Reproduced with permission. Lipsitz LA, Storch HA, Minaker KL, et al: *Clin Sci* 1985;69:337.)

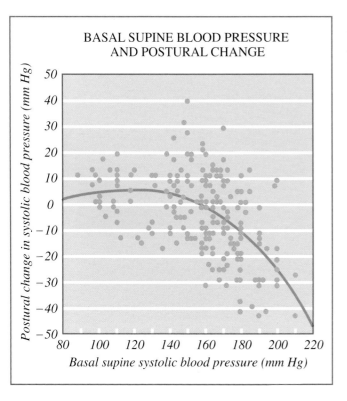

BASAL SUPINE BLOOD PRESSURE AND POSTURAL CHANGE

OFFICE AND AMBULATORY DIASTOLIC BLOOD PRESSURE

Patients with diastolic pressure at beginning ≤ 90 mm Hg
n = 17

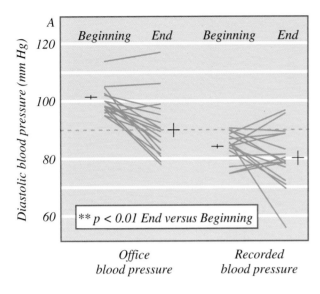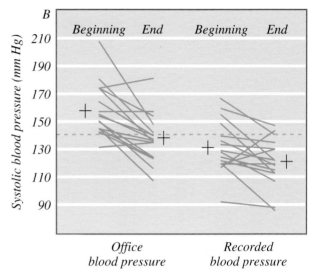

FIGURE 7.6 • Office and ambulatory (recorded) diastolic blood pressure at beginning and end of study in 17 patients with ambulatory diastolic blood pressure of 90 mm Hg or lower at beginning despite office readings above 95 mm Hg. (Reproduced with permission. Waeber B, Scherrer U, Petrillo A, et al: *Lancet* 1987;2:732.)

FIGURE 7.7 • Proposed schema of blood pressure measurement for patients with apparently resistant hypertension. (Reproduced with permission. Pickering TG: *Hypertension* 1988;11(Suppl II):II-96 and the American Heart Association.)

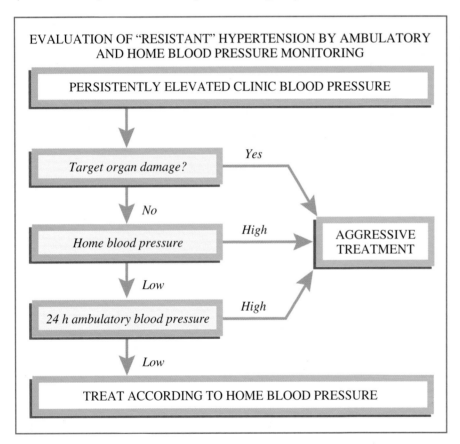

Hypertension

90 mm Hg in 17 of 34 patients (Figure 7.6). Additional therapy, given on the basis of the higher office readings, lowered office values to an average of 90 mm Hg for the 17, although some individuals still had higher than 90 mm Hg office levels following the period of additional therapy. The out-of-the-office readings, already below 90 mm Hg before additional therapy in these 17 patients, fell in some to potentially hazardous levels.

Patients who are apparently resistant to therapy—their office diastolic pressures remaining above 95 mm Hg despite treatment with two or three drugs—should be evaluated in a stepwise fashion (Figure 7.7). If target organ damage is not present, home readings should be obtained. If they average less than 90 mm Hg, ambulatory recordings may be indicated to ensure that more aggressive therapy is not warranted. Much of the information needed can be provided by pressures taken by the patient or another person with readily accessible and easy-to-use semiautomatic devices that cost around $50 (Table 7.1). The physician should keep a few in the office to loan out for the 4 to 6 weeks needed to ascertain the usual level of pressure. Once the diagnosis is made and therapy begins, all patients who can afford to purchase a home device should monitor their course in this manner.

Increasingly, 24-hr ambulatory recordings will be obtained with devices that are rapidly becoming easier to use and less expensive. A typical tracing (Figure 7.8) on a normotensive subject shows moderate variation during the daytime and a marked fall in pressure during the first three fourths of sleep. Note the rather marked rise in pressure upon awakening and arising from bed. This early morning spontaneous rise in pressure precedes, and is very likely at least to be partially responsible for, the significant incidence of cardiovascular catastrophes—strokes, heart attacks, and sudden death—that have been repeatedly documented during the hours from 6 to 10 AM.[3]

Recordings of pressure during sleep may also be useful to identify pressure levels too low or too high. On the one side, the naturally lower levels during the first three quarters of sleep may be joined by therapy-induced further reductions to invoke hypoperfusion of vital organs, in particular the heart. On the other side, failure of pressure to fall normally may be as-

---

TABLE 7.1 • INDICATIONS FOR HOME BLOOD PRESSURE MONITORING

For diagnosis:
Recognize initial, short-term elevations in blood pressure
Identify persistent "white-coat" hypertension
Determine usual blood pressure levels in borderline hypertension

For prognosis:
Inadequate data except for relation to left ventricular hypertrophy (LVH)

For therapy:
Monitor response to therapy
- Ensure adequate blood pressure control during awake hours
- Evaluate effects of increasing or decreasing amounts of therapy
- Ascertain whether poor office blood pressure response to increasing treatment represents overtreatment or true resistance
- Identify periods of poor control when office readings are normal but target organ damage progresses
- Identify the relationship of blood pressure levels to presumed side effects of therapy
- Involve patient to improve adherence

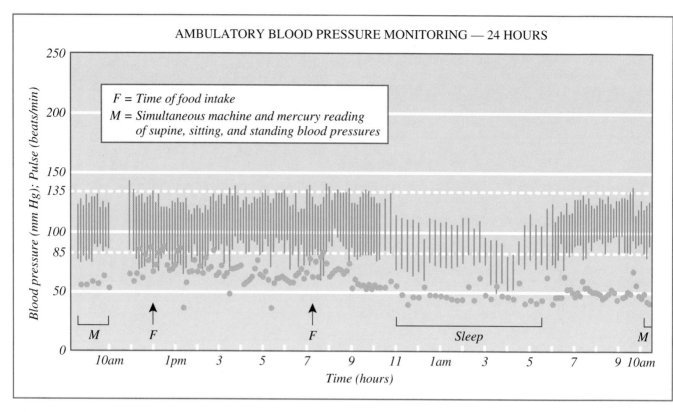

FIGURE 7.8 • Ambulatory blood pressure monitoring for 24 hrs beginning at 10 a.m. in a normal 40-year-old man with no evidence of hypertension or other cardiovascular disease. (Reproduced with permission. Zachariah PK, Sheps SG, Smith RL: *Diagnosis* 1988A;10:39.)

FIGURE 7.9 • Relationship between left ventricular mass index (LVMI) and night systolic blood pressure in treated hypertensive patients. (Reproduced with permission. Gosse P, Campello G, Roudaut R, Dallocchio M: *Am J Hypertens* 1988;1:195S.)

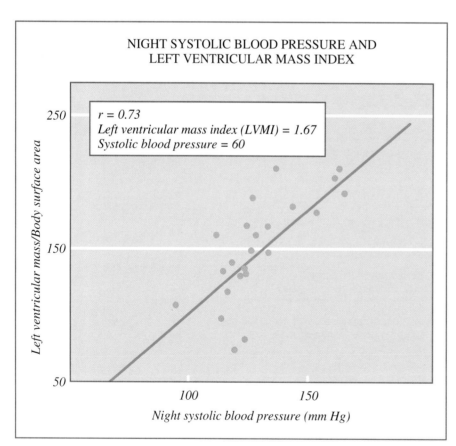

sociated with more left ventricular hypertrophy (LVH)[4] (Figure 7.9). The higher nocturnal pressures could either be responsible for or induced by the left ventricular hypertrophy. Either way, measuring blood pressure during sleep may become a widely utilized technique to ensure adequate but not overzealous control of hypertension. Other indications for ambulatory readings are presented in Table 7.2.

As more ambulatory recordings and multiple self-taken readings are obtained, the usual variability of the blood pressure will have to be recognized and dealt with. As seen in Figure 7.10, almost all subjects who were normotensive by an office reading had a few elevated pressures during a 24-hr recording. Similarly, almost all patients who were considered "fixed" hypertensives will have some normal readings, more so while asleep, but often during the daytime as well. As expected, those with "labile" office readings will have varying percentages of normal and high readings.

Ambulatory readings are on the average lower than those obtained at home or in the clinic (Table 7.3). However, average ambulatory readings in this study included those taken during sleep. If only the daytime (awake) readings are included, they come out very close to those taken at home and both of these, in turn, are usually lower than those taken in the office setting.

Prognosis

A shadow lingers over the increasing use of out-of-the-office readings to establish the diagnosis. Almost all of the considerable data that established the risk of hypertension were based on one or two sets of office readings. Therefore, even one isolated high office reading cannot be disregarded.

However, increasingly strong evidence points to the likelihood that ambulatory pressures predict the risk for target organ damage and cardiovascular events better than do casual or office readings. As for target organ damage, most of the data are cross-sectional—the extent of left ventricular hypertrophy revealed by echocardiography is more closely correlated to 24-hr ambulatory pressure than to casual pressure.[5] This closer correlation with ambulatory pressure has also been shown for

---

TABLE 7.2 • INDICATIONS FOR AMBULATORY BLOOD PRESSURE MONITORING

For diagnosis: same as for home blood pressure measurements (refer to Table 7.1) plus:

Patients unable to obtain self (home)-measurements

Need for immediate ascertainment

Measure sleep blood pressure levels

For prognosis:

Provide better correlation with target organ damage

Identify role of sleep blood pressure

For therapy:

Same as for home measurements (refer to Table 7.1) plus identification of effects during sleep

Establish duration and degree of effect of new agents

---

other indices of target organ damage, including changes in the optic fundi and renal function.[6,7]

Even more supportive of the prognostic value of ABPM are the data of Perloff et al.[8] They examined 1,076 patients, both with multiple office blood pressures on three visits and with ambulatory readings taken every 30 minutes while the patients were awake over a 1- to 2-day period. The average office readings for all patients were 161/101 mm Hg, whereas the ambulatory readings averaged 146/92 mm Hg. Ambulatory readings were lower in 78% of the patients. These patients were followed for up to 16 years, with the mean duration being 5 years. Life table analyses of their massive set of data showed a significantly greater cumulative 10-year incidence of both fatal and nonfatal cardiovascular events among patients with higher ambula-

tory and office blood pressure than among those with ambulatory blood pressures lower than their office readings.

The evidence, then, strongly suggests that the usual, longer-term out-of-the-office blood pressure levels are more closely correlated to future risk than are single office readings. As will be described in the next section, the risks of any degree of high pressure are not uniform. If 100 people had a diastolic blood pressure of 95 mm Hg, perhaps one third will suffer a cardiovascular complication over the next 20 to 30 years. Obviously, risk for the entire group is increased because of the higher level of pressure. However, for the majority of individuals with such mild hypertension, no obvious complications will arise and no increased cardiovascular morbidity or mortality will supervene even if no therapy is given. Out-of-the-of-

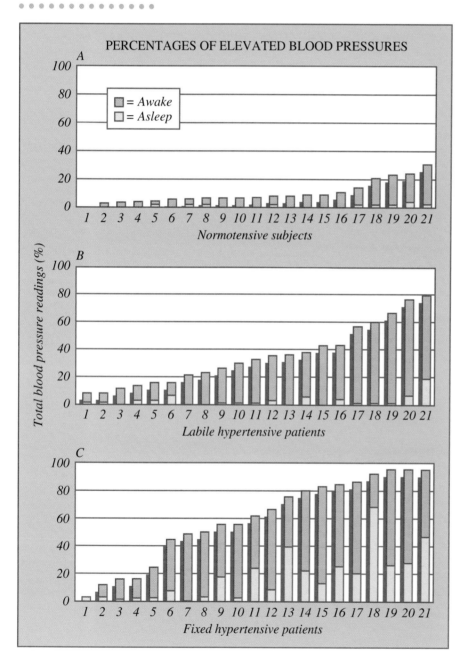

FIGURE 7.10 • Distribution of percentages of elevated blood pressures—systolic blood pressure > 140 mm Hg or diastolic blood pressure > 90 mm Hg—in normotensive (A), borderline (B), and fixed hypertensive (C) patients while awake or asleep during recordings of 24-hr ambulatory blood pressure. (Reproduced with permission. Horan MJ, Kennedy HL, Padgett NE: *Ann Intern Med* 1981;94:466.)

fice readings seem to predict better than office readings which patients are at risk. Those whose out-of-the-office readings are considerably lower are less likely to develop target organ damage and overt cardiovascular complications. Nonetheless, no elevated pressure, even an isolated, one time reading should be disregarded. But, unless the level is so high as to mandate immediate intervention, no patient should be called "hypertensive" or started on therapy until multiple readings are taken, preferably including many out of the office.

CRITERIA FOR DIAGNOSIS

The diagnosis of hypertension should be based upon the presence of a usual blood pressure level that is known to be associated with a significant increase in cardiovascular risk. As noted above, that usual level of blood pressure can be accurately ascertained for the larger population but much less accurately for the individual patient. Nonetheless, it is reasonable to identify and label a person as "hypertensive" because that person's usual blood pressure is at a level that is associated with a significantly increased risk for the larger population, even if that person would not be

harmed if left undiagnosed and untreated. Our ability to determine future risk remains incomplete, so we must include some who might best be left alone in order to protect the overall population. As we shall see, making the diagnosis of hypertension need not lead to active drug therapy. It, at the least, should serve as a motivation to improve overall lifestyle and to monitor the course of the blood pressure. For many with mild hypertension, no target organ damage, and low overall cardiovascular risk, simple surveillance may be all that is needed.

Population Risks

Since each individual's risk cannot be exactly determined, the criteria for the diagnosis must be based on the experience gained from long-term observations of large populations. The best single database is that of the Framingham Heart Study.[9] These data are based on biennial measurements over a 30-year follow-up. The incidence of coronary heart disease rises progressively with increasing levels of either systolic or diastolic blood pressure, at a higher rate for the older than the younger and for men than for women at any given blood pres-

TABLE 7.3 • AVERAGE PRESSURES IN HYPERTENSIVE SUBJECTS AS DETERMINED BY THREE METHODS OF MEASUREMENT COMPARED OVER A 2 WEEK PERIOD[1]			
Measurement	**Ambulatory (Awake and asleep)**	**Home**	**Clinic**
Systolic blood pressure (mm Hg)			
Initial	134 ± 11	140 ± 14	158 ± 23[2]
Second	132 ± 12	143 ± 13	152 ± 20
Diastolic blood pressure (mm Hg)			
Initial	85 ± 10	86 ± 12	93 ± 11
Second	86 ± 10	87 ± 12	91 ± 10

[1]Values are average ± standard deviation.

[2]< 0.05, significantly different from second reading.

(Reproduced with permission. James GD, Pickering TG, Yee LS, et al: *Hypertension* 1988;11:545.)

sure level (Figure 7.11). The risk for myocardial infarction is three times greater among the men in Framingham than the women with "definite" hypertension—blood pressure equal to or above 160/95 mm Hg (Figure 7.12). Note that about one fourth of all myocardial infarctions were unrecognized and these too are closely correlated to the degree of blood pressure.

A much larger population than the Framingham cohort has been prospectively monitored. A meta-analysis of all of these data, performed by MacMahon et al,[10] includes all available major prospective observational studies relating blood pressure levels to the development of stroke and coronary heart disease (CHD). These nine studies involved almost 420,000 people who were followed for 6 to 24 years. Among this group, 599 fatal strokes and 4,260 CHD deaths were recorded. In this analysis, the associations were examined for diastolic blood pressure, which has been the usual index. The overall results demonstrate "direct, continuous and apparently independent associations" with "no evidence of any *threshold* level of diastolic blood pressure below which lower levels of diastolic blood pressure were not associated with lower risks of stroke and CHD" (Figure 7.13).

MacMahon et al took into account the common practice seen in the nine studies of measuring diastolic blood pressure on only one occasion, which leads to a substantial underestimation of the true association of the usual or long-term average diastolic blood pressure with disease. This arises because of the strong tendency on repeated readings for both lower and higher readings to regress toward the middle. Since there are relatively few events associated with the lower readings and a much greater number associated with the higher readings, this "regression dilution bias" makes it appear that the risk is greater with higher readings than in fact exists over the longer term. Since most events occur in people whose first reading is higher than subsequent readings, it appears that the events develop at higher diastolic blood pressure than at the significantly lower levels actually present over the longer term. By applying a correction to all nine sets of data, based upon the three sets of readings over 4 years in the Framingham study, MacMahon's group came up with estimates of risk that are about 60% greater than those previously published using uncorrected data. They estimate that a persistently higher diastolic blood pressure of 5.0 mm Hg is associated with at least a 34% increase in stroke risk and at least a 21% increase in CHD risk.

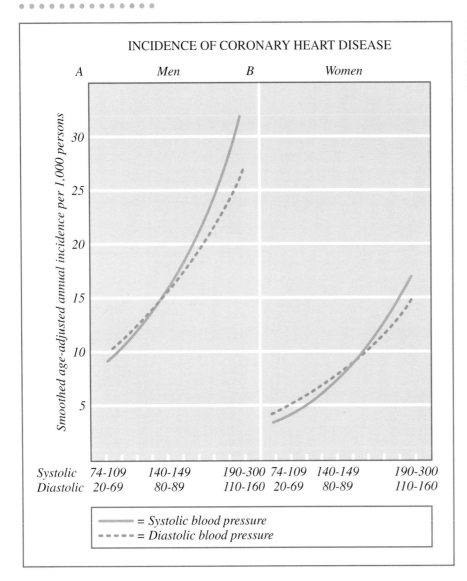

FIGURE 7.11 • The incidence of coronary heart disease according to systolic vesus diastolic blood pressure in men (A) and women (B) aged 45 to 74 in the Framingham study over a 20-year follow-up. (Reproduced with permission. Castelli WP: *Am J Med* 1984;76:4.)

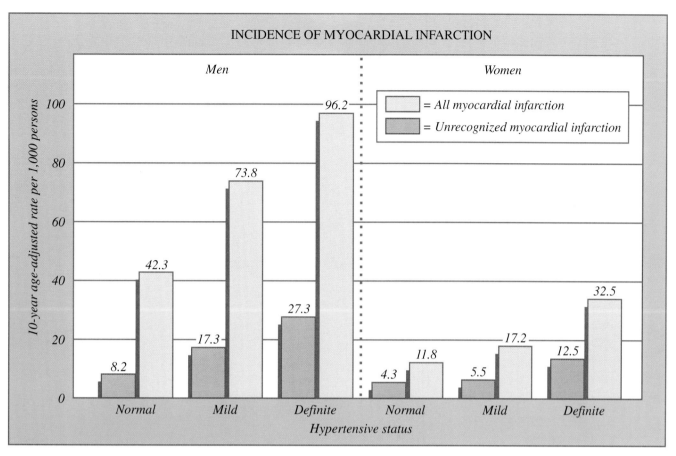

FIGURE 7.12 • Incidence of myocardial infarction by sex and hypertensive status in a 30-year follow-up of Framingham cohort subjects (ages 33 to 90) free of coronary heart disease at examination. (Reproduced with permission. Kannel WB, Dannenberg AL, Abbott RD: *Am Heart J* 1985;109:581.)

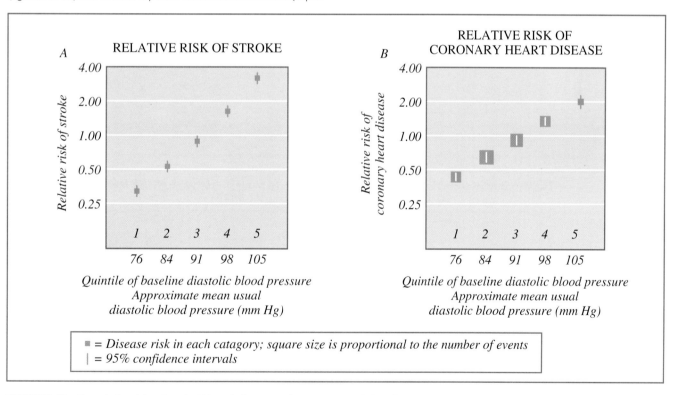

FIGURE 7.13 • The relative risks of stroke (A) and of coronary heart disease (B) estimated from the combined results of the prospective observational studies for each of the five categories of diastolic blood pressure. Estimates of the usual diastolic blood pressure in each baseline catagory are taken from mean diastolic blood pressure values 4 years postbaseline in the Framingham study. (Reproduced with permission. MacMahon S, Peto R, Cutler J, et al: *Lancet* 1990;335:765.)

Levels for the Individual

From these data, it is clear that the risk is greater at a diastolic blood pressure of 84 mm Hg than at 76 mm Hg. Yet, the recommendations of all "official" authorities is to consider a diastolic blood pressure of 90 mm Hg as the lower limit for the diagnosis of hypertension[11] (Table 7.4). Those with diastolic blood pressure between 85 and 89 mm Hg are defined as "high-normal," but only those at 90 mm Hg or above are diagnosed as hypertensive.

The reasons for this difference mainly revolve around the relatively small *absolute* risk associated with diastolic blood pressures in the 80 to 89 mm Hg range, even though the relative risk is increased (Table 7.5). In this prospective study—included in the meta-analysis by MacMahon et al shown in Figure 7.13—the relative risk for coronary disease increased 52% among white men with an initial diastolic blood pressure between 80 and 87 mm Hg, compared those with diastolic blood pressures below 80 mm Hg. The 52% increase is derived by taking the rate per 1,000 persons with actual coronary events in the two groups, 100.6 versus 66.0, and dividing the difference (34.6) by the rate for those with the lower diastolic blood pressure (66.0). Therefore, this 52% increase in relative risk reflects a 3.5% increase in absolute risk—

• • • • • • • • • • • • • • •

TABLE 7.4 • FOURTH JOINT NATIONAL COMMITTEE CLASSIFICATION OF BLOOD PRESSURE[1]

Range (mm Hg)	Category[2]
Diastolic	
< 85	Normal blood pressure
85–89	High normal blood pressure
90–104	Mild hypertension
105–114	Moderate hypertension
≥ 115	Severe hypertension
Systolic (when diastolic blood pressure < 90 mm Hg)	
< 140	Normal blood pressure
140–159	Borderline isolated systolic hypertension
≥ 160	Isolated systolic hypertension

[1]Classification based on the average of two or more readings on two or more occasions.

[2]A classification of borderline isolated systolic hypertension (systolic blood pressure, 140 to 159 mm Hg) or isolated systolic hypertension (systolic blood pressure ≥ 160 mm Hg) takes precedence over a classification of high normal blood pressure (diastolic blood pressure, 85 to 89 mm Hg) when both occur in the same person. A classification of high normal blood pressure (diastolic blood pressure, 85 to 89 mm Hg) takes precedence over a classification of normal blood pressure (systolic blood pressure < 140 mm Hg) when both occur in the same person.

TABLE 7.5 RISK (8.6-YEAR) FOR MAJOR CORONARY EVENTS IN 7,054 WHITE MEN BY DIASTOLIC BLOOD PRESSURE AT ENTRY

Diastolic blood pressure at entry[1]	Adjusted rate of major coronary events/1,000 persons	Relative risk	Absolute excess risk/1,000 persons
Below 80 (Quintiles 1 and 2)	66.0	1.0	
80–87 (Quintile 3)	100.6	1.52	34.6
88–95 (Quintile 4)	109.4	1.66	43.4
Above 95 (Quintile 5)	143.3	2.17	77.3

[1]The blood pressure ranges varied slightly for various 5-year age groups: 40 to 44, 45 to 49, etc.

(Reprinted with permission. The Pooling Project Research Group: *J Chronic Dis* 1978;31:201 and the American Heart Association.)

34.6/1,000 persons. The importance of this greater risk with higher pressure should not be ignored if one uses the smaller change in absolute risk numbers rather than the larger change in relative risk numbers, but caution is needed when applying epidemiologic statistics to individual patients.

If there were no risks of therapy, either financial, psychological or related to adverse effects, the argument could be made that those with levels of pressure below 90 mm Hg should be diagnosed and treated. But, as will be described later, all therapies—even nondrug—have risks and costs. Consequently, a diastolic blood pressure median of 95 mm Hg has been established for initiating drug treatment for most patients[12] (Figure 7.14). For some at low overall risk, such as older women without other risk factors, a higher level might be

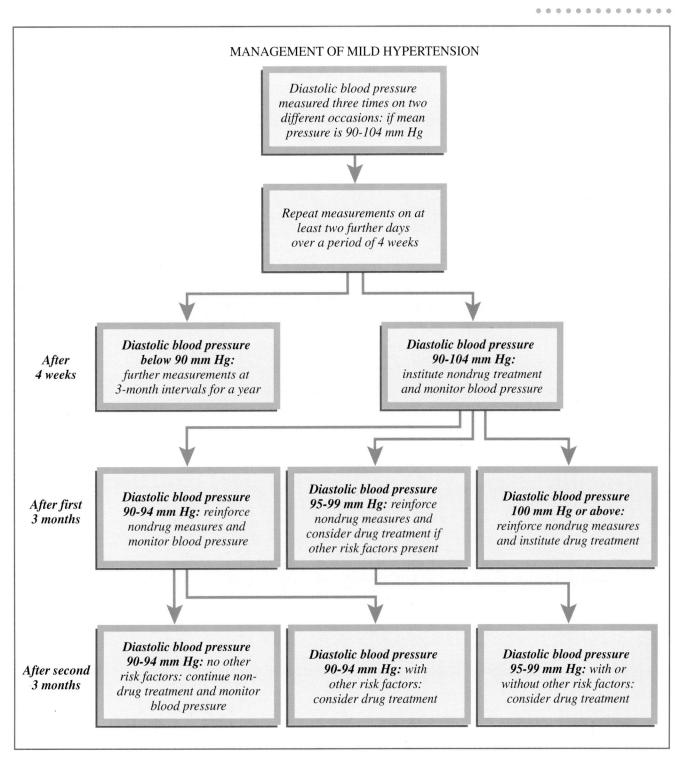

MANAGEMENT OF MILD HYPERTENSION

FIGURE 7.14 • Recommendations for the definition and management of mild hypertension by participants at the Third Mild Hypertension Conference of the World Health Organization and the International Society of Hypertension. (Reproduced with permission. World Health Organization/International Society of Hypertension: *J Hypertens* 1989;7:689.)

more appropriate. For others at higher risk—a young diabetic with microalbuminuria—an even lower level might be taken as indicating the need for therapy.

Despite the usual attention to diastolic levels, systolic pressures are equally if not more predictive of future risk (refer to Figure 7.11). Particularly in the older population, where isolated elevations in systolic pressure are quite common, attention must be given to these pressures because they are associated with significant increases in cardiovascular risk (Figure 7.15).

It should be noted that most hypertension is mild:

- About 80% of all people with a diastolic blood pressure of 90 mm Hg or higher will be in the "mild" category (diastolic blood pressure, 90 to 104 mm Hg).
- Approximately 15%, "moderate" (diastolic blood pressure 105 to 114 mm Hg).
- Only 5% or less, "severe" (diastolic blood pressure, 115 mm Hg and higher).

As increased attention has been directed toward improving the management of hypertension, more and more people identified with "mild" hypertension have been brought into therapy. This is because when examining the overall population, this segment contributes to most of the excess morbidity and mortality associated with hypertension (Figure 7.16). However, as will be noted, it has been difficult to document protection against coronary disease by treating mild and moderate groups.

Therefore, the criteria for institution of therapy remains unsettled. In the U.S., therapy is often given even at levels of diastolic blood pressure below 90 mm Hg,[13] whereas the 1988 JNC-4 Report and the 1989 WHO/ISH report recommend treatment at 95 mm Hg for most and 90 mm Hg for some (refer to Figure 7.14). In 1989, the British Hypertension Society[14] recommended a more conservative therapy only—treat most individuals with blood pressures of 100 mm Hg or higher.

EVALUATION OF THE NEWLY DIAGNOSED PATIENT

Beyond proceeding to therapy, patients found to be hypertensive need a thorough evaluation, limited as to procedures and laboratory testing, but covering all important aspects of the history (Table 7.6) and physical examination (Table 7.7).

Most patients are asymptomatic when first found to be hypertensive. However, not infrequently, the label of hypertension invokes considerable anxiety leading to various symptoms often through recurrent episodes of hyperventilation (Figure 7.17). Not only does hyperventilation induce numerous symptoms often ascribed to hypertension, such as dizziness, palpitations, and headaches, but it also can induce significant vascular contractions which decrease blood flow to the brain and heart. Care should be taken when patients are advised of an elevated blood pressure. The ability of proper management to prevent the potential adverse consequences must be emphasized and a reasonable perspective placed on the overall risk status of the patient.

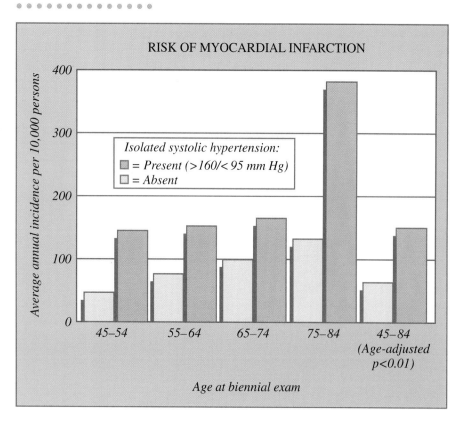

FIGURE 7.15 • Risk of myocardial infarction with isolated systolic hypertension (>160/<95 mm Hg) in men aged 45 to 84—Framingham Study, 24-year follow-up. (Reproduced with permission. Kannel WB: *J Am Coll Cardiol* 1990;15:206.)

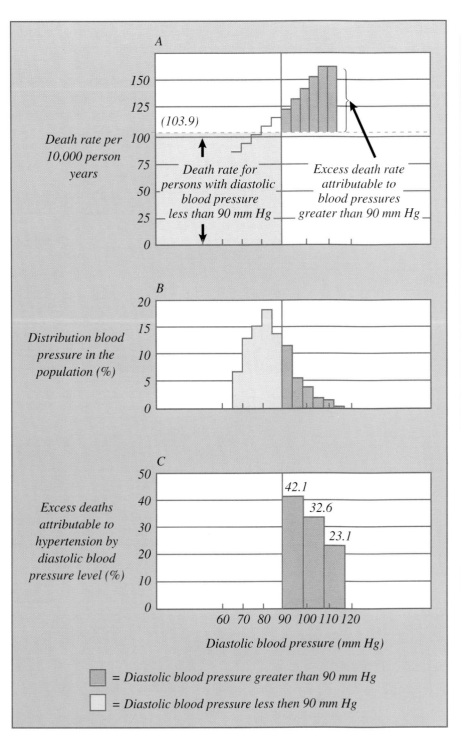

A

Death rate per 10,000 person years

150
125
100 (103.9)
75
50
25
0

Death rate for persons with diastolic blood pressure less than 90 mm Hg

Excess death rate attributable to blood pressures greater than 90 mm Hg

B

Distribution blood pressure in the population (%)

20
15
10
5
0

C

Excess deaths attributable to hypertension by diastolic blood pressure level (%)

50
42.1
40
32.6
30
23.1
20
10
0

60 70 80 90 100 110 120

Diastolic blood pressure (mm Hg)

☐ = *Diastolic blood pressure greater than 90 mm Hg*

☐ = *Diastolic blood pressure less then 90 mm Hg*

FIGURE 7.16 • The percentage of excess deaths attributable to hypertension by diastolic blood pressure level (C), based upon the death rate observed in Framingham (A) and the distribution of the blood pressure (B) found in the Hypertension Detection and Follow-up Program (HDFP) population. The percentage of excess deaths was calculated as follows: **Death rate x Distribution = % Excess deaths** (Reproduced with permission. The Hypertension Detection and Follow-up Program Cooperative Group: *Circ Res* 1977;40(Suppl 1):106 and the American Heart Association.)

Search for Secondary Causes

Part of the initial medical evaluation should be directed to the recognition of a potential secondary cause which might be relieved by specific therapy rather than controlled by lifelong medication. The list of possibilities for secondary causes of systemic arterial hypertension is long (Table 7.8). However, the percentage of patients who have a secondary cause is small (Table 7.9). Nonetheless, considering the large number of hypertensive patients—40 million or more in the U.S.—a 0.2% frequency represents 80,000 people. So, reasonable efforts should be made to rule out secondary causes.

Most secondary causes can be excluded relatively easily by the history, physical exam and routine initial laboratory testing, such as a CBC, urine analysis, automated blood chemistry (glucose, creatinine, potassium, total cholesterol and high density lipoprotein-cholesterol) and an electrocardiogram. When features

TABLE 7.7 • IMPORTANT ASPECTS OF THE PHYSICAL EXAMINATION	
Accurate measurement of blood pressure	Heart: size, rhythm
General appearance: distribution of body fat, skin lesions, muscle strength, alertness	Lungs: rhonchi, rales
Fundoscopic	Abdomen: renal masses, bruits over aorta or renal arteries, femoral pulses
Neck: palpation and auscultation of carotids, thyroid	Extremities: peripheral pulses, edema

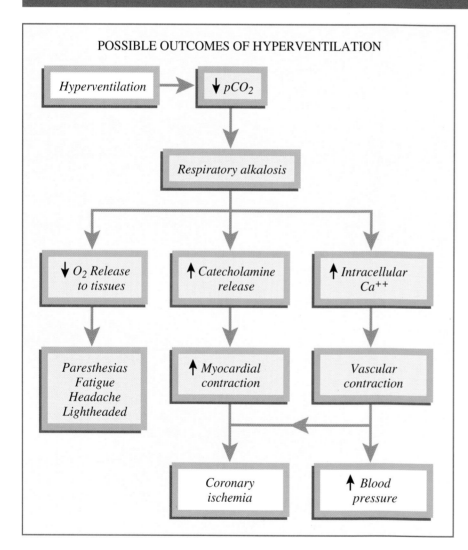

FIGURE 7.17 • The mechanisms by which acute hyperventilation may induce various symptoms, coronary ischemia, and a rise in blood pressure.

TABLE 7.8 • TYPES OF HYPERTENSION

I. Systolic and diastolic hypertension

Primary, essential, or idiopathic

Secondary

- Renal

    Renal parenchymal disease

      Acute glomerulonephritis

      Chronic nephritis

      Polycystic disease

      Connective tissue diseases

      Diabetic nephropathy

      Hydronephrosis

    Renovascular

    Renin-producing tumors

    Renoprival

    Primary sodium retention (Liddle's syndrome, Gordon's syndrome)

- Endocrine

    Acromegaly

    Hypothyroidism

    Hyperthyroidism

    Hypercalcemia (Hyperparathyroidism)

    Adrenal

Cortical

  Cushing's syndrome

  Primary aldosteronism

  Congenital adrenal hyperplasia

Medullary: Pheochromocytoma

Extra-adrenal chromaffin tumors

Carcinoid

Exogenous hormones

  Estrogen

  Glucocorticoids

  Mineralcorticoids: licorice

  Sympathomimetics

  Tyramine-containing foods and monamine oxidase inhibitors

- Coarctation of the aorta
- Pregnancy-induced hypertension
- Neurologic disorders

    Increased intracranial pressure

      Brain tumor

      Encephalitis

      Respiratory acidosis

    Sleep apnea

    Quadriplegia

    Acute prophyria

Familial dysautonomia

Lead poisoning

Guillain-Barré syndrome

- Acute stress, including surgery

    Psychogenic hyperventilation

    Hypoglycemia

    Burns

    Pancreatitis

    Alcohol withdrawal

    Sickle cell crisis

    Postresuscitation

    Postoperative

- Increased intravascular volume
- Alcohol, drugs, etc.

II. Systolic hypertension

Increased cardiac output

  Aortic valvular insufficiency

  AV fistula, patent ductus

  Thyrotoxicosis

  Paget's disease of bone

  Beriberi

  Hyperkinetic circulation

Rigidity of aorta

TABLE 7.9 • FREQUENCY OF VARIOUS DIAGNOSES IN HYPERTENSIVE SUBJECTS

Diagnosis	Rudnick KV, et al, 1977	Danielson M, Dammstrom B, 1981	Sinclair AM, et al, 1987
Essential hypertension	94%	95.3%	92.1%
Chronic renal disease	5%	2.4%	5.6%
Renovascular disease	0.2%	1.0%	0.7%
Coarctation of aorta	0.2%		
Primary aldosteronism		0.1%	0.3%
Cushing's syndrome	0.2%	0.1%	0.1%
Pheochromocytoma		0.2%	0.1%
Oral contraceptive-induced	0.2%	0.8%	1.0%
Number of patients	665	1,000	3,783

(Adapted with permission. Rudnick KV, Sackett DL, Hirst S, et al: *Canad Med Assoc J* 1977;117;492. Danielson M, Dammstrom B: *Acta Med Scand* 1981;209:451. Sinclair AM, Isles CG, Brown I, et al: *Arch Intern Med* 1987;47:1289.)

suggest a secondary cause, relatively simple diagnostic procedures may be indicated (Table 7.10). If the initial procedures are abnormal, additional ones should be performed to establish the diagnosis with certainty.[15]

Evaluation for Target Organ Damage

The second major goal of initial evaluation is to ascertain the extent of target organ damage, thereby to determine the need for therapy in general and individual choices of drugs in particular. The various complications of hypertension can be broadly considered as "hypertensive" or "atherosclerotic" (Table 7.11).

Hypertension per se is more closely connected to the former and is one of many risk factors of the latter.

Funduscopic Examination • Only in the optic fundi can small blood vessels be seen with ease, but this requires dilation of the pupil, a procedure that should be more commonly practiced (Figure 7.18). With the use of the short-acting mydriatic, tropicamide 1%, excellent dilation can be achieved in almost 90% of patients within 15 minutes. The presence of retinopathy is an independent indicator of mortality and should be determined in every hypertensive patient during the initial examination, followed by annual exams.

• • • • • • • • • • • • • • • • •

TABLE 7.10 • OVERALL GUIDE TO WORKUP OF HYPERTENSION

Diagnosis	Diagnostic procedure	
	Initial	Additional
Chronic renal disease	Urinalysis, serum creatinine, sonography	Isotopic renogram, renal biopsy
Renovascular disease	Bruit, plasma renin before and 1 hr after captopril	Aortogram, isotopic renogram 1 hr after captopril
Coarctation	Blood pressure in legs	Aortogram
Primary aldosteronism	Plasma potassium, plasma renin and aldosterone (ratio)	Urinary potassium, plasma or urinary aldosterone after saline load
Cushing's syndrome	AM plasma cortisol after 1 mg dexamethasone at bedtime	Urinary cortisol after variable doses of dexamethasone
Pheochromocytoma	Spot urine for metanephrine	Urinary catechols; plasma catechols, basal and after 0.3 mg clonidine

TABLE 7.11 • COMPLICATIONS OF HYPERTENSION

Hypertensive
- Accelerated-malignant hypertension (Grades III and IV retinopathy)
- Encephalopathy
- Cerebral hemorrhage
- Left ventricular hypertrophy
- Congestive heart failure
- Renal insufficiency
- Aortic dissection

Atherosclerotic
- Cerebral thrombosis
- Myocardial infarction
- Coronary artery disease
- Claudication syndromes

(Reproduced with permission. Smith WM: *Circ Res* 1977;40(Suppl 1):I-98 and the American Heart Association.)

Two separate, but related vascular diseases, are demonstrable. These are hypertensive neuroretinopathy (hemorrhages, exudates, and papilledema) and arteriosclerotic retinopathy (diffuse narrowing, arteriovenous nicking, and silver wiring). The retinopathy of diabetes—punctate hemorrhages and hard exudates—is seen in twice as many individuals with diabetes with hypertension as without.

Mild and Moderate Hypertension • Changes in light reflex, vessel caliber and tortuosity, and arteriovenous crossing defects reflect thickening of the walls of retinal arterioles, which narrows the column of bloodflow (refer to Figure 7.18A).

Severe Hypertension • The group III and IV changes, flame-shaped hemorrhages, soft exudates, and papilledema, are indicative of severe hypertension (refer to Figure 7.18 B,C,D)

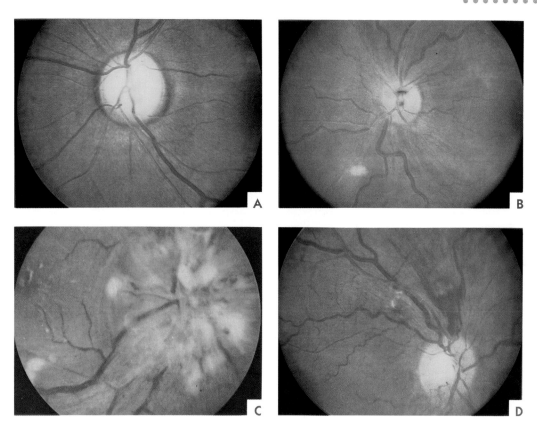

FIGURE 7.18 • Retinal changes associated with systemic hypertension. The retina of a 49-year-old black woman with asymptomatic essential hypertension of at least 10 years' duration displays arteriolar narrowing and straightening, increased light reflex, irregular caliber, loss of small arteriolar branches, and early arteriovenous crossing changes (A). A 42-year-old black woman with essential hypertension and blood pressure levels averaging 260/130 mm Hg was asymptomatic except for headaches (B). Retinal examination reveals severe vascular sclerosis, seen as marked irregularity of arteriolar caliber, "sheathing," and nearly complete loss of the arterioles. A "cotton wool" exudate is seen at seven o'clock. The nasal disk margin is blurred, which may occur normally. A 38-year-old black man with malignant hypertension, bilateral papilledema, and azotemia had no visual disturbance (C). Retinal examination reveals massive edema, hemorrhages, and exudates completely obscuring the disk and burying the blood vessels. The veins are congested, and the arterioles show diffuse thickening "copper wire". There are hard exudates (edema residues) forming in the nerve bundle grooves in the macular region at ten o'clock. (D) The retina of a 50-year-old black woman with severe hypertension of 25 years' duration shows evidence of arteriosclerosis: marked narrowing, irregular caliber, increased light reflex, and arteriovenous crossing changes (D). Atherosclerosis is also suggested by the large fan-shaped superficial hemorrhage, due to occlusion of a branch of the superior temporal vein as it enters the disk region. (Reproduced with permission. Hurst JW, Anderson RH, Becker AE, et al: *Atlas of the Heart* New York, NY: Gower Medical Publishing; 1988:12.4.)

Cardiac • Hypertension accelerates the development of atherosclerosis within the coronary vessels and puts increased tension on the myocardium, which causes it to hypertrophy (Figure 7.19). These in turn may result in myocardial ischemia, and this ischemia coupled with hypertrophy may lead to congestive heart failure, arrhythmias, and sudden death[16] (Figure 7.20).

The presence of hypertension is associated with multiple factors that accelerate coronary artery disease, including:
• Acceleration of atherosclerotic narrowing of larger coronary arteries (Figure 7.21).
• Abnormally high resistance of the coronary microvasculature.
• "Limited coronary reserve," such as a reduced capacity for the

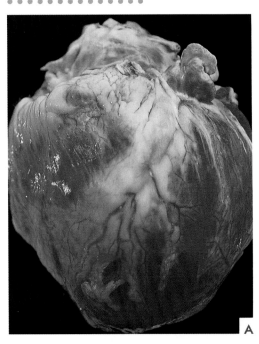
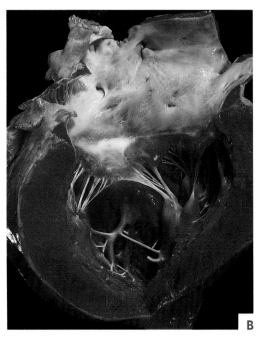

FIGURE 7.19 • Globular heart (A) is opened (B) to reveal left ventricular wall hypertrophy, an adaptive phenomenon to long-standing systemic hypertension. (Reproduced with permission. Hurst JW, Anderson RH, Becker AE, et al: *Atlas of the Heart* New York, NY: Gower Medical Publishing; 1988:12.4.)

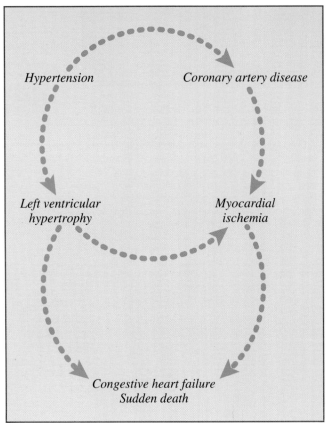

FIGURE 7.20 • The probable interrelationships between hypertension, left ventricular hypertrophy (LVH), and the various manifestations of hypertensive heart disease. The probable synergism between LVH and myocardial ischemia related to coronary artery disease is emphasized and is likely to be responsible for many of the cases of congestive heart failure (CHF) and sudden death. (Reproduced with permission. Massie BM, Tubau JF, Szlachcic J, et al: *J Cardiovasc Pharmacol* 1989;13(Suppl 1):S18.)

coronary bed to vasodilate, which reduces the expected increase in coronary blood flow in response to various stimuli. This impairment is ordinarily related to three events:

- Myocardial hypertrophy that outstrips the vascular bed.
- Thickened coronary arteries that are less able to dilate.
- The higher cavitary pressures within the left ventricle that impede flow through these vessels.[17]

Clinical Manifestations • These multiple mechanisms render hypertensives more susceptible to silent ischemia, unrecognized myocardial infarction, and sudden death (refer to Figure 7.12). The increased prevalence of sudden death among hypertensives most likely involves left ventricular hypertrophy (Figure 7.22), and is possibly mediated through an increased frequency of high-grade ventricular ectopy.

As will be noted in detail, the treatment of hypertension has not been found to reduce the incidence of coronary disease in most controlled trials. Beyond other possible reasons, Cruickshank[18] has presented evidence that treatment-induced reduction in perfusion pressures, through coronary vessels either narrowed or having impaired vasodilatory reserve, may invoke ischemic events. Therefore, the presence of coronary artery disease may present additional difficulties in the treatment of hypertension.

One of the mechanisms for myocardial ischemia is the increased demand for blood supply from a hypertrophied left ventricle. Hypertrophy as a response to the increased afterload of elevated systemic vascular resistance can be viewed as protective up to a certain point. Beyond that point, a variety of dysfunctions accompany left ventricular hypertrophy.

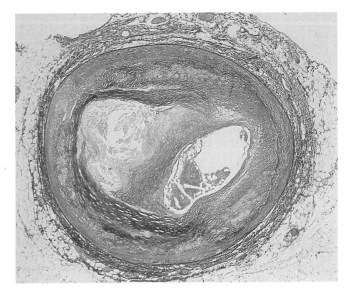

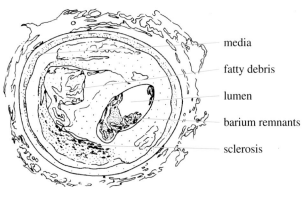

FIGURE 7.21 • Histologic section of the coronary artery showing classical artherosclerotic lesion. Fatty debris is the major plaque constituent. (Reproduced with permission. Swales JD, Sever PS, Peart S: *Clinical Atlas of Hypertension* London, England: Gower Medical Publishing; 1991:4.8.)

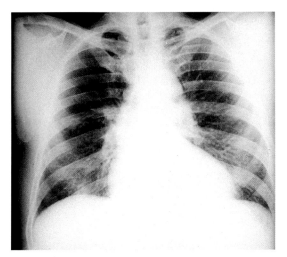

FIGURE 7.22 • Chest film from a hypertensive patient shows a large heart due to left ventricular hypertrophy. (Reproduced with permission. Swales JD, Sever PS, Peart S: *Clinical Atlas of Hypertension* London, England: Gower Medical Publishing; 1991:8.6.)

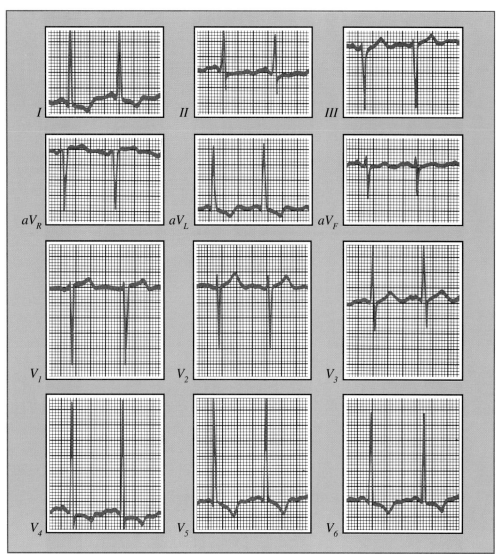

FIGURE 7.23 • This ECG from a 61-year-old patient with essential hypertension illustrates left ventricular hypertrophy. (Reproduced with permission. Hurst JW, Anderson RH, Becker AE, et al: *Atlas of the Heart* New York, NY: Gower Medical Publishing; 1988:12.5.)

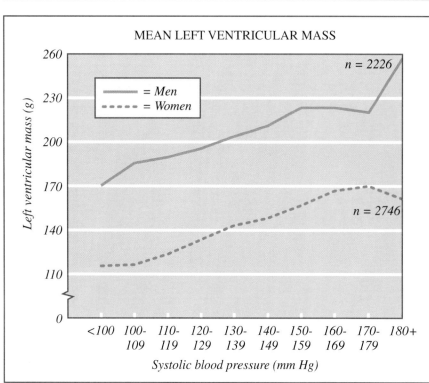

FIGURE 7.24 • Mean left ventricular mass by sex and by systolic pressure, including participants taking antihypertensive medications, aged 17 to 90 years. Data were obtained by M-mode echocardiograms taken on 2,226 men and 2,746 women in the Framingham Study between the years 1979 to 1983—cohort examination 16 and offspring cycle 3. (Reproduced with permission. Savage DD, Levy D, Dannenberg AL, Garrison RJ, Castelli WP: *Am J Cardiol* 1990;65:371.)

Whereas left ventricular hypertrophy is identified by electrocardiography (Figure 7.23) in only 5% to 10% of hypertensives, reports have documented left ventricular hypertrophy by echocardiography in between 19% and 80% of hypertensives.[19] Its prevalence is closely correlated with systolic blood pressure (Figure 7.24). In addition, independent correlations are seen with increasing body weight and age.

The configuration of ventricular hypertrophy can vary, presumably dependent upon the relative degree of volume or pressure load as well as other factors (Figure 7.25). Changes in both systolic and diastolic function accompany left ventricular hypertrophy[20] (Figure 7.26). Those with minimally increased left ventricular muscle mass may have supernormal contractility reflecting an increased inotropic state with a high percentage of

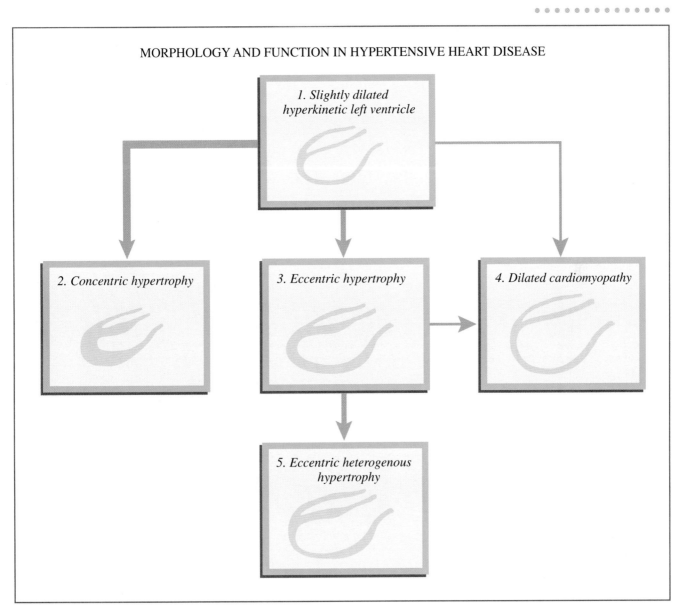

FIGURE 7.25 • A classification of morphology and function in hypertensive heart disease based on echocardiography. (Reproduced with permission. Nielsen I: *Scand J Clin Lab Invest* 1989;49(Suppl 1):16.)

fractional shortening and increased wall stress. Those with substantial concentric left ventricular hypertrophy may have high ejection fractions, reflecting small left ventricular end-diastolic cavity dimensions (refer to Figure 7.26B). A group of such patients with "hypertensive hypertrophic cardiomyopathy," all elderly and mostly female and black, presented with chest pain or dyspnea that suggested heart failure.[21] Their status worsened with vasodilator medications that reduced afterload and caused hypotension by further increasing the already excessive left ventricular emptying and by reducing diastolic filling.

Patients with eccentric left ventricular hypertrophy are often obese, which apparently presents a volume load to the left ventricle. There is normal cardiac output but increased left ventricular wall stresses, especially during exercise.

As noted in Figure 7.26A, the various alterations of systolic and diastolic function seen with left ventricular hypertrophy could obviously progress into left ventricular pump failure or congestive heart failure (CHF). Hypertension is responsible for a large portion of CHF episodes. Although its contribution to CHF may be receding with more widespread therapy, hypertension remains the major preventable factor in the disease that involves over 200,000 deaths and almost 2 million events each year in the United States. Data suggest that antihypertensive treatment does not completely prevent CHF but postpones its development by several decades.[22] Angiotensin-con-

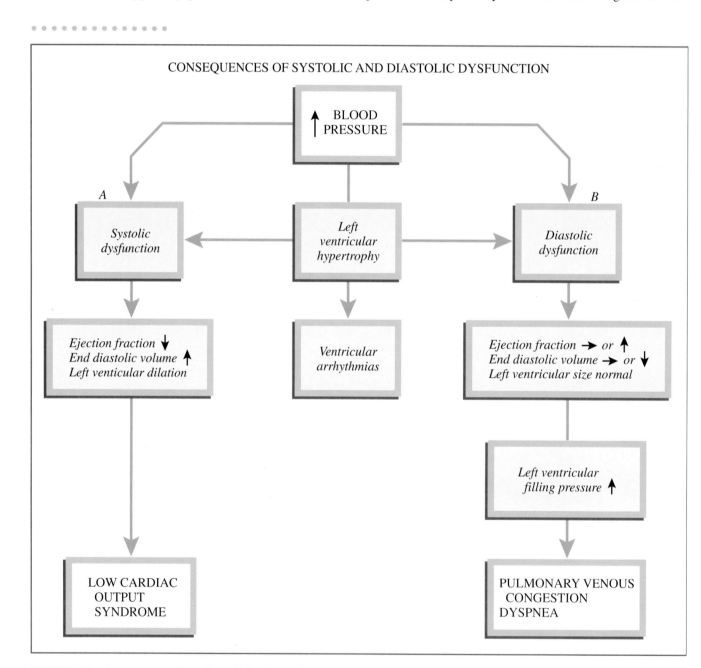

FIGURE 7.26 • Consequences of systolic and diastolic dysfunction related to hypertension. Systolic dysfunction and congestive heart failure may occur late in the evolution of hypertensive heart disease, because of impaired ventricular contraction (A). Diastolic dysfunc-

tion is the most common manifestation of the effect of hypertension on cardiac function and also can lead to congestive heart failure due to increased filling pressures (B). (Reproduced with permission. Shepherd RFJ, Zachariah PK, Shub C: *Mayo Clin Proc* 1989;64:1521.)

verting enzyme (ACE) inhibitors prolong survival of normotensive patients with CHF and these agents may be even more beneficial in hypertensive patients with CHF.

Most episodes of CHF in hypertensive patients are associated with dilated cardiomyopathy and a reduced ejection fraction. Recall, however, the presence of pulmonary congestion with intact or even supernormal systolic function but marked diastolic dysfunction associated with severe concentric LVH seen particularly among selected hypertensive patients, especially older women.[21]

Cerebral • Cerebral function should be evaluated, but it is seldom possible to relate cerebral dysfunction to the severity of the hypertension. Even more than heart disease, hypertension is the major cause of strokes and transient ischemic attacks (TIA). These pathological features of cerebrovascular disease are found at a higher rate among hypertensive patients:

• Increased formation of atheroma, both in larger arteries and in smaller penetrating vessels.

• Hyaline arteriosclerosis.
• Microaneurysms of Charcot-Bouchard.
• Lacunae, small 0.5- to 1.5-cm cavities that are found in 10% of normotensive elderly people but 90% of hypertensive patients (Figure 7.27). They likely represent multiple infarcts.
• Multi-infarct dementia (Figure 7.28).
• Subcortical arteriosclerotic encephalopathy—Binswanger's disease.
• Hypertensive encephalopathy.

Perhaps of greatest importance, because more can be done to prevent progression of the disease to stroke, is the recognition of extracranial vascular disease, which is also more common in hypertensive patients.[23] Atherosclerotic disease in extracranial arteries may be responsible for asymptomatic carotid bruits, transient ischemic attacks (TIAs), and other clinical syndromes (Table 7.12).

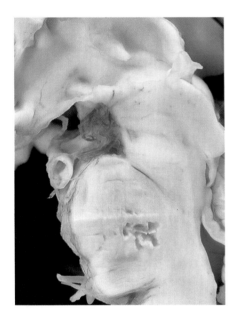

FIGURE 7.27 • Median section through the pons reveals a clustering of multiple lacunar infarcts due to hypertension. (Reproduced with permission. Hurst JW, Anderson RH, Becker AE, et al: *Atlas of the Heart* New York, NY: Gower Medical Publishing; 1988:12.6.)

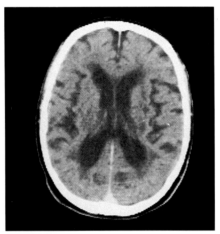

FIGURE 7.28 • CT scan of the brain of a hypertensive patient shows multi-infarcts. In some hypertensive patients, cerebrovascular disease manifests itself as a progressive multi-infarct dementia. (Reproduced with permission. Swales JD, Sever PS, Peart S: *Clinical Atlas of Hypertension* London, England: Gower Medical Publishing; 1991:4.17.)

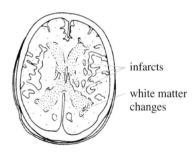

TABLE 7.12 • CLINICAL FEATURES OF EXTRACRANIAL VASCULAR DISEASE	
Recurrent transient ischemic attacks	Involvement of central retinal artery
• Weakness or paresthesias in arms	• Decreased intracular pressure by ophthalmodynamometry
• Unilateral blindness	• Retinal emboli
Reduced pulsation in carotid arteries	Dilated collateral vessels over forehead
• Localized bruit	Unilateral headache
• Murmur on either side	

Renal • Renal dysfunction, both structural (Figure 7.29) and functional, is almost always demonstrable in hypertensive patients, even those with minimally elevated pressures. Pathologically, the changes of milder degrees of hypertension are mainly hyalinization and sclerosis of the walls of the afferent arterioles, referred to as arteriolar nephrosclerosis. Renal in-volvement may be asymptomatic and not demonstrable by usual clinical testing. The earliest usual symptom is nocturia and the earliest abnormal lab test is microalbuminuria, reflecting intraglomerular hypertension.

The loss of renal function is progressively greater the higher the blood pressure[24] but only a minority of hypertensive pa-

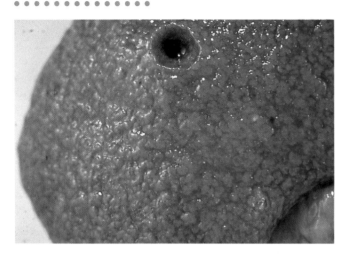

FIGURE 7.29 • Macroscopic view of a kidney from a patient with essential hypertension. The size of the kidney is normal, but there is an adherent capsule with a slightly granular appearance. (Reproduced with permission. Swales JD, Sever PS, Peart S: *Clinical Atlas of Hypertension* London, England: Gower Medical Publishing; 1991:4.21.)

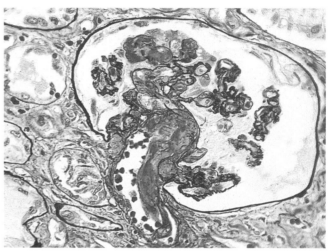

FIGURE 7.30 • Fibrinoid necrosis of a glomerular afferent arteriole and the capillary tufts is evident in a patient with the malignant phase of hypertension. (Reproduced with permission. Hurst JW, Anderson RH, Becker AE, et al: *Atlas of the Heart* New York, NY: Gower Medical Publishing; 1988:12.7.)

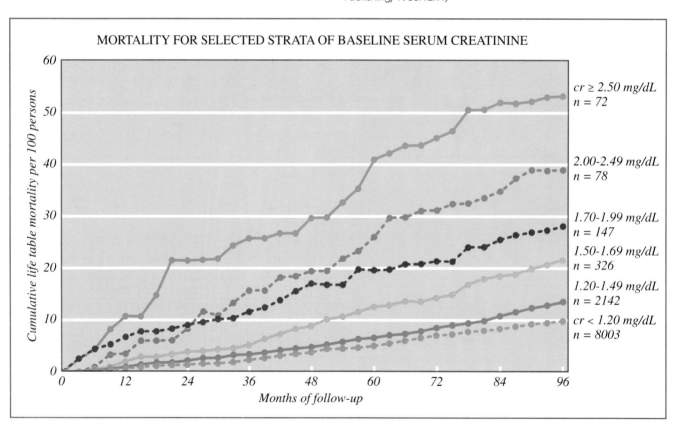

FIGURE 7.31 • Cumulative 8-year life table mortality curves (percentage at months of follow-up) for selected strata of baseline serum creatinine. The sample size (n) and the creatinine stratum limits (mg/dL) are noted to the right of each curve. (Reproduced with permission. Shulman NB, Ford CE, Hall WD, et al: *Hypertension* 1989;13(Suppl I): I-80 and the American Heart Association.)

tients die as a result of renal failure. Those with malignant hypertension almost always have extensive fibrinoid necrosis (Figure 7.30). Hypertension remains a leading risk for end-stage renal disease, being largely responsible for the twice higher incidence in blacks than in whites in the eastern United States. Despite good control of the hypertension, renal function may deteriorate and this, too, is more common among blacks. Among the 10,940 patients treated in the Hypertension Detection and Follow-up Program (HDFP), mortality rates increased progressively with increasing levels of serum creatinine at baseline[25] (Figure 7.31). Despite better overall control of hypertension, the incidence of end-stage renal disease as a consequence of hypertensive nephrosclerosis seems to be increasing.[26]

An Overview of the Natural History • A broad overview of the natural history of untreated hypertension is shown in Figure 7.32. Obviously, the presence of various target organ complications reflects a failure to detect the elevated pressure in the early stages and to provide therapy that might stop the progress of its complications. Even more desirable would be the recognition of the prehypertensive phase and successful intercession to prevent the development of sustained hypertension.

ASSESSMENT OF OVERALL CARDIOVASCULAR RISK

The third reason for an initial evaluation is to assess overall risk. The interaction of hypertension with the other major cardio-

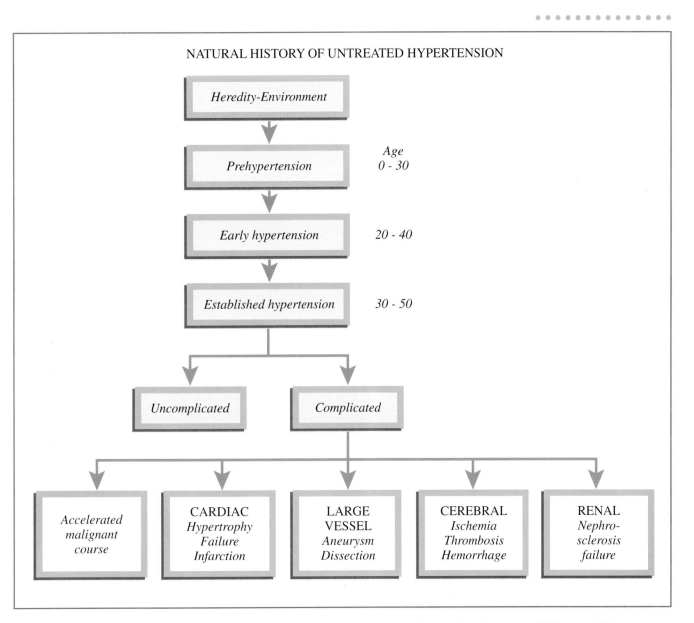

FIGURE 7.32 • A representation of the natural history of untreated essential hypertension. (Reproduced with permission. Kaplan NM: *Clinical Hypertension* 4th ed. Baltimore, Md: Williams and Wilkins; 1986:124.)

vascular risk factors is clearly shown in the data from Framingham, which demonstrate the increased probability of cardiovascular diseases with varying levels of systolic blood pressure as influenced by the presence of other risk factors (Figure 7.33).

Now that the various aspects of the diagnosis and evaluation of the individual patient have been examined, we will turn to a brief review of the pathogenesis of hypertension in order to be able to fashion the most effective plan for its management.

MECHANISMS OF HYPERTENSION

As noted in Table 7.9, 90% to 95% of all hypertension is of unknown cause—idiopathic or primary. The term "essential," usually used to identify this state, seems both inappropriate and misleading and the term "primary" will be used hereafter.

As more knowledge has been gained about the pathophysiology of hypertension, bits and pieces of the whole have been identified as being caused by a specific mechanism—

renovascular disease. However, despite numerous leads, no single defect has been recognized among the majority of patients whose hypertension, therefore, remains primary.

PRIMARY HYPERTENSION

Persistent hypertension can only develop in response to an increase in cardiac output (CO) or a rise in peripheral vascular resistance (PR). Therefore, defects may be present in one or more of the multiple factors that affect these two forces[15] (Figure 7.34). An interplay of derangements in multiple factors affecting cardiac output and peripheral resistance may precipitate the disease, and these may differ in both type and degree in different patients. Looking for a single defect in all patients with essential hypertension may be a mistake. The following sage advice was presented in an editorial in *The Lancet*:

Blood pressure is a measurable end product of an exceedingly complex series of factors, including those which control blood vessel caliber and responsiveness, those which control fluid volume within and outside the vascular bed, and those which control cardiac output. None of these fac-

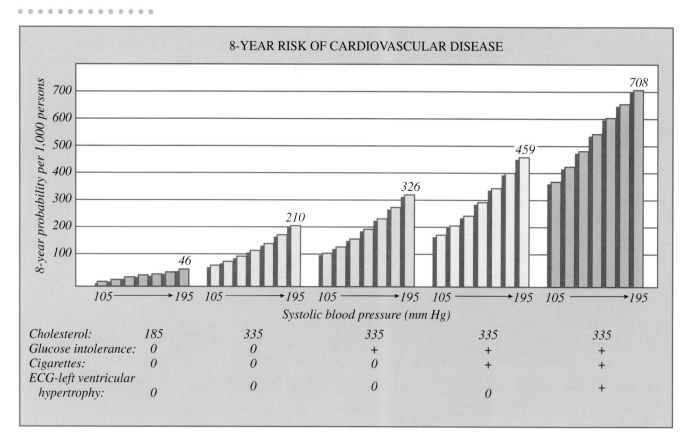

FIGURE 7.33 • The 8-year risk of cardiovascular disease for 40-year-old men in Framingham according to progressively higher systolic blood pressure at specified levels of other risk factors. (Reproduced with permission. Kannel WB: In: Kaplan NM, Stamler J, eds. *Prevention of Coronary Heart Disease* Philadelphia, Pa: WB Saunders Co.; 1983.)

tors is independent, they interact with each other and respond to changes in blood pressure. It is not easy, therefore, to dissect out cause and effect. Few factors which play a role in cardiovascular control are completely normal in hypertension: indeed, normality would require explanation, since it would suggest a lack of responsiveness to increased pressure.[27]

Before considering the various factors shown in Figure 7.34 which affect the basic equation:

Blood pressure = Cardiac output x Peripheral resistance

let us consider the hemodynamic patterns that have been measured in patients with hypertension. One caution is needed—the

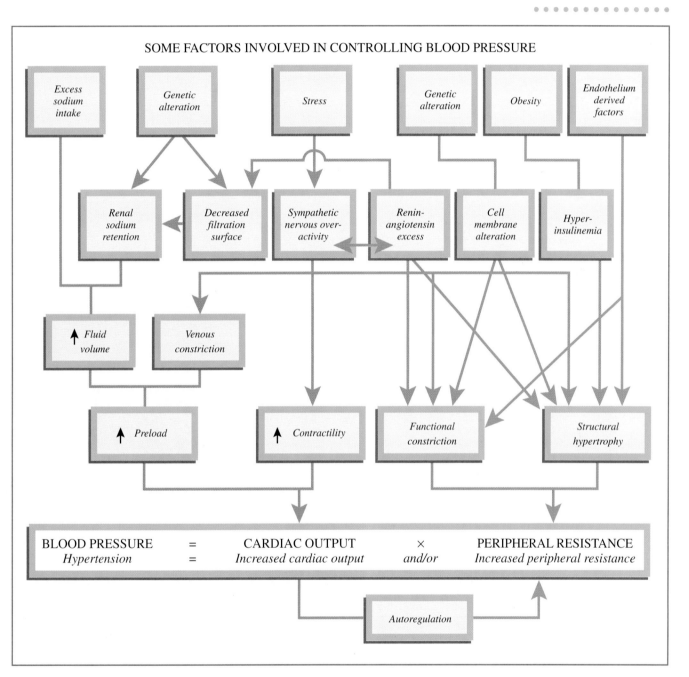

FIGURE 7.34 • Some of the factors involved in the control of blood pressure that affect the basic equation:
Blood pressure = Cardiac output x Peripheral resistance

pathogenesis of the disease is probably a slow and gradual process. By the time blood pressure becomes elevated, the initiating factors may no longer be apparent, since they may have been "normalized" by the compensatory interactions alluded to above. Nonetheless, when a group of untreated, young hypertensive patients was initially studied, cardiac output was normal or slightly increased and peripheral resistance was normal[28] (Figure 7.35). Over the next 20 years, cardiac output progressively fell and peripheral resistance rose.

Regardless of how hypertension begins, the eventual primacy of increased resistance can be shown even in models of hypertension that feature an initial increase in fluid volume and cardiac output[29] (Figure 7.36). The same pattern has been seen in humans—patients with primary aldosteronism whose disease was completely controlled with the aldosterone antagonist, spironolactone, were followed after this drug was discontinued and the syndrome was allowed to recur in its natural manner.[30] Initially, plasma volume was expanded, however, it returned toward normal as peripheral resistance rose progressively.

Genetic Predisposition

As seen in Figure 7.34, genetic alterations may initiate the cascade to permanent hypertension. Clearly, heredity plays a role

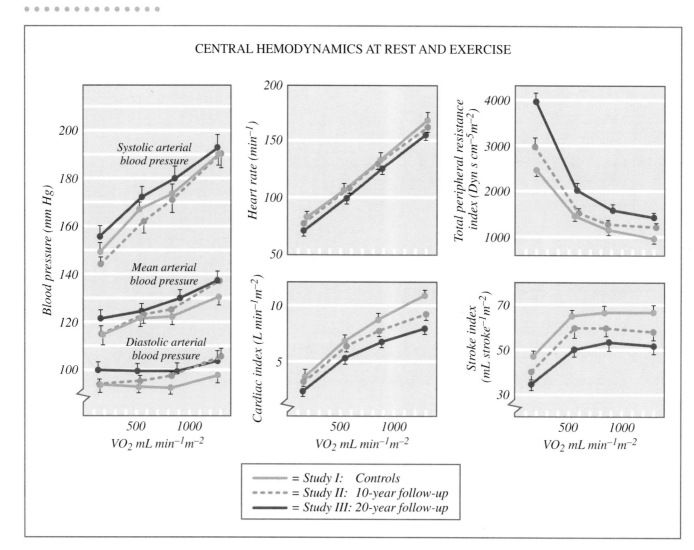

FIGURE 7.35 • Central hemodynamic at rest and during exercise in age group 1 (17 to 29 years) at first study and at restudies after 10 and 20 years. Note the marked increase in the total peripheral resistance index from study I to study III and also the reduction in the stroke and cardiac index from study I to study III. (Reproduced with permission. Lund-Johansen P: *J Hypertens* 1989;7(Suppl 6):S52.)

Hypertension

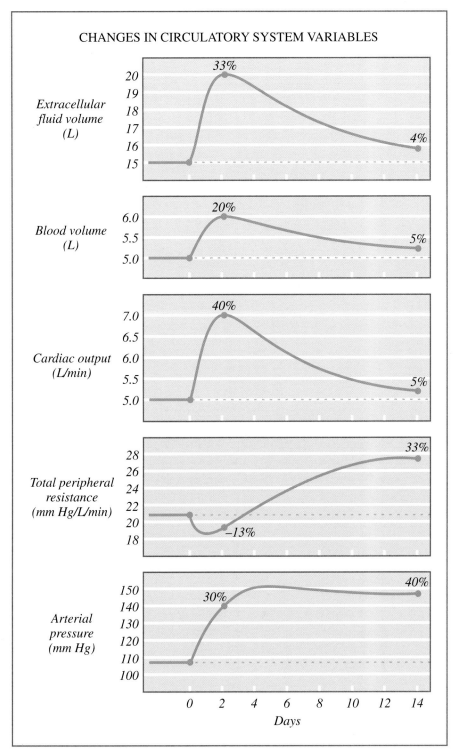

CHANGES IN CIRCULATORY SYSTEM VARIABLES

Extracellular fluid volume (L)

Blood volume (L)

Cardiac output (L/min)

Total peripheral resistance (mm Hg/L/min)

Arterial pressure (mm Hg)

Days

FIGURE 7.36 • Progressive changes in important circulatory system variables during the first few weeks of volume-loading hypertension. The initial rise in cardiac output is the basic cause of the hypertension. Subsequently, the autoregulation mechanism returns the cardiac output almost to normal while at the same time causing a secondary increase in total peripheral resistance. (Reproduced with permission. Guyton AC: *Textbook of Medical Physiology* 7th ed. Philadelphia, Pa: WB Saunders; 1986:265.)

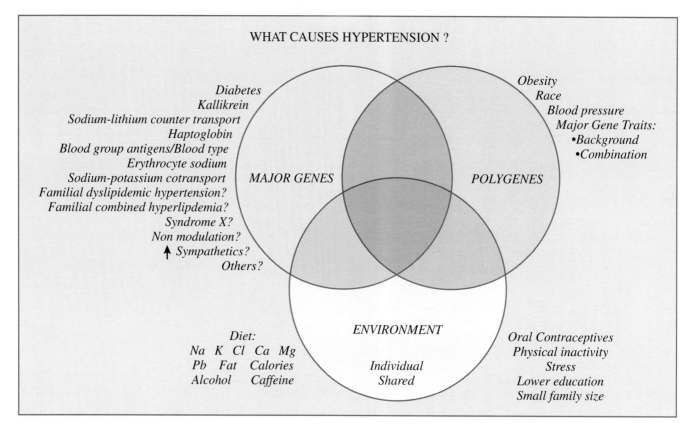

WHAT CAUSES HYPERTENSION ?

Diabetes
Kallikrein
Sodium-lithium counter transport
Haptoglobin
Blood group antigens/Blood type
Erythrocyte sodium
Sodium-potassium cotransport
Familial dyslipidemic hypertension?
Familial combined hyperlipdemia?
Syndrome X?
Non modulation?
↑ *Sympathetics?*
Others?

MAJOR GENES

POLYGENES

Obesity
Race
Blood pressure
Major Gene Traits:
•*Background*
•*Combination*

Diet:
Na K Cl Ca Mg
Pb Fat Calories
Alcohol Caffeine

ENVIRONMENT

Individual
Shared

Oral Contraceptives
Physical inactivity
Stress
Lower education
Small family size

FIGURE 7.37 • A model showing overlapping contributions from major genes, polygenes and environmental factors to the multifactorial susceptibility to hypertension. (Reproduced with permission. Williams RR, Hunt SC, Hasstedt SJ, et al: *J Hypertens* 1989;7 (Suppl 6):S8.)

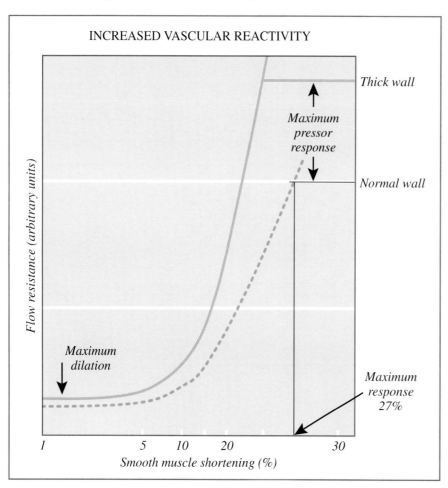

INCREASED VASCULAR REACTIVITY

Thick wall

Maximum pressor response

Normal wall

Maximum dilation

Maximum response 27%

Flow resistance (arbitrary units)

1   5   10   20   30
Smooth muscle shortening (%)

FIGURE 7.38 • Increased vascular reactivity in hypertension explained by structural changes. The differences in flow resistance are calculated in a mathematical model assuming a 30% increased wall thickness as the only difference between hypertensive and normal vessels. (Modified and adapted with permission. Folkow B: *Am Heart J* 1987;114:938 and Westerhof N, Huisman RM: *Clin Sci* 1987;72:391.)

although no discriminatory gene markers are currently available.[31] In studies of twins and family members in which the degree of familial aggregation of blood pressure levels is compared with the closeness of genetic sharing, the genetic contributions have been estimated to range from 30% to 60%. As Williams et al[31] portray, hypertension may be caused by the interaction of a large number of genetic and environmental factors (Figure 7.37).

Vascular Hypertrophy

Since an increased peripheral resistance is both necessary and sufficient to perpetuate hypertension, even if it starts with an increased cardiac output, we will focus on factors known to increase peripheral resistance (PR) (refer to Figure 7.34). Although functional constriction is portrayed as a possible mechanism, it appears that the high PR in hypertension is determined mainly by structural hypertrophy, which in turn gives rise to a generalized increase in contractility[32] (Figure 7.38). Data from human subjects support the hypothesis proposed by Folkow[32] of a "positive-feedback interaction" wherein even mild functional pressor influences—if repeatedly exerted—may lead to structural hypertrophy that reinforces and perpetuates the elevated pressure (Figure 7.39A). Lever[33] added two hypotheses to Folkow's first: A reinforcement of the hypertrophic response to stimuli that

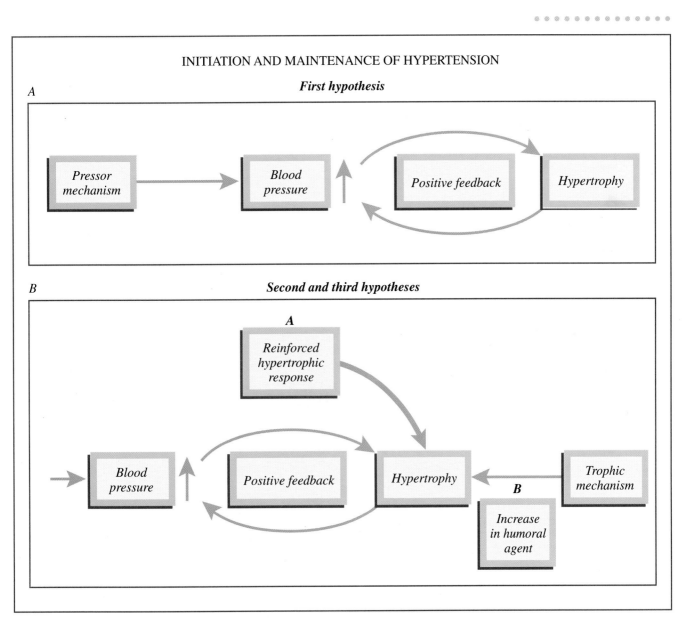

FIGURE 7.39 • Hypotheses for the initiation and maintenance of hypertension. Folkow's first proposal that a minor overactivity of a pressor mechanism raises blood pressure slightly, initiating positive feedback and a progressive rise of blood pressure (A). (B) is similar to (A) with an additional two signals: an abnormal or "reinforced" hypertrophic response to pressure (A) and increase of a humoral agent causing hypertrophy directly (B). (Reproduced with permission. Lever AF: *J Hypertension* 1986;4:515.)

initially raises the pressure—defects in the vascular cell membrane—and the action of various trophic mechanisms that may cause vascular hypertrophy directly for which Lever refers to as the "slow pressor mechanism" (Figure 7.39B).

Therefore, Lever's scheme contains both a fast pressor mechanism and a slow hypertrophic effect, which can be induced by a number of pressor-growth promotors. Lever uses renovascular hypertension as one model in which hypertension is initiated by a fast acting pressor (angiotensin II) and maintained by the trophic action of the hormone to induce vascular hypertrophy (Figure 7.40). The evidence for the model derives, first, from the fact that the direct, immediate pressor actions of angiotensin II are less than the degree of chronic hypertension that occurs with equal concentrations of the hormone. This suggests an additional contribution of a "slow mechanism." Secondly, lower concentrations of an-giotensin II are needed to maintain hypertension than to initiate it. Thirdly, angiotensin II is a known trophin for vascular smooth muscle.

The immediate pressor effect is mediated by increased free intracellular calcium. The slowly developing vascular hypertrophy is postulated to involve phosphatidylinositol metabolism in the cell membrane (Figure 7.41). The binding of angiotensin II to its receptor activates the enzyme phospholipase C, which hydrolyzes the membrane phosphatidylinositol 4,5-biphosphate (PIP_2), and releases inositol triphosphate (IP_3) into the cytosol and diacylglycerol (DG) in the plane of the membrane. The cytosolic IP_3 mobilizes calcium from its intracellular stores and causes an immediate contraction. The DG in the membrane activates protein kinase C, which increases the activity of an amiloride-sensitive Na+/H+ exchanger. Thereby, sodium enters the cell down an electrochemical gradient and protons are ex-

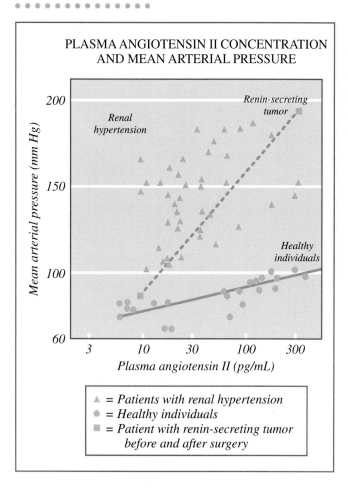

FIGURE 7.40 • Relation of plasma angiotensin II concentration and mean arterial pressure in patients with renal hypertension mostly caused by renal artery stenosis as compared with healthy subjects before and during infusion of angiotensin II. Shown separately are values from a patient with renin-secreting tumor before and after surgery. In all these patients, arterial pressure is higher than can be explained by the direct vasoconstrictor effect of angiotensin II as assessed by infusion of the peptide in normal subjects. (Reproduced with permission. Lever AF: *J Hypertens* 1986;4:515.)

truded so that the cell becomes more alkaline. Increased cell alkalinity is believed to initiate DNA synthesis and hence promoting cell hypertrophy.

This scheme to explain the immediate pressor action and the slow hypertrophic effect of angiotensin II is thought to be common to the action of pressor-growth promotors.[34] When present in high concentrations over long periods, as with angiotensin II in renal artery stenosis, each of these pressor-growth promotors causes hypertension. Moreover, when the source of the excess pressor-growth promotor is removed, hypertension may recede slowly, presumably reflecting the time needed to reverse vascular hypertrophy.

In the majority of hypertensive patients, no marked excess of any known pressor hormones is identifiable. Nonetheless, a lesser excess of one or more may have been responsible for initiation of a process sustained by the positive feedback postulated by Folkow[32] and the trophic effects emphasized by Lever.[33] This sequence encompasses a variety of specific initiating mechanisms that accentuate and maintain the hypertension by a nonspecific feedback-trophic mechanism (Figure 7.42). If this double process is fundamental to the pathogenesis of essential hypertension, the difficulty in recognizing the initiating, causal factor is easily explained. As formulated by Lever[33]:

The primary cause of hypertension will be most apparent in the early stages. In the later stages, the cause will be concealed by an increasing contribution from hypertrophy. A particular form of hypertension may wrongly be judged to have "no known cause" because each mechanism considered is insufficiently abnormal by itself to produce hypertension. The cause of essential hypertension may have been considered already but rejected for this reason.

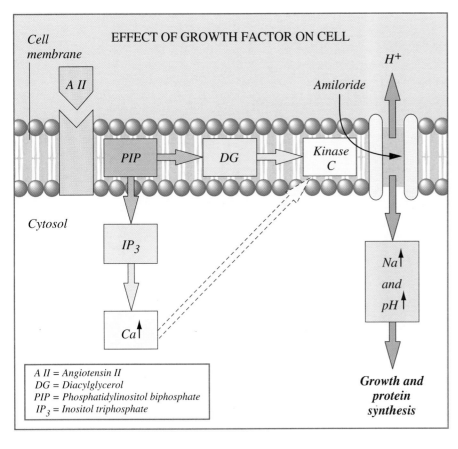

FIGURE 7.41 • The main events in a signaling system activated by growth factors. Angiotensin II occupies a membrane receptor and phosphatidylinositol biphosphate (PIP) is hydrolyzed by phosphodiesterase in the membrane. Inositol triphosphate (IP_3) is released into the cytosol and diacylglycerol (DG) in the plane of the membrane. The latter activates protein kinase C linked to an amiloride-sensitive Na^+/H^+ exchanger whose activity increases. Sodium enters the cell down an electrochemical gradient and protons are extruded. The increased intracellular pH that results promotes growth and protein synthesis. (Reproduced with permission. Lever AF: *J Hypertens* 1986;4:515.)

In order to examine the various possible pressor-growth promoters, we will go back to the individual factors shown in Figure 7.34.

Sodium Excess and Intracellular Calcium

A considerable body of circumstantial evidence supports a role for sodium, acting either as an expander of preload volume in concert with renal sodium retention or as an intracellular modulator of calcium-induced vasoconstriction (Table 7.13).

In a study of over 10,000 subjects in 52 centers throughout the world[35] (Figure 7.43), dietary sodium intake assessed by urinary sodium excretion has been correlated to the rise in diastolic blood pressure with age. In almost all of these populations, daily sodium intake averaged over 100 mmol/24 hr, which is likely above the threshold at which sodium intake is closely related to the development of hypertension (Figure 7.44). Those who consume more than the threshold amount would be expected to show little increase in the prevalence of hypertension

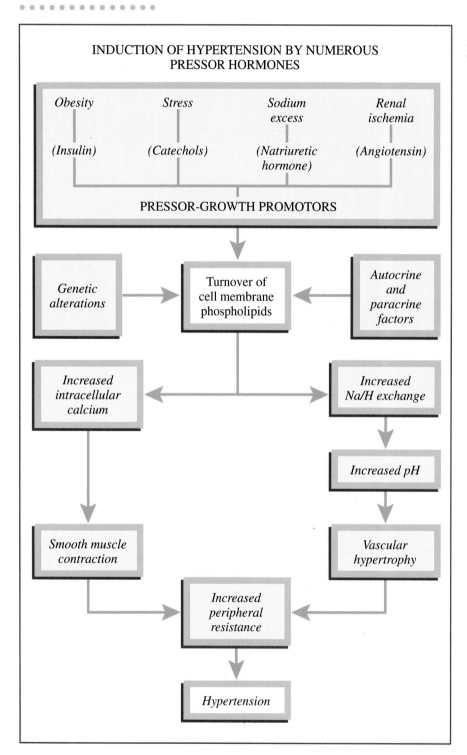

FIGURE 7.42 • The induction of hypertension by numerous pressor hormones that act as vascular growth promoters.

TABLE 7.13 • EVIDENCE FOR A ROLE OF SODIUM IN PRIMARY (ESSENTIAL) HYPERTENSION

In multiple populations the rise in blood pressure with age is directly correlated with increasing levels of sodium intake.

Multiple, scattered groups who consume little sodium (less than 50 mmol/d) have little or no hypertension. When they consume more sodium, hypertension appears.

Animals given sodium loads, if genetically predisposed, develop hypertension.

Some people, when given large sodium loads over short periods, develop an increase in vascular resistance and blood pressure.

An increased concentration of sodium is present in the vascular tissue and blood cells of most hypertensives.

Sodium restriction to a level of 60 to 90 mmol/d will lower blood pressure in most people. The antihypertensive action of diuretics requires an initial natriuresis.

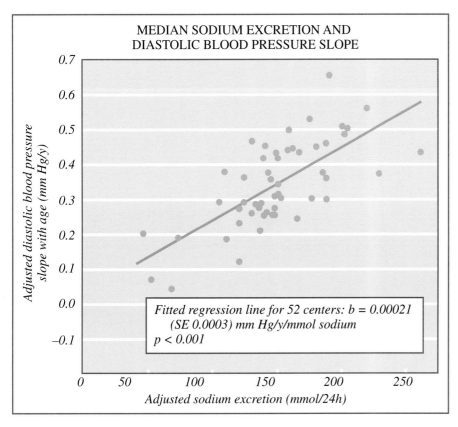

MEDIAN SODIUM EXCRETION AND DIASTOLIC BLOOD PRESSURE SLOPE

Fitted regression line for 52 centers: b = 0.00021 (SE 0.0003) mm Hg/y/mmol sodium p < 0.001

FIGURE 7.43 • Cross center plots of diastolic blood pressure slope with age, median sodium excretion and fitted regression line for 52 centers, also adjusted for body mass index and alcohol intake. (Reproduced with permission. Intersalt Cooperative Research Group: *Br Med J* 1988;297:319.)

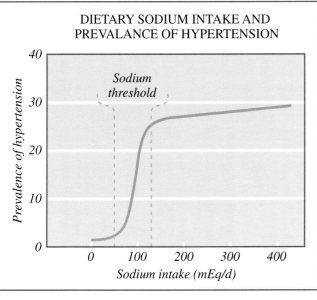

DIETARY SODIUM INTAKE AND PREVALANCE OF HYPERTENSION

FIGURE 7.44 • The probable association between usual dietary sodium intake and the prevalence of hypertension in large populations. (Reproduced with permission. Kaplan NM: *JAMA* 1984;251:142.)

with progressively more sodium intake. As seen in Figure 7.43, almost all populations were above the threshold level, except those four groups who consumed less than 70 mmol/d and in whom blood pressure levels and age-related increases were considerably lower.

Since almost everyone in Western countries ingests a high sodium diet, the fact that only 20% or so develop hypertension suggests a variable degree of sodium sensitivity. Obviously, heredity and other environmental exposures may be major determinants. Short periods of high sodium intake, in most studies involving 200 to 400 mmol/d for 10 to 30 days, will cause the blood pressure to rise in some, but not all normotensive or borderline hypertensive people. Those whose blood pressure rises by 10% or by 10 mm Hg are usually called "sodium sensitive," the others "sodium resistant." Weinberger et al.[36] define sodium sensitivity as a 10 mm Hg or greater decrease in mean blood pressure the morning after 1 day of a 10 mEq sodium diet during which three oral doses of

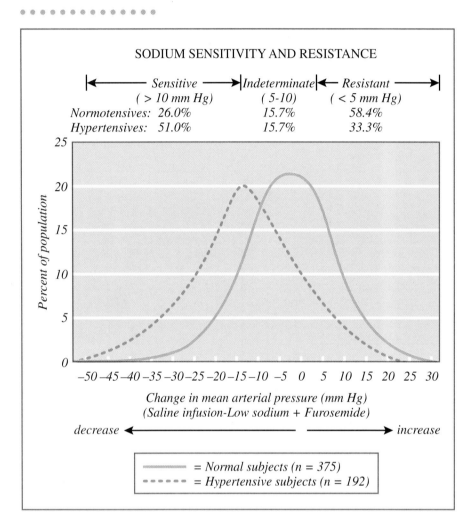

FIGURE 7.45 • Blood pressure responses to the maneuvers in normotensive and hypertensive subjects. The hypertensive individuals are significantly more sodium sensitive than the normotensives. The distributions are Gaussian. (Reproduced with permission. Weinberger MH, Miller JZ, Luft FC, et al: *Hypertension* 1986;8(Suppl II):II-127 and the American Heart Association.)

furosemide were given at 1000, 1400, and 1800 . They found that half of hypertensive individuals were sodium sensitive, twice more than seen among normotensives (Figure 7.45). Whether the world can be divided neatly into two such populations remains to be seen. The more likely situation is that a continuously progressing responsiveness may be heightened with increasing age.

The manner by which high sodium intake leads to hypertension in those who are sodium sensitive may involve the elaboration of a digitalis-like natriuretic hormone, presumably of hypothalamic origin, which inhibits the Na+,K+-ATPase pump, thereby increasing the concentration of sodium within cells[37] (Figure 7.46). Although inhibition of the sodium pump increases renal sodium excretion and restores vascular volume, the increase in intracellular sodium would be expected to increase the concentration of free intracellular calcium as well.[38] With increased intracellular sodium, sodium/calcium exchange mechanisms would presumably extrude less calcium,

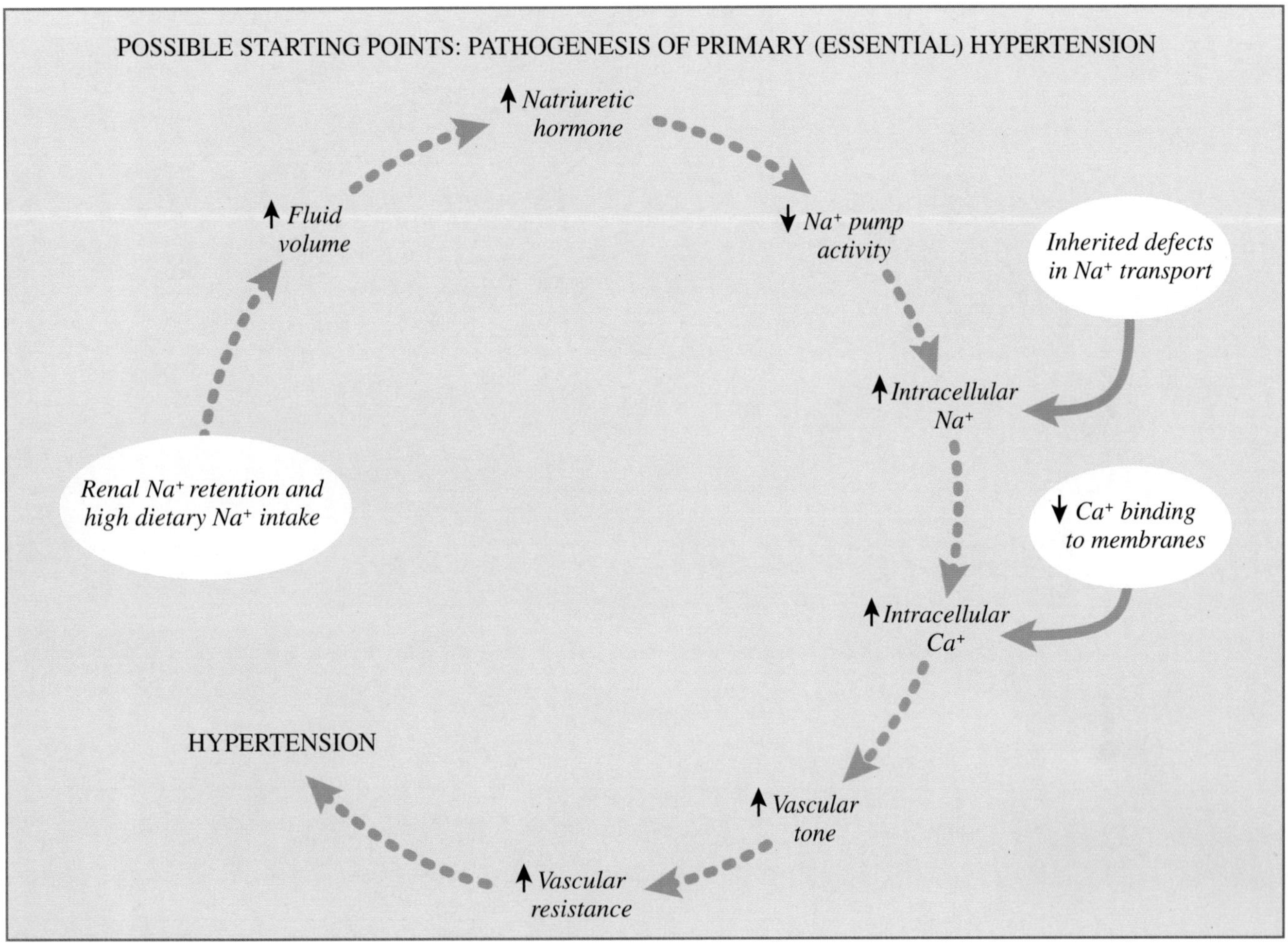

POSSIBLE STARTING POINTS: PATHOGENESIS OF PRIMARY (ESSENTIAL) HYPERTENSION

FIGURE 7.46 • Hypothesis for the pathogenesis of primary essential hypertension, starting from one of three points. The combination of high sodium intake and renal sodium retention which induces an increase in the hypothalamic natriuretic hormone and thereby inhibits sodium transport. An inherited defect in sodium transport is invoked to induce an increase in intracellular sodium. A primary membrane defect directly leads to increased free intracellular calcium.

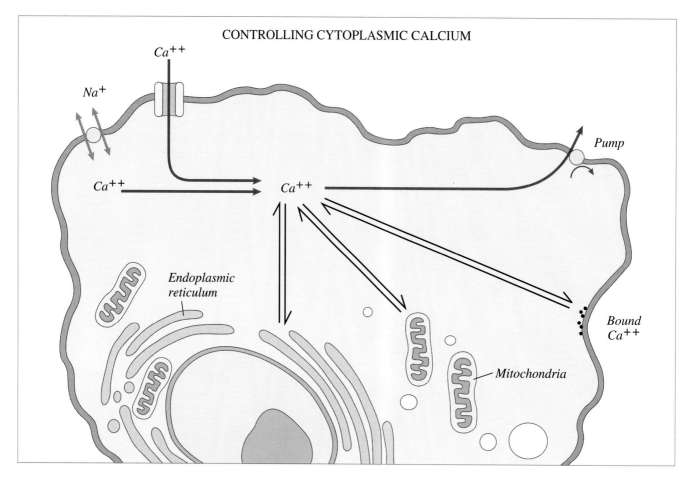

FIGURE 7.47 • Mechanisms controlling cytosolic Ca++. Entry is mainly via calcium channels and the Na+/Ca++ exchange. Binding is to the cell membrane, mitochondria, and endoplasmic reticulum. Exit is via the Na++/Ca++ exchange and the Ca++ ATPase pump. (Reproduced with permission. Exton JH: *Kidney Int* 1987;32(Suppl 23):S-68.)

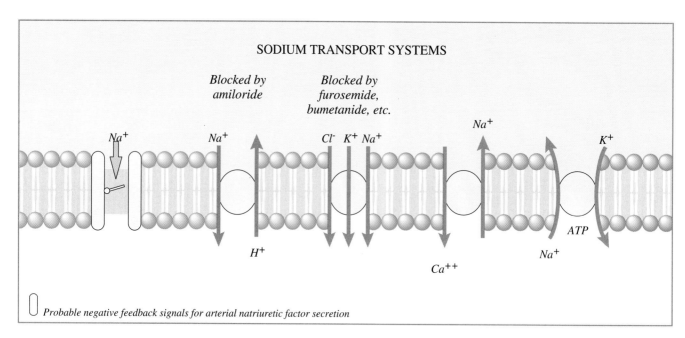

FIGURE 7.48 • Sodium transport systems. From left to right, these include the sodium channel, Na+/H+ antiport exchange, Na-K cotransport, Na+-Ca++ exchange, and the Na+-K+ ATPase pump. (Reproduced with permission. Lazdunski M: *Am J Med* 1988;84(Suppl 1B):3.)

leading to higher intracellular free calcium levels (Figure 7.47). According to Blaustein,[38] as little as a 5% increase in intracellular sodium would inhibit sodium/calcium exchange sufficiently to raise intracellular calcium enough to increase resting tone of vascular smooth muscle by as much as 50%.

As shown in Figure 7.46, increased intracellular sodium concentrations may be caused by inherited defects in sodium transport, including one or more of those shown in Figure 7.48. Defects in these sodium transport mechanisms have been observed in various experimental models of hypertension, and in some people with hypertension, but it is uncertain whether they play a causal role or serve simply as markers.[39]

A third mechanism has been proposed to explain the higher intracellular calcium levels found in cells of hypertensive persons—a primary defect in the binding of calcium to membranes within the cell,[40] shown on the right side of Figure 7.46. At this time, uncertainty remains as to the function of a number of possible mechanisms that could be responsible for the high intracellular sodium and calcium levels measured in cells from hypertensive animals and people.

While the search for the putative pressor natriuretic hormone has been to date unsuccessful, a natriuretic hormone from the cardiac atria has been identified and widely studied. Atrial natriuretic factor (ANF) or peptide is vasodilatory and appears to be involved in the normal regulation of body fluid volume (Figure 7.49). Atrial natriuretic factor appears to be involved in the pressure-natriuresis that occurs with acute volume expansion, but its role in the pathogenesis of hypertension has not been defined.

Defects in Renal Sodium Excretion

In concert with excess sodium intake, a subtle and nondiscernable decrease in renal sodium excretion could over time lead to volume excess that might start the cascade to hypertension. Three hypotheses proposed involve a defect in renal sodium excretion:

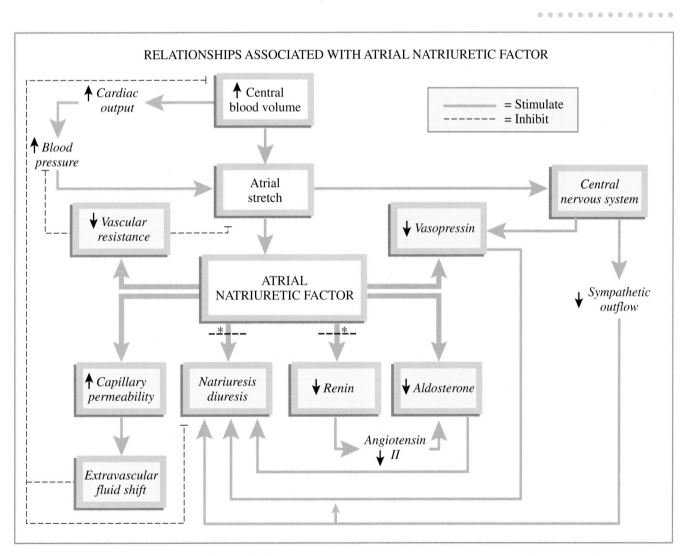

FIGURE 7.49 • Schematic representation showing the following:
• The regulation of atrial natriuretic factor (ANF) secretion.
• The major target organ actions of ANF.
• The relationship between ANF and the reflex inhibition of central sympathetic outflow during expansion of central blood volume.

(Reproduced with permission. Atlas SA, Laragh JH: Atrial natriuretic factor and its involvement in hypertensive disorders. In: Laragh JH, Brenner BM, eds. *Hypertension. Pathophysiology, Diagnosis, and Management*, Volume 1 New York, NY: Raven Press; 1990.)

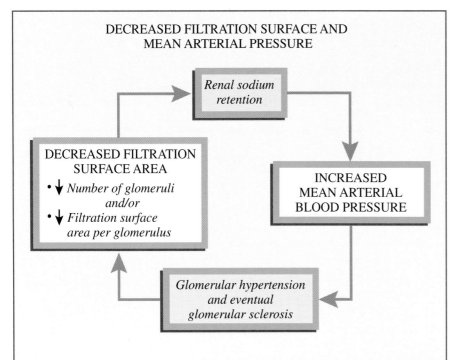

FIGURE 7.50 • Relationship between decreased filtration surface area (FSA) and mean arterial pressure. Decreased FSA, due to decreased nephron number and/or FSA per glomerulus, leads to renal sodium retention, and thereby to increased mean arterial pressure. Systemic hypertension in turn promotes glomerular hypertension and eventual sclerosis, further decreasing the functioning filtration surface area. (Reproduced with permission. Brenner BM, Garcia DL, Anderson S: *Am J Hypertens* 1988;1:335.)

TABLE 7.14 • HYPOTHESIS: THERE IS NEPHRON HETEROGENEITY IN ESSENTIAL HYPERTENSION

There are ischemic nephrons with impaired sodium excretion intermingled with adapting hyperfiltering hypernatriuretic nephrons.

Renin secretion is high from ischemic nephrons and very low from hyperfiltering nephrons.

The inappropriate circulating renin-angiotensin level impairs sodium excretion because:

• In the adapting hypernatriuretic nephrons:

It increases tubular sodium reabsorption.

It enhances tubuloglomerular feedback-mediated afferent constriction.

• As the circulating renin level is diluted by nonparticipation of adapting nephrons it becomes inadequate to support efferent tone in hypoperfused nephrons.

A loss of nephron number with age and from ischemia further impairs sodium excretion.

(Reproduced with permission.Sealey JE, Blumenfeld JD, Bell GM, et al: *J Hypertens* 1988;6:763.)

- An inherited or acquired decrease in filtration surface area (FSA)[41] (Figure 7.50).
- Nephron heterogeneity with intermingling of ischemic and hyperfiltering nephrons[42] (Table 7.14).
- Nonmodulation of renal sodium excretion in response to high sodium intake, presumably secondary to an inability to change target tissue responsiveness to angiotensin.[43] Such nonmodulators, when given sodium loads, fail to increase renal blood flow, thereby retaining more and more sodium over time (Figure 7.51).

One or more of these mechanisms may be responsible for renal sodium retention. They all relate to another basic mechanism for sodium and blood pressure control—the renin-angiotensin system.

The Renin-Angiotensin System

The renin-angiotensin mechanism may also be involved in the pathogenesis of hypertension, both as a direct pressor and as a growth promotor. All functions of renin are mediated through the synthesis of angiotensin II. This system is the primary stimulus for the secretion of aldosterone and hence mediates the mineralocorticoid responses to varying sodium intakes and volume loads (Figure 7.52). When sodium intake is reduced or effective plasma volume shrinks, the increase in renin-angiotensin II stimulates aldosterone secretion, which, in turn, is responsible for a portion of the enhanced renal retention of sodium and water.

As will be described, hypertension may develop either from renin levels that are suppressed, such as by an adrenal adenoma that causes mineralocorticoid excess, or when renin levels are elevated—from a kidney made ischemic by renovascular

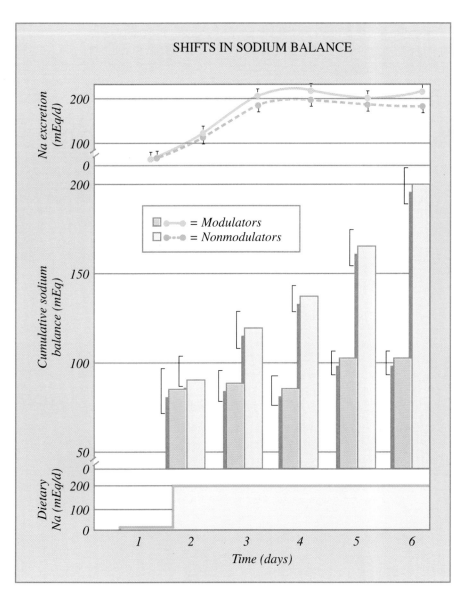

SHIFTS IN SODIUM BALANCE

FIGURE 7.51 • Documented shifts in sodium balance in patients with essential hypertension, classified as to modulating status, with a shift in sodium intake from 10 to 200 mEq/d. Note that the nonmodulators take a longer time to achieve external sodium balance and show more positive sodium balance when they do so. The weight gain in each group was congruent with the degree of positive sodium balance. The nonmodulators increased their blood pressure significantly, whereas the modulators did not. (Reproduced with permission. Hollenberg NK, Moore T, Shoback D, et al: *Am J Med* 1986;81:412.)

stenosis. The fact that renin levels may be either low or high in patients with primary hypertension has led some to believe that an excess of mineralocorticoid activity on the one hand, or a more subtle, diffuse intrarenal ischemia on the other, may be involved in the pathogenesis of primary hypertension.

The renin-angiotensin system is probably active in multiple individual organs, more from *in situ* synthesis of various components rather than by transport from renal J-G cells through the circulation. The complete system has been found, among other places, in endothelial cells, the brain and adrenal cortex, potentially broadening roles for this system beyond previously accepted boundaries.

Stress and Catecholamines

Catecholamines arising in response to stress shown in Figure 7.42 are pressor-growth promoters. Evidence incriminating a role for increased sympathetic activity is summarized in Table 7.15. As seen in Figure 7.34, increased sympathetic nervous activity could raise blood pressure in a number of ways—either alone or in concert with stimulation of renin release by catecholamines—by causing arteriolar and venous constriction,

by increasing cardiac output, or by altering the normal renal pressure-volume relationships.

Obesity and Hyperinsulinemia

Hypertension is two to three times more common in the obese, and blood pressure rises and falls in concert with weight gain and loss. The associations are most striking in people whose excess weight is predominantly located in the abdomen and upper body, a localization that is under the direct influence of androgens. Thus, as most men gain weight, they deposit the fat in the upper body, giving rise to typical "middle-aged" spread. This upper body obesity is associated with an increased prevalence not only of hypertension but also of hyperlipidemia and diabetes mellitus and all of these, in turn, appear to be interrelated by way of hyperinsulinemia (Figure 7.53). Hyperinsulinemia is common to all forms of obesity, but even more so in upper body obesity wherein the release of free fatty acids during lipolysis impairs the normal extraction and utilization of insulin by the liver so that more insulin bathes the periphery.

Insulin receptors are present on endothelial and arterial smooth muscle cells and insulin is a potent trophic hormone. In-

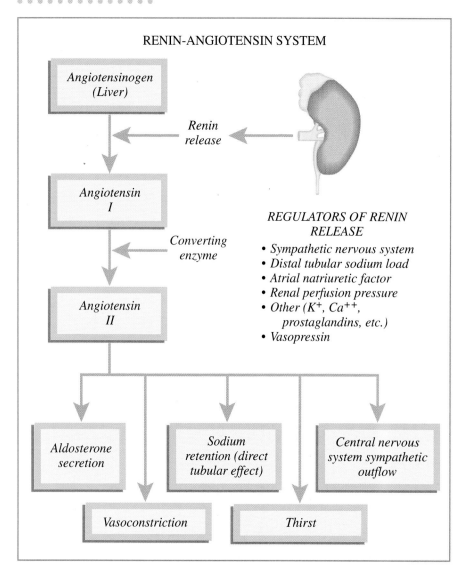

RENIN-ANGIOTENSIN SYSTEM

Angiotensinogen (Liver)

Renin release

Angiotensin I

Converting enzyme

Angiotensin II

REGULATORS OF RENIN RELEASE
- *Sympathetic nervous system*
- *Distal tubular sodium load*
- *Atrial natriuretic factor*
- *Renal perfusion pressure*
- *Other (K^+, Ca^{++}, prostaglandins, etc.)*
- *Vasopressin*

Aldosterone secretion

Sodium retention (direct tubular effect)

Central nervous system sympathetic outflow

Vasoconstriction

Thirst

FIGURE 7.52 • The renin angiotensin system showing major regulators of renin release, the biochemical cascade leading to angiotensin II, and the major effects of angiotensin II. (Reproduced with permission. Dzau VJ, Pratt RE: In: Fozzard HA et al, eds. *The Heart and Cardiovascular System* New York, NY: Raven Press; 1986.)

TABLE 7.15 • EVIDENCE FOR SYMPATHETIC NERVOUS ACTIVATION IN PRIMARY (ESSENTIAL) HYPERTENSION

In animals, acute hypertension can be induced by release of catecholamines in response to discrete brain lesions.

In rats bred to become hypertensive spontaneously, alerting stimuli invoke greater discharges from central autonomic centers.

Some hypertensive people have high plasma catecholamine levels that correlate with blood pressure.

Hypertensives with high plasma catechols (and high plasma renin levels) display greater suppressed hostility on psychometric testing.

Some hypertensives overrespond to stress, and hypertension occurs more often in persons exposed to high levels of psychogenic stress.

Drugs that inhibit adrenergic nervous activity lower blood pressure.

EFFECTS OF UPPER BODY OBESITY

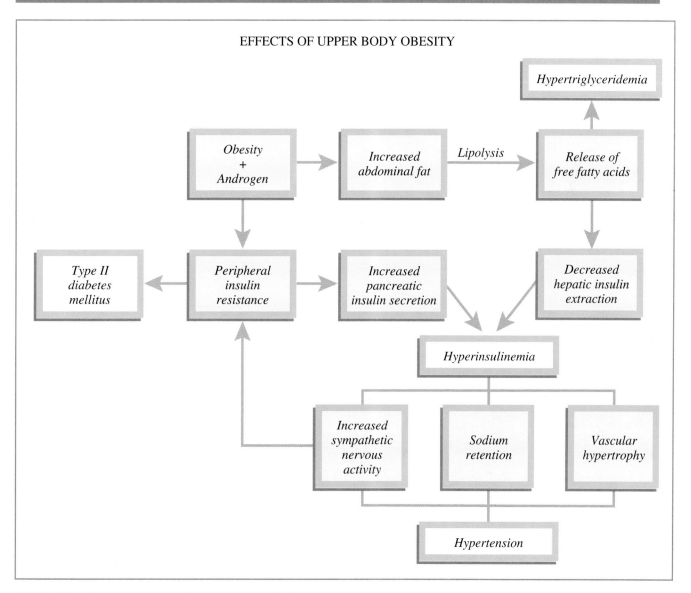

FIGURE 7.53 • The mechanism by which upper body obesity can promote glucose intolerance, hypertriglyceridemia, and hypertension via hyperinsulinemia.

sulin activates the amiloride-sensitive Na+/H+ exchanger noted in Figure 7.42 to be the putative switch for protein synthesis and hypertrophy. In addition to its trophic action, insulin can raise the blood pressure by at least two other mechanisms—a rise in circulating catecholamines and a stimulation of renal sodium reabsorption.

The presence of hyperinsulinemia in obesity and its potential causal role in the hypertension of upper body obesity is rather obvious (refer to Figure 7.53). Less obvious, but of even greater possible importance, is the fact that hyperinsulinemia is also common in nonobese patients with primary hypertension[44,45] (Figure 7.54). The hyperinsulinemia is attributable to peripheral insulin resistance, but the reason for this resistance is unknown. Regardless of how it occurs, insulin re-

sistance with resultant hyperinsulinemia is likely to be a pressor-growth promoter involved in the pathogenesis of primary hypertension, both in the obese and the nonobese.

Endothelium-Derived Factors

The last putative mechanism involved in the pathogenesis of hypertension shown in Figure 7.34 is the action of one or more of a rapidly expanding number of endothelium-derived factors that have only recently been identified (Figure 7.55). The exact role of these vasoactive substances is unknown but some, such as the vasoconstrictor endothelin[46] and the endothelium-derived relaxing factors, have significant effects upon vascular tone[47] and could play a role in the development or sustainment of systemic arterial hypertension.

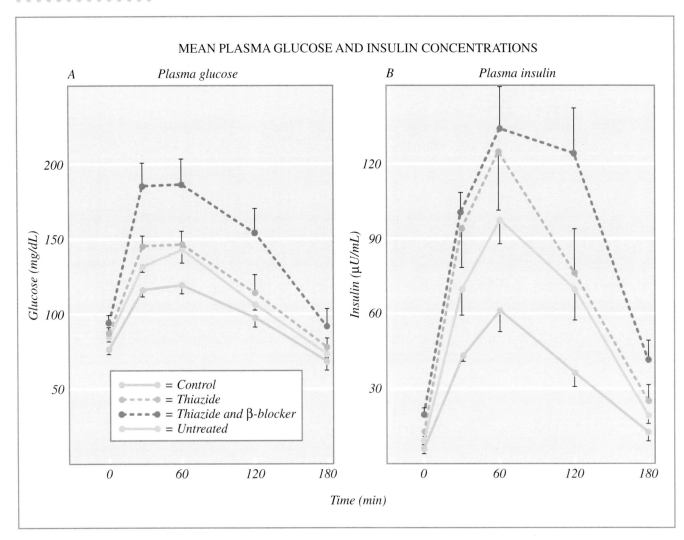

FIGURE 7.54 • Mean plasma glucose (A) and insulin concentrations (B) before and after the 75 oral glucose challenge in the four experimental groups. The controls were normotensive and were well-matched for age and body mass index with the untreated and treated hypertensive subjects (Reproduced with permission. Swislocki AL, Hoffman BB, Reaven GM: *Am J Hypertens* 1989;2:419.)

Associated Conditions

Beyond the possible involvement of these multiple factors, certain extrinsic factors are closely associated with hypertension but obviously are not involved in the majority of patients. Perhaps, the most important is alcohol abuse. Even in small quantities, alcohol may raise blood pressure; in larger quantities, alcohol may be responsible for a significant number of cases of hypertension. Some researchers have found a linear, progressively increasing level of blood pressure with increasing consumption of alcohol, but most report a threshold effect[48] (Figure 7.56). On the other hand, some find lower levels of blood pressure among those who drink small amounts of ethanol—5

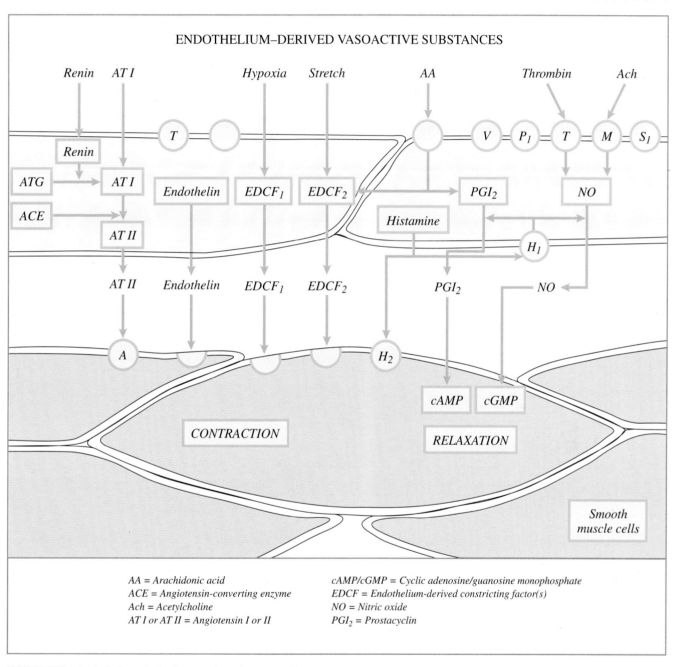

FIGURE 7.55 • Endothelium-derived vasoactive substances. (Reproduced with permission. Luscher TF, Yang Z, Diedrich D, et al: *J Cardiovasc Pharmacol* 1989;14(Suppl 6):S63.)

to 15 mL/d—than among those who drink none at all.[49] The latter pattern more clearly parallels the association with total and coronary mortality[50] as well as ischemic stroke.[51]

SECONDARY CAUSES

In addition to alcohol abuse, a number of other mechanisms may lead secondarily to hypertension. These include sleep apnea, polycythemia, lead intoxication, and others listed in Table 7.8. Some of these deserve additional attention either because they are fairly common, such as oral contraceptive use, or because they frequently need to be excluded, such as primary aldosteronism in hypokalemic hypertensives.

Oral Contraceptive Use

Estrogen-containing oral contraceptive pills are likely the most common cause of secondary hypertension in women. Most women using these contraceptives experience a slight rise in blood pressure. Approximately 5% will develop hypertension within 5 years of starting oral contraceptive use, more than twice the incidence seen among women of the same age who do not use them.[52] Although the hypertension is usually mild, it may persist after the oral contraceptive is discontinued, it can be severe, and

it is almost certainly a factor in the increased cardiovascular mortality seen among young women who take these agents.

The likelihood of women who use oral contraceptives developing hypertension is much greater among those who are over age 35, obese, or who drink large quantities of alcohol. In most women, the hypertension is mild; however, in some it may accelerate rapidly and cause severe renal damage.[53] When the pill is discontinued, in about half the cases, blood pressure falls to normal within 3 to 6 months. Whether the pill caused permanent hypertension in the other half or just uncovered primary hypertension at an earlier time is not clear.

Women given the pill should be properly monitored as follows:

- The supply should be limited initially to 3 months and thereafter to 6 months.
- They should be required to return for a blood pressure check before an additional supply is provided.
- If blood pressure has risen, an alternative contraceptive should be offered.

If the pill remains the only acceptable contraceptive method, the elevated blood pressure can be reduced with appropriate

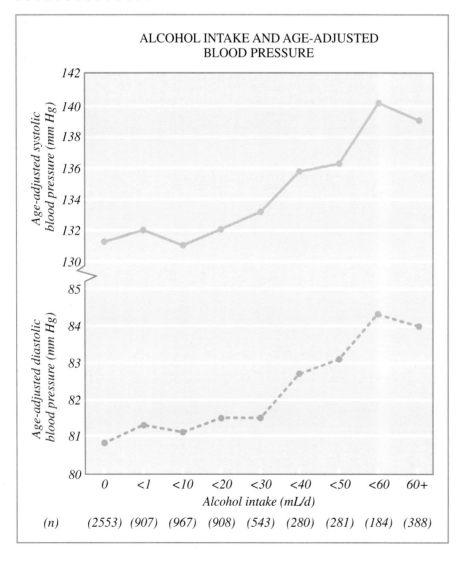

FIGURE 7.56 • Age-adjusted systolic and diastolic blood pressures by alcohol intake category. Numbers of patients for each category of alcohol intake are shown in parentheses. (Reproduced with permission. Criqui MH, Langer RD, Reed DM: *Circulation* 1989;80:609.)

therapy. In view of the probable role of aldosterone in pill-induced hypertension, use of a diuretic-spironolactone combination seems appropriate. In those who stop taking oral contraceptives, evaluation for secondary hypertensive diseases should be postponed for at least 3 months to allow remission of the renin-aldosterone changes induced by the estrogen.

Postmenopausal estrogen use does not appear to induce hypertension even though it does induce various changes in the renin-aldosterone mechanism similar to those noted with oral contraceptives. Moreover, the majority of case-control studies have shown a significantly *lower* mortality rate from coronary heart disease among postmenopausal estrogen users than nonusers.[54]

Renal Parenchymal Disease

Renal parenchymal disease is the most common cause of secondary hypertension, responsible for 2% to 5% of cases seen in unselected adult populations (refer to Table 7.9). As chronic glomerulonephritis becomes less common, hypertensive nephrosclerosis and diabetic nephropathy have become the most common causes of end-stage renal disease (ESRD). The hypertension that is usual in diabetic nephropathy contributes significantly to the progression of renal damage. The higher prevalence of hypertension among American blacks is probably responsible for their significantly higher rate of ESRD, with hypertension as the underlying cause in as many as one-half of these patients.[26]

Not only does hypertension cause renal failure and renal failure cause hypertension, but more subtle renal dysfunction may be involved in patients with primary hypertension. As discussed earlier, the kidneys may initiate the hemodynamic cascade eventuating in primary hypertension. As that disease progresses, some renal dysfunction is demonstrable in most patients. Progressive renal damage is the end result and is the cause of death in at least 10% of hypertensive individuals. Since early treatment of hypertension will likely protect against nephrosclerosis, there is hope that improved control of hypertension will slow the progression and reduce the frequency of ESRD.

In view of the increasing evidence that glomerular capillary hypertension is responsible for the progressive loss of renal function once renal damage begins[55] (Figure 7.57), aggressive reduction of intraglomerular hypertension to prevent further renal loss is being studied. Preliminary experimental evidence suggests that angiotensin converting enzyme (ACE) in-

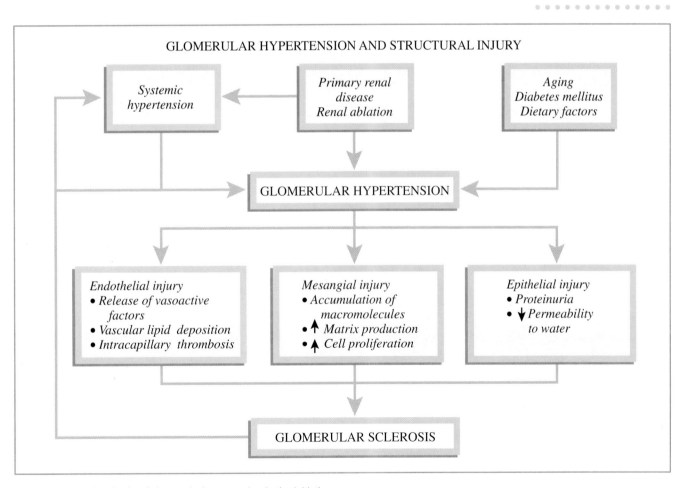

FIGURE 7.57 • Pivotal role of glomerular hypertension in the initiation and progression of structural injury. (Reproduced with permission. Anderson S, Brenner BM: *Q J Med* 1989;70:185.)

hibitors may be particularly effective in this regard.[56] However, the best long-term protection has been obtained with drugs other than ACE inhibitors[57] (Figure 7.58).

Renovascular Hypertension

No more than 1% of all adults with hypertension have renovascular hypertension (refer to Table 7.9), but the prevalence is much higher in those with sudden onset of severe hypertension and other suggestive features[58] (Table 7.16). In particular, significant renal artery stenosis was found in 23% of 118 patients with hypertension and/or renal insufficiency undergoing coronary angiography.[59]

The two major types of renovascular disease tend to appear at different times and in different sexes. Atherosclerotic disease affecting mainly the proximal third of the main renal artery is seen mostly in older men (Figure 7.59). Fibroplastic disease involving mainly the distal two thirds of the renal arteries and their branches appears most commonly in younger women (Figure 7.60). Overall, about two thirds of cases are caused by atherosclerotic disease and one third by fibroplastic disease.

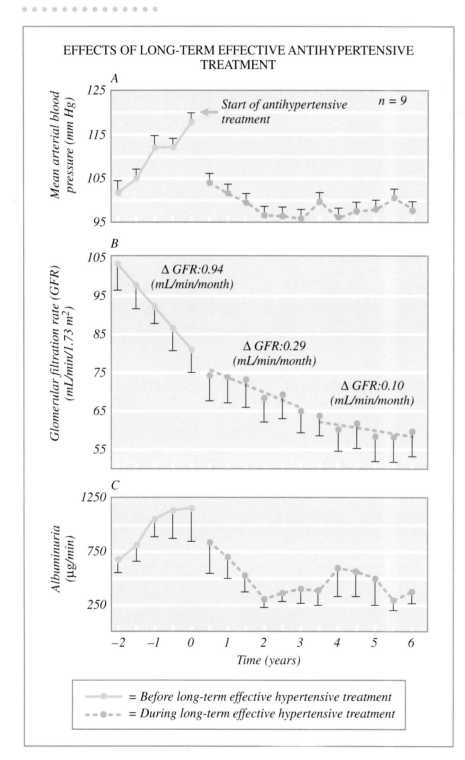

EFFECTS OF LONG-TERM EFFECTIVE ANTIHYPERTENSIVE TREATMENT

FIGURE 7.58 • Average course of mean arterial blood pressure (A), glomerular filtration rate (B), and albuminuria (C) before and during long-term effective antihypertensive treatment of nine insulin-dependent diabetic patients who had nephropathy. Therapy included furosemide, metoprolol, and hydralazine in most patients. (Reproduced with permission. Parving H-H, Andersen AR, Smidt UM, et al: *Br Med J* 1987;294:1443.)

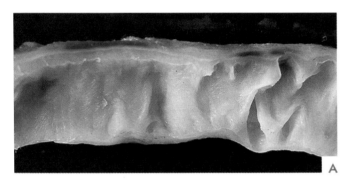

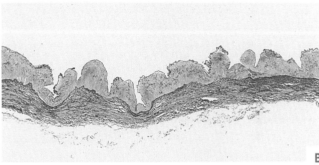

FIGURE 7.59 • Fibromuscular dysplasia of the renal artery, as seen in this specimen, is characterized by transverse, thickened, muscular ridges and localized saccular pouches with a thin wall (A). Longitudinal section through such an artery shows the distinct structural abnormality of the media (B). Fibromuscular dysplasia may be a cause of renovascular hypertension, particularly in young adults. (Reproduced with permission. Hurst JW, Anderson RH, Becker AE, et al: *Atlas of the Heart* New York, NY: Gower Medical Publishing; 1988:12.9.)

FIGURE 7.60 • Renal arteriogram in a 68-year-old male with hypertension shows a small kidney on the left and extreme narrowing of the renal artery due to atherosclerosis. (Reproduced with permission. Hurst JW, Anderson RH, Becker AE, et al: *Atlas of the Heart* New York, NY: Gower Medical Publishing; 1988:12.9.)

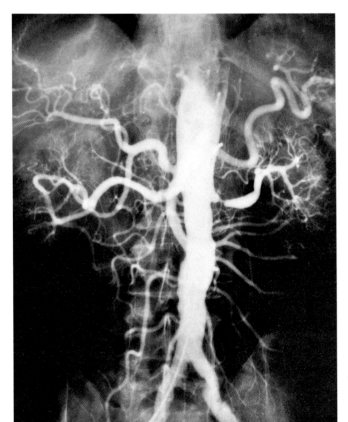

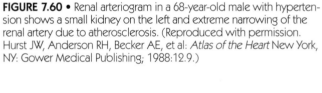

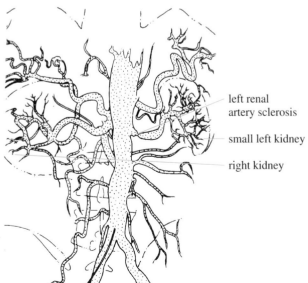

left renal artery sclerosis

small left kidney

right kidney

Renovascular disease is often bilateral, although usually one side is clearly predominant. The possibility of bilateral disease should be suspected in those with renal insufficiency, particularly if rapidly progressive oliguric renal failure develops without evidence of obstructive uropathy and, even more so, if it develops after start of ACE inhibitor therapy.[60]

The presence of the clinical features shown in Table 7.16 indicates the need for a screening test for renovascular hypertension in perhaps 10% of all hypertensive individuals. A positive screening test, or very strong clinical features, calls for more definitive confirmatory tests. Some patients have renovascular hypertension but may have none of the clinical features described in Table 7.16, clinically resembling patients with mild primary hyper-

tension. Nonetheless, these features should be used to exclude the majority of hypertensives from additional workup and to identify the 10% or so who should undergo a complete evaluation.

As shown in Figure 7.61, a reasonable initial test in people with suggestive clinical features may be isotopic renography and plasma renin measurements after an oral captopril challenge, to be followed by renal arteriography and then renal vein renin assays. The last procedure may not be needed if isotopic renography after captopril indicates significant renal ischemia in the kidney with renal artery disease revealed by arteriography.

Experience with measurement of peripheral blood renin activity (PRA) before and one hour after a single 50 mg dose of the ACE inhibitor, captopril, suggests that this approach may

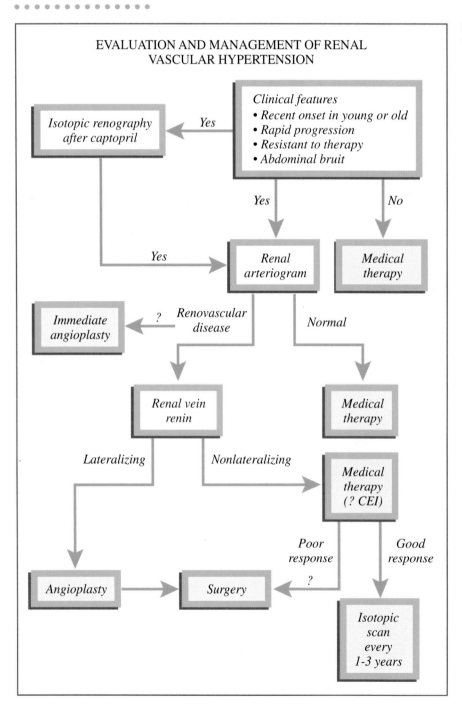

FIGURE 7.61 • The evaluation and management of renal vascular hypertension.

provide an easy, noninvasive way to establish the functional significance of a lesion, either after or preferably before arteriography[61] (Table 7.17).

A combination of isotopic renography with plasma renin measurements one hour after the oral captopril dose provides additional diagnostic information. Either labelled hippurate to measure renal blood flow, or dietheylenetriamine penta-acetic acid (DTPA) to measure the glomerular filtration rate (GFR) may be used[62] (Figures 7.62, 7.63). If the postcaptopril test shows a significant difference, the procedure should be repeated without captopril to document the ischemic origin of the differences in blood flow or GFR.

TABLE 7.17 • CRITERIA FOR THE CAPTOPRIL SCREENING TEST

Method

- The patient should maintain a normal salt intake and receive no diuretics
- If possible, all antihypertensive medications should be withdrawn 3 weeks prior to the test
- The patient should be seated for at least 30 minutes. Then, a venous blood sample is drawn to measure baseline plasma renin activity
- Captopril, 50 mg diluted in 10 mL of water immediately before the test, is administered orally
- At 60 minutes, a venous blood sample is drawn for measurement of stimulated plasma renin activity

Interpretation: A positive test requires:

- Stimulated plasma renin activity of 12 ng/mL/hr or more and
- Absolute increase in plasma renin activity of 10 mg/mL/hr or more and
- Increase in plasma renin activity of 150% or more, or 400% or more if baseline plasma renin activity is less than 3 ng/mL/hr

(Reproduced with permission. Muller FB, Sealey JE, Case DB, et al: *Am J Med* 1986;80:633

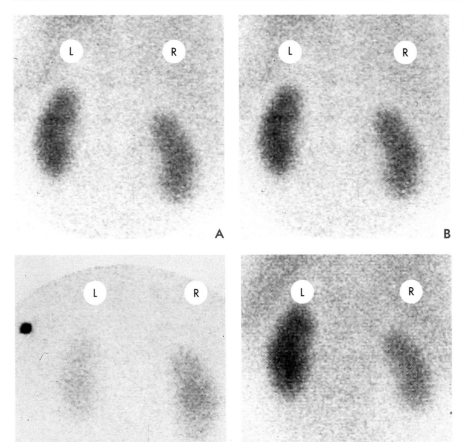

FIGURE 7.62 • ⁹⁹ᵐTc diethylenetriamine penta-acetic acid (DTPA) renal scans before (A) and 1 hr (B) after oral captopril, 25 mg. Results show that there is a marked reduction of function on the right following captopril. This indicates a significant renal artery stenosis. (Reproduced with permission. Swales JD, Sever PS, Peart S: *Clinical Atlas of Hypertension* London, England: Gower Medical Publishing; 1991:8.18.)

Since so little is known about the natural history of untreated renovascular disease, it is difficult to assess the results of therapy. Advances in medical therapy have made it easier to control the hypertension, and the availability of transluminal angioplasty offers another "curative" approach, but current evidence supports surgical repair as being more likely to provide relief of hypertension and preserve renal function.

Angiotensin-converting enzyme inhibitors may provide better control of renovascular hypertension compared to other antihypertensive medications, but these drugs may expose the already ischemic kidney to a further loss of blood flow by removing the high levels of angiotensin II that were supporting its circulation.[60] Calcium-entry blockers and other antihypertensive drugs may be almost as effective as ACE inhibitors and considerably safer.

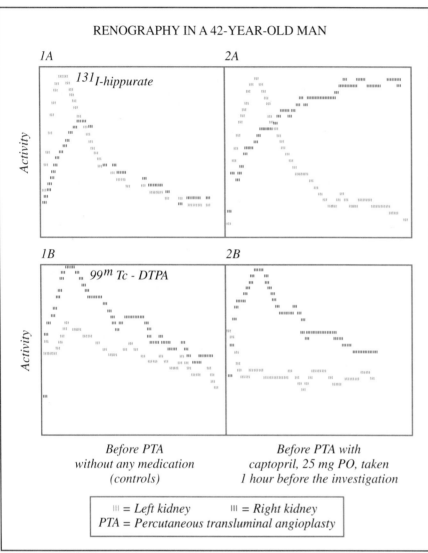

FIGURE 7.63 • Renography of a 42-year-old man with hypertension and stenosis of the left renal artery. After percutaneous transluminal angioplasty (PTA), his hypertension was cured. ^{131}I-hippurate (A) and the lower ^{99m}Tc-diethylenetriamine penta-acetic acid (DTPA) (B). Time-activity curves in two different circumstances: Before PTA without any medication—control (1), and before PTA but with 25 mg of captopril taken orally 1 hr before the investigation (2). Before PTA, captopril slowed down the excretion of [131]hippurate and reduced the uptake of ^{99m}Tc-DTPA only in the left kidney. After PTA this effect disappeared. (Reproduced with permission. Geyskes GG, Oei HY, Puylaert CBAJ, et al: *Hypertension* 1987;9:451 and the American Heart Association.)

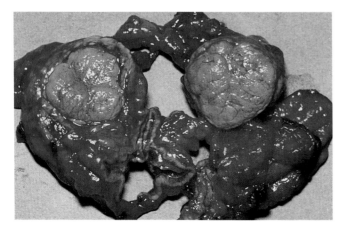

FIGURE 7.64 • An adrenal adenoma causing primary aldosteronism—Conn's syndrome. This was removed from a hypertensive patient with hypokalemia. (Reproduced with permission. Swales JD, Sever PS, Peart S: *Clinical Atlas of Hypertension* London, England: Gower Medical Publishing; 1991:5.18.)

Adrenal Causes of Hypertension

The three major adrenal causes of hypertension—primary aldosteronism (Figure 7.64), pheochromocytoma, and Cushing's syndrome—together comprise less than 1% of all hypertension (refer to Table 7.9). Primary aldosteronism will usually be suspected in patients found to be hypokalemic, particularly if this occurs spontaneously [63] (Figure 7.65).

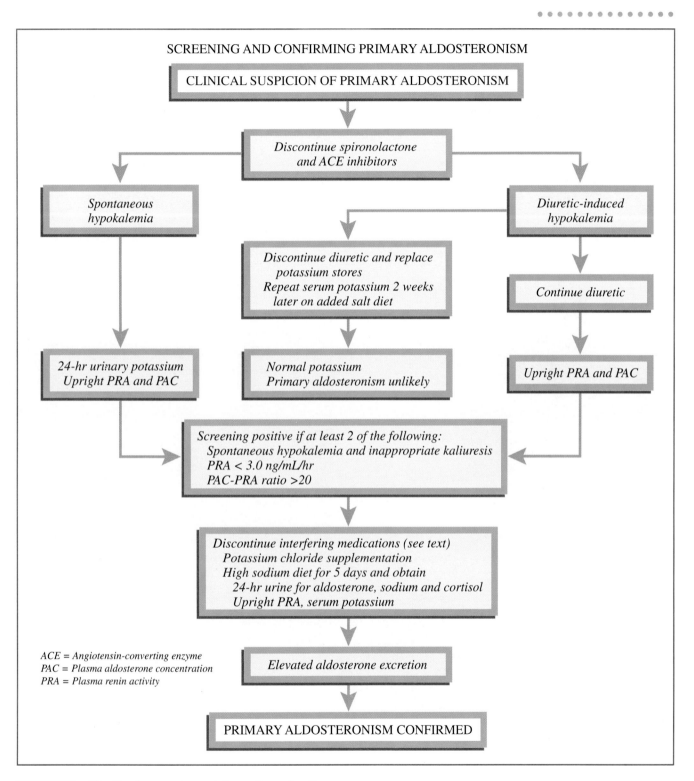

FIGURE 7.65 • Algorithm for screening and diagnostic confirmation of primary aldosteronism. (Reproduced with permission. Young WF, Hogan MJ, Klee GG, et al: *Mayo Clin Proc* 1990;65:96.)

Pheochromocytomas (Figure 7.66) should be suspected in those patients with suggestive features of episodic catecholamine discharge (Table 7.18). The diagnosis can usually be easily made by measurements of urinary catecholamine excretion, with metanephrine being most reliable and least susceptible to interference (Table 7.19). Labetalol will cause falsely elevated levels of all three urinary and blood catecholamine tests.

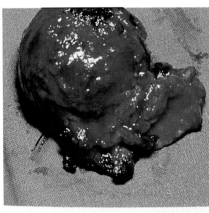

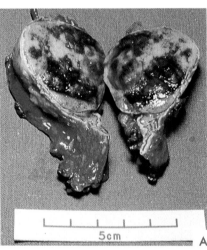

5cm

5cm

A

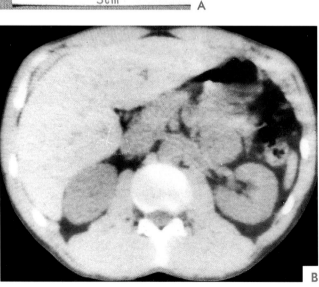

B

FIGURE 7.66 • Large hemorrhagic pheochromocytoma removed from a hypertensive patient (A). CT scan of a patient with labile hypertension and a high plasma norepinephrine level show pheochromocytoma resting on the vessels of the left kidney (B). It was subsequently removed successfully with cure. (Reproduced with permission. Swales JD, Sever PS, Peart S: *Clinical Atlas of Hypertension* London, England: Gower Medical Publishing; 1991:5.21, 8.15.)

TABLE 7.18 • FEATURES SUGGESTIVE OF PHEOCHROMOCYTOMA

Hypertension: Persistent or paroxysmal
- Markedly variable blood pressures (± orthostatic hypotension)
- Sudden paroxysms (± subsequent hypertension) in relation to:

  Stress: anesthesia, angiography, parturition

  Pharmacologic provocation: histamine, nicotine, caffeine, ß-blockers, glucocorticoids, tricyclic antidepressants
- Rare patients persistently normotensive
- Manipulation of tumors: abdominal palpation, urination
- Unusual settings

  Childhood

  Pregnancy

  Familial

  Multiple endocrine adenomas: medullary carcinoma of thyroid (MEN-2a), mucosal neuromas (MEN-2b)

  Neurocutaneous lesions: neurofibromatosis

Associated symptoms
- Sudden spells with headache, sweating, palpitations, nervousness, nausea, and vomiting
- Pain in chest or abdomen

Associated signs
- Sweating
- Tachycardia
- Arrhythmia
- Pallor
- Weight loss

Cushing's syndrome should be suspected in hypertensive patients with easy bruising, myopathy, plethora, hirsutism, red striae, and truncal obesity[64] (Figure 7.67). The workup involves steroid suppression tests[65] (Figure 7.68).

Miscellaneous Causes

Coarctation of the aorta should be evaluated by palpation of femoral pulses and measurement of blood pressure in the legs, particularly in younger patients. Reduced or absent

TABLE 7.19 • URINARY TESTS FOR PHEOCHROMOCYTOMA

	Urinary excretion (mg/d or μg/mg creatinine)		Number of patients with tumor	Patients with tumor correctly identified (%)
	Normal adults	Pheochromo-cytoma		
Free catecholamines	< 0.1	0.1 - 10.0	179	85
Metanephrine and normetanephrine	< 1.2	1.0 - 100.0	282	96
Vanillylmandelic acid	< 6.5	5 - 600	294	84

(Reproduced with permission Manu P, Runge, LA: *Am J Epidemiol* 1984;120:788.)

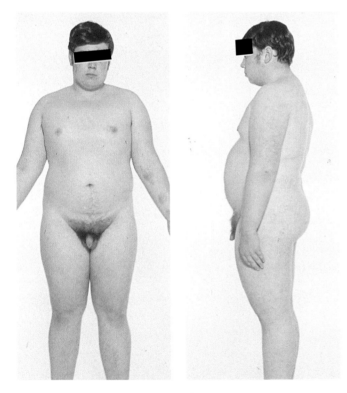

FIGURE 7.67 • A man with hypertension associated with Cushing's syndrome. Obesity is largely truncal in types with a "buffalo" hump. The face is rounded and the patient bruised readily. (Reproduced with permission. Swales JD, Sever PS, Peart S: *Clinical Atlas of Hypertension* London, England: Gower Medical Publishing; 1991:5.20.)

femoral artery pulses and a blood pressure lower in both legs than in the arms is suggestive of a coarctation of the aorta (Figure 7.69).

Hypertension may appear postoperatively for multiple reasons, including pain, excitement, hypoxia, hypercapnia, and excessive volume loads.[66] The problem has been particularly frequent immediately following coronary bypass surgery,[67] and is especially serious following cardiac transplantation. Cyclosporine is often responsible for the hypertension experienced by those undergoing this procedure.[68]

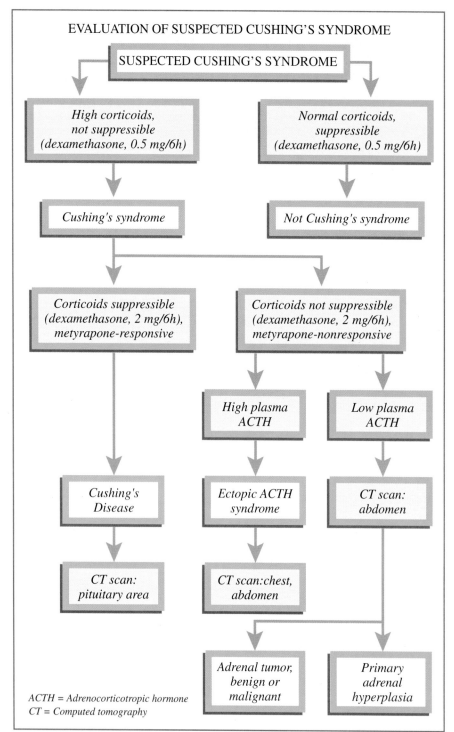

EVALUATION OF SUSPECTED CUSHING'S SYNDROME

SUSPECTED CUSHING'S SYNDROME

High corticoids, not suppressible (dexamethasone, 0.5 mg/6h)

Normal corticoids, suppressible (dexamethasone, 0.5 mg/6h)

Cushing's syndrome

Not Cushing's syndrome

Corticoids suppressible (dexamethasone, 2 mg/6h), metyrapone-responsive

Corticoids not suppressible (dexamethasone, 2 mg/6h), metyrapone-nonresponsive

High plasma ACTH

Low plasma ACTH

Cushing's Disease

Ectopic ACTH syndrome

CT scan: abdomen

CT scan: pituitary area

CT scan: chest, abdomen

Adrenal tumor, benign or malignant

Primary adrenal hyperplasia

ACTH = Adrenocorticotropic hormone
CT = Computed tomography

FIGURE 7.68 • Evaluation of patients with suspected Cushing's syndrome. Because some medications alter adrenocorticotropic hormone (ACTH) production rate, patients should be medication free before initiation of assessment. (Reproduced with permission. Carpenter PC: *Mayo Clin Proc* 1986;61:49.)

FIGURE 7.69 • Coarctation presenting as hypertension in a young woman. The ascending aorta is dilated and the collateral vessels produce a "notching" of the under surface of the ribs. (Reproduced with permission. Swales JD, Sever PS, Peart S: *Clinical Atlas of Hypertension* London, England: Gower Medical Publishing; 1991:5.20.)

GENERAL PRINCIPLES OF THERAPY

With this background, therapy of hypertension can be based upon more than empiricism. Before covering the specific modes of therapy and indicating how they may reverse the various pathogenetic mechanisms shown in Figure 7.34, more general guidelines must be drawn for the rationale of such therapy and for its most effective use.

THE RATIONALE FOR THERAPY

The number of people worldwide now being *continuously* treated for hypertension represents the largest use of long-term drug therapy in recorded history. Since most of these people have fairly mild, asymptomatic hypertension it is pertinent to examine the rationale for this massive therapeutic

exercise. In brief, this has occurred over the past few years as a result of the confluence of three events:

- Even minimally elevated pressures have been shown to increase the overall risk for premature cardiovascular disease (refer to Figure 7.13).
- Trials have shown that progression of hypertension, strokes, and, probably, heart failure can be reduced by drug therapy.
- The availability of medications that are easier to take.

The widespread use of antihypertensive therapy has been vigorously defended and credited for at least some of the reduction in coronary and stroke mortality seen in the United States since 1968 (Figure 7.70). However, the wisdom of such aggressive treatment of hypertension is now being seriously questioned for numerous reasons, including:

- Awareness that the risks of relatively mild hypertension, although apparent for the aggregate, are not shared by all.
- Inability to confirm that drug therapy has been protective

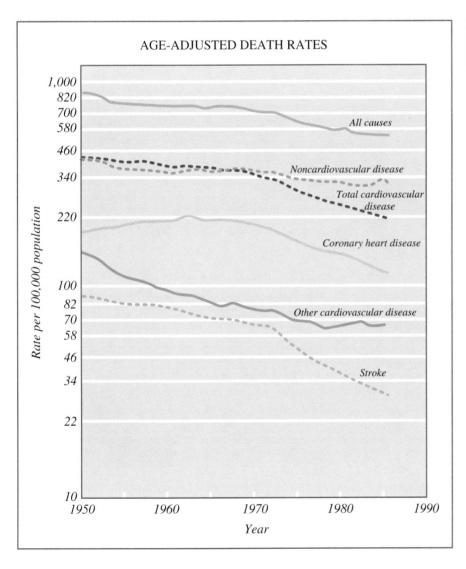

FIGURE 7.70 • Age-adjusted death rates for selected causes of death in the United States, 1950 to 1986. (Reproduced with permission. Kannel WB: *J Cardiovasc Pharmacol* 1989;13(Suppl 1):S4.)

NINE TRIALS — EFFECTS OF TREATMENT

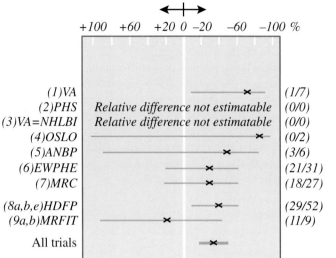
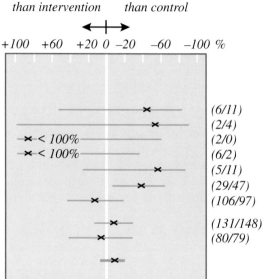

FATAL STROKE

Control better than intervention — *Intervention better than control*

+100   +60   +20   0   –20   –60   –100 %

Trial	Events
(1)VA	(1/7)
(2)PHS — *Relative difference not estimable*	(0/0)
(3)VA=NHLBI — *Relative difference not estimable*	(0/0)
(4)OSLO	(0/2)
(5)ANBP	(3/6)
(6)EWPHE	(21/31)
(7)MRC	(18/27)
(8a,b,e)HDFP	(29/52)
(9a,b)MRFIT	(11/9)
All trials	

FATAL CORONARY HEART DISEASE

Control better than intervention — *Intervention better than control*

+100   +60   +20   0   –20   –60   –100 %

Events
(6/11)
(2/4)
(2/0) < 100%
(6/2) < 100%
(5/11)
(29/47)
(106/97)
(131/148)
(80/79)

(VA) = Veterans Administration Cooperative Study Group on Antihypertensive Agents, 1970
(PHS) = US Public Health Service Hospitals Cooperative Study, 1977
(VA-NHLBI) = Veterans Administration Heart, Lung, and Blood Institute Feasibility Study, 1978
(OSLO) = Oslo Study, 1980
(ANBP) = Australian National Blood Pressure Study, 1980
(EWPHE) = European Working Party on Hypertension in the Elderly, 1985
(MRC) = British Medical Research Council Trial, 1985
(HDFP) = Hypertension Detection and Follow-up Program, 1979
(MRFIT) = Multiple Risk Factor Intervention Trial, 1982

⊢—— *95% confidence interval* ——⊣
——×——
mean

FIGURE 7.71 • Bar graph showing estimates with approximate 95% confidence intervals of the relative difference in fatal coronary heart disease (CHD) and nonfatal myocardial infarction (MI) between intervention and control groups. The numbers in parentheses are the numbers of events (intervention/control). Note that the data from the European Working Party on Hypertension in the Elderly (EWPHE) trial are reported only for total cardiac mortality. (Reproduced with permission. Cutler JA, MacMahon SW, Furberg CD: *Hypertension* 1989;13(Suppl. I):I-36.)

References (1) Veterans Administration Cooperative Study Group on Anti-hypertensive Agents: Effects of treatment on morbidity in hypertension. II. Results of patients with diastolic blood pressure averaging 90 through 114 mm Hg. *JAMA* 1970;213:1143. (2) Smith WM, for the US Public Health Service Hospitals Cooperative Study Group: Treatment of mild hypertension: Results of a ten-year intervention trial. *Circ Res* 1977;40(suppl I):I-98. (3) Perry HM, Goldman AI, Lavin MA, et al: Evaluation of drug treatment in mild hypertension: VA-NHLBI feasibility trial. *Ann NY Acad Sci* 1978;304:267. (4) Helgeland A: Treatment of mild hypertension: A five year controlled drug trial. *Am J Med* 1980;69:725. (5) Report by the Management Committee: The Australian therapeutic trial in mild tension. *Lancet* 1980;1:1261. (6) Amery A, Birkenhager W, Brixko P, et al: Mortality and morbidity results from the European Working Party on high blood pressure in the elderly trial. *Lancet* 1985;1:1349. (7) Medical Research Council Working Party: MRC trial of treatment of mild hypertension: Principal results. *Br Med J* 1985;291:97. (8a) Hypertension Detection and

Follow-up Program Cooperative Group: Five-year findings of the Hypertension Detection and Follow-up Program. I. Reduction in mortality of persons with high blood pressure, including mild tension. *JAMA* 1979;242:2562. (8b) Hypertension Detection and Follow-up Program Cooperative Group: Five-year findings of the Hypertension Detection and Follow-up Program. III. Reduction in stroke incidence among other persons with high blood pressure. *JAMA* 1982;247:633-638. (9a) Hypertension Detection and Follow-up Program Cooperative Group: Five-year findings of the Hypertension Detection and Follow-up Program. V. Effects of stepped care treatment on the incidence of myocardial infarction and angina pectoris. *Hypertension* 1984;6(suppl I):I-198. (9b) Multiple Risk Factor Intervention Trial Research Group: Multiple Risk Factor Intervention Trial: Risk factor changes and mortality results. *JAMA* 1982;248:1465. (9c) Multiple Risk Factor Intervention Trial Research Group: Coronary heart disease death, nonfatal acute myocardial infarction and other clinical outcomes in the Multiple Risk Factor Intervention Trial. *Am J Cardiol* 1986;58:1.

against coronary mortality in nine clinical trials involving more than 41,000 patients[69] (Figure 7.71). This has raised concerns about the drugs used in these trials inducing biochemical changes that may increase risk by lowering potassium, raising lipids, or altering glucose tolerance.

- Concerns about the adverse effects of therapy, not only biochemical markers but the quality of life and, more dramatically, the potential for too great a reduction in blood pressure to lead to additional coronary ischemia.[18]
- Recognition by cost/benefit analysis that the financial cost is much larger than anticipated to protect the relatively few who benefit.[70]

RESULTS OF CLINICAL TRIALS

The failure to find clear protection against coronary disease by reduction of the blood pressure in the nine controlled clinical trials, which compared active therapy with placebo (refer to Figure 7.71), may not reflect a failure of the therapy, but a misguided attempt. In two of the larger trials, the Hypertension Detection and Follow-up Program (HDFP)[71] and Multiple Risk Factor Intervention Trial (MRFIT)[72], a greater reduction of the blood pressure did protect some of the participants (Table 7.20). Therapy was given to all patients, but more to one half than the other half. In both of these large trials, the patients who had normal elec-

trocardiograms at entry were protected by more intensive therapy, whereas those with abnormal entry electrocardiograms suffered higher coronary mortality with more therapy. These data fit with those from other less well-controlled studies which have shown a hazard for increasing coronary ischemia when pressures are lowered below a critical level—a J-curve with a threshold of 85 to 90 mm Hg diastolic.[18] In light of the potential importance of the J-curve, particularly in hypertensives with pre-existing coronary disease, it will be more thoroughly described when the goal of therapy is considered.

Since a diuretic, often given in relatively high doses, was the first, and often the only drug administered in all the trials, except for half of the treated patients in the Medical Research Council (MRC) trial,[73] the presence of diuretic-induced biochemical derangements may explain the lack of coronary protection. A different approach, specifically the use of a ß-blocker as first drug, was used in the other half of the treated patients in the MRC trial. Beta-blockers also failed to provide overall protection against coronary disease, other than in those men who did not smoke. In two other trials, the International Prospective Primary Prevention Study in Hypertension (IPPPSH)[74] and the Heart Attack Primary Prevention in Hypertension (HAPPHY),[75] ß-blockers were compared against diuretics, and they too failed to demonstrate any clear advantage

TABLE 7.20 • CORONARY MORTALITY RATES PER 1,000 PERSON-YEARS IN PATIENTS WITH OR WITHOUT ECG ABNORMALITIES AT ENTRY

Trial	Number of subjects	Coronary hear disease rate/1,000 person-years		
		Less therapy	More therapy	Difference (%)
HDFP, 1984				
Normal ECG	3210	3.1	2.0	–35
Abnormal ECG	1963	3.5	4.3	+23
MRFIT, 1985				
Normal ECG	5593	3.4	2.6	–24
Abnormal ECG	2418	2.9	4.9	+70

The HDPF (Hypertension and Follow-up Program) patients consisted of men with diastolic blood pressure of between 90 and 104 mm Hg not on antihypertensive therapy at baseline, who were similar to the MRFIT (Multiple Risk Factor Intervention Trial) population.

of either drug[76] (Figure 7.72). Unfortunately, there are no data on coronary protection with any other drugs than diuretics and ß-blockers but, as we shall see, there is a strong likelihood that they will be more protective.

GUIDELINES FOR TREATMENT

Current evidence supports the view that the risks of mild hypertension are not so great as to warrant active therapy for all cases. A more aggressive course could be justified if there were no risks or problems associated with active therapy. However, in all trials, 20% to 40% of patients given drug therapy experienced some adverse effects, seldom life-threatening but often enough to interfere with the quality of life.[77]

In view of the legitimate concerns arising from the evidence now available, a reconsideration of the common practice of treating all patients with any degree of blood pressure elevation seems appropriate. The need for active drug therapy for those with moderate or severe hypertension—diastolic

blood pressure above 105 mm Hg—is incontrovertible. Nonetheless, there is a need to insure that their pressure is persistently elevated. Even among the patients enrolled in the Australian Therapeutic Trial, whose diastolic blood pressure was between 105 and 109 mm Hg after two sets of readings 4 weeks apart, 11% of those given only placebo pills had diastolic blood pressure persistently below 90 mm Hg for the next 4 years[78] (Figure 7.73). Their blood pressure fell mostly during the first 4 months. Therefore, unless there is an obvious need for more immediate institution of drug therapy, such as progressive target organ damage or blood pressures so high as to present immediate danger, all patients should be allowed to achieve a spontaneous reduction of initially high pressures over at least a 3 to 4 month interval. During that time, they should have their pressure carefully monitored. If pressures increase, as in the 10% to 15% of the placebo-treated patients in the various trials shown in Figure 7.71, immediate institution of drug therapy may be indicated.

• • • • • • • • • • • • • • •

MAIN TRIALS COMPARING PREDOMINANTLY DIURETIC-BASED THERAPY WITH PREDOMINANTLY β-BLOCKER-BASED THERAPY

| | Number of events | | Odd ratios and confidence limits |
Endpoint and trial	Diuretic based therapy	β-blocker-based therapy	
Stroke			
MRC	18/4297	42/4403	
IPPPSH	46/3172	45/3185	
HAPPHY	41/3272	32/3297	
All stroke:	105/10741	119/10885	0.89 Sd 0.13
Coronary heart disease			
MRC	119/4297	103/4403	
IPPPSH	74/3172	61/3185	
HAPPHY	116/3272	132/3297	
All coronary heart disease	309/10741	296/10885	1.06 Sd 0.08
Vascular death			
MRC	69/4297	65/4403	
IPPPSH	56/3172	45/3185	
HAPPHY	60/3272	57/3297	
All vascular death:	185/10741	167/10885	1.12 Sd 0.11

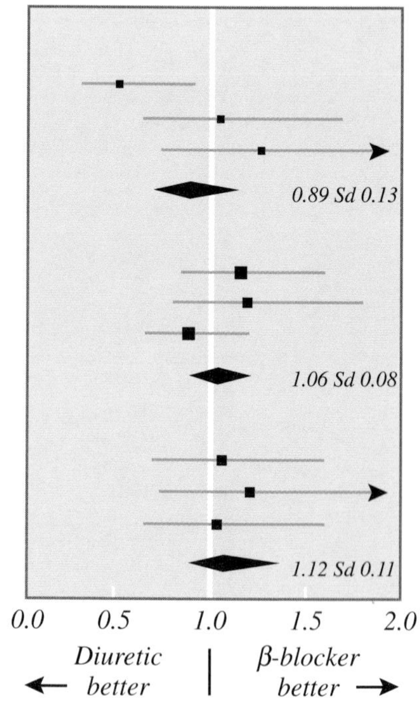

MRC = British Medical Research Council Trial
IPPPSH = International Primary Prevention Study in Hypertension
HAPPHY = Heart Attack Primary Prevention in Hypertension

FIGURE 7.72 • Effects on stroke, coronary heart disease, and vascular death in the the large randomized trials comparing predominantly diuretic-based therapy with predominantly ß-blocker-based therapy. In the Medical Research Council (MRC) trial, diastolic blood pressure was an average of 1 mm Hg lower in the diuretic group, while in IPPPSH and Heart Attack Primary Prevention in Hypertension (HAPPHY), diastolic blood pressure was 1 mm Hg lower in the ß-blocker group. (Reproduced with permission. Collins R, Peto R, MacMahon S, et al: *Lancet* 1990;335:827.)

Monitoring of the blood pressure can be done at home. For some patients, ambulatory 24-hr monitoring may provide, in a condensed manner, better prognostic evidence than multiple blood pressure measurements taken in the office. While the blood pressure is being monitored, appropriate nondrug therapies may help lower the pressure even more, without risk and with relatively little inconvenience. Such nondrug therapies may not only lower the blood pressure, but also reduce overall cardiovascular risk by relief of such conditions as hyperlipidemia, glucose intolerance, and alcohol abuse.

The Level of Blood Pressure to Treat

Successful reduction of elevated blood pressure will protect against progression of hypertension, stroke, and probably, congestive heart failure and renal damage. Therefore, drug therapy is indicated in all with diastolic blood pressure persistently above 100 mm Hg, in many with diastolic blood pressure above 95 mm Hg, and in some with diastolic blood pressure above 90 mm Hg or an even lower level, as noted in Figure 7.14.

Recall that the risks associated with elevations of systolic pressure have been shown to be equally strong and even more lin-

ear than seen with elevations of diastolic pressure. Most trials have mainly considered diastolic blood pressure levels, so that there is less evidence concerning the levels of systolic blood pressure that mandate therapy. This is particularly true among the large segment of elderly people with predominant or pure systolic hypertension. Results of the Systolic Hypertension in the Elderly Program (SHEP) document protection against strokes, coronary events, and congestive heart failure by gentle reduction of systolic pressures with small doses of diuretics and ß-blockers[79]. Therefore, elevations of systolic pressure above 170 mm Hg, at any age, deserve gradual reduction by appropriate nondrug and drug therapies. As for the elderly with both systolic and diastolic elevations, the data are quite similar as for middle-aged subjects, with excellent protection against strokes but only suggestive evidence against CHD (Figure 7.74).

Rationale for Use of Different Levels

The benefit of treating all patients with persistent diastolic blood pressure above 100 mm Hg seems well established on the basis of the clinical trials shown in Figure 7.71. The evidence for benefit of those with diastolic blood pressure

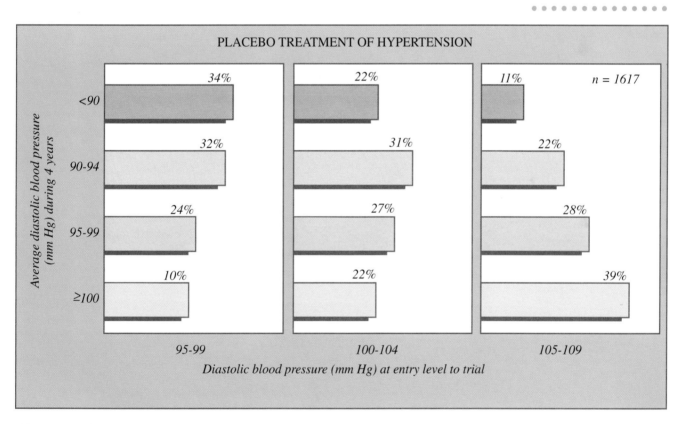

FIGURE 7.73 • The average diastolic blood pressure over 4 years in the 1617 hypertensive patients treated without drugs in the Australian Therapeutic Trial. Note that the majority of those with initial diastolic blood pressure from 95 mm Hg all the way up to 109 mm Hg ended with diastolic blood pressure below 100 mm Hg and that excess complications were noted only in those whose end diastolic blood pressure was above 100 mm Hg. (Composed from data in Management Committee: *Lancet* 1980;1:1261.)

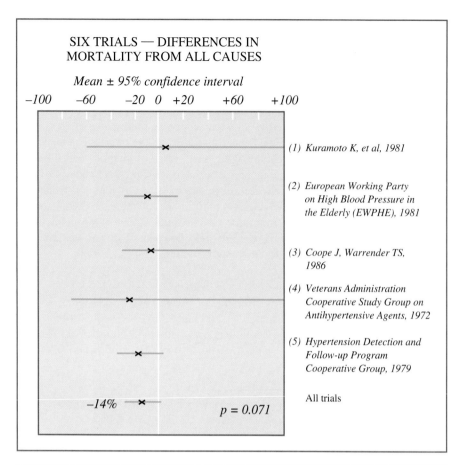

SIX TRIALS — DIFFERENCES IN MORTALITY FROM ALL CAUSES

Mean ± 95% confidence interval

−100   −60   −20 0 +20   +60   +100

(1) *Kuramoto K, et al, 1981*

(2) *European Working Party on High Blood Pressure in the Elderly (EWPHE), 1981*

(3) *Coope J, Warrender TS, 1986*

(4) *Veterans Administration Cooperative Study Group on Antihypertensive Agents, 1972*

(5) *Hypertension Detection and Follow-up Program Cooperative Group, 1979*

All trials

−14%   *p = 0.071*

FIGURE 7.74 • Differences in mortality from all causes between the actively treated group and the control group, in different trials of patients over age 60 with diastolic hypertension. For each trial, the difference and the 95% confidence limits are illustrated. A negative sign means a decrease in events in the actively treated group compared with the control group. None of these trials showed a statistically significant reduction, nor when the data from all trials were combined. (Reproduced with permission. Staessen J, Fagard R, Van Hoof R, et al: J Cardiovasc Pharmacol 1988a;12(Suppl 8):S33.)

References (1) Kuramoto K, Matsushita S, Kuwajima I, et al: Prospective study on the treatment of mild hypertension in the aged. *Jpn Heart J* 1981;22:75. (2) Sprackling ME, Mitchell JRA, Short AH, et al: Blood pressure reduction in the elderly: A randomized controlled trial of methyldopa. *Br Med J* 1981;283:1151. (3) Coope J, Warrender TS: Randomized trial of treatment of hypertension in elderly patients in primary care. *Br Med J* 1986;293:1145. (4) Veterans Administration Cooperative Study Group on Antihypertensive Agents. Effects of treatment on morbidity in hypertension. *Circulation* 1972;45:991. (5) Hypertension Detection and Follow-up Program Cooperative Group. Five-year findings of the Hypertension Detection and Follow-up Program. *JAMA* 1979;242:2562.

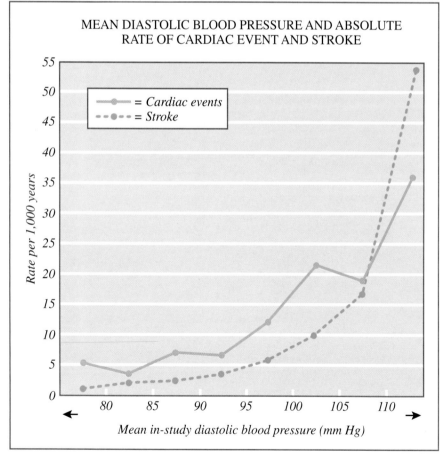

MEAN DIASTOLIC BLOOD PRESSURE AND ABSOLUTE RATE OF CARDIAC EVENT AND STROKE

Rate per 1,000 years

= *Cardiac events*
= *Stroke*

Mean in-study diastolic blood pressure (mm Hg)

FIGURE 7.75 • Absolute rate of cardiac events and stroke related to diastolic blood pressure during antihypertensive treatment. The extremes of the diastolic pressure scale include all values at or below 80 and above 110 mm Hg. (Reproduced with permission. IPPPSH Collaborative Group: *J Hypertens* 1985;3:388.)

above 95 mm Hg is less certain but reasonably strong (Figure 7.75). These curves from the IPPPSH trial[74] show progressive falls in both cardiac events and stroke when blood pressures were reduced from above 110 to below 95 mm Hg. Below 95 mm Hg, no significant falls in the already quite low event rates were observed. Similar protection in those whose initial readings were above 95 mm Hg was demonstrated in the Australian[78] and the MRC[73] trials.

Those with diastolic blood pressures between 90 and 95 mm Hg, who constitute 40% of the entire hypertensive population, have not been found to benefit from drug therapy in the controlled trials (refer to Figure 7.71). Part of this may reflect the finding that many of the patients in these trials were not, in fact, hypertensive since none of the trials required more than a 2-month run-in period before randomization to active or placebo therapy. It has been shown that as many as one third to one half of patients with diastolic blood pressures above 95 mm Hg will be persistently below 90 mm Hg after 4 to 6 months on no therapy.

Moreover, the risks are relatively small at such low levels of elevated blood pressure, and the trials, despite their size and duration, may not have been adequate to show protection with so little pre-existing risk. Moreover, the trials mainly involved low-risk, otherwise healthy patients, unlike many seen in clinical practice. In the HDFP trial,[71] those patients with initial diastolic blood pressures between 90 and 95 mm Hg whose pressures were lowered more aggressively (the stepped-care group) had fewer cardiovascular events than did those whose pressures were lowered less. However, the more intensively treated **special intervention** half of the patients in MRFIT whose initial diastolic blood pressures were between 90 and 94 mm Hg had a higher total and coronary death rate than did those given less therapy or what was termed **usual care**. The evidence from these two large non-placebo-controlled trials done in the United States remains contradictory.

In hopes of documenting further the benefits of antihypertensive therapy for the millions with mild to moderate hypertension, additional analysis of the subsequent mortality among MRFIT participants[80] and meta-analysis of trials involving more severe hypertensives[76] have been performed. Unfortunately, they shed little light on the issue of coronary protection for mild-moderate hypertension. In particular, the meta-analysis by Collins et al[76] may be misleading since unlike other meta-analyses, such as the one performed by Cutler et al,[69] they include data from patients with severe hypertension—diastolic blood pressure above 115 mm Hg. Their analysis showed statistically impressive reductions in overall CHD morbidity (Figure 7.76) but, despite inclusion of data from severe hypertensives, overall CHD mortality remained insignificantly reduced and was less than half that expected from the degree of blood pressure reduction achieved in the trials.

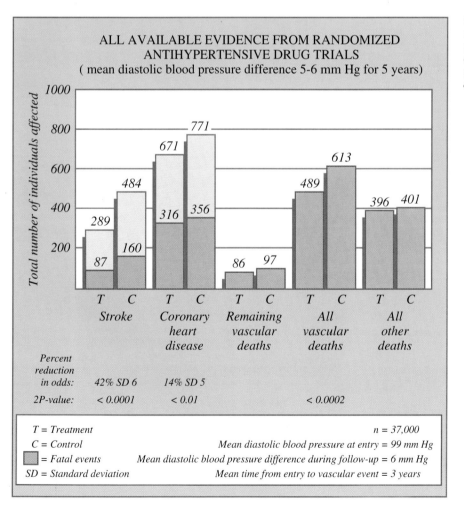

ALL AVAILABLE EVIDENCE FROM RANDOMIZED ANTIHYPERTENSIVE DRUG TRIALS
(mean diastolic blood pressure difference 5-6 mm Hg for 5 years)

T = Treatment
C = Control
= Fatal events
SD = Standard deviation

n = 37,000
Mean diastolic blood pressure at entry = 99 mm Hg
Mean diastolic blood pressure difference during follow-up = 6 mm Hg
Mean time from entry to vascular event = 3 years

FIGURE 7.76 • Combined results of the 14 unconfounded randomized trials of antihypertensive drug therapy in patients with all degrees of hypertension. (Reproduced with permission. Collins R, Peto R, MacMahon S, et al: *Lancet* 1990;335:827.)

There is, then, legitimate cause for the disagreement among the experts as to at what level to institute active drug therapy. Some believe that drug therapy should be given to all individuals with diastolic blood pressures above 90 mm Hg, while others believe that it should be given only to those with a diastolic blood pressure above 100 mm Hg. The disagreement is not only of academic interest. As many as 40 million persons in the United States alone are in the 90 to 100 mm Hg range. Thus, the issue has great clinical relevance.

Based on available data, the position adopted by a conference sponsored by the World Health Organization and the International Society of Hypertension seems an appropriate compromise (refer to Figure 7.14). It states that, after 3 to 6 months of observation, a diastolic blood pressure of 95 mm Hg should be used as the level for instituting drug therapy. Some patients at high overall risk should probably be treated even if they have lower diastolic blood pressures. Included in this group are diabetics who have early evidence of glomerulosclerosis that will surely progress if untreated. For such patients, active drug therapy may be indicated at diastolic blood pressure levels even below 90 mm Hg. More clinical trials are needed among such patients, but those at high risk may need the potential benefits from a lower blood pressure, despite the risks attendant to the therapy. On the other hand, women with relatively lower risk at every level of pressure may be less in need of therapy than are men. The level for instituting therapy in most women may appropriately be a diastolic blood pressure of 100 mm Hg, rather than the level of 95 mm Hg for most men.

Although it has not been possible to predict with certainty which patients will develop complications, the larger the number of other cardiovascular risk factors present, the larger the number of complications observed, and the greater the potential for protection by amelioration of other risks as well. The importance of cessation of cigarette smoking has been particularly

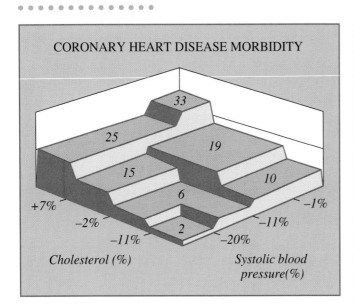

CORONARY HEART DISEASE MORBIDITY

FIGURE 7.77 • Coronary heart disease morbidity during the 4th to 12th year of antihypertensive treatment in relationship to relative change during initial 4 years of follow-up of both systolic blood pressure and serum cholesterol levels divided into quartiles. Rates adjusted for risk at entry. (Reproduced with permission. Samuelsson O, Wilhelmsen L, Andersson OK, et al: *JAMA* 1989;258:1768 and American Medical Association.)

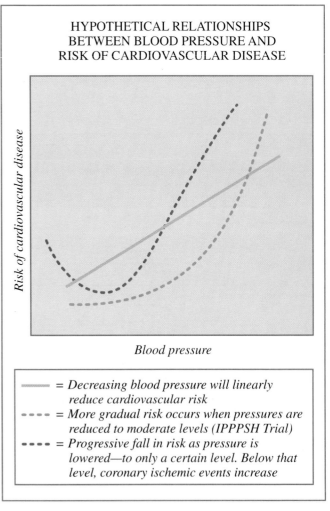

HYPOTHETICAL RELATIONSHIPS BETWEEN BLOOD PRESSURE AND RISK OF CARDIOVASCULAR DISEASE

= *Decreasing blood pressure will linearly reduce cardiovascular risk*

= *More gradual risk occurs when pressures are reduced to moderate levels (IPPPSH Trial)*

= *Progressive fall in risk as pressure is lowered—to only a certain level. Below that level, coronary ischemic events increase*

FIGURE 7.78 • Three models representing hypothetical relationships between levels of blood pressure and risk of cardiovascular disease. (Reproduced with permission. Epstein FH: Proceedings of the XVth International Congress of Therapeutics, September 5-9, 1979. Brussels: *Excerpta Medica*, 1980.)

emphasized.[73] Similarly, reduction of serum cholesterol along with reduction of the blood pressure has been shown to provide more protection against CHD than either alone[81] (Figure 7.77).

The Goal of Therapy

Having decided to treat, the clinician must consider the goal of therapy. Until recently, most assumed that the effects of blood pressure reduction on cardiovascular risk would fit a straight line downward (refer to solid line in Figure 7.78).[82] However, data from large trials indicate a more gradual decline in risk when pressures are reduced to moderate levels (refer to lighter dotted line in Figure 7.78), which was approximately 95 mm Hg in the IPPPSH trial (refer to Figure 7.75). Subsequently, Cruickshank[18] has called attention to a J-curve (refer to darker dotted line in Figure 7.78), reflecting a progressive fall in risk as pressure is lowered, but only to a certain level. Below that level, the risk for coronary ischemic events increases. Cruick-

shank added data of his own to that of five other studies, all indicating a rise in coronary events when treatment reduced diastolic blood pressure levels below a J-point that was usually between 85 and 90 mm Hg (Figure 7.79). More recently, Alderman et al[83] have provided additional confirmation—a rise in coronary events when diastolic blood pressure is lowered, on average, to below 85 mm Hg. The data from the HDFP and MRFIT studies (refer to Table 7.20) shows higher coronary mortality rates among patients with baseline ECG abnormalities if they are given more intensive therapy. The apparent propensity to induce coronary ischemia when pressures are lowered below a certain critical threshold may not apply to other vital organs. Therefore, maximal protection against stroke or renal damage may require greater falls in pressure than the coronary circulation can safely tolerate. Moreover, the problem may not occur with antihypertensive drugs, unlike diuretics and ß-blockers, that dilate the coronary vessels.

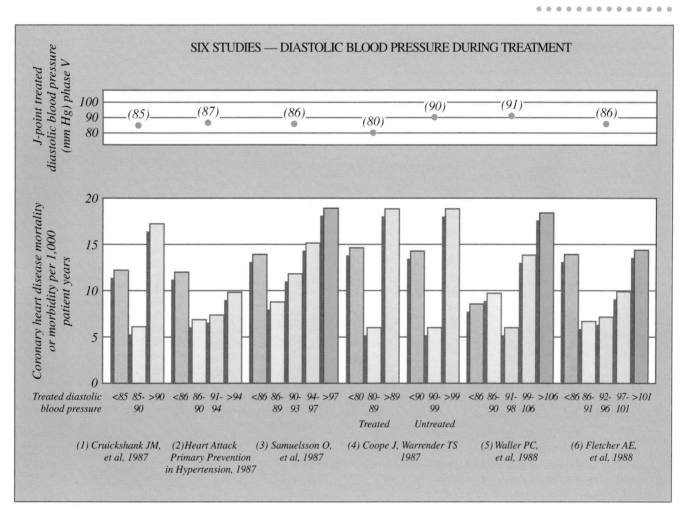

FIGURE 7.79 • Relation of diastolic blood pressure (phase V) during treatment to mortality or morbidity from coronary heart disease. The six studies included 14,536 patients. Information from the Heart Attack Primary Prevention in Hypertension (HAPPHY) trial is by personal communication—Wilhelmsen L. (Reproduced with permission. Cruickshank JM: *Br Med* J 1988;297:1227.)

References (1) Cruickshank JM, Thorp JM, Zacharias FJ: Benefits and potential harm of lowering high blood pressure. *Lancet* 1987;1:581. (2) Wilhelmsen L, Berglund G, Elmfeldt D, et al: Beta-blockers versus diuretics in hypertensive men: Main results from the HAPPHY trial. *J Hypertension* 1987;5:561. (3) Samuelsson O, Wilhelmsen L, Andersson OK, et al: Cardiovascular morbidity in relation to change in blood pressure and serum cholesterol levels in treated hypertension: Results from the primary prevention trial in Goteborg, Sweden. *JAMA* 1987; 258:1768. (4) Coope J, Warrender TS: Randomised trial of treatment of hypertension in elderly patients in primary care. *Br Med J* 1986; 293:1145. (5) Waller PC, Isles CG, Lever AF, et al: Does therapeutic reduction of diastolic blood pressure cause death from coronary heart disease? *J Human Hypertension* 1988;2:7. (6) Fletcher AE, Beevers DG, Bulpitt CJ, et al: The relationship between a low treated blood pressure and IHD mortality: A report from the DHSS hypertension care computing project (DHCCP). *J Human Hypertension* 1988;2:11.

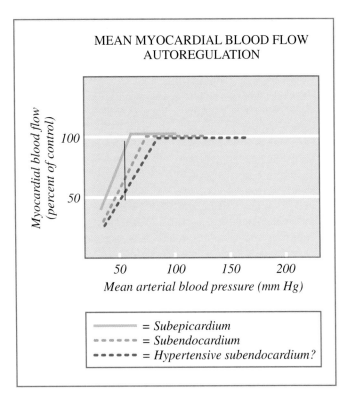

MEAN MYOCARDIAL BLOOD FLOW
AUTOREGULATION

Myocardial blood flow (percent of control)

100

50

50   100   150   200

Mean arterial blood pressure (mm Hg)

——————— = Subepicardium
- - - - - - = Subendocardium
•----•----• = Hypertensive subendocardium?

FIGURE 7.80 • Mean myocardial blood flow autoregulation curves are shown for subepicardium and corresponding subendocardial layers of the left ventricle in canine hearts, modified from Haunso. The autoregulatory curve of subendocardial blood flow in hypertensive hearts is suggested. During low arterial pressure (vertical line), when autoregulation is exhausted in both myocardial layers, subendocardial blood flow is lower than in the more superficial layers of the left ventricle. Note that the fall in myocardial blood flow is abrupt and marked when systemic pressure is reduced below the lower limit of autoregulation. (Reproduced with permission. Strandgaard S, Haunso S: *Lancet* 1987;2:658.)

TABLE 7.21 • 5-YEAR INCIDENCE OF HYPERTENSION IN 201 YOUNG MEN AND WOMEN WITH BASELINE BLOOD PRESSURE AVERAGING 122/82 MM HG

	Weight (kg)	Urinary sodium (mmol/d)	Alcohol intake (g/d)	Incidence of hypertension (Diastolic blood pressure > 90 mm Hg)
Intervention	−2.0	−41	−9.9	9/102 (8.8%)
Monitor only	+0.8	−11	−7.7	19/99 (19.2%)

(Reproduced with permission. Stamler R, Stamler J, Gosch FC, et al: *JAMA* 1989;262:1801.)

TABLE 7.22 • DIET VERSUS DRUGS IN OBESE HYPERTENSIVES

Patient population:
• 61 men
• Average age = 54
• Average BMI = 31
• Average blood pressure = 154/97 mm Hg

Diet:
• A decrease of 500 kcal/d induced a 7.6 kg weight loss
• A decrease of 42 mmol Na⁺/d led to an average sodium excretion of 127 mmol/d

Drug:
• Atenolol, 50-100 mg qd plus diuretic or calcium channel blocker prn

Results:	Blood pressure	Diastolic blood pressure < 90 mm Hg	Cholesterol	High Density Lipoprotein-Cholesterol
Diet	4/3	9/31	−13 mg/dL	+4 mg/dL
Drug	−16/11	22/30	+2 mg/dL	−5 mg/dL

(Reproduced with permission. Berglund A, Andersson OK, Berglund G, et al: *Med J Br* 1989;299:480.)

The special vulnerability of the coronary circulation when the blood pressure is lowered in patients with hypertension may have multiple explanations, including:

- The myocardium is usually hypertrophied, requiring even more nutrients.
- Oxygen delivery to the myocardium is near maximal even in nonhypertrophied hearts so that little more can be extracted when perfusion pressure is lowered.
- Coronary arteries do not autoregulate as well as cerebral arteries, particularly if they are sclerotic[84] (Figure 7.80).
- Coronary vascular reserve is limited, so that a fall in perfusion pressure may not be tolerated.[85]

Having achieved good control, it may be possible to reduce or withdraw drug therapy. Perhaps, one fourth of patients with initially mild hypertension who achieve good control with therapy will remain normotensive for at least 1 year after their therapy is discontinued.[86] Such patients need to remain under observation.

From this evidence, it is clear that there is no single answer to the questions of whom to treat with drugs for mild hypertension and how low the pressure should be reduced. Each patient must be considered separately, taking various factors into account. The foregoing discussion should indicate the wisdom of withholding drug therapy from many of these patients, at least until the effects of time and nondrug therapies have been given a chance, and to avoid too fast and too great falls in blood pressure.

NONDRUG THERAPY

As larger numbers of patients with mild hypertension are being identified and the importance of reducing other cardiovascular risks is appreciated, awareness of the value of nondrug therapies is increasing.

Data from long-term controlled studies of multifaceted nondrug therapy document a relatively small but significant reduction in blood pressure both in normotensives who are especially prone to develop hypertension[87,88] (Table 7.21) and in hypertensive individuals whose therapy has been discontinued.[89,90] Of equal, if not greater, benefit is the concomitant reduction in other risk factors even if the pressure fall is less than provided by drug therapy[91] (Table 7.22).

All hypertensive patients should benefit from mild restriction of dietary salt, reduction of excess body weight, and moderation of alcohol intake. Although high blood lipid levels and cigarette smoking may have little direct effect on blood pressure, patients with hypertension should be encouraged to eliminate risk factors that predispose to cardiovascular disease. This is particularly necessary due to a significantly higher prevalence of dyslipidemia in hypertensive individuals, a problem which may be further aggravated by therapy (Figure 7.81). Evidence for the effectiveness of individual nondrug therapies will now be considered (Table 7.23).

• • • • • • • • • • • • • • • •

FIGURE 7.81 • Serum cholesterol (mg/dL and mmol/L) in relation to diastolic blood pressure in three age groups of healthy men. (Reproduced with permission. Hjermann I, Helgeland A, Holme I, et al: *J Epidemiol Comm Health* 1978;32:117.)

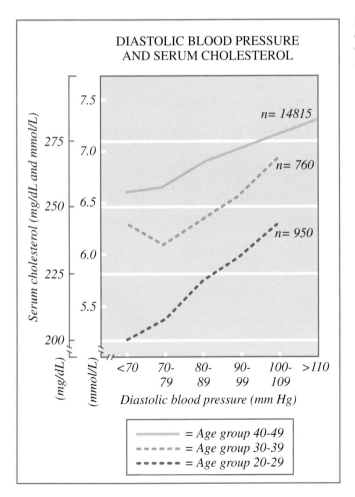

DIASTOLIC BLOOD PRESSURE AND SERUM CHOLESTEROL

n= 14815
n= 760
n= 950

Serum cholesterol (mg/dL and mmol/L)

Diastolic blood pressure (mm Hg)

——— = Age group 40-49
- - - - - = Age group 30-39
- - - - - = Age group 20-29

WEIGHT REDUCTION

In most published studies, weight loss has been shown to reduce blood pressure[92] (Figure 7.82). In this review of adequately controlled intervention studies published through 1985, a 1.0 kg decrease in body weight was accompanied by an average reduction of 1.6/1.3 mm Hg in blood pressure. Weight loss may reduce the sensitivity of blood pressure to sodium[93] further improving the response to nondrug therapy. Although the rate of recidivism among obese people may be high, an attempt at weight reduction in all obese hypertensive patients should be made, using whatever level of caloric restriction the patient is able to maintain.

DIETARY SODIUM RESTRICTION

Modest salt restriction may help lower the blood pressure. In Staessen et al[92] review of 24 intervention studies, an average reduction in sodium intake of 100 mmol per day decreased blood pressure 5.4/6.5 mm Hg (Figure 7.83). In a controlled study, the fall in blood pressure was shown to be greater at a daily sodium intake of 50 mmol/d than at 100 mmol/d.[94] However, not all hypertensive people will respond to a moderate degree of sodium restriction from 70 to 100 mmol/d or 2 g/d. Blacks tend to be more sodium sensitive, and elderly patients may be particularly responsive to sodium restriction, perhaps because of their usually lower renin responsiveness.

Although there is no assurance that moderate sodium restriction will help, there is no evidence that it will hurt. For examples, neither the intake of other vital nutrients nor exercise tolerance in a hot environment is reduced by a lower sodium intake. Therefore, moderate sodium restriction should be useful for all persons, as a preventive measure in those who are normotensive and, more certainly, as partial therapy in those who are hypertensive. The easiest way to accomplish such moderate sodium restriction is to substitute natural foods low in sodium and high in potassium for processed foods, which have sodium added and potassium removed.

POTASSIUM SUPPLEMENTATION

Some of the advantages of a lower sodium intake may relate to its tendency to increase body potassium content, both by a coincidental increase in dietary potassium intake and by a decrease in potassium wastage if diuretics are being used. Potassium deficiency has multiple effects that may increase blood pressure and there is growing evidence that blood pressure will be lowered by correction of hypokalemia or by addition of potassium to diets of patients who are normokalemic.[95] Nonetheless, diuretic-induced hypokalemia may be more of a danger than many suspect, especially for the development of ventricular arrhythimias, so that hypertensive patients should be protected from potassium depletion. Moreover, extra dietary potassium intake may protect against vascular damage and strokes.[96]

MAGNESIUM SUPPLEMENTATION

In controlled trials, little effect on the blood pressure is seen with magnesium supplements.[97] However, those who are magnesium depleted may not be able to replete concomitant potassium deficiency.

CALCIUM SUPPLEMENTATION

An increase in free intracellular calcium may be a final step in the pathogenesis of primary hypertension. Nonetheless, some hypertensive patients have a lower calcium intake and higher urinary calcium excretion than do normotensive patients.[98] About one

- - - - - - - - - - - - - - - -

TABLE 7.23 • NONDRUG THERAPIES FOR HYPERTENSION

Stop smoking (not for blood pressure but for cardiovascular health)

Lose weight, particularly for upper body obesity

Reduce sodium intake (2 g/d or 88 mmol/d)

Moderate alcohol intake (no more than 3 usual portions/d)

Regular aerobic, isotonic exercise

Relax and relieve stress

Less saturated fat, more fish oils

Maintain adequate potassium, calcium, and magnesium intake

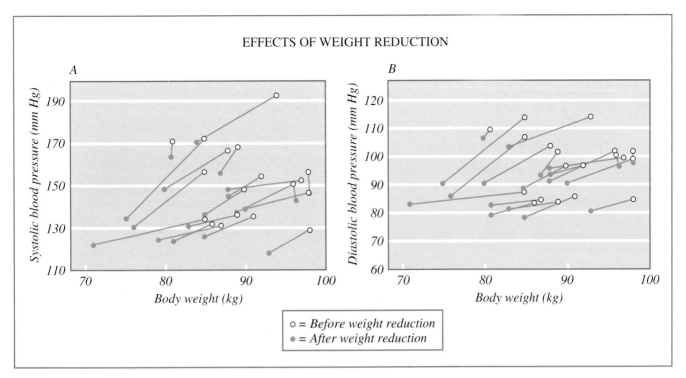

FIGURE 7.82 • Systolic (A) and diastolic (B) blood pressure before and after body weight reduction. (Reproduced with permission.

Staessen J, Fagard R, Lijnen P, et al: *J Hypertens* 1989;7(Suppl. 1):S19.)

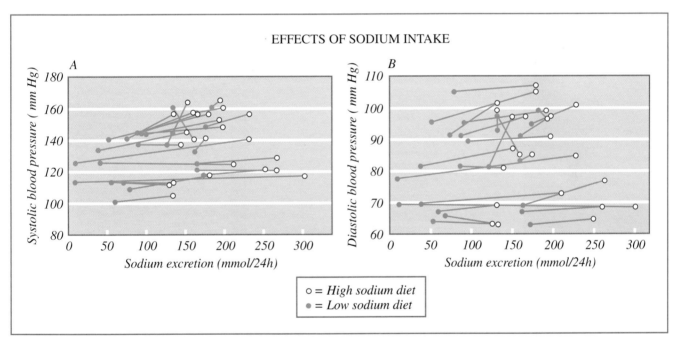

FIGURE 7.83 • Systolic (A) and diastolic blood pressure (B) on a high and low sodium intake in 16 studies published from 1973 to

1987 involving 24 groups. (Reproduced with permission. Staessen J, Fagard R, Lijnen P, et al: *J Hypertens* 1989;7(Suppl 1):S19.)

third of hypertensive people given 1 to 2 g/d of supplemental calcium show a decrease in blood pressure[99] (Figure 7.84), while others given calcium supplements have a rise in blood pressure. Because of this disparity, the best course is not to give supplemental calcium, but to insure that calcium intake is not inadvertently reduced despite restrictions of milk and cheese in an attempt to reduce saturated fat and sodium intake.

OTHER DIETARY CHANGES

Studies have noted some lowering of the blood pressure by a lacto-ovo-vegetarian diet[100] and high doses of polyunsaturated fish oil[101] (Figure 7.85). Neither decreases in total dietary fat[102] nor increases in dietary fiber[103] alter blood pressure. In an attempt to reduce calories and overall coronary risk, substitution of carbohydrate for fat may further aggravate the hyperinsulinemia often present in primary hypertension and therefore be counterproductive.[104]

When consumed by noncoffee drinkers, caffeine equivalent to the amount in two cups of coffee will increase blood pressure, probably by activation of the sympathetic nervous system.[105] However, chronic caffeine ingestion is not associated with significant rises in blood pressure because of tolerance to the hemodynamic effects.

MODERATION OF ALCOHOL

Moderate alcohol consumption, less than 1 oz/d of ethanol, does not increase the prevalence of hypertension. Heavier drinking clearly exerts a pressor effect that makes alcohol abuse the most common cause of reversible hypertension.[106] One to two portions of alcohol-containing beverages a day, containing 0.5 to 1.0 oz of ethanol, need not be prohibited, particularly since fewer coronary events have been noted in those who consume that amount.[107]

ISOTONIC EXERCISE

Regular isotonic exercise results in a 5 to 10 mm Hg reduction in blood pressure, accompanied by and probably related to a fall in sympathetic nervous activity[108] (Figure 7.86). Isometric exercises, such as weight-lifting, pushing, and pulling, may be harmful to the hypertensive patient. This is because during an isometric contraction, blood pressure often rises to high levels by a reflex mechanism.

RELAXATION TECHNIQUES

Various forms of relaxation—transcendental meditation, yoga, biofeedback, psychotherapy—have reduced the blood pressure of some hypertensive patients. Responders tend to be those with overt signs of sympathetic nervous over-activity.[109]

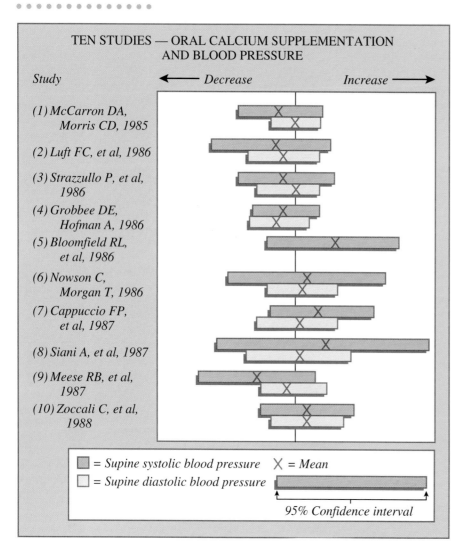

TEN STUDIES — ORAL CALCIUM SUPPLEMENTATION AND BLOOD PRESSURE

Study   ← *Decrease*   *Increase* →

(1) McCarron DA, Morris CD, 1985

(2) Luft FC, et al, 1986

(3) Strazzullo P, et al, 1986

(4) Grobbee DE, Hofman A, 1986

(5) Bloomfield RL, et al, 1986

(6) Nowson C, Morgan T, 1986

(7) Cappuccio FP, et al, 1987

(8) Siani A, et al, 1987

(9) Meese RB, et al, 1987

(10) Zoccali C, et al, 1988

■ = *Supine systolic blood pressure*   X = *Mean*
□ = *Supine diastolic blood pressure*

95% *Confidence interval*

FIGURE 7.84 • Mean and 95% confidence intervals of the differences in supine systolic and diastolic blood pressure after oral calcium supplementation. (Reproduced with permission. Cappuccio FP, Siani A, Strazzullo P: *J Hypertens* 1989;7:941.)

References (1) McCarron DA, Morris CD: Blood pressure response to oral calcium in persons with mild to moderate hypertension. *Ann Intern Med* 1985;103:825. (2) Luft FC, Aronoff GR, Sloan RS, et al: Short-term augmented calcium intake has no effect on sodium homeostasis. *Clin Pharmacol Ther* 1986;39:414. (3) Strazzullo P, Siani A, Guglielmi S, et al: Controlled trial of long-term oral calcium supplementation in essential hypertension. *Hypertension* 1986;8:1084. (4) Grobbee DE, Hofman A: Effect of calcium supplementation on diastolic blood pressure in young people with mild hypertension. *Lancet* 1986;11:703. (5) Bloomfield RL, Young LD, Zurek G, et al: Effects of oral calcium carbonate on blood pressure in subjects with mildly elevated arterial pressure. *J Hypertens* 1986;4(suppl 5):S351. (6) Nowson C, Morgan T: Effect of calcium carbonate on blood pressure. *J Hypertens* 1986;4(suppl 5):S673. (7) Cappuccio FP, Markandu ND, Singer DRJ, et al: Does oral calcium supplementation lower high blood pressure? A double-blind study. *J Hypertens* 1987;5:67. (8) Siani A, Strazzullo P, Guglielmi S, et al:Clinical studies of the effects of different oral calcium intakes in essential hypertension. *J Hypertens* 1987;5(suppl 5):S311. (9) Meese RB, Gonzales DG, Casparian JM, et al: The inconsistent effects of calcium supplements upon blood pressure in primary hypertension. *Am J Med Sci* 1987;294:219. (10) Zoccali C, Mallamaci F, Delfino D, et al: Double-blind randomized, crossover trial of calcium supplementation in essential hypertension. *J Hypertens* 1988;6:451.

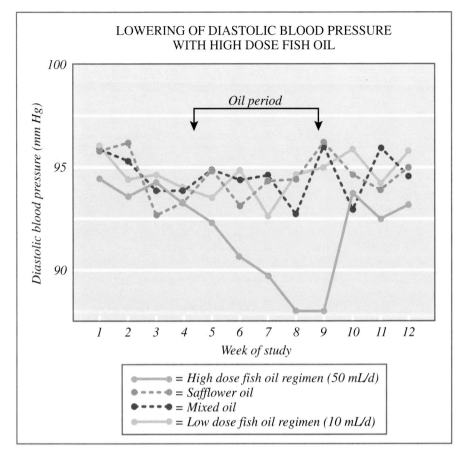

LOWERING OF DIASTOLIC BLOOD PRESSURE
WITH HIGH DOSE FISH OIL

Oil period

= High dose fish oil regimen (50 mL/d)
= Safflower oil
= Mixed oil
= Low dose fish oil regimen (10 mL/d)

FIGURE 7.85 • Changes in diastolic blood pressure in the four treatment groups during the 12 weeks of study. The values are group means; the coefficients of variation ranged from 8% to 12%. The high-dose fish-oil regimen (50 mL/d) had a significant effect on both systolic pressure ($p < 0.002$ by repeated-measures analysis of variance) and diastolic pressure ($p < 0.02$). The low-dose fish-oil regimen and the safflower-oil and mixed-oil regimens had no significant effect. (Reproduced with permission. Knapp H, Fitzgerald GA: *N Engl J Med* 1989;320:1037.)

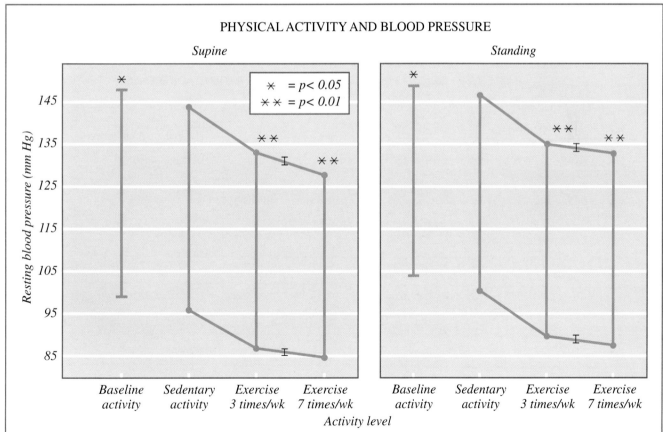

PHYSICAL ACTIVITY AND BLOOD PRESSURE

Supine

$* = p < 0.05$
$** = p < 0.01$

Standing

FIGURE 7.86 • Resting supine and standing blood-pressure at three levels of physical activity that were sequenced in a random fashion by a Latin square design. Baseline measurement, sedentary activity, 3 times/wk exercise, and 7 times/wk exercise. $p < 0.05$ = difference from sedentary value for both systolic and diastolic blood pressure. (Reproduced with permission. Nelson L, Jennings GL, Esler MD, et al: *Lancet* 1986;2:473.)

ANTIHYPERTENSIVE DRUG THERAPY

If the nondrug therapies described above are not followed, prove ineffective, or if the level of hypertension at the onset is so high that immediate drug therapy is deemed necessary, the general guidelines listed in Table 7.24 should help improve patient adherence to lifelong treatment.

GENERAL GUIDELINES
Gradual Reduction in Pressure

I recommend, as stated in Table 7.24, to start with small doses of medication, aiming for a reduction of 5 to 10 mm Hg in blood pressure at each step. Some physicians attempt to control a patient's hypertension rapidly and completely. Regardless of which drugs are used, this approach often leads to easy fatigability, weakness, postural dizziness, and feeling of being washed out, that many patients find intolerable, particularly when they felt well before therapy was begun. Although hypokalemia and other electrolyte abnormalities may be responsible for some of these symptoms, a more likely explanation has been provided by the studies of Strandgaard and Haunso[84] (Figure 7.87). They demonstrated the constancy of cerebral blood flow by autoregulation over a range of mean arterial pressures from approximately 60 to 120 mm Hg in normal subjects and from 110 to 180 mm Hg in patients with hypertension. This shift to the right protects the hypertensive patient from a surge of blood flow, which could cause cerebral edema. However, the shift also predisposes the hypertensive patient to cerebral ischemia when blood pressure is lowered.

Note that the lower limit of autoregulation necessary to preserve a constant cerebral blood flow in hypertensive patients is a mean of approximately 110 mm Hg. Thus, acutely lowering the pressure from 160/110 mm Hg (mean = 127 mm Hg) to 140/85 mm Hg (mean = 102 mm Hg) may induce cerebral hypoperfusion, although hypotension in the accepted sense has not been produced. This provides an explanation for the symptoms that many patients experience at the start of antihypertensive therapy—manifestations of cerebral hypoperfusion even though blood pressure levels do not seem inordinately low. Fortunately, as shown in the middle of Figure 7.87, if therapy is continued for a period of time, the curve of cerebral autoregulation shifts back toward normal, allowing patients to tolerate greater reductions in blood pressure without experiencing symptoms.

Individualized Therapy

The addition of drugs, stepwise, in sufficient doses will enable one to achieve the intended goal of therapy. Over the past 30 years, the purely empirical basis for the use of antihypertensive drugs has been replaced by a stepped-care approach, which involves use of a diuretic or an adrenergic-blocking drug first, followed by a stepwise addition of other drugs as needed.

Rather than always starting with the same drug and following a rigid step-care approach, a more scientific and rational approach has been recommended for selecting the initial drug

---

TABLE 7.24 • GENERAL GUIDELINES TO IMPROVE PATIENT ADHERENCE TO ANTIHYPERTENSIVE THERAPY

- Be aware of the problem and be alert to signs of patient nonadherence.
- Establish the goal of therapy: to reduce blood pressure to near normotensive levels with minimal or no side effects.
- Educate the patient about the disease and its treatment.
  - Involve the patient in decision making.
  - Encourage family support.
- Maintain contact with the patient.
  - Encourage visits and calls to allied health personnel.
  - Allow the pharmacist to monitor therapy.
  - Give feedback to the patient via home BP readings.
  - Make contact with patients who do not return.
- Keep care inexpensive and simple.
  - Do the least workup needed to rule out secondary causes.
  - Obtain follow-up laboratory data only yearly unless indicated more often.

Use home blood pressure readings.
Use nondrug, no-cost therapies.
Use the fewest daily doses of drugs needed.
If appropriate, use combination tablets.
Tailor medication to daily routines.
- Prescribe according to pharmacological principles.
  - Add one drug at a time.
  - Start with small doses, aiming for 5- to 10-mm Hg reductions at each step.
  - Prevent volume overload with adequate diuretic and sodium restriction.
  - Be willing to stop unsuccessful therapy and try a different approach.
  - Anticipate side effects.
  - Adjust therapy to ameliorate side effects that do not spontaneously disappear.
  - Continue to add effective and tolerated drugs, stepwise, in sufficient doses to achieve the goal of therapy.

based on patient's individual needs and demographics[11] (Figure 7.88). Individualized therapy involves three considerations:
- The patient's race—blacks responding less well to ß-blockers and perhaps to angiotensin-converting enzyme (ACE) inhibitors.
- The patient's age—the elderly responding a bit better to diuretics and calcium blockers.

- The patient's concomitant conditions as portrayed in a recent survey by Stewart et al[110] (Table 7.25).

Some of the comorbid conditions point toward a choice, such as the use of a calcium blocker in a patient with angina. Other conditions point away from certain choices, for instance, avoidance of a ß-blocker in a patient with bronchospastic lung disease.

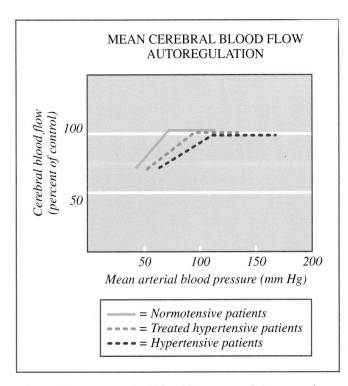

FIGURE 7.87 • Mean cerebral blood flow autoregulation curves from normotensive, severely hypertensive, and effectively treated hypertensive patients are shown to reflect a less marked fall in blood flow when arterial pressure is lowered. (Reproduced with permission. Strandgaard S, Haunso S: *Lancet* 1987;2:658.)

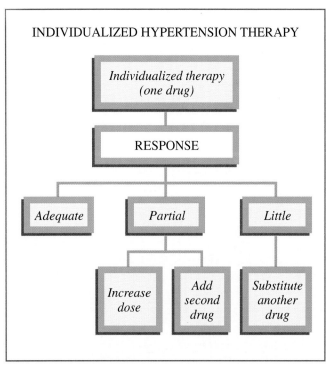

FIGURE 7.88 • Individualized approach to the therapy of hypertension. The choice of initial therapy is based on multiple clinical features.

TABLE 7.25 • COMORBID CONDITIONS AMONG 2,706 HYPERTENSIVE PATIENTS	
Diabetes	18.1%
Arthritis	36.1%
Back problems	4.4%
Chronic lung disease	7.4%
Angina	8.0%
Myocardial infarction	2.2%
Congestive heart failure	5.8%
None	37.3%

(Reproduced with permission. Stewart AL, Greenfield S, Hays RD: *JAMA* 1989;262:907.)

For those with more severe hypertension, in whom the first choice can be expected to be only partially effective, the stepped-care approach makes good scientific sense. A diuretic will enhance the effectiveness of most other drugs used, preventing the "pseudotolerance" that develops because of the fluid retention that frequently follows the use of some adrenergic blocking drugs and vasodilators. An ACE inhibitor or calcium-entry blocker is increasingly being chosen as the second or third drug when triple therapy is needed.

As a result of the individualized approach, the use of diuretics has been falling, whereas the use of calcium-entry blockers and ACE inhibitors has been growing rapidly (Figure 7.89).

DIURETICS

Diuretics useful in the treatment of hypertension may be divided into four major groups by their primary site of action within the tubule, starting in the proximal portion and moving to the collecting duct:

- Agents acting on the proximal tubule, such as carbonic anhydrase inhibitors, which have limited antihypertensive efficacy.
- Loop diuretics.
- Thiazides and related sulfonamide compounds.
- Potassium-sparing agents (Figure 7.90).

A thiazide is the usual choice, often in combination with a potassium-sparing agent. Loop diuretics should be reserved for those patients with renal insufficiency or resistant hypertension.

All diuretics initially lower the blood pressure by increasing urinary sodium excretion and by reducing plasma volume, extracellular fluid volume, and cardiac output. Within 6 to 8

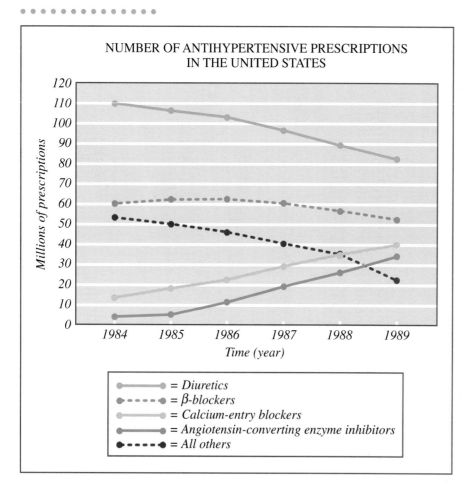

FIGURE 7.89 • Number of prescriptions written for antihypertensive drugs in millions in the United States from 1984 to 1988 (Reproduced with permission. *National Prescription Audit* Ambler, Pa: IMS; 1989.)

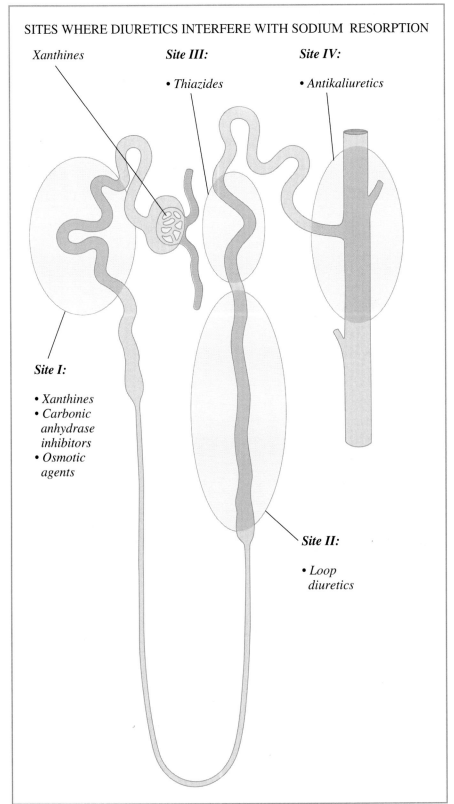

SITES WHERE DIURETICS INTERFERE WITH SODIUM RESORPTION

Xanthines

Site III:

• *Thiazides*

Site IV:

• *Antikaliuretics*

Site I:

• *Xanthines*
• *Carbonic anhydrase inhibitors*
• *Osmotic agents*

Site II:

• *Loop diuretics*

FIGURE 7.90 • Nephron showing the four main tubular sites where diuretics interfere with sodium reabsorption. The main action of xanthines on the kidney is upon vascular perfusion of the glomerulus though some effect on sodium reabsorption at site I is also likely. (Reproduced with permission. Lant A: *Drugs* 1986;31(Suppl 4):40.)

weeks the lowered plasma, extracellular fluid volume, and cardiac output return toward normal (Figure 7.91). At this point and beyond, the lower blood pressure is related to a fall in peripheral resistance, thereby improving the underlying hemodynamic defect of hypertension.

With continuous diuretic therapy, blood pressure usually falls about 10 mm Hg, although the degree depends on various factors, including the initial height of the pressure, the quantity of sodium ingested, the adequacy of renal function, and the intensity of the counterregulatory renin-aldosterone response. The antihypertensive effect of the diuretic persists indefinitely, although it may be overwhelmed by dietary sodium intake above 8 g/d.

If other drugs are used, a diuretic may also be needed. Without a concomitant diuretic, antihypertensive drugs that do not block the renin-aldosterone mechanism may cause sodium retention (Figure 7.92). This mechanism probably reflects the success of the drugs in lowering the blood pressure and may involve the abnormal renal pressure-natriuresis relationship that is presumably present in primary hypertension. The critical need for adequate diuretic therapy to keep intravascular volume diminished has been repeatedly documented. Therefore, diuretics are likely to continue to be wide-ly used in antihypertensive therapy. Drugs which inhibit the renin-aldosterone mechanism, such as ACE inhibitors, or which induce some natriuresis themselves, such as calcium-entry blockers, may continue to work without the need for concomitant diuretics. However, a diuretic will enhance the effectiveness of all other types of drugs, including calcium-entry blockers.[111]

Dosage and Choice of Agent

Most patients with mild to moderate hypertension and reasonably intact renal function—serum creatinine below 2.0 mg/dL—will respond to an amount equivalent to 12.5 mg of hydrochlorothiazide. Larger doses will have some additional antihypertensive effect, but at the price of additional potassium wastage.[112] The nonthiazide agent, indapamide, has special properties which make it an attractive choice. This agent seldom disturbs lipid or glucose levels,[113] and may exert an additional vasodilatory action by increasing prostacyclin generation in the vascular smooth muscle cells.[114]

With renal insufficiency, manifested by a serum creatinine level above 2.0 mg/dL or creatinine clearance below 25 mL/min, thiazides are usually not effective. Multiple doses of furosemide or a single dose of metolazone will be needed.

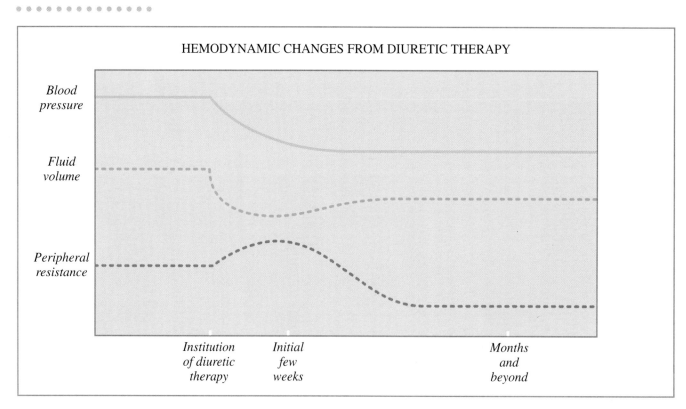

FIGURE 7.91 • Hemodynamic changes responsible for the antihypertensive effects of diuretic therapy.

Side Effects

A number of biochemical changes often accompany successful diuresis. These include a decrease in plasma potassium and increases in glucose, insulin, and cholesterol (Figure 7.93).

Hypokalemia • Serum potassium falls an average of 0.67 mmol/L after institution of continuous, daily diuretic therapy for hypertension.[115] This reduction in serum concentration may precipitate potentially hazardous ventricular ectopic activity, even in patients not known to be susceptible because of concomitant digitalis therapy or myocardial irritability.[116] The arrhythmogenic effect of diuretic-induced hypokalemia may become manifest only at times of stress, when catecholamines may lower the plasma potassium level another 0.5 to 1.0 mmol/L or when β_2-agonists are used as bronchodilators.[117]

Prevention of hypokalemia is preferable to correction of potassium deficiency. The following maneuvers should help prevent diuretic-induced hypokalemia:
- Use the smallest amount of diuretic needed.
- Use a moderately long-acting (12- to 18-hr) diuretic, such as hydrochlorothiazide, since longer-acting drugs like chlorthalidone may increase potassium loss.
- Restrict sodium intake to less than 100 mmol/d, or 2 g.
- Increase dietary potassium intake.
- Restrict concomitant use of laxatives.
- Use a combination of a thiazide with a potassium-sparing agent. If the latter is prescribed, avoid supplemental potassium, since dangerous hyperkalemia may supervene if these drugs are given together.
- The concomitant use of a ß-blocker or an ACE inhibitor may diminish potassium loss, by presumably blunting the diuretic-induced rise in renin-aldosterone.

Hypomagnesemia • Concomitant diuretic-induced magnesium deficiency may prevent the restoration of intracellular deficits of potassium, so that hypomagnesemia should be corrected.

Hyperuricemia • The serum uric acid level is elevated in as many as one third of untreated hypertensive patients. With chronic diuretic therapy, hyperuricemia appears in another third of patients, probably as a consequence of increased proximal tubular reabsorption accompanying volume contraction. Diuretic-induced hyperuricemia precipitates acute gout most frequently in those who are obese and who consume large amounts of alcohol.[118]

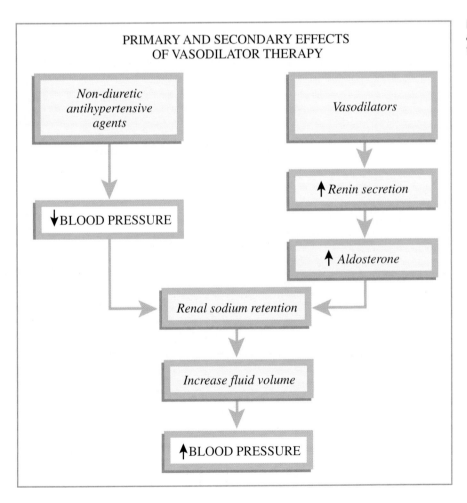

PRIMARY AND SECONDARY EFFECTS
OF VASODILATOR THERAPY

FIGURE 7.92 • Manner by which nondiuretic antihypertensive agents may lose their effectiveness by reactive renal sodium retention.

POSSIBLE COMPLICATIONS: CHRONIC DIURETIC THERAPY

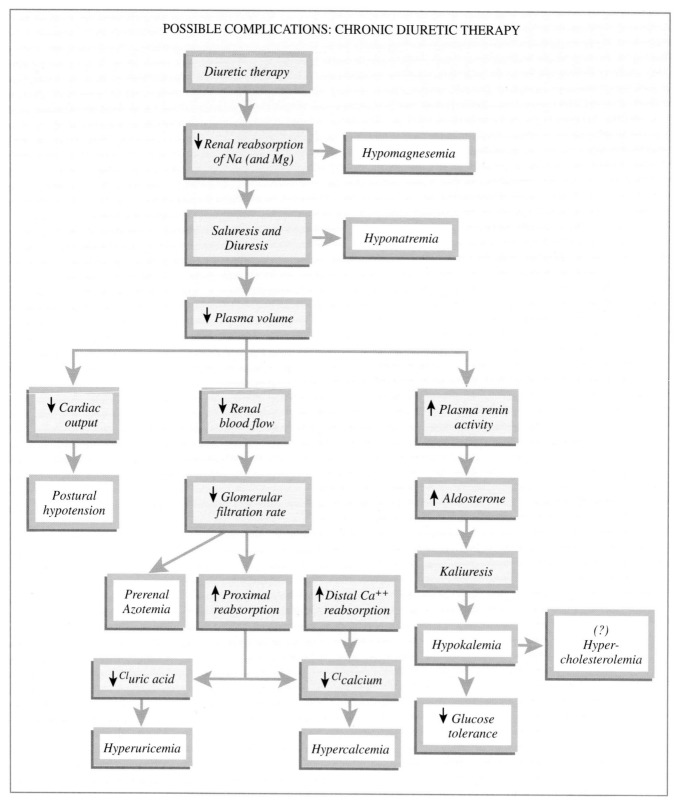

FIGURE 7.93 • Mechanisms by which chronic diuretic therapy may lead to various complications. The mechanism for hypercholes-terolemia remains in question, although it is shown as arising via hypokalemia.

Hyperlipidemia • Serum cholesterol levels often rise after diuretic therapy[119] (Figure 7.94). Although the rise in lipids can be prevented by a diet low in saturated fat, the propensity to worsen the lipid profile may reduce the potential for diuretic therapy to reduce the incidence of coronary disease while it lowers blood pressure.

Hyperglycemia and Insulin Resistance • Diuretics may impair glucose tolerance and rarely may precipitate diabetes mellitus. Perhaps of even greater concern, diuretics are associated with additional insulin resistance and hyperinsulinemia.[120] The manner by which diuretics reduce insulin sensitivity is uncertain but, in view of the multiple potential pressor actions of hyperinsulinemia noted previously, this could be a significant problem.

Hypercalcemia • A slight rise in serum calcium, less than 0.5 mg/dL, is frequently seen with thiazide diuretic therapy, at least in part because increased calcium reabsorption accompanies the increased sodium reabsorption in the proximal tubule induced by contraction of extracellular fluid volume. The di-uretic-induced positive calcium balance is associated with a reduction in the incidence of hip fractures in the elderly.[121]

Other Problems • A high rate of impotence—22.6%—was found among men taking 10 mg of bendroflumethiazide per day, compared with a rate of 10.1% among those on placebo and 13.2% among those on propranolol in the large British Medical Research Council (MRC) trial.[122]

Nonsteroidal anti-inflammatory drugs (NSAIDS) may inhibit the antihypertensive effects of both thiazides and loop diuretics, presumably by inhibiting the synthesis of vasodilatory prostaglandins in the kidney.

Loop Diuretics

Loop diuretics are usually needed in the treatment of hypertensive patients with renal insufficiency, defined as a serum creatinine above 2.0 mg/dL. Furosemide has been most widely used, although metolazone may work as well and requires only a single daily dose.

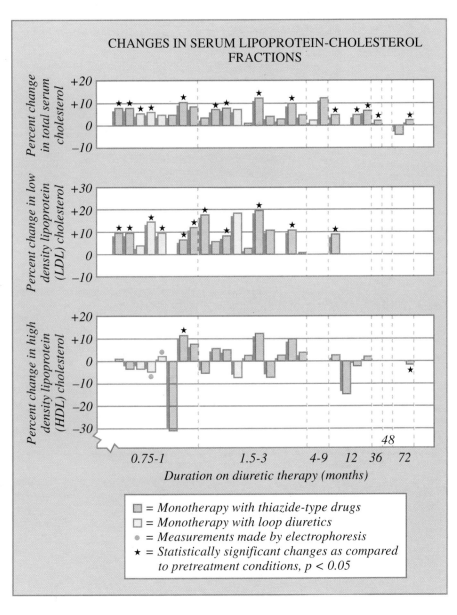

CHANGES IN SERUM LIPOPROTEIN-CHOLESTEROL FRACTIONS

Duration on diuretic therapy (months)

☐ = Monotherapy with thiazide-type drugs
☐ = Monotherapy with loop diuretics
• = Measurements made by electrophoresis
★ = Statistically significant changes as compared to pretreatment conditions, p < 0.05

FIGURE 7.94 • Percentage of changes in serum lipoprotein-cholesterol fractions as related to the duration of a monotherapy with thiazide-type or loop diuretics. The data shown are from published studies with a minimum number of 10 subjects and a minimum duration of 4 weeks.(Reproduced with permission. Weidmann P, Uehlinger DE, Gerber A: *J Hypertens* 1985;3:297.)

Potassium-sparing Agents

These drugs are normally used in combination with a diuretic. Of the three currently available, spironolactone is an aldosterone antagonist, while the other two, dyrenium and amiloride, are direct inhibitors of potassium secretion.

An Overview of Diuretics in Hypertension

Diuretics have been effective for the treatment of millions of hypertensive patients during the past 30 years. They reduce diastolic blood pressure and maintain it below 90 mm Hg in about half of all hypertensive patients, providing the same degree of effectiveness as most other antihypertensive drugs.[111] In two groups that constitute a rather large portion of the hypertensive population, the elderly and blacks, diuretics may be particularly effective. One diuretic tablet per day is usually all that is needed, minimizing cost and maximizing adherence to therapy.

The side effects of diuretic therapy are usually not overtly bothersome, but the hypokalemia, hypercholesterolemia, hyperinsulinemia, and worsening of glucose tolerance that often accompany prolonged diuretic therapy have given rise to increasing concerns about their long-term benignity. This concern has been fueled by the failure of diuretic-based therapy to reduce coronary mortality in the major trials of the therapy of mild hypertension (refer to Figure 7.71). Therefore, the use of diuretics will likely continue to diminish in the future. When they are used, they will be given in smaller doses and more care will be taken to monitor and prevent the various biochemical changes they may induce.

ADRENOCEPTOR BLOCKING DRUGS

A number of adrenoceptor blocking drugs are available, including some that act centrally on vasomotor center activity, peripherally on neuronal catecholamine discharge or by blocking α- and/or ß-adrenoceptors (Table 7.26), and some that act at multiple sites.

Drugs that Act within the Neuron

Reserpine, guanethidine, and related compounds act to inhibit the release of norepinephrine from peripheral adrenergic neurons, each in a different manner.

Reserpine • Reserpine, the most active and widely used of the derivatives of the rauwolfia alkaloids, depletes the postganglionic adrenergic neurons of norepinephrine by inhibiting its uptake into storage vesicles. The drug has certain advantages:

- Only one dose a day is needed.
- In combination with a diuretic, the antihypertensive effect is significant.
- Little postural hypotension is noted.
- Many patients experience no side effects.

A dose of only 0.05 mg/d will give almost as much antihypertensive effect as 0.125 or 0.25 mg/d, but with fewer side effects.[123] However, the psychological depression that occurs in perhaps 2% of patients may be severe, but difficult to recognize and treat. Although it remains popular in some places, the use of reserpine has declined progressively.

Guanethidine • Guanethidine and a series of related guanidine compounds, including guanadrel, bethanidine, and debrisoquine, act by inhibiting the release of norepinephrine from the adrenergic neurons. Blood pressure is reduced further when the patient is upright, owing to gravitational pooling of blood in the legs, since compensatory sympathetic nervous system-mediated vasoconstriction is blocked. This results in the most common side effect, postural hypotension. As other drugs have become available, guanethidine has been mainly relegated to the treatment of severe hypertension unresponsive to all other agents.

TABLE 7.26 • ADRENERGIC INHIBITORS USED IN TREATMENT OF HYPERTENSION

Peripheral neuronal inhibitors	Central adrenergic inhibitors	α-Receptor blockers	ß-Receptor blockers	α- and ß-receptor blocker:
Reserpine	Methyldopa (Aldomet)	α_1- and α_2-receptor • Phenoxybenzamine (Dibenzyline)	Acebutolol (Sectral) Atenolol (Tenormin)	Labetalol (Normodyne, Trandate)
Guanethidine (Ismelin)	Clonidine (Catapres)	• Phentolamine (Regitine)	Betaxolol (Kerlone) Carteolol (Cartrol)	
Guanadrel (Hylorel)	Guanabenz (Wytensin)	α_1-receptor • Doxazosin (Cardura)	Dilevalol (Unicard) Metoprolol (Lopressor)	
Bethanidine (Tenathan)	Guanfacine (Tenex)	• Prazosin (Minipress)	Nadolol (Corgard) Penbutolol (Levatol)	
		• Terazosin (Hytrin)	Pindolol (Visken) Propranolol (Inderal) Timolol (Blocadren)	

Drugs that Act upon Receptors

Predominantly Central α-Agonists Until recently, methyldopa was the most widely used of the adrenoceptor blockers, but its use has fallen off as ß-blockers and other drugs have become more popular. In addition, three other drugs, clonidine, guanabenz, and guanfacine, which act similarly to methyldopa but have fewer serious side effects, have become available.

Central α-agonists act primarily within the central nervous system where they stimulate α-adrenoreceptors, reducing the sympathetic outflow from the central nervous system (Figure 7.95). The blood pressure mainly falls due to a decrease in peripheral resistance with little effect on cardiac output. On the other hand, methyldopa, probably in concert with other antihypertensive agents that decrease sympathetic activity, may reduce the degree of left ventricular hypertrophy as noted by echocardiography.[124] Renal blood flow is well maintained, and significant postural hypotension is unusual. Therefore, the drug has been widely used in hypertensive patients with renal insufficiency or cerebrovascular disease.

These agents need be given no more than twice daily and guanfacine only once daily. As in the case of the other adrenoceptor blockers and peripheral vasodilators that may cause reactive fluid retention, they are best used in combination with a diuretic.

Side effects include some that are common to all centrally acting drugs that reduce sympathetic outflow: sedation, dry mouth, orthostatic hypotension, impotence, and galactorrhea. However, methyldopa causes some unique side effects that are probably of an autoimmune nature, since a positive antinuclear antibody test is seen in about 10% of patients who take the drug and red cell autoantibodies in about 20%. Inflammatory diseases in various organs have been reported with methyldopa, most commonly involving the liver with diffuse parenchymal injury similar to viral hepatitis.[125]

Clonidine, because of its fairly short biological half-life, has a propensity to be followed by rapid rebound of the blood pressure to pretreatment levels when it is abruptly discontinued, which occasionally results in withdrawal symptoms, including tachycardia, restlessness, and sweating. Rarely, the blood pressure increases beyond the pretreatment level. Similar overshoots have been reported less commonly after the discontinuation of a variety of other antihypertensives.[126] If the rebound requires treatment, the α-agonist may be reintroduced or α-adrenoreceptor antagonists given.

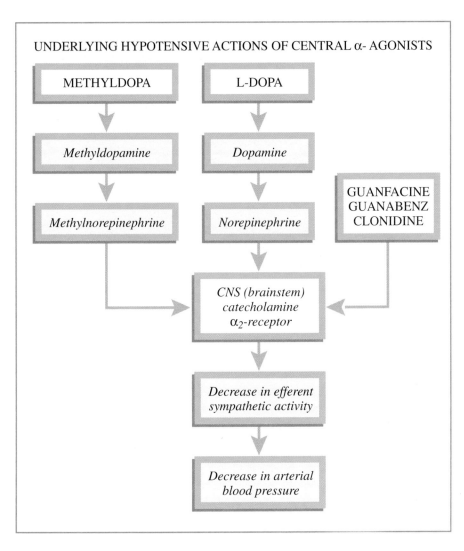

FIGURE 7.95 • The common mechanism probably underlying the hypotensive actions of methyldopa, L-dopa, clonidine, guanabenz, and guanfacine. (Reproduced with permission. Henning M. In: van Zwieten PA, ed. *Handbook of Hypertension. Pharmacology of Antihypertensive Drugs* Volume 3 Amsterdam: Elsevier; 1984:156.)

UNDERLYING HYPOTENSIVE ACTIONS OF CENTRAL α- AGONISTS

METHYLDOPA → *Methyldopamine* → *Methylnorepinephrine*

L-DOPA → *Dopamine* → *Norepinephrine*

GUANFACINE GUANABENZ CLONIDINE

CNS (brainstem) catecholamine α₂-receptor

Decrease in efferent sympathetic activity

Decrease in arterial blood pressure

Clonidine is available in a transdermal preparation that may provide smoother blood pressure control for as long as 7 days with fewer side effects. However, bothersome skin rashes preclude its use in perhaps one fourth of patients.[127]

Clonidine has been used to treat severe hypertension with hourly doses of 0.1 and 0.2 mg.[128] In addition, it may suppress withdrawal symptoms from opiates and nicotine and may have wider use in various psychiatric disorders.[129]

α-Adrenoceptor Antagonists

Prazosin was the first of a group of selective antagonists of the postsynaptic α_1-receptors and others, such as terazosin and doxazosin, are now available. By blocking α-mediated vasoconstriction, these agents induce a fall in peripheral resistance with both venous and arteriolar dilation. Because the presynaptic α-adrenoceptor is left unblocked, the feedback loop for the inhibition of norepinephrine release is intact, an action which is also certainly responsible for the antihypertensive effect greater than is seen with nonselective α-blockers, such as dibenzyline, and the absence of concomitant tachycardia, tolerance, and renin release (Figure 7.96).

The α_1-blockers are as effective as other first-line antihypertensives and are similarly aided by concomitant use of a diuretic. The favorable hemodynamic changes—a fall in peripheral resistance with maintenance of cardiac output—make them an attractive choice for patients who wish to remain physically active. Patients who may have trouble with ß-blockers, including those with asthma or peripheral vascular disease, should be able to tolerate alpha blockade. In addition, blood lipids are not adversely altered and may actually improve with α-blockers, unlike the adverse effects observed with diuretics and ß-blockers.[130] Moreover, improved insulin sensitivity, with lesser rises in plasma glucose and insulin levels after a glucose load, has been observed with prazosin.[131]

Side effects, beyond first-dose postural hypotension, include the nonspecific effects of lower blood pressure, such as dizziness, weakness, fatigue, and headaches. Most patients, however, find the drug easy to take, and experiences little sedation, dry mouth, or impotence.

ß-Adrenoceptor Antagonists

In the 1980s, ß-adrenoceptor blockers became the most popular form of antihypertensive therapy after diuretics (refer to Figure 7.89). Their popularity reflects their relative effectiveness and freedom from many bothersome side effects. However, they are no more effective in lowering blood pressure than

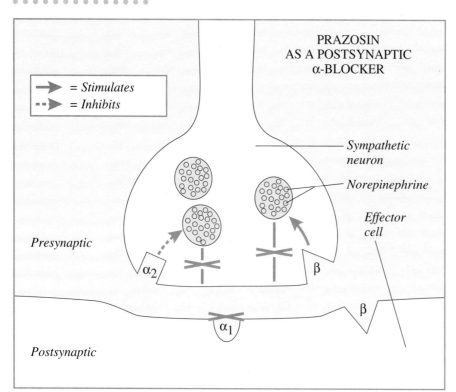

= Stimulates
= Inhibits

PRAZOSIN AS A POSTSYNAPTIC α-BLOCKER

Presynaptic

α_2

β

Sympathetic neuron

Norepinephrine

Effector cell

β

α_1

Postsynaptic

FIGURE 7.96 • The action of prazosin as a postsynaptic α-blocker. By blocking the α_1-adrenergic receptor on the vascular smooth muscle, catecholamine-induced vasoconstriction is inhibited. The α_2-receptor on the neuronal membrane is not blocked. Therefore, inhibition of additional norepinephrine release by the short feedback mechanism is maintained.

are other adrenoceptor blocking agents, and side effects occur in a significant number of patients. Some of these side effects, including fatigue, bronchospasm, peripheral vasospasm, and depression, may be quite bothersome. For the majority of patients who do not develop such side effects, ß-blockers are usually easy to take, since somnolence, dry mouth, and impotence are seldom encountered. Because ß-blockers have been found to reduce mortality when taken after acute myocardial infarction—secondary prevention—it was assumed that they might offer special protection against initial coronary events—primary prevention. In three large clinical trials (refer to Figure 7.72), a ß-blocker provided no more protection than a diuretic. In the metoprolol portion of the HAPPHY trial, the coronary mortality rate was lower for those on metoprolol than for those who were on a diuretic, whose mortality rate rose considerably during the last period of the trial.[132]

The Variety of ß-Blockers

The ß-blockers now available in the United States are shown in Figure 7.97 along with others available in other countries or under investigation. A number of agents with additional vasodilatory effects will likely soon be approved for use in the United States, and they may overcome many of the unfavorable hemodynamic and adverse effects of currently available

agents. Pharmacologically, the three most important differences affecting their clinical use are cardioselectivity, intrinsic sympathomimetic activity, and lipid solubility. Despite these differences, they seem to be equally effective as antihypertensives.

Cardioselectivity • Beta-blockers differ as to their degree of cardioselectivity relative to their blocking effect on the β_1-adrenoceptors in the heart compared to that on the β_2-adrenoceptors in the bronchi, peripheral blood vessels, and elsewhere (refer to Figure 7.97). Such cardioselectivity can be easily shown using small doses in acute studies; with the rather high doses used to treat hypertension, much of this effect is lost.

Intrinsic Sympathomimetic Activity • Some ß-blockers have intrinsic sympathomimetic activity, interacting with ß-receptors to cause a measurable agonist response, but at the same time blocking the greater agonist effects of endogenous catecholamines. As a result, while in usual doses they lower the blood pressure to about the same degree as other ß-blockers, they cause a smaller decline in heart rate, cardiac output, and renin levels.

Lipid Solubility • Atenolol and nadolol are among the least lipid-soluble of the ß-blockers. This could translate into two clinically important advantages. First, because they escape hepatic inactivation and are excreted virtually unchanged

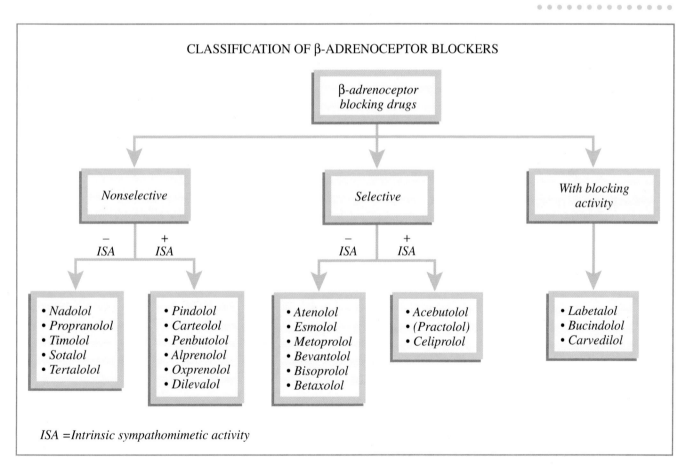

CLASSIFICATION OF β-ADRENOCEPTOR BLOCKERS

β-adrenoceptor blocking drugs

Nonselective
Selective
With blocking activity

− ISA + ISA − ISA + ISA

- Nadolol
- Propranolol
- Timolol
- Sotalol
- Tertalolol

- Pindolol
- Carteolol
- Penbutolol
- Alprenolol
- Oxprenolol
- Dilevalol

- Atenolol
- Esmolol
- Metoprolol
- Bevantolol
- Bisoprolol
- Betaxolol

- Acebutolol
- (Practolol)
- Celiprolol

- Labetalol
- Bucindolol
- Carvedilol

ISA = Intrinsic sympathomimetic activity

FIGURE 7.97 • Classification of ß-adrenoceptor blockers based on cardioselectivity and intrinsic sympathomimetic activity.

through the kidneys (Figure 7.98), they remain as active drugs in the plasma much longer, allowing once-a-day dosage. Second, because they do not enter the brain as readily, they may cause fewer central nervous system (CNS) side effects.[134]

At the same time ß-blockers lower blood pressure through various means, their blockade of peripheral ß-adrenoceptors inhibits vasodilation, leaving α-adrenoceptors open to catecholamine-mediated vasoconstriction with an acute rise in peripheral vascular resistance[135] (Figure 7.99). Over time, vascular resistance tends to return to normal, which presumably preserves the antihypertensive effect of a reduced cardiac output. As seen in Figure 7.99, the eventual level of vascular resistance differs and some vasoconstriction may persist with agents such as timolol and atenolol.

Clinical Effects • Even in small doses, ß-blockers begin to lower the blood pressure within a few hours, although their maximal effect may not be noted for some weeks. Even though progressively higher doses have usually been given, careful study has shown a near-maximal effect from smaller doses. In a double-blind crossover study involving 24 patients, 40 mg of propranolol twice a day provided the same antihypertensive effects as 80, 160, or 240 mg twice a day.[136] The degree of blood pressure reduction is at least comparable to that noted with other antihypertensive drugs. Duration of action is well beyond the drugs' plasma half-life so that most can be used once daily. One of the attractions of these agents is the constancy of their antihypertensive action, altered little by changes in activity, posture, or temperature. Because the sympathetic nervous system is blocked, the hemodynamic responses to stress are reduced, probably enough to interfere with athletic performance.[137]

Beta-blockers may be particularly well suited for hypertensive individuals with coexisting coronary disease, migraine, glaucoma, hyperkinetic circulation, or marked anxiety. These agents have been particularly useful in patients needing therapy with direct vasodilators, such as minoxidil, or during perioperative stress.

Side Effects • Most of the side effects of ß-blockers relate to their major pharmacologic action, the blockade of ß-adrenoceptors. Patients with certain concomitant problems may have them worsen when ß-adrenoceptors are blocked. These include peripheral vascular disease, bronchospasm, and congestive heart failure.

Diabetics may have additional problems with ß-blockers, more so with nonselective ones. The responses to hypoglycemia, both the symptoms and the counterregulatory hormonal changes that raise blood sugar levels, are partially dependent on sympathetic nervous activity. Diabetics who are susceptible to hypoglycemia may not be aware of the usual warning signals and may not rebound as quickly.

The most common side effects are fatigue and depression. Fatigue may reflect the decrease in cerebral blood flow that may accompany successful lowering of the blood pressure by any drug (refer to Figure 7.87). More direct effects on the CNS—depression, insomnia, nightmares, and hallucinations—occur in some patients.[134] The more common side effects of central agonists sedation, depression, and dry mouth are rare.

When a ß-blocker is discontinued, angina pectoris and myocardial infarction may occur.[138] Since patients with hypertension are more susceptible to coronary disease, they should

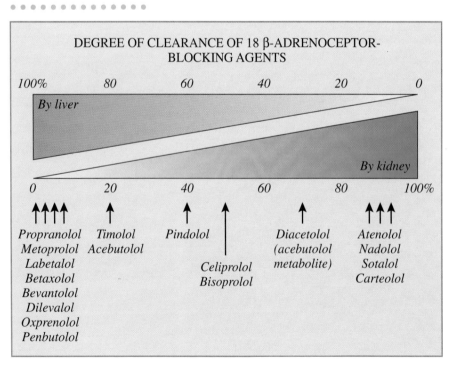

DEGREE OF CLEARANCE OF 18 β-ADRENOCEPTOR-BLOCKING AGENTS

FIGURE 7.98 • Relative degree of clearance by hepatic uptake and metabolism (liver) and renal excretion (kidney) of 18 ß-adrenoceptor blocking agents. The differences largely reflect differences in lipid solubility, which progressively diminishes from left to right. (Reproduced with permission. Meier J: *Cardiology* 1979;64(Suppl 1):1.)

be weaned gradually and given appropriate coronary vasodilator therapy. Perturbations of lipoprotein metabolism accompany the use of ß-blockers. Nonselective agents cause greater falls in cardioprotective high-density lipoprotein-cholesterol levels, whereas intrinsic sympathomimetic activity agents cause less or no effect and some agents, such as celiprolol, may raise HDL-cholesterol levels. Patients with renal insufficiency may take ß-blockers without additional hazard, although modest drops in renal blood flow and glomerular filtration rate have been measured, presumably from renal vasoconstriction. Dosage of the lipid-insoluble atenolol and nadolol should be reduced in patients with renal insufficiency.

α- and ß-Blockers

It is likely that ß-blockers will continue to be popular in the treatment of hypertension. If a ß-blocker is chosen, those that have intrinsic sympathomimetic activity, are more cardioselective and lipid-insoluble offer the likelihood of fewer perturbations of lipid and carbohydrate metabolism and greater patient adherence to therapy, since only one dose a day will be needed and side effects are likely minimized.

The combination of an α- and a ß-blocker in one molecule is available in the form of labetalol, which combines both α-and ß-blocking actions, in a ratio between 1:3 and 1:7. The fall in pressure mainly results from a decrease in peripheral resistance, with little or no fall in cardiac output[139] (Figure 7.100).

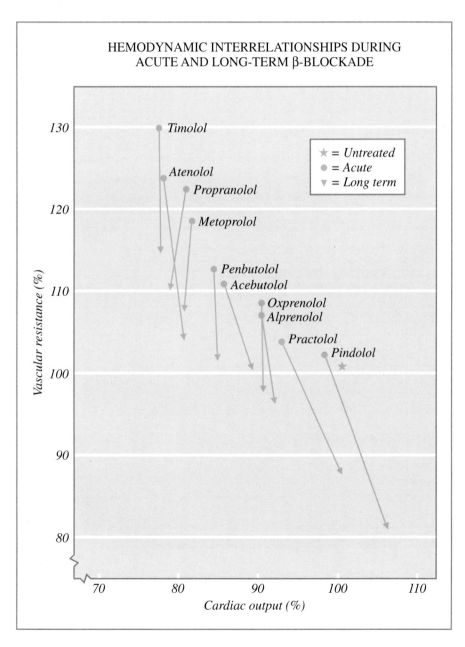

FIGURE 7.99 • Hemodynamic interrelationships during acute and long-term ß-blockade in hypertension. (Reproduced with permission. Man in't Veld AJ, Van den Meiracker AH, Schalekamp MA: *Am J Hypertens* 1988;1:91.)

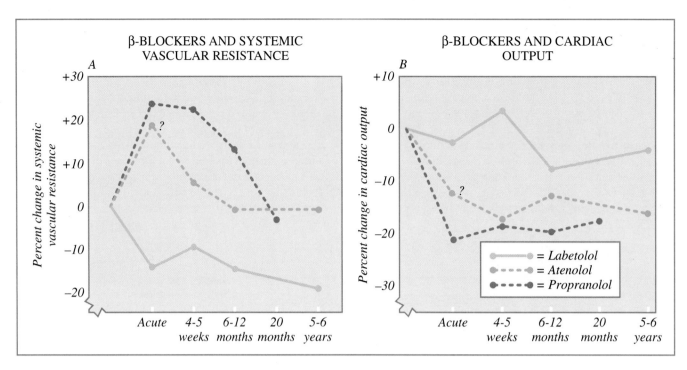

FIGURE 7.100 • Systemic vascular resistance after acute therapy (A), after approximately 1 month of therapy, after 6 to 12 months, and after 5 to 6 years of therapy with labetalol, atenolol, or propranolol. For acute labetalol, data comes from Jokes AM, Thompson FD: *Br J Clin Pharmacol* 1976;3(Suppl):789. Tsukiyama H, Otsuka K, Higuma K: *Br J Clin Pharmacol* 1982;13:269S for 4 to 5 weeks; and Lund-Johansen P: *Am J Med* 1983;75:24 for 1 to 6 years of labetalol. For atenolol, acute data estimated from Holtzman JL, Finley D, Johnson B, et al: *Clin Pharmacol Ther* 1986;40:268. The 4- to 5-week data averaged from

Tsukiyama H, Otsuka K, Higuma K: *Br J Clin Pharmacol* 1982;13:269S and Dreslinski GR, Messerli FH, Dunn FG, et al: *Circulation* 1982;65:1365. The 1- to 5-year data adapted from Lund-Johansen P: *J Cardiovasc Pharmacol* 1979;1:487. For propranolol data, refer to Tarazi RC, Dustan HP: *Am J Cardiol* 1972;29:633. For 5-week data, refer to Tsukiyama H, Otsuka K, Higuma K: *Br J Clin Pharmacol* 1982;13:269S. Cardiac output or cardiac index (B) for same groups as in (A), with same data sources. (Reproduced with permission. Opie LH: *Cardiovasc Drugs Ther* 1988;2:369.)

TABLE 7.27 • VASODILATOR DRUGS USED TO TREAT HYPERTENSION

Drug	Relative action on arteries (A) or veins (V)
Direct	
Hydralazine	A >> V
Minoxidil	A >> V
Nitroprusside	A = V
Diazoxide	A > V
Nitroglycerin	V > A
Calcium entry blockers	A >> V
Converting enzyme inhibitors	A > V
Alpha blockers	A = V

The most bothersome side effects are related to postural hypotension. Intravenous labetalol and its optical isomer, dilevalol, have been used successfully to treat hypertensive emergencies.

DIRECT VASODILATORS

Until recently, direct-acting arteriolar vasodilators were mainly used as third drugs, when a diuretic and adrenergic blocker did not control the blood pressure. However, with the availability of vasodilators of different types that can be easily tolerated when used as first or second drugs (Table 7.27), a wider and earlier application of vasodilators in therapy of hypertension has begun.

Hydralazine (Apresoline) is the only direct vasodilator available for routine use. Minoxidil (Loniten) is more potent, but it is usually reserved for patients with severe, refractory hypertension associated with renal insufficiency. Diazoxide and ni-

troprusside are given intravenously for hypertensive crises and are discussed later in this chapter.

Hydralazine

Since the early 1970's, hydralazine, in combination with a diuretic and a ß-blocker, has been used increasingly to treat more severe hypertension. The drug acts directly to relax the smooth muscle in precapillary resistance vessels with little or no effect on postcapillary venous capacitance vessels. As a result, blood pressure falls by a reduction in peripheral resistance, but in doing so a number of reactive processes activated by the arterial baroreceptor arc that blunt the decrease in pressure and cause side effects. When a diuretic is used to overcome fluid retention, and an adrenergic inhibitor is used to prevent the reflex increase in sympathetic activity and rise in renin, the vasodilator is more effective and causes few, if any, side effects (Figure 7.101).

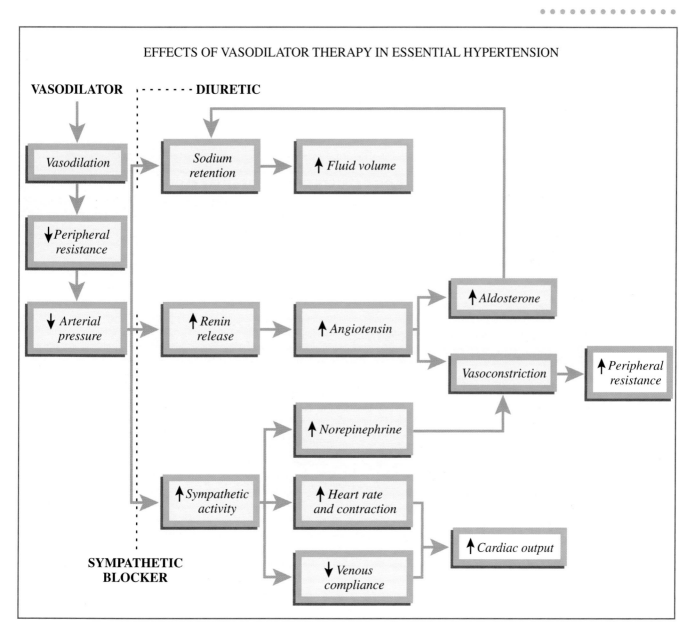

FIGURE 7.101 • Primary and secondary effects of vasodilator therapy in essential hypertension and the manner by which diuretic and ß-adrenergic blocker therapy can overcome the undesirable secondary effects. (Reproduced with permission. Koch-Weser J: *Arch Intern Med* 1974;133:1017.)

Hydralazine is given only twice a day. Its daily dosage should be kept below 400 mg to prevent the lupus-like syndrome that appears in 10% to 20% of patients who receive more. This reaction, although uncomfortable to the patient, is almost always reversible.

Minoxidil

Minoxidil, unrelated to other vasodilators, acts in a manner similar to hydralazine, but is even more effective and may be used once a day. It has been found to be particularly useful in managing patients with severe hypertension and renal insufficiency. Even more than with hydralazine, diuretics and adrenoceptor blockers must be used with minoxidil to prevent the reflex increase in cardiac output and fluid retention. The drug also causes hair to grow profusely, and the facial hirsutism precludes use of the drug in most women.

CALCIUM-ENTRY BLOCKERS

Calcium-entry blockers are being increasingly used in the treatment of hypertension. They differ in both their sites and their mode of action[140] (Table 7.28). Nifedipine and other dihydropyridine derivatives have the most attractive hemodynamic profile—the greatest peripheral vasodilatory action with little effect on cardiac conduction. However, comparative trials have shown verapamil and diltiazem to also be effective antihypertensives, with fewer side effects.

Calcium-entry blockers may cause at least an initial natriuresis, probably by causing renal vasodilation, which may obviate the need for concurrent diuretic therapy. In fact, unlike all other antihypertensive agents, their effectiveness may be reduced rather than enhanced by concomitant dietary sodium restriction, whereas most careful studies show an enhancement of their effect by concomitant diuretic therapy.[111] These agents may be particularly effective in elderly hypertensives but blacks may be somewhat less responsive.[140] Concerns about their possible effects on various hormonal and other secretory processes that involve calcium-entry seem largely unfounded and they appear to be neutral in their effects on lipids and insulin sensitivity.[141] Renin and aldosterone secretion may be reduced which may contribute to the lack of fluid retention seen with their use. Calcium-entry blockers will reduce left ventricular mass and ectopy. Nifedipine has been effectively used to reduce high levels of blood pressure quickly. Doses of 10 to 20 mg provide almost uniform reduction of blood pressure by 25% within 30 minutes.[142]

In addition to their increasing use for treatment of angina and hypertension, calcium-entry blockers have a large number of possible uses, based largely on their ability to dilate various spastic vessels and organs (Table 7.29). One of their major at-

TABLE 7.28 • PHARMACOLOGIC EFFECTS OF CALCIUM-ENTRY BLOCKERS

	Diltiazem	Verapamil	Nifedipine	Nicardipine
Heart rate	↓	↓	↑	↑
Myocardial contractility	↓	↓↓	↓	–
Nodal conduction	↓	↓↓	–	–
Peripheral vasodilation	↑	↑	↑↑	↑↑

↓ = Decrease   ↑ = Increase   – = No change

TABLE 7.29 • PROSPECTIVE USES FOR CALCIUM-ENTRY BLOCKERS

Cardiovascular	Noncardiovascular
Migraine	Asthma
Raynaud's phenomenon	Esophageal motility disorders
Nocturnal leg cramps	Myometrial hyperactivity
Subarachnoid hemorrhage	Biliary or renal colic
Ischemic stroke	Prevention of neural loss with age
Hypertrophic cardiomyopathy	
Pulmonary hypertension	
Possibly reduce platelet activation	

tributes is the virtual absence of any contraindication to their use and the relative benignity of their side effects. Except for potential conduction problems when verapamil or diltiazem is given to patients on a ß-blocker, there are almost no serious concerns about the use of calcium-entry blockers.

RENIN-ANGIOTENSIN INHIBITORS

The renin-angiotensin system may now be inhibited in four ways (Figure 7.102), three of which can now be applied clinically. The first, use of adrenergic blockers to inhibit the release of renin, was discussed earlier in this chapter. Secondly, direct inhibition of renin activity by specific renin inhibitors is being actively investigated.[143] Thirdly, blockade of angiotensin's actions by a competitive blocker is feasible in the form of saralasin, but this requires intravenous administration. Finally,

inhibition of the enzyme that converts the inactive decapeptide angiotensin I to the active octapeptide angiotensin II, is now being widely utilized with orally effective angiotensin converting enzyme (ACE) inhibitors.[144]

The first ACE inhibitor, captopril, was synthesized as a specific inhibitor of the converting enzyme that breaks the peptidyldipeptide bond in angiotensin I, preventing the enzyme from attaching to and splitting the angiotensin I structure. Because angiotensin II cannot be formed and angiotensin I is inactive, the ACE inhibitor paralyzes the renin-angiotensin system, thereby removing the effects of endogenous angiotensin II as both a vasoconstrictor and a stimulant to aldosterone synthesis. Enalapril and lisinopril, differing primarily by the absence of a sulfhydryl group, work in a similar manner but with a slower onset and a longer duration of action.

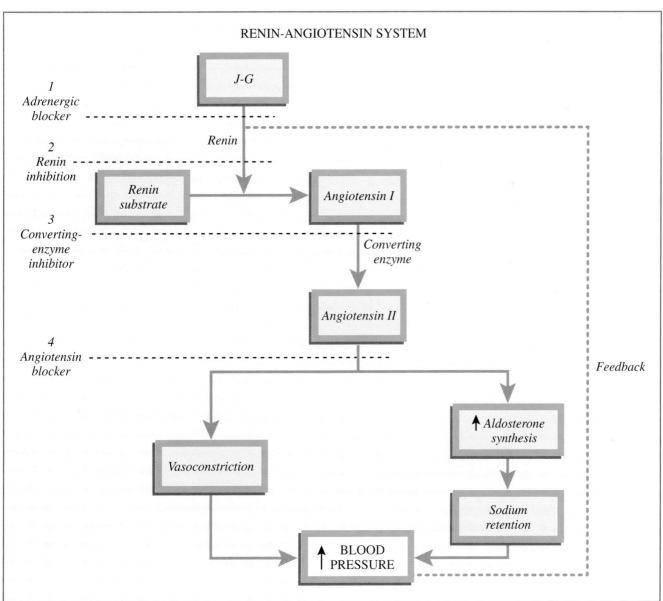

FIGURE 7.102 • Renin-angiotensin system and four sites where its activity may be inhibited.

The plasma angiotensin II levels actually come back up with chronic use of ACE inhibitors while the blood pressure remains lowered[145] suggesting that the antihypertensive effect may involve other mechanisms. The same enzyme which converts angiotensin I to angiotensin II is also responsible for inactivation of the vasodepressor hormone bradykinin. By inhibiting the breakdown of bradykinin, ACE inhibitors may increase the concentration of a vasodepressor hormone while they decrease the concentration of a vasoconstrictor hormone (Figure 7.103). Levels of vasodilatory prostaglandins may be increased simultaneously. In whatever manner they work, ACE inhibitors lower blood pressure mainly by reducing peripheral

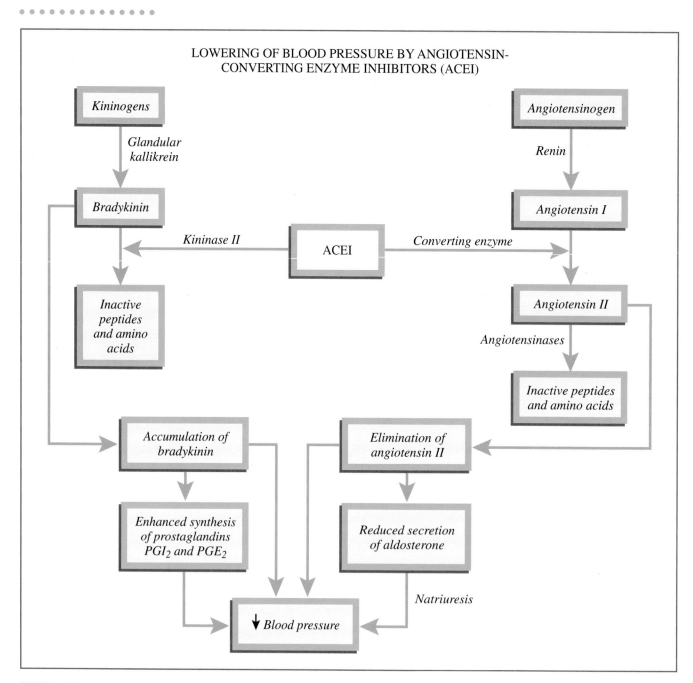

FIGURE 7.103 • Mechanisms by which angiotensin-converting enzyme inhibitors (ACEI) may lower the blood pressure.

resistance with little, if any, effect on heart rate, cardiac output, or body fluid volumes.

In patients with uncomplicated primary hypertension, ACE inhibitors provide equal or greater antihypertensive effects as a diuretic or a ß-blocker. They may be somewhat less effective in blacks[146] perhaps because blacks tend to have lower renin levels but they are equally effective in elderly and younger hypertensive patients.[147]

The initial dose of ACE inhibitor may precipitate a rather dramatic but transient fall in blood pressure, and the initial dosage should be as little as 12.5 mg bid of captopril or 5 mg once a day of enalapril or lisinopril. The response to an ACE inhibitor is usually well maintained, possibly because its suppression of aldosterone mitigates the tendency toward volume expansion that often antagonizes the effects of other antihypertensives. Nonetheless, concomitant use of a diuretic will significantly enhance the effectiveness of these agents.

ACE inhibitors may find wider use if the inability to modulate adrenal and renal responses to different levels of sodium intake, ascribed to fixed high angiotensin II levels within these tissues, turns out to be a common defect in normal and high-renin hypertensives. The defect appears to be corrected by ACE inhibitor therapy, holding the promise for a more specific form of therapy for a large portion of the hypertensive population. Similarly, ACE inhibitors may prove especially useful for patients with intraglomerular hypertension, specifically those with diabetic nephropathy or reduced renal functional mass, who may especially benefit from the reduction in efferent arteriolar resistance that follows reduction in angiotensin II. The experimental evidence for this protection is strong and the clinical evidence, although now limited, is supportive.[148]

These drugs have been a mixed blessing for patients with renovascular hypertension. On the one hand, they usually control the blood pressure effectively.[149] On the other hand, their removal of the high levels of angiotensin II may deprive the stenotic kidney of the hormonal drive to its blood flow, thereby causing a marked fall of renal perfusion. Those with solitary kidneys or bilateral disease may develop renal failure.[150]

In most studies, patients have significantly fewer adverse effects from an ACE inhibitor than from other agents.[151] The major advantages are related to the absence of effects in sites affected by other drugs. No CNS side effects, no reduction in cardiac output, and no interference with sympathetic activity are noted. Beyond the decrease in bothersome overt side effects, ACE inhibitor therapy does not produce biochemical changes that may be of even more concern, even though they are not so obvious. There are no increases in lipids, glucose,

or uric acid nor falls in potassium levels and insulin sensitivity may improve.[120]

ACE inhibitors may cause both specific and nonspecific adverse effects. Among the specific ones are rash, loss of taste, glomerulopathy manifested by proteinuria, and leukopenia. In addition, these drugs may cause a hypersensitivity reaction with angioneurotic edema or, much more commonly, a cough which, although often persistent, is not associated with pulmonary dysfunction.[152] Patients on potassium supplements or sparing agents may not be able to excrete potassium loads, and therefore may develop hyperkalemia.

These drugs are being widely used for all degrees and forms of hypertension. Their use will increase further if their particular ability to decrease intrarenal hypertension experimentally is translated into greater protection from progressive renal damage clinically. Moreover, their increasing use as unloaders in patients with congestive heart failure may be accompanied by their use in patients after myocardial infarction, if the preliminary evidence of their attenuating the development of left ventricular enlargement is confirmed.[144]

OTHER DRUGS

Other forms of antihypertensive therapy are under investigation. One that has been widely studied is the serotonin S_2-receptor blocker, ketanserin. The reduction in HMG-CoA reductase activity noted in cultured skin fibroblasts may explain the fall in low density lipoprotein (LDL) cholesterol levels reported with its use.[153] The observation that a single injection of interleukin-2 controlled the blood pressure in SHR rats for at least 6 months[154] was not confirmed in another study.[155]

SPECIAL CONSIDERATIONS IN THERAPY

The rigid, diuretic-first stepped-care approach has been broadened to include other classes of drugs for initial monotherapy following the overall individualized approach[11] (refer to Figure 7.88). A drug from any class other than direct vasodilators can be chosen. There is little overall difference in their effectiveness, but black patients tend to respond less well to ß-blockers and ACE inhibitors, whereas older ones may respond somewhat better to calcium entry blockers and diuretics.[147] The choice is then logically made on the basis of the good or bad effects of the drugs on concomitant conditions (refer to Table 7.25).

For initial therapy, vasodilatory drugs that reduce peripheral resistance are generally preferable to those that reduce cardiac output (Figure 7.104). If the first choice does not work adequately, a drug of a different class is added. For the second drug, a diuretic may be used, if it was not the first choice. If a third drug is needed, a vasodilator will usually be added. In the past, this was usually hydralazine; increasingly, it will be a calcium-entry blocker or an ACE inhibitor.

RESISTANT HYPERTENSION

Some patients do not respond well because they do not take their medications. On the other hand, what appears to be a poor response based on office of blood pressure readings may turn out to be an adequate response when home readings are used.[156] However, a number of factors may be responsible for a poor response even if the appropriate medication is taken regularly (Table 7.30). Most common is volume overload owing to either inadequate diuretic or excessive dietary sodium intake. Larger doses or more potent diuretics often bring resistant hypertension under control. On the other hand, there are a few patients whose blood pressure is resistant to therapy because of overly vigorous diuresis, which contracts vascular volume and activates both renin and catecholamines.

THE ELDERLY

In this increasingly large population, few long-term controlled data are available as to the indications for therapy and the appropriate choice of drugs. If both systolic and diastolic pressures are elevated, elderly patients should be treated in a manner similar to that for younger persons since they seem to respond as well and have no additional problems with medications.[157] Drugs with a propensity to cause postural hypotension should be avoided, and all drugs should be given in slowly increasing doses to prevent excessive lowering of the pressure. Thereby, the occasional episodes of serious cerebral ischemia and stroke related to antihypertensive therapy should be avoidable. The elderly may have many features that contribute to an increased risk of therapy (Table 7.31). Beyond all else, they must be treated slowly and gently to avoid serious adverse drug reactions.

Isolated systolic hypertension in the elderly presents a risk, particularly for strokes. Data on the effectiveness of therapy for isolated systolic hypertension have been provided by the Systolic Hypertension in the Elderly Program (SHEP) trial.[79] These data show that judicious lowering of the pressure will protect against and not precipitate cardiovascular catastrophes.

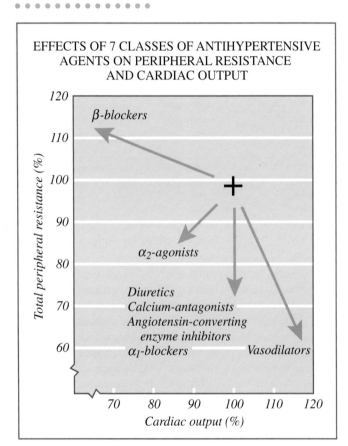

EFFECTS OF 7 CLASSES OF ANTIHYPERTENSIVE AGENTS ON PERIPHERAL RESISTANCE AND CARDIAC OUTPUT

FIGURE 7.104 • The major action of the seven classes of antihypertensive agents on peripheral resistance and cardiac output. (Reproduced with permission. Man in't Veld et al: *Am J Hypertens* 1988:1:91.)

The vessels may not be able to dilate as well as the functionally constricted, more pliant vessels of young people, so that the goal of therapy should be a systolic pressure of 150 mm Hg for people over 60 years of age.

HYPERTENSION WITH CONGESTIVE HEART FAILURE

In hypertensive patients who are in heart failure, cardiac output may fall so markedly that their blood pressure is reduced, obscuring the degree of hypertension; often, however, the diastolic pressure is elevated by intense vasoconstriction while the systolic pressure declines as a result of the reduced stroke volume. Lowering the blood pressure may, by itself, relieve the heart failure. Chronic unloading has been most efficiently accomplished with ACE inhibitors which may at the same time reduce renal function[158] (Figure 7.105). Antihypertensive agents that primarily decrease cardiac output, particularly ß-blockers, remove the heart's needed sympathetic support, and may be dangerous in the presence of heart failure.

● ● ● ● ● ● ● ● ● ● ● ● ● ● ●

TABLE 7.30 • CAUSES OF POOR RESPONSE TO ANTIHYPERTENSIVE DRUGS

Nonadherence to therapy

Drug related

Doses too low

Inappropriate combinations (for example, two centrally-acting adrenergic inhibitors)

Rapid inactivation (e.g., hydralizine)

Effects of other drugs

Sympathomimetics

Antidepressants

Adrenal steroids

Nonsteroidal anti-inflammatory drugs

Nasal decongestants

Oral contraceptives

Associated conditions

Increasing obesity

Excess alcohol intake: >30 mL/d

Renal insufficiency

Renovascular hypertension

Malignant or accelerated hypertension

Other causes of hypertension

Volume overload

Inadequate diuretic therapy

Excess sodium intake

Fluid retention from reduction of blood pressure

Progressive renal damage

(Reproduced with permission. Joint National Committee: *Arch Intern Med* 1988;148:1023.)

TABLE 7.31 • FACTORS THAT MIGHT CONTRIBUTE TO INCREASED RISK OF PHARMACOLOGIC TREATMENT OF HYPERTENSION IN THE ELDERLY

Factors	Potential complications
Diminished baroreceptor activity	Orthostatic hypotension
Decreased intravascular volume	Orthostatic hypotension, dehydration
Sensitivity to hypokalemia	Arrhythmia, muscle weakness
Decreased renal and hepatic function	Drug accumulation
Polypharmacy	Drug interactions
Central nervous system changes	Depression, confusion

HYPERTENSION WITH ISCHEMIC HEART DISEASE

The coexistence of ischemic heart disease makes antihypertensive therapy even more essential, since relief of the hypertension may ameliorate the coronary disease. Beta blockers and calcium-entry blockers are particularly useful if angina or arrhythmias are present. Caution is needed to avoid the decreased coronary perfusion that is likely responsible for the J-curve seen in multiple trials with diuretic and ß-blocker based therapy.[18] Hopefully, this problem will not occur when agents that vasodilate the coronary vessels are used in their place.

During the early phase of an acute myocardial infarction, markedly high levels of blood pressure may reflect sympathet-ic nervous hyperreactivity to pain. Cautious use of antihypertensive drugs that do not decrease cardiac output may be useful in the immediate postinfarct period, and ß-blockers without intrinsic symptommetric activity have been shown to provide long-term benefit. ACE inhibitors may turn out to prevent progressive myocardial dilation and dysfunction, especially in patients with anterior Q-wave myocardial infarction.[159]

REGRESSION OF LEFT VENTRICULAR HYPERTROPHY

In view of the multiple risks associated with significant left ventricular hypertrophy (LVH) as described earlier in this chapter, increasing interest has been directed to effects of various anti-

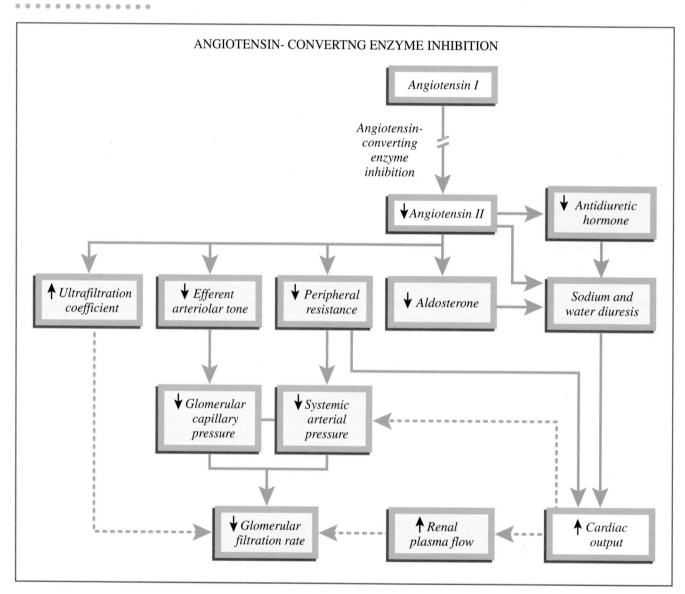

FIGURE 7.105 • Consequences of angiotensin-converting enzyme (ACE) inhibition, and compensatory events that may result. (Reproduced with permission. Suki WN: *Arch Intern Med* 1989;149:669.)

hypertensive agents on this frequent finding. Clearly, not all drugs are equal[160] (Figure 7.106). In general, diuretics and direct vasodilators have not been found to reverse left ventricular hypertrophy, whereas most other agents have done so and the degree of regression generally relates to the degree of blood pressure reduction. In a study published after Devereux's review, the calcium-entry blocker, verapamil, was shown to reduce left ventricular hypertrophy more frequently than the ß-blocker, atenolol, despite equal antihypertensive efficacy of the two agents.[161] This study in elderly hypertensive patients found that the regression of left ventricular hypertrophy increased diastolic filling and did not impair systolic function.

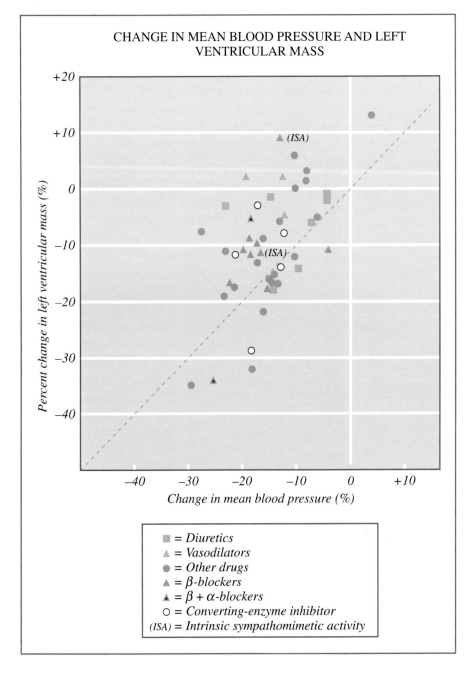

CHANGE IN MEAN BLOOD PRESSURE AND LEFT VENTRICULAR MASS

Percent change in left ventricular mass (%)

Change in mean blood pressure (%)

■ = Diuretics
▲ = Vasodilators
● = Other drugs
▲ = β-blockers
▲ = β + α-blockers
○ = Converting-enzyme inhibitor
(ISA) = Intrinsic sympathomimetic activity

FIGURE 7.106 • A significant relation exists between change in mean blood pressure and left ventricular mass induced by antihypertensive drug treatment in 47 published trials in patients with essential hypertension. Subdivision of the results by the class of antihypertensive drug used reveals that α- and/or ß-adrenoceptor blockers and angiotensin converting enzyme inhibitors were particularly likely to reduce both blood pressure and left ventricular mass. (Reproduced with permission. Devereux RB: Hypertensive Cardiac Hypertrophy. In: Laragh JH, Brenner BM eds. *Hypertension. Pathophysiology, Diagnosis, and Management, Volume 1.* New York, NY: Raven Press; 1990:359.)

THERAPY FOR HYPERTENSIVE CRISIS

Rapidly progressive damage to the arterial vasculature is demonstrable experimentally when the diastolic blood pressure exceeds 140 mm Hg, and a surge of cerebral blood flow may rapidly lead to encephalopathy (Figure 7.107). If such high pressure persists or there are signs of encephalopathy, the pressure should be lowered using parenteral agents in patients considered to be in immediate danger, or with oral agents in those who are alert and in no other acute distress (Table 7.32).

A number of drugs for this purpose are now available (Table 7.33). If diastolic blood pressure exceeds 140 mm Hg, and the patient has any complications, such as a dissecting aneurysm, a constant infusion of nitroprusside is most effective and will almost always lower the pressure to the desired level. Constant monitoring, preferably with an intra-arterial line, is mandatory. A slightly excessive dose may abruptly lower the pressure to levels that will induce hazardous hypoperfusion to vital organs. The potency and rapidity of action of nitroprusside have made it the treatment of choice for life-threatening hypertension. However, nitroprusside acts as a venous and arteriolar dilator, so that venous return and cardiac output are lowered and intracranial pressures may increase. Therefore, other parenteral agents are being more widely used, including labetalol[139] and the calcium-

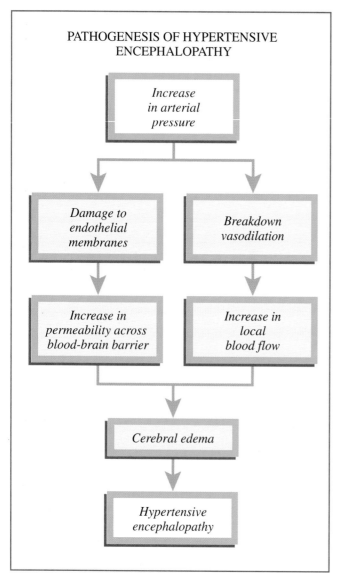

FIGURE 7.107 • The pathogenesis of hypertensive encephalopathy.

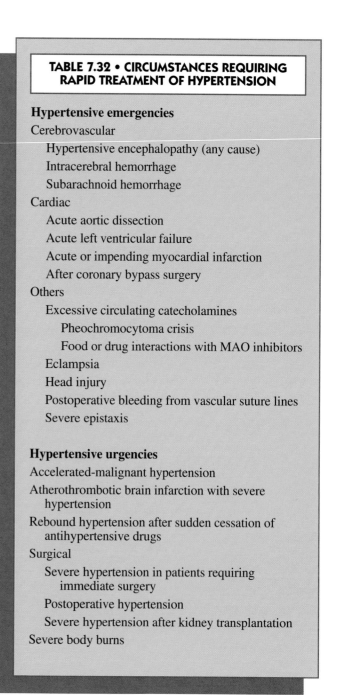

TABLE 7.32 • CIRCUMSTANCES REQUIRING RAPID TREATMENT OF HYPERTENSION

Hypertensive emergencies
Cerebrovascular
    Hypertensive encephalopathy (any cause)
    Intracerebral hemorrhage
    Subarachnoid hemorrhage
Cardiac
    Acute aortic dissection
    Acute left ventricular failure
    Acute or impending myocardial infarction
    After coronary bypass surgery
Others
    Excessive circulating catecholamines
        Pheochromocytoma crisis
        Food or drug interactions with MAO inhibitors
    Eclampsia
    Head injury
    Postoperative bleeding from vascular suture lines
    Severe epistaxis

Hypertensive urgencies
Accelerated-malignant hypertension
Atherothrombotic brain infarction with severe hypertension
Rebound hypertension after sudden cessation of antihypertensive drugs
Surgical
    Severe hypertension in patients requiring immediate surgery
    Postoperative hypertension
    Severe hypertension after kidney transplantation
Severe body burns

entry blocker nicardipine.[162] As the experimental evidence of different effects of various antihypertensive drugs on cerebral blood flow and autoregulation is translated into clinical practice, more changes in the management of patients with severe hypertension will likely be made.[163]

Oral therapy may be used for patients in less immediate danger. Almost every drug has been used and most with repeated doses will reduce high pressures, but three are now most popular (Table 7.34). The current preference is nifedipine, 5 to 10 mg by mouth or sublingually repeated in 30 minutes if need-

TABLE 7.33 • PARENTERAL DRUGS FOR TREATMENT OF HYPERTENSIVE EMERGENCY (IN ORDER OF RAPIDITY OF ACTION)			
Drug	**Dosage**	**Onset of Action**	**Adverse Effects**
Vasodilators			
• Nitroprusside (Nipride, Nitropress)	0.25–10 μg/kg/min as IV infusion	Instantaneous	Nausea, vomiting, muscle twitching, sweating, thiocyanate intoxication
• Nitroglycerin	5–100 μg/min as IV infusion	2-5 min	Tachycardia, flushing, headache, vomiting, methemoglobinemia
• Diazoxide (Hyperstat)	50–100 mg/IV bolus repeated, or 15–30 mg/min by IV infusion	2–4 min	Nausea, hypotension, flushing, tachycardia, chest pain
• Hydralazine (Apresoline)	10–20 mg IV 10–50 mg IM	10–20 min 20–30 min	Tachycardia, flushing, headache, vomiting, aggravation of angina
• Enalaprilat (Vasotec IV)	1.25–5 mg q 6 hr	15 min	Precipitous fall in blood pressure in high renin states; response variable
Adrenergic inhibitors			
• Phentolamine (Regitine)	5–15 mg IV	1–2 min	Tachycardia, flushing
• Trimethaphan (Arfonad)	0.5–5 mg/min as IV infusion	1–5 min	Paresis of bowel and bladder, orthostatic hypotension, blurred vision, dry mouth
• Esmolol (Brevifloc)	500 μg/kg/min for 4 min, then 150–300 μg/kg/min IV	1–2 min	Hypotension
• Propranolol (Inderal)	1–10 mg load; 3 ng/hr	1–2 min	ß-blocker side effects—bronchospasm, decrease cardiac output
• Labetalol (Normodyne, Trandate)	20-80 mg IV bolus every 10 min 2 mg/min IV infusion	5-10 min	Vomiting, scalp tingling, burning in throat, postural hypotension, dizziness, nausea
• Nicardipine	5-10 mg/hr IV	10 min	Tachycardia, headache, flushing, local phlebitis

ed.[142] The sublingual route provides a slower and probably, therefore, safer route. The pressure almost always falls about 25% within the first 30 minutes. Rarely, and not unexpectedly, a few patients may suffer tissue ischemia with such rapid and marked falls in pressure. A safer course for some patients, particularly if the current high pressure is simply a reflection of stopping previously effective oral medication, is simply to restart that medication, and monitor their response closely. If their nonadherence to therapy was caused by side effects, appropriate changes should be made.

Fewer patients in a hypertensive crisis are being seen, presumably because more hypertensive individuals are being recognized and treated before the disease enters this malignant course. It is hoped that the continued successful treatment of many more hypertensive patients will prevent the subtler, but more frequent, long-range sequelae of hypertension, including coronary heart disease.

THE FUTURE DIRECTION FOR THE MANAGEMENT OF HYPERTENSION

The present recognition that past therapy of hypertension has not provided protection against its major cardiovascular complications—coronary heart disease—will undoubtedly lead to considerable changes in the future management of hypertension. These changes will include the following:

- More careful measurement of the blood pressure both for diagnosis and monitoring of therapy. This will include routine use of home measurements and more widespread use of automatic ambulatory devices.

- Attention to all of the major risk factors for premature coronary disease, in particular those which may be worsened by therapy of hypertension. This will particularly include dyslipidemias and hyperinsulinemia.
- The presence of left ventricular hypertrophy and diastolic dysfunction will be more carefully assessed and therapy more directed toward their reversal.
- More aggressive use of nondrug therapies, including moderate sodium restriction and regular aerobic exercise.
- A change from the fast and furious pace of therapy now followed by many physicians to a more gradual and gentle approach using an individualized choice of therapy which will be provided in a manner to titrate the pressure down slowly to avoid hypoperfusion of vital organs.
- This gradual and gentle approach will become particularly critical as an increasing portion of elderly people with predominately systolic hypertension are begun on drug therapy based on the results of the Systolic Hypertension in the Elderly Program (SHEP) trial of 1991.
- The goal of therapy will be more carefully considered, no longer aiming for as low a pressure as can be obtained but carefully bringing the pressure down to one that will not reduce coronary perfusion. As the J curve becomes increasingly recognized, data will hopefully become available showing that the occurrence of coronary ischemia at pressures below 145/85 mmHg can be reduced with drugs which vasodilate the coronary circulation rather than using diuretics and ß-blockers, which reduce coronary blood flow.

All in all, the future of the management of hypertension looks both interesting and productive, no longer empiric and loosely controlled, but rationally and carefully monitored to ensure maximal protection against the cardiovascular complications that bedevil the hypertensive patient.

TABLE 7.34 • ORAL DRUGS FOR HYPERTENSIVE URGENCIES				
Drug	**Class**	**Dose**	**Onset**	**Duration**
Nifedipine (Procardia, Adalat)	Calcium-entry blocker	5–10 mg sublingual or swallowed	5–15 min	3–5 hr
Captopril (Capoten)	Angiotensin-converting enzyme inhibitor	6.5–50 mg	15 min	4–6 hr
Clonidine (Catapres, others)	Central sympatholytic	0.2 mg initial then 0.1 mg/hr, up to 0.8 mg total	1/2–2 hr	6–8 hr

REFERENCES

1. Pickering TG, James GD, Boddie C, et al: How common is white coat hypertension? *JAMA* 1988;259:225.

2. Waeber B, Scherrer U, Petrillo A, et al: Are some hypertensive patients overtreated? A prospective study of ambulatory bloodpressure recording. *Lancet* 1987;2:732.

3. Argentino C, Toni D, Rasura M, et al: Circadian variation in the frequency of ischemic stroke. *Stroke* 1990;21:387.

4. Gosse P, Campello G, Roudaut R, et al: High night blood pressure in treated hypertensive patients: Not harmless. *Am J Hypertens* 1988;1:195S.

5. Devereux RB, Pickering TG: Relationship between ambulatory and exercise blood pressure and cardiac structure. *Am Heart J* 1988;116:1124.

6. Floras JS, Jones JV, Hassan MO, et al: Cuff and ambulatory blood pressure in subjects with essential hypertension. *Lancet* 1981;2:107.

7. Parati G, Pomidossi G, Albini F, et al: Relationship of 24-hour blood pressure mean and variability to severity of target organ damage in hypertension. *J Hypertens* 1987;5:93.

8. Perloff D, Sokolow M, Cowan R: The prognostic value of ambulatory blood pressure. *JAMA* 1983;249:2792.

9. Levy D, Wilson PWF, Anderson KM, et al: Stratifying the patient at risk from coronary disease: New insights from the Framingham Heart Study. *Am Heart J* 1990;119:712.

10. MacMahon S, Peto R, Cutler J, et al: Blood pressure, stroke, and coronary heart disease. Part 1: Prolonged differences in blood pressure: Prospective observational studies corrected for the regression dilution bias. *Lancet* 1990;335:765.

11. 1988 Joint National Committee: The 1988 report of the Joint National Committee on Detection, Evaluation, and Treatment of High Blood Pressure. *Arch Intern Med* 1988;148:1023.

12. WHO/ISH Mild Hypertension Liaison Committee: 1989 guidelines for the management of mild hypertension: Memorandum from a WHO/ISH meeting. *J Hypertens* 1989;7:689-693.

13. McClellan W, Neel J, Owen S: Correlates of drug therapy of diastolic blood pressure between 80-89 mm Hg by physicians in the community. *Am J Hypertens* 1989;2:869.

14. British Hypertension Society: Treating mild hypertension. Agreement from the large trials. *Br Med J* 1989;298:694-98.

15. Kaplan NM: *Clinical Hypertension* 5th edition. Baltimore, Md: Williams and Wilkins; 1990.

16. Massie BM, Tubau JF, Szlachcic J, et al: Hypertensive heart disease: The critical role of left ventricular hypertrophy. *J Cardiovasc Pharmacol* 1989;13(Suppl 1):S18.

17. Dellsperger KC, Marcus ML: The effects of pressure-induced cardiac hypertrophy on the functional capacity of the coronary circulation. *Am J Hypertens* 1988;1:200.

18. Cruickshank JM: Coronary flow reserve and the J curve relation between diastolic blood pressure and myocardial infarction. *Br Med J* 1988;297:1227.

19. Savage DD, Levy D, Dannenberg AL, et al: Association of echocardiographic left ventricular mass with body size, blood pressure and physical activity (the Framingham Study). *Am J Cardiol* 1990;65:371.

20. Shepherd BFJ, Zachariah PK, Shub C: Hypertension and left ventricular diastolic function. *Mayo Clin Proc* 1989;64:1521.

21. Topol EJ, Traill TA, Fortuin NJ: Hypertensive hypertrophic cardiomyopathy of the elderly. *N Engl J Med* 1985;312:277.

22. Yusuf S, Thom T, Abbott RD: Changes in hypertension treatment and in congestive heart failure mortality in the United States. *Hypertension* 1989;13(Suppl I):I74.

23. Lusiani L, Visona A, Pagnan A: Noninvasive study of arterial hypertension and carotid atherosclerosis. *Stroke* 1990;21:410.

24. Lindeman RD, Tobin JD, Shock NW: Hypertension and the kidney. *Nephrol* 1987;47(Suppl 1):62.

25. Shulman NB, Ford CE, Hall WD, et al: Prognostic value of serum creatinine and effect of treatment of hypertension on renal function: Results from the Hypertension Detection and Follow-up Program. *Hypertension* 1989;13(Suppl 1):I80.

26. Whelton PK, Klag MJ: Hypertension as a risk factor for renal disease: review of clinical and epidemiological evidence. *Hypertension* 1989A;13(Suppl 1):I19.

27. Editorial: Catecholamines in essential hypertension. *Lancet* 1977;1:1088.

28. Lund-Johansen P: Central haemodynamics in essential hypertension at rest and during exercise: A 20-year follow-up study. *J Hypertens* 1989;7(Suppl 6):S52.

29. Guyton AC: Dominant role of the kidneys and accessory role of whole-body autoregulation in the pathogenesis of hypertension. *Am J Hypertens* 1989;2:575.

30. Wenting GJ, Man In'T Veld AJ, Schalekamp MADH: Time-course of vascular resistance changes in mineralocorticoid hypertension of man. *Clin Sci* 1981;61:97.

31. Williams RR, Hunt SC, Hasstedt SJ, et al: Current knowledge regarding the genetics of human hypertension. *J Hypertens* 1989;7(Suppl 6):S8.

32. Folkow B: Structure and function of the arteries in hypertension. *Am Heart J* 1987;114:938.

33. Lever AF: Slow pressor mechanisms in hypertension: A role for hypertrophy of resistance vessels? *J Hypertens* 1986;4:515.

34. Berridge MJ: The Croonian Lecture, 1988. Inositol lipids and calcium signalling. *Proc R Soc Lond* 1988;B234:359.

35. Intersalt Cooperative Research Group: Intersalt: An international study of electrolyte excretion and blood pressure. Results for 24-hour urinary sodium and potassium excretion. *Br Med J* 1988;297:319.

36. Weinberger MH, Miller JZ, Luft FC, et al: Definitions and characteristics of sodium sensitivity and blood pressure resistance. *Hypertension* 1986;8(Suppl 2):II127.

37. Haddy FJ: Digitalis-like circulating factor in hypertension: potential messenger between salt balance and intracellular sodium. *Cardiovasc Drug Ther* 1990;4:343.

38. Blaustein MP: Sodium/calcium exchange and the control of contractility in cardiac muscle and vascular smooth muscle. *J Cardiovasc Pharmacol* 1988;12(Suppl 5):S56.

39. Garay R: Topology of Na+ transport abnormalities in erythrocytes from essential hypertensive patients. A first step towards the diagnosis and specific treatment of different forms of primary hypertension. *Cardiovasc Drug Ther* 1990;4:373.

40. Postnov YV: An approach to the explanation of cell membrane alteration in primary hypertension. *Hypertension* 1990;15:332.

41. Brenner BM, Garcia DL, Anderson S: Glomeruli and blood pressure. Less of one, more the other? *Am J Hypertens* 1988;1:335.

42. Sealey JE, Blumenfeld JD, Bell GM, et al: On the renal basis of essential hypertension: Nephron heterogeneity with discordant renin secretion and sodium excretion causing a hypertensive vasoconstriction-volume relationship. *J Hypertens* 1988;6:763.

43. Hollenberg NK, Williams GH: Abnormal renal function, sodium-volume homeostasis, and renin system behavior in normal-renin essential hypertension. In: Laragh JH, Brenner BM, eds. *Hypertension. Pathophysiology, Diagnosis, and Management.* New York: Raven Press; 1990:1349.

44. Ferrannini E, Buzzigoli G, Bonadonna R, et al: Insulin resistance in essential hypertension. *N Engl J Med* 1987;317:350.

45. Swislocki ALM, Hoffman BB, Reaven GM: Insulin resistance, glucose intolerance and hyperinsulinemia in patients with hypertension. *Am J Hypertens* 1989;2:419.

46. Bobik A, Grooms A, Millar JA, et al: Growth factor activity of endothelin on vascular smooth muscle. *Am J Physiol* 1990;258:C408.

47. Luscher TF, Yang Z, Diederich D, et al: Endothelium-derived vasoactive substances: potential role in hypertension, atherosclerosis, and vascular occlusion. *J Cardiovasc Pharmacol* 1989;14(Suppl 6):S63-S69.

48. Criqui MH, Langer RD, Reed DM: Dietary alcohol, calcium, and potassium. Independent and combined effects on blood pressure. *Circulation* 1989;80:609.

49. Witteman JCM, Willett WC, Stampfer MJ, et al: Relation of moderate alcohol consumption and risk of systemic hypertension in women. *Am J Cardiol* 1990;65:633.

50. Klatsky AL, Armstrong MA, Friedman GD: Alcohol and cardiovascular deaths. *Circulation* 1989;80(Suppl II):II-614.

51. Camargo CA Jr: Moderate alcohol consumption and stroke. The epidemiologic evidence. *Stroke* 1989;20:1611.

52. Woods JW: Oral contraceptives and hypertension. *Hypertension* 1988;11(Suppl II):II-11.

53. Lim KG, Isles CG, Hodsman GP, et al: Malignant hypertension in women of childbearing age and its relation to the contraceptive pill. *Br Med J* 1987;294:1057.

54. Knopp RH: The effects of postmenopausal estrogen therapy on the incidence of arteriosclerotic vascular disease. *Obstet Gynecol* 1988;72:23S.

55. Anderson S, Brenner BM: Progressive renal disease: A disorder of adaptation. *Q J Med* 1989;70:185.

56. Parving H-H, Hommel E, Smidt UM: Protection of kidney function and decrease in albuminuria by captopril in insulin dependent diabetics with nephropathy. *Br Med J* 1988;297:1086.

57. Parving H-H, Andersen AR, Smidt, UM, et al: Effect of antihypertensive treatment on kidney function in diabetic nephropathy. *Br Med J* 1987;294:1443.

58. Working Group on Renovascular Hypertension: Detection, evaluation, and treatment of renovascular hypertension. *Arch Intern Med* 1987;147:820.

59. Vetrovec GW, Landwehr DM, Edwards VL: Incidence of renal artery stenosis in hypertensive patients undergoing coronary angiography. *J Interven Cardiol* 1989;2:2.

60. Hricik DE: Angiotensin-converting enzyme inhibitor in renovascular hypertension: the narrowing gap between functional renal failure and progressive renal atrophy. *J Lab Clin Med* 1990;115:8.

61. Muller FB, Sealey JE, Case DB, et al: The captopril test for identifying renovascular disease in hypertensive patients. *Am J Med* 1986;80:633.

62. Geyskes GG, Oei HY, Puylaert CBAJ, et al: Renovascular hypertension identified by captopril-induced changes in the renogram. *Hypertension* 1987;9:451.

63. Young WF Jr, Hogan MJ, Klee GG, et al: Primary aldosteronism: Diagnosis and treatment. *Mayo Clin Proc* 1990;65:96.

64. Ross EJ, Lynch DC: Cushing's syndrome-killing disease: Discriminatory value of signs and symtoms aiding early diagnosis. *Lancet* 1982;2:642.

65. Carpenter PC: Cushing's Syndrome: Update of diagnosis and management. *Mayo Clin Proc* 1986;61:49.

66. Heuser D, Guggenberger H, Fretschner R: Acute blood pressure increase during the perioperative period. *Am J Cardiol* 1989;63:26C.

67. Weinstein GS, Zabetakis PM, Clavel A, et al: The renin-angiotensin system is not responsible for hypertension following coronary artery bypass grafting. *Ann Thorac Surg* 1987;43:74.

68. Starling RC, Cody RJ: Cardiac transplant hypertension. *Am J Cardiol* 1990;65:106.

69. Cutler JA, MacMahon SW, Furberg CD: Controlled clinical trials of drug treatment for hypertension. A review. *Hypertension* 1989; 13(Suppl. I):1.

70. Littenberg B, Garber AM, Sox HC Jr: Screening for hypertension. *Ann Intern Med* 1990;112:192.

71. Hypertension Detection and Follow-up Program Cooperative Research Group: The effect of antihypertensive drug treatment on mortality in the presence of resting electrocardiographic abnormalities at baseline: The HDFP experience. *Circulation* 1984;70:99.

72. Multiple Risk Factor Intervention Trial Research Group: Baseline rest electrocardiographic abnormalities, antihypertensive treatment, and mortality in the Multiple Risk Factor Intervention Trial. *Am J Cardiol* 1985;55:1.

73. Medical Research Council Working Party: MRC trial of treatment of mild hypertension: Principal results. *Br Med J* 1985;291:97.

74. IPPPSH Collaborative Group: Cardiovascular risk and risk factors in a randomized trial of treatment based on the beta-blocker oxprenolol: The International Prospective Primary Prevention Study in Hypertension (IPPPSH). *J Hypertens* 1985.3:379.

75. Wilhelmsen L, Berglund G, Elmfeldt D, et al: Beta-blockers versus diuretics in hypertensive men: Main results from the HAPPHY trial. *J Hypertens* 1987;5:561.

76. Collins R, Peto R, MacMahon S, et al: Blood pressure, stroke and coronary heart disease. Part II, short-term reductions in blood pressure: Overview of randomised drug trials in their epidemiological context. *Lancet* 1990;335:827.

77. Curb JD, Schneider K, Taylor JO, et al: Antihypertensive drug side effects in the hypertension detection and follow-up program. *Hypertension* 1988;11(Suppl. II):11.

78. Management Committee: The Australian therapeutic trial in mild hypertension. *Lancet* 1980;1:1261.

79. SHEP Research Group: Prevention of stroke by antihypertensive drug treatment in older persons with isolated systolic hypertension. *JAMA* 1991; 265:3255.

80. Multiple Risk Factor Intervention Trial Research Group: Mortality rates after 10.5 years of participants in the Multiple Risk Factor Intervention Trial. Findings related to a priori hypotheses of the trial. *JAMA* 1990;263:1795.

81. Samuelsson O: Experiences from hypertension trials. Impact of other risk factors. *Drugs* 1988;36(Suppl. 3):9.

82. Epstein FH: Proceedings of the XVth International Congress of Therapeutics, September 5-9, 1979. Brussels: *Excerpta Medica.*

83. Alderman MH, Ooi WL, Madhavan S, et al: Treatment-induced blood pressure reduction and the risk of myocardial infarction. *JAMA* 1989;262:920.

84. Strandgaard S, Haunso S: Why does antihypertensive treatment prevent stroke but not myocardial infarction? *Lancet* 1987;2:658.

85. Pepi M, Alimento M, Maltagliati A, et al: Cardiac hypertrophy in hypertension. Repolarization abnormalities elicited by rapid lowering of pressure. *Hypertension* 1988;11:84.

86. Alderman MH, Lamport B: Withdrawal of drug therapy in the treatment of hypertension. In: Kaplan NM, Brenner BM, Laragh JH, eds. *Perspectives in Hypertension, Volume 3, New Therapeutic Strategies in Hypertension.* New York: Raven Press 1989:171.

87. Stamler R, Stamler J, Gosch FC, et al: Primary prevention of hypertension by nutritional-hygienic means. *JAMA* 1989;262:1801.

88. Hypertension Prevention Trial Research Group: The hypertension prevention trial: Three-year effects of dietary changes on blood pressure. *Arch Intern Med* 1990;150:153.

89. Stamler R, Stamler J, Grimm R, et al: Nutritional therapy for high blood pressure. Final report of a four-year randomized controlled trial-the hypertension control program. *JAMA* 1987;257:1484.

90. Oberman A, Wassertheil-Smoller S, Langford HG, et al: Pharmacologic and nutritional treatment of mild hypertension: Changes in cardiovascular risk status. *Ann Intern Med* 1990;112:89.

91. Berglund A, Andersson OK, Berglund G, et al: Antihypertensive effect of diet compared with drug treatment in obese men with mild hypertension. *Br Med J* 1989;299:480.

92. Staessen J, Fagard R, Lijnen P, et al: Body weight, sodium intake and blood pressure. *J Hypertens* 1989;7(Suppl. 1):S19.

93. Rocchini AP, Key J, Bondie D, et al: The effect of weight loss on the sensitivity of blood pressure to sodium in obese adolescents. *N Engl J Med* 1989;321:580.

94. MacGregor GA, Markandu ND, Sagnella GA, et al: Double-blind study of three sodium intakes and long-term effects of sodium restriction in essential hypertension. *Lancet* 1989;2:1244.

95. Cappuccio FP.MacGregor GA: Does potassium supplementation lower blood pressure? A meta-analysis of published trials. *J Hypertens* 1991; 9:465.

96. Khaw K- T, Barrett-Connor E: Dietary potassium and stroke-associated mortality. A 12-year prospective population study. *N Engl J Med* 1987;316:235.

97. Whelton PK, Klag MJ: Magnesium and blood pressure: Review of the epidemiologic and clinical trial experience. *Am J Cardiol* 1989b;63:26G.

98. Zoccali C, Mallamaci F, Cuzzola F, et al: Mechanisms of hypercalciuria in essential hypertension. *J Hypertens* 1989; 7(Suppl. 6):S406.

99. Cappuccio FP, Siami A, Strazzullo P: Oral calcium supplementation and blood pressure: An overview of randomized controlled trials. *J Hypertens* 1989;7:941.

100. Rouse IL, Beilin LJ, Mahoney DP, et al: Nutrient intake, blood pressure, serum and urinary prostaglandins and serum thromboxane B2 in a controlled trial with a lacto-ovo-vegetarian diet. *J Hypertens* 1986;4:241.

101. Knapp HR, FitzGerald GA: The antihypertensive effects of fish oil. A controlled study of polyunsaturated fatty acid supplements in essential hypertension. *N Engl J Med* 1989;320:1037.

102. Sacks FM: Dietary fats and blood pressure: A critical review of the evidence. *Nutr Rev* 1989;47:291.

103. Swain JF, Rouse IL, Curley CB, et al: Comparison of the effects of oat bran and low-fiber wheat on serum lipoprotein levels and blood pressure. *N Engl J Med* 1990;322:147.

104. Parillo M, Coulston A, Hollenbeck C, et al: Effect of a low fat diet on carbohydrate metabolism in patients with hypertension. *Hypertension* 1988;11:244.

105. Sharp DS, Benowitz NL: Pharmacoepidemiology of the effect of caffeine on blood pressure. *Clin Pharmacol Ther* 1990;47:57.

106. Moore RD, Levine DM, Southard J, et al: Alcohol consumption and blood pressure in the 1982 Maryland hypertension survey. *Am J Hypertens* 1990;3:1.

107. Jackson R, Scragg R, Beaglehole R: CHD risk associated with regular and acute consumption of alcohol. *Circulation* 1990;81:9.

108. Nelson L, Jennings GL, Esler MD, et al: Effect of changing levels of physical activity on blood-pressure and haemodynamics in essential hypertension. *Lancet* 1986;2:473.

109. McGrady A, Higgins JT Jr: Prediction of response to biofeedback-assisted relaxation in hypertensives: Development of a hypertensive predictor profile (HYPP). *Psychosomatic Med* 1989;51:277.

110. Stewart AL, Greenfield S, Hays RD, et al: Functional status and well-being of patients with chronic conditions. Results from the Medical Outcomes study. *JAMA* 1989;262:907.

111. Burris JF, Weir MR, Oparil S, et al: An assessment of diltiazem and hydrochlorothiazide in hypertension. *JAMA* 1990;263:1507.

112. McVeigh G, Galloway D, Johnston D: The case for low dose diuretics in hypertension: Comparison of low and conventional doses of cyclopenthiazide. *Br Med J* 1988;297:95.

113. Prisant LM, Beall SP, Nichoalds GE, et al: Biochemical, endocrine, and mineral effects of indapamide in black women. *J Clin Pharmacol* 1990;30:121.

114. Uehara Y, Shirahase H, Nagata T, et al: Radical scavengers of indapamide in prostacyclin synthesis in rat smooth muscle cell. *Hypertension* 1990;15:216.

115. Morgan DG, Davidson C: Hypokalemia and diuretics: An analysis of publications. *Br Med J* 1980;280:905.

116. Holland OB, Kuhnert L, Pollard J, et al: Ventricular ectopic activity with diuretic therapy. *Am J Hypertens* 1988;1:380.

117. Lipworth BJ, McDevitt DG, Struthers AD: Electrocardiographic changes induced by inhaled salbutamol after treatment with bendrofluazide: Effects of replacement therapy with potassium, magnesium and triamterene. *Clin Sci* 1990;78:255.

118. Waller PC, Ramsay LE: Predicting acute gout in diuretic-treated hypertensive patients. *J Human Hypertension* 1989;3:457.

119. Weidmann P, Uehlinger DE, Gerber A: Antihypertensive treatment and serum lipoproteins. *J Hypertens* 1985;3:297.

120. Pollare T, Lithell H, Berne C: A comparison of the effects of hydrochlorothiazide and captopril on glucose and lipid metabolism in patients with hypertension. *N Engl J Med* 1989a;321:868.

121. LaCroix AZ, Wienpahl J, White LR, et al: Thiazide diuretic agents and the incidence of hip fracture. *N Engl J Med* 1990;322:286.

122. Medical Research Council Working Party on Mild to Moderate Hypertension: Adverse reactions to bendrofluazide and propranolol for the treatment of mild hypertension. *Lancet* 1981;2:539.

123. Participating Veterans Administration Medical Centers: Low doses v standard dose of reserpine. *JAMA* 1982;248:2471.

124. Fouad FM, Nakashima Y, Tarazi RC, et al: Reversal of left ventricular hypertrophy in hypertensive patients treated with methyldopa. *Am J Cardiol* 1982;49:795.

125. Kaplowitz N, Aw TY, Simon FR, et al: Drug-induced hepatotoxicity. *Ann Intern Med* 1986;104:826.

126. Houston MC: Abrupt cessation of treatment in hypertension: Consideration of clinical features, mechanisms, prevention and management of the discontinuation syndrome. *Am Heart J* 1981;102:415.

127. Schmidt GR, Schuna AA, Goodfriend TL: Transdermal clonidine compared with hydrochlorothiazide as monotherapy in elderly hypertensive males. *J Clin Pharmacol* 1989;29:133.

128. Zeller KR, Kuhnert LV, Matthews C: Rapid reduction of severe asymptomatic hypertension. A prospective, controlled trial. *Arch Intern Med* 1989;149:2186.

129. Franks P, Harp J, Bell B: Randomized, controlled trial of clonidine for smoking cessation in a primary care setting. *JAMA* 1989;262:3011.

130. Grimm RH Jr: α_1-antagonists in the treatment of hypertension. *Hypertension* 1989;13(Suppl. I):1.

131. Pollare T, Lithell H, Selinus I, Berne C: Application of prazosin is associated with an increase of insulin sensitivity in obese patients with hypertension. *Diabetologia* 1988;31:415.

132. Wikstrand J, Warnold I, Olsson G, et al: Primary prevention with metoprolol in patients with hypertension. Mortality results from the MAPHY study. *JAMA* 1988;259:1976.

133. Parati G, Ravogli A, Bragato R, et al: Clinical and hemodynamic effects of celiprolol in essential hypertension. *J Cardiovasc Pharmacol* 1989;14(Suppl.7):S14.

134. Dahlof C, Dimenas E: Side effects of β-blocker treatments as related to the central nervous system. *Am J Med Sci.* 1990;229:236.

135. Man in't Veld AJ, Van den Meiracker AH, Schalekamp MA: Do beta-blockers really increase peripheral vascular resistance? Review of the literature and new observations under basal conditions. *Am J Hypertens* 1988;1:91.

136. Serlin MM, Orme ML'E, Baber NA, et al: Propranolol in the control of blood pressure: A dose-response study. *Clin Pharmacol Ther* 1980;27:586.

137. Duncan JJ, Vaandrager H, Farr JE, et al: Effect of intrinsic sympathomimetic activity on the ability of hypertensive patients to derive a cardiorespiratory training effect during chronic β-blockade. *Am J Hypertens* 1990;3:302.

138. Psaty BM, Koepsell TD, Wagner EH, et al: The relative risk of incident coronary heart disease associated with recently stopping the use of β-blockers. *JAMA* 1990;263:1653.

139. Goa KL, Benfield P, Sorkin EM: Labetalol: A reappraisal of its pharmacology, pharmacokinetics and therapeutic use in hypertension and ischaemic heart disease. *Drugs* 1989;37:583.

140. Kaplan NM: Calcium entry blockers in the treatment of hypertension. Current status and future prospects. *JAMA* 1989;26:817.

141. Pollare T, Lithell H, Morlin C, et al: Metabolic effects of diltiazem and atenolol: Results from a randomized, double-blind study with parallel groups. *J Hypertens* 1989b;7:551.

142. Jaker M, Atkin S, Soto M, et al: Oral nifedipine vs oral clonidine in the treatment of urgent hypertension. *Arch Intern Med* 1989;149:260.

143. Bursztyn M, Gavras I, Tifft CP, et al: Effects of a novel renin inhibitor in patients with essential hypertension. *J Cardiovasc Pharmacol* 1990;15:493.

144. Gavras H: Angiotensin converting enzyme inhibition and its impact on cardiovascular disease. *Circulation* 1990;81:381.

145. Waeber B, Nussberger J, Juillerat L, et al: Angiotensin converting enzyme inhibition: Discrepancy between antihypertensive effect and suppression of enzyme activity. *J Cardiovasc Pharmacol* 1989;14(Suppl. 4):S53.

146. Weinberger MH: Blood pressure and metabolic responses to hydrochlorothiazide, captopril, and the combination in black and white mild-to-moderate hypertensive patients. *J Cardiovasc Pharmacol* 1985;7:S52.

147. Kaplan NM: Critical comments on recent literature. Age and the response to antihypertensive drugs. *Am J Hypertens* 1989;2:213.

148. Keane WF, Anderson S, Aurell M, et al: Angiotensin converting enzyme inhibitors and progressive renal insufficiency. *Ann Intern Med* 1989;111:503.

149. Hollenberg NK: The treatment of renovascular hypertension: Surgery, angioplasty, and medical therapy with converting-enzyme inhibitors. *Am J Kid Dis* 1987;10(Suppl.1):52.

150. Wenting GJ, Derkx FHM, Tan-Tjiong L, et al: Risks of angiotensin converting enzyme inhibition in renal artery stenosis. *Kidney Int* 1987;31(Suppl. 20):S-180.

151. Schoenberger JA, Testa M, Ross AD, et al: Efficacy, safety, and quality-of-life assessment of captopril antihypertensive therapy in clinical practice. *Arch Intern Med* 1990;150:301.

152. Boulet L-P, Milot J, Lampron N, Lacourciere Y: Pulmonary function and airway responsiveness during long-term therapy with captopril. *JAMA* 1989;261:413.

153. Suzukawa M, Nakamura H: Effects of ketanserin tartrate on 3-hydroxy, 3-methylglutaryl coenzymea reductase activity in cultured human skin fibroblasts. *Cardiovasc Drugs Ther* 1990;4:69.

154. Tuttle RS, Boppana DP: Antihypertensive effect of interleukin-2. *Hypertension* 1990;15:89.

155. Pascual DW, Jin H, Bost KL, et al: Interleukin-2 does not attenuate hypertension in spontaneously hypertensive rats. *Hypertension* 1990;16:468.

156. Mejia AD, Egan BM, Schork NJ, et al: Artefacts in measurement of blood pressure and lack of target organ involvement in the assessment of patients with treatment-resistant hypertension. *Ann Intern Med* 1990;112:270.

157. Goldstein G, Materson BJ, Cushman WC, et al: Treatment of hypertension in the elderly: II. Cognitive and behavioral function. Results of a Department of Veterans Affairs Cooperative Study. *Hypertension* 1990;15:361.

158. Suki WN: Renal hemodynamic consequences of angiotensin-converting enzyme inhibition in congestive heart failure. *Arch Intern Med* 1989;149:669.

159. Moss AJ, Benhorin J: Prognosis and management after a first myocardial infarction. *N Engl J Med* 1990;322:743.

160. Devereux RB: Hypertensive cardiac hypertrophy: In: Laragh JH, Brenner BM, eds. *Hypertension. Pathophysiology, Diagnosis, and Management.* New York: Raven Press 1990:359.

161. Shulman SP, Weiss JL, Becker LC, et al: The effects of antihypertensive therapy on left ventricular mass in elderly patients. *N Engl J Med* 1990;322:1350.

162. Wallin JD: Intravenous nicardipine hydrochloride: Treatment of patients with severe hypertension. *Am Heart J* 1990;119:434.

163. Barry DI: Cerebrovascular aspects of antihypertensive treatment. *Am J Cardiol* 1989;63:14C.

index

Aspergillosis, after cardiac transplantation, 6.69
Aspirin
    after aortocoronary bypass surgery, 6.12
    and atrial fibrillation, 3.40
    for non-Q-wave infarcts, 1.60
    for pericarditis, 1.74
    in PTCA, 5.8, 5.24
    for stable angina, 1.25–1.26
        cyclooxygenase inhibition, **1.26**
        side effects, *1.27*
    See also Thrombolytic therapy.
Asystole, ventricular, hypersensitive carotid sinus syndrome, 3.35
Atenolol, lipid solubility, 7.87–7.88
Atherectomy, 5.28–5.32, **5.30–5.32**
Atherogenesis, and lipoproteins, 4.18–4.20, **4.18–4.21**
Atheroma, in hypertension, 7.27
Atherosclerosis
    in angina, 1.3
    and aortocoronary bypass surgery, 6.12
    and hypertension, 7.22, **7.22**
Athletes, heart block, 3.68
ATPase
    myosin, in heart failure, 2.12, 2.14
    Na$^+$,K$^+$-
        digoxin effects, 2.27
        in hypertension, 7.41
Atrial natriuretic factor, 7.43, **7.43**
    in heart failure, 2.15, 2.19, 2.22, *2.22*
    in hypertension, 7.43, **7.43**
Atrial septal defect, balloon catheterization, 5.41
Atrioventricular (AV) node
    anatomy, 3.3, **3.5**
    beta-blockers, 1.19
    calcium antagonists, 1.20
    junction escape beats, 3.44–3.45, **3.44**
    junctional rhythm, 3.45
    nonparoxysmal junctional tachycardia, 3.45, **3.45**
    tachycardia
        reentrant, 3.45–3.48, **3.46**, 3.47
        temporary pacemakers, 3.27
Atrium
    fibrillation, 3.39–3.43, **3.39–3.42**
        septal defect, 3.39
    flutter, 3.38–3.39, **3.38**
    tachycardia, 3.43–3.44, **3.43**
Atropine
    for hypersensitive carotid sinus syndrome, 3.36
    for sinus bradycardia, 3.34
Australian Therapeutic Trial, 7.64
Azothioprine, after cardiac transplantation, 6.65

*b*acterial infections, after cardiac transplantation, 6.69
Balloon
    dilatation. *See* Angioplasty, percutaneous transluminal coronary (PTCA).
    pump, intra-aortic (IABP), for left ventricular dysfunction, 6.44–6.46, **6.46**, *6.45*
Baroreceptor reflexes
    in heart failure, 2.18, 2.21
    and hypertension, 7.3
Beta-blockers. *See* Adrenoceptor blocking drugs.

Bethanidine, 7.84
Bigeminy, 3.58
Bile acids
    in cholesterol metabolism, 4.3–4.4
    sequestrant drugs, 4.49–4.50, **4.49**, 4.50
        for hypercholesterolemia, 4.59–4.61
    See also Hyperlipidemia.
Binswanger's disease, 7.27
Biofeedback, and hypertension, 7.74
Biopsy, myocardial, 6.67
Bjork-Shiley valve, **6.14**
Blood flow, coronary, nitrate effects, 1.12
Blood groups in cardiac transplantation, 6.55
Blood pressure
    in hypertension, 7.65–7.69, **7.64–7.68**
    and infarct expansion, **1.76**
    measurement, 7.3–7.11, **7.3–7.5**
        out-of-office readings, 7.3–7.9, **7.6, 7.8**, *7.7–7.11*
    nitrate effects, 1.28
Blood urea nitrogen (BUN), aspirin effects, 1.26
Bradycardia, sinus nodal, 3.34–3.35, **3.35**
Bradykinin, and ACE inhibitors, 7.94
Brain
    death, 6.54–6.55, *6.55*
    in hypertension, 7.27
Bretylium, 3.12, 3.20–3.21
Bucindolol, 2.47
Bundle branch block
    in myocardial infarction, 1.77–1.78
    reentrant ventricular tachycardia, 3.66
Bypass Angioplasty Revascularization Investigation (BARI), 5.12
Bypass graft surgery, and PTCA. *See* Angioplasty, percutaneous transluminal coronary (PTCA)

*C*affeine
    and hypertension, 7.74
    and premature atrial complexes, 3.38
    and tachycardias, 3.33, 3.34
Calcium
    binding, in heart failure, 2.12
    in cardiac electrophysiology, 3.3
    channel blockers
        and antiarrhythmic drugs, 3.12
        and heart failure, 2.10
        in hypertension, 7.92–7.93, *7.92*
        for hypertrophic cardiomyopathy, 2.62, **2.62**, 2.73
        and infarct expansion, 1.76
        for left ventricular hypertrophy, 7.99
        for non-Q-wave infarcts, 1.60
        for preexcitation syndrome, 3.55
        for pulmonary hypertension, 2.75
        sinus bradycardia, 3.34
        for stable angina, 1.20–1.25, **1.20–1.23**, *1.24*
            side effects, *1.25*
        for unstable angina, 1.29
        for variant angina, 1.34
    and diuretic therapy, 7.83
    kinetics, in heart failure, 2.12–2.14, **2.13, 2.14**
    in primary hypertension, 7.38–7.43, **7.42, 7.43**
    supplementation, 7.72–7.74, **7.74**
    in vascular hypertrophy, 7.36

for sinus bradycardia, 3.34
Isosorbide dinitrate
    for heart failure, 2.35–2.38
    for stable angina, 1.16
    for unstable angina, 1.28

*K*ent bundles, 3.50
Ketanserin, 7.95
Kidney
    and ACE inhibitors, 2.45–2.46
    failure, and constrictive pericarditis, 2.65
    in hypertension, 7.28–7.29, **7.28**
    See also Renal.

*L*abetalol, for hypertensive crisis, 7.100
Laser ablation of plaque, 5.32–5.36, **5.32–5.35**
Lauric acid, 4.40
Lead intoxication, and hypertension, 7.50
Lecithin-cholesterol acyl transferase (LCAT), 4.13
Left ventricular
    diastolic function, 2.60–2.66
        hypertrophic cardiomyopathy, 2.61–2.62, **2.60–2.63**
            restrictive cardiomyopathy and constrictive pericarditis, 2.62–2.65, **2.63–2.65**
    hypertrophy, and hypertension, 7.23–7.26, 7.98–7.99, **7.26, 7.99**
    outflow tract obstruction (LVOTO), 6.21–6.23, **6.22–6.24**
    systolic dysfunction, 2.25–2.49, **2.25**
        ACE inhibitors, 2.41–2.47, **2.42–2.45**, *2.41–2.46*
        adrenoceptor antagonists, 2.47–2.48, **2.47**, 2.48, *2.49*
        calcium channel blocking drugs, 2.39–2.41, **2.40**, 2.41, *2.39*
        diuretics, 2.31–2.34, **2.31–2.34**, *2.30–2.33*
        flosequinan, 2.38–2.39, **2.38**, 2.39
        neurohormonal antagonists, 2.41
        nitrates and hydralazine, 2.35–2.38, **2.35–2.37**, *2.37*
        pharmacologic treatment of stable heart failure, 2.26, 2.27
        positive inotropic agents, 2.26–2.31
            digoxin, 2.26–2.29, **2.27–2.29**, *2.27–2.29*
            cyclic AMP-dependent, 2.29–2.31, **2.30**, *2.29–2.31*
            vasodilators, 2.34–2.35
Legionella pneumonia, 6.69
Leukotrienes, and angina, 1.3
Levarterenol, 2.58, 2.59
Lidocaine
    antiarrhythmic actions, 3.11, 3.17
    and heart failure, 2.10
Lillehei-Kaster valves, **6.14**
Linoleic acid, 4.40, 4.42–4.43
Lipid Research Clinics Coronary Primary Prevention Trial, 4.28–4.29, **4.28**
    bile acid sequestrants, 4.49
Lipoprotein lipase, 4.7, 4.11
    in high-carbohydrate diets, 4.43
    in hypertriglyceridemia, 4.36
Lipoproteins
    alcohol effects, 4.45, **4.45**
    and atherogenesis, 4.18–4.20, **4.18–4.21**
    and beta-blockers, 7.89
    in hypertriglyceridemia, 4.62

metabolism, 4.4–4.13
    apolipoproteins, 4.6–4.7, **4.7**, *4.7*
    chylomicrons, 4.7–4.9, **4.7–4.9**
    high density lipoproteins (HDL), 4.12–4.13, **4.15–4.17**
    low density lipoproteins (LDL), 4.12, **4.12–4.14**
    and dietary cholesterol, 4.37–4.38, **4.38**
    and drug therapy, 4.49–4.51, 4.56–4.59
    very low density lipoproteins (VLDL), 4.11, **4.10, 4.11**
        familial dysbetalipoproteinemia, 4.70–4.71
    in obesity, 4.40–4.41
    profile analysis, 4.31–4.33, **4.32, 4.33**, *4.33*
    structure, 4.6
Liquid protein diet, and ventricular tachycardia, 3.65
Lisinopril
    for heart failure, 2.42
    for hypertension, 7.93
Lithium, and sinus bradycardia, 3.34
Liver
    cholesterol metabolism, 4.3–4.4
    and hyperlipidemia, 4.35
Long QT syndrome, 3.7
    and ventricular tachycardia, 3.63–3.65, **3.64**
Lovastatin, 4.50, 4.51
    for familial combined hyperlipidemia, 4.66
    for familial dysbetalipoproteinemia, 4.71
    for hypoalphalipoproteinemia, 4.73
Lown-Ganong-Levine syndrome, 3.51
Lysolecithin, in cholesterol metabolism, 4.3

*M*agnesium
    in diuretic therapy, 7.81
    in hypertension, 7.72
Magnetic resonance imaging, and cardiac transplantation, 6.70
Mammary arteries, in aortocoronary bypass surgery, 6.11–6.12
Mannitol in cardioplegia, 6.5
Marfan's syndrome, aortic regurgitation, 2.70
Medical Research Council (MRC) trial, 7.63
Meditation, transcendental, and hypertension, 7.74
Medtronic-Hall valve, **6.14**
Membranes, in cardiac electrophysiology, 3.3–3.7
Menses, and arrhythmias, 3.33
Meperidine, 1.61
Mephentermine, 2.59
Metarminol, 2.59
    for AV nodal reentrant tachycardia, 3.48
Methotrexate, after cardiac transplantation, 6.67
Methoxamine
    for AV nodal reentrant tachycardia, 3.48
    for cardiogenic shock, 2.59
Methylchloro ketone, and restenosis in PTCA, 5.24
Methyldopa, for hypertension, 7.85, **7.85**
Metolazone
    for heart failure, 2.33
    for hypertension, 7.80, 7.83
Metoprolol
    antiarrhythmic actions, 3.19
    for heart failure, 2.47
    after myocardial infarction, 1.64, **1.62**
Mevastatin, 4.50
Mevinolin, 5.24

antiarrhythmic actions, 3.12, 3.20
for atrial flutter, 3.39
after myocardial infarction, 1.64, **1.63**
for premature atrial complexes, 3.38
for sinus nodal reentry, 3.37
Prospective Randomized Flosequinan Longevity Evaluation
(PROFILE), 2.39
Prospective Randomized Milrinone Survival Evaluation
(PROMISE), 2.31, **2.30**
Prostacyclin
and angina, 1.10
aspirin effects, 1.25, **1.26**
Prostaglandins
and angina, 1.3
in heart failure, 2.15, 2.19, 2.22–2.23, **2.23**
for pulmonary hypertension, 2.75
Prosthesis, valvular, 6.13–6.15, **6.13–6.15**
Protein kinase C, in vascular hypertrophy, 7.36
Pseudoxanthoma elasticum, 2.64
Psychotherapy, and hypertension, 7.74
PTCA (percutaneous transluminal coronary artery angioplasty)
as alternative to thrombolytic therapy, 1.60, **1.61**
in cardiogenic shock, 1.64
for unstable angina, 1.32, 1.34
for variant angina, 1.34
See also Angioplasty.
Pulmonary
capillary wedge pressure
in cardiogenic shock, 2.56–2.57
in heart failure, 2.19, 2.53, *2.19*
chronic obstructive, beta-blocker therapy, 1.19
edema
pharmacologic treatment, 2.49–2.59
diuretics, 2.51, **2.51**
morphine, 2.50–2.52, 2.59
nitroprusside and nitroglycerin, 2.51–2.53, 2.59,
2.52, *2.53*
positive inotropic agents, 2.53–2.56, **2.54**, 2.55
hypertension, 2.71–2.75, **2.71**
anesthesia and pregnancy, 2.72
anti-inflammatory drugs, 2.73
anticoagulants, 2.73
digitalis and diuretics, 2.73
heart-lung transplantation, 2.75
oxygen administration, 2.72–2.73, **2.72**
vasodilators, 2.73–2.75, *2.74*
valvuloplasty, 5.36, **5.36**, 5.37
veno-occlusive disease, and pulmonary hypertension, 2.71
Pumps, extracorporeal centrifugal, 6.46–6.48, **6.47**

*q*RS complex
in premature ventricular complexes, 3.56–3.58
See also Electrocardiography (ECG).
Quadrigeminy, 3.58
Quality of life, and cardiac transplantation, 6.53
Quinidine
antiarrhythmic actions, 3.11, 3.14–3.16
for atrial fibrillation, 3.40
for atrial flutter, 3.39
for AV nodal reentrant tachycardia, 3.48
and ventricular tachycardia, 3.65

*r*acial differences, ACE inhibitors and beta-blockers, 7.77,
7.95
Radiofrequency ablation therapy, 3.23
future developments, 3.72
for ventricular tachycardia, 3.66, **3.62**
Radiography in heart failure, 2.10, **2.10, 2.11**
Rapamycin, 6.70
Rastan-Konno operation, 6.21–6.23
Receptors
for antiarrhythmic agents, 3.13, 3.20, 3.21
low density lipoproteins, 4.12, **4.13,** 4.37–4.38
bile acid sequestrants, 4.49
in familial hypercholesterolemia, 4.35
and HMG-CoA reductase inhibitors, 4.51
Recipients in cardiac transplantation
heterotopic technique, 6.57–6.62, **6.62–6.64**
management, 6.56–6.57
orthotopic technique, 6.57, **6.58–6.61**
selection, 6.56, *6.56*
Registry of PTCA, 5.4
early data, 5.4
indications, 5.9
success rates, 5.14–5.16, 5.21
Rejection, myocardial, 6.66–6.68, **6.67,** 6.68, *6.66*
Relaxation techniques, in hypertension, 7.74
Renal failure
and hypercholesterolemia, 4.35
and hypertriglyceridemia, 4.36
parenchymal disease, and hypertension, 7.51–7.52, **7.51,**
7.52
Renin-angiotensin
in heart failure, 2.15
in primary hypertension, 7.45–7.46, **7.46**
inhibitors, 7.93–7.95, **7.93,** 7.94
Renovascular hypertension, 7.52–7.56, **7.53–7.56,** *7.53*
ACE inhibitors, 7.95
Reperfusion, and ventricular function, **1.48,** 1.49
Reserpine, 7.84
Retinopathy, and hypertension, 7.20–7.21
Revascularization, coronary artery
in unstable angina, 1.29, **1.29**
for variant angina, 1.34
See also Angioplasty, percutaneous transluminal coronary
(PTCA).
Rheumatic fever
aortic incompetence, 6.17
aortic regurgitation, 2.70
atrial fibrillation, 3.39
heart failure, 2.8
mitral stenosis and regurgitation, 6.17
tricuspid valve disease, 6.38
Risk factors
for coronary heart disease, 4.30
for dyslipidemia, 4.30–4.31, **4.31**
for hypercholesterolemia, 4.59–4.62
for hypertension
individual, 7.14–7.16, **7.15–7.17,** *7.14*
population, 7.11–7.12, **7.12,** 7.13
for hypoalphalipoproteinemia, 4.72
infarct extension, *1.76*
Rotoblator for atherectomy, 5.32, **5.32**
Rub, friction, in pericarditis, 1.74